Visceral and Non-Vascular Therapy

A Teaching File

Visceral and Non-Vascular Percutaneous Therapy

A Teaching File

Volume II

Renan Uflacker, M.D., M.Sc.
Professor of Radiology
Director of Division of Vascular and Interventional Radiology
Department of Radiology
Medical University of South Carolina
Charleston, South Carolina

LIPPINCOTT WILLIAMS & WILKINS
A **Wolters Kluwer** Company
Philadelphia • Baltimore • New York • London
Buenos Aires • Hong Kong • Sydney • Tokyo

Acquisitions Editor: Beth K. Barry
Developmental Editor: Selina M. Bush
Production Editor: Patrick Carr
Manufacturing Manager: Tim Reynolds
Marketing Manager: Kimberly Cifone
Cover Designer: Jeane Norton
Compositor: Maryland Composition
Printer: Maple Press

530 Walnut Street
Philadelphia, PA 19106 USA
LWW.com

Printed in the USA

ISBN: 0-7817-3666-8

10 9 8 7 6 5 4 3 2 1

This book is dedicated
To my wife
Helena
To my son
André
To my daughter
Alice

And
To our patients and coworkers

CONTENTS

CONTRIBUTING AUTHORS

Valeria Cardoso de Souza, MD
Interventional Radiology, Hospital Osvaldo Cruz, São Paulo, SP, Brazil
— Case Report: 9.2

Bahri Üztünsöz, MD
Associate Professor, Chief of Vascular and Interventional Radiology, GATA Medical Faculty, Ankara, Turkey. Currently, Interventional Radiology, Department of Radiology, LSU Health Sciences Center, New Orleans, Louisiana.
— Case Reports: 9.1, 15.6.1, 15.7.1, 15.7.2,15.7.3, 16.6.1, 16.7.1

Carlos Abath, MD
Director, Angiorad, Hospital Memorial, Recife, Brazil
— Case Report: 16.1.2

Michael Wholey, MD, MBA
Assistant Professor of Radiology, Chief of Clinical Cardiovascular and Special Interventions, Department of Radiology, University of Texas Health, Science Center, San Antonio, Texas.
— Case Reports: 16.5.1, and 16.5.2

Renan Uflacker, MD
Professor of Radiology, Director, Division of Vascular and Interventional Radiology, Department of Radiology, Medical University of South Carolina, Charleston, South Carolina.

PUBLISHER'S FOREWORD

Teaching Files are one of the hallmarks of education in radiology. There has long been a need for a comprehensive series of books, using the Teaching File format, that would provide the kind of personal consultation with the experts normally found only in the setting of a teaching hospital. Lippincott Williams & Wilkins is proud to have created such a series; our goal is to provide the resident and practicing radiologist with a useful resource that answers this need.

Actual cases have been culled from extensive teaching files in major medical centers. The discussions presented mimic those performed on a daily basis between residents and faculty members in all radiology departments.

We hope that this series will become a valuable and trusted teaching tool for radiologists at any stage of training or practice, and that it will also be a benefit to clinicians whose patients undergo these imaging studies.

–The Publisher

PREFACE

Visceral and Non-Vascular Percutaneous Therapy: A Teaching File, is the second of two volumes on percutaneous therapy. As in the first volume, case reports are presented in an organized fashion, giving elements of the patient problem and reasons for the intervention, figures obtained during the performance of the procedure, detailed descriptive legends, and discussion of the disease, procedure techniques, and outcomes. Again, the organization of the book is procedure-oriented, and the reader will be able to find the areas of interest in chapters organized according to procedure or group of techniques.

Being involved in the area of image-guided percutaneous procedures for more than 24 years, it still amazes me how much things have changed. What was just a percutaneous access for diagnostic catheter placement and contrast media injection, evolved into a powerful tool for minimally invasive treatment of an increasing list of diseases. When we began planning for this book, things looked easier than they turned out to be. More effort was necessary to summarize the general knowledge of the techniques and outcomes of percutaneous invasive procedures. The menu of procedures and variations is so great that a much larger two-volume publication was necessary. While the first volume covered vascular procedures, this second volume is dedicated to a variety of occlusive procedures, (including embolizations and drug infusions), and techniques of drainage and catheter/needle treatment of organs throughout the body for obstruction and infection.

As the manuscript developed, we kept in mind the trainee. It is relatively difficult to replicate a "hand-on" procedure in the pages of a textbook, and some will learn faster than others. This book is designed to provide the foundations for the decision-making process, as well as hints for conducting the procedure itself.

There is a saying regarding surgeons: Sometimes wrong; never in doubt. The same applies for anyone conducting image-guided percutaneous procedures. Every day we are faced with uncertainties, and no procedure can be taken for granted. But decisions must be made, and procedures performed, and as in any other field, skill, judgment, and confidence are learned through experience. On the whole, surgeons tend to speak of the importance of practice, not talent, in determining expertise. Personally, I believe that practice only enhances talent. With practice, conscious learning becomes unconscious knowledge, and once cannot say precisely when and how.

As expected, some procedures described here came and went. Some changed forever patient care standards, and a few, although useful, never made the impact that was initially expected. There is no fixed body of knowledge, and the illusion of perfect training is always undone by the need for additional training and the mastering of new technologies. As Interventional Radiologists, at least three-quarters of what we do today was not learned in training. Most of the procedures we perform today were built upon skills we already had, though some did not. Progress—and the necessary learning and relearning it requires—is continuous. Commitment is the key to remaining current in such a climate.

The management and responsibility for care of some types of patients and diseases changed hands a few times. More frequently than not, percutaneous procedures and devices developed and championed by interventionalists, tended to switch hands to other medical specialties as the techniques evolved and proved successful. However, interventional radiologists are not alone in this transitional environment, and other professionals suffer the same frustrations of shifting practice patterns. Nevertheless, transition and change may represent an opportunity for fair competition, as long as we adapt. Competition results from freedom of choice and the best-trained professionals usually prevail in the views of patients and colleagues.

—Renan Uflacker, M.D.

Visceral and Non-Vascular Therapy

A Teaching File

PART I

Visceral Therapeutic Embolization And Blood Flow Reduction

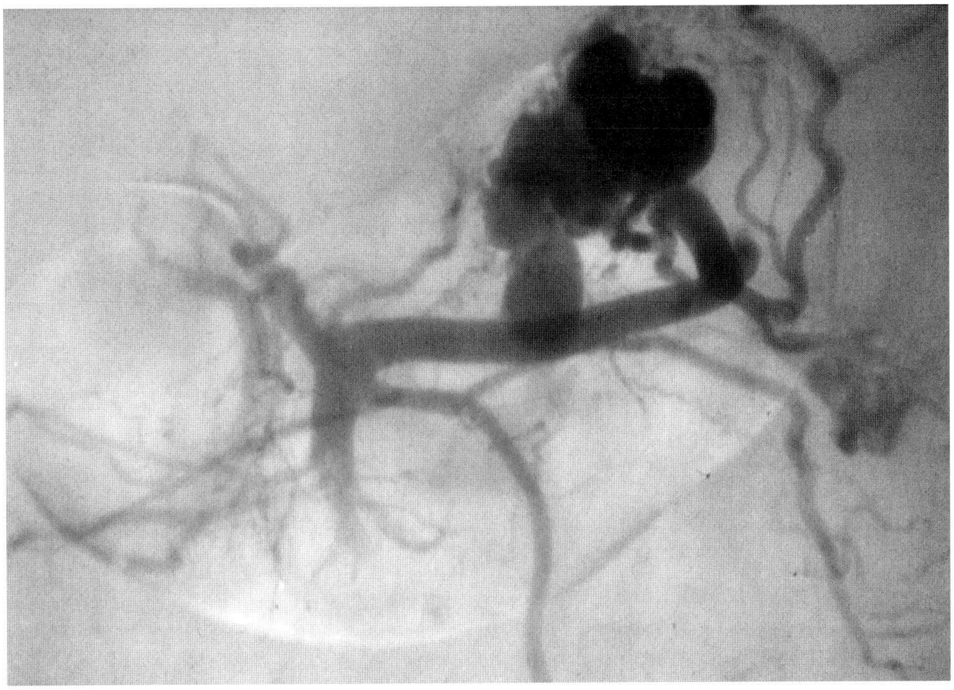

CHAPTER 1

Embolization And Blood Flow Reduction In Gastrointestinal Bleeding And Portal Hypertension

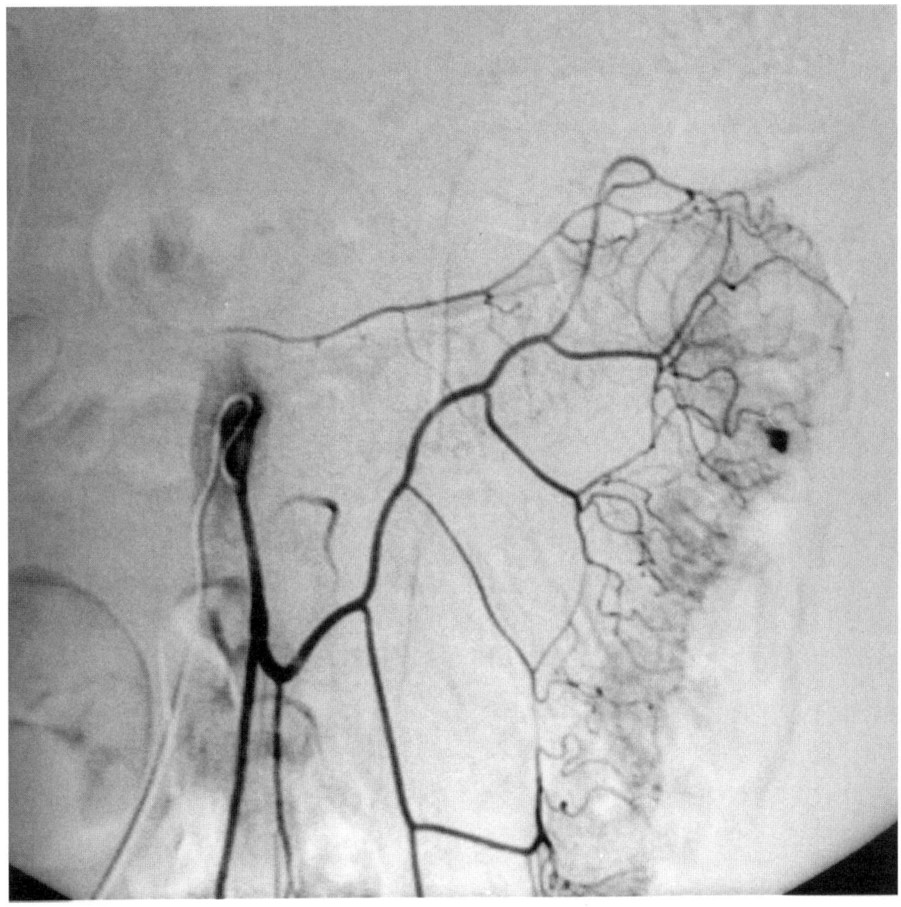

1.1 Embolization In Gastrointestinal Bleeding

Case 1.1:

Lower gastrointestinal (GI) bleeding from a diverticulum in the colon of a 67-year-old male patient with massive rectal bleeding.

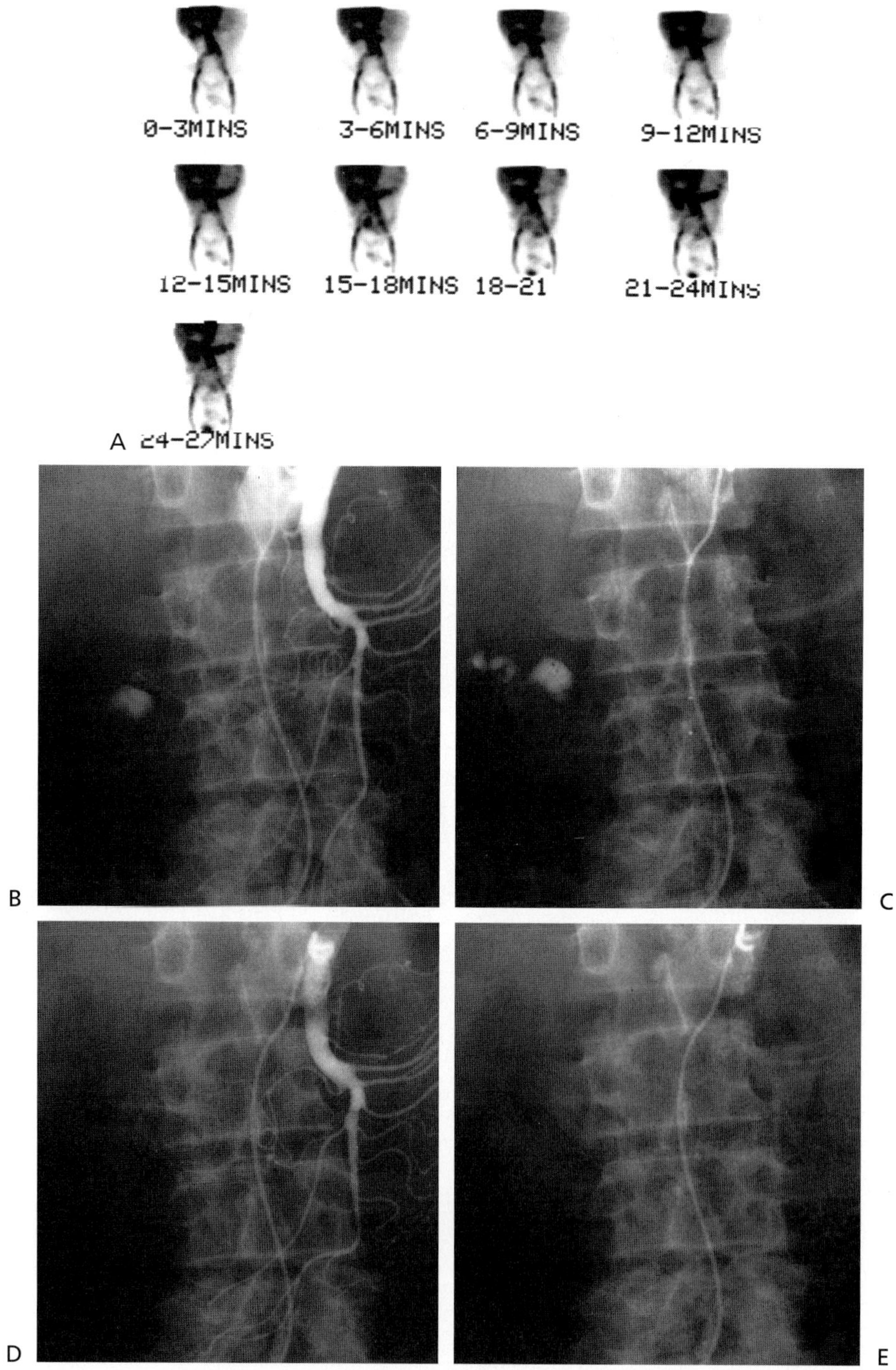

Figure 1.1

Bleeding diverticulum of the right colon. **A:** Technetium-99m–labeled red blood cell scan. Note accumulation of activity in the right colon moving through the transverse and descending colon. **B:** Superior mesenteric artery (SMA) injection was performed and showed a point of extravasation in a diverticulum in the right colon. **C:** Late-phase SMA angiogram shows some diffusion of contrast in the lumen of the colon. **D,E:** Arteriogram after infusion of vasopressin into the SMA (0.4 IU/min for 20 minutes) shows no extravasation.

Comment: Lower GI bleeding by definition originates below the ligament of Treitz. Bleeding in the colon is the most frequent origin of acute lower GI bleeding. Bleedings are more frequent and more massive from diverticula of the right colon. Lower GI bleeding from the colon frequently is intermittently massive but may be chronic low grade, making the angiographic diagnosis more difficult. In elderly patients, the mortality for lower GI bleeding may reach 26%. Radionuclide imaging is extremely sensitive for lower GI bleeding. Bleedings as low as 0.1 mL/min are detected, but the technique is less specific in identifying cause or location. Intraarterial vasopressin infusion should be started at 0.2 IU/min for 20 minutes. If not effective, infusion should be increased to 0.4 IU/min for another 20 minutes. If effective, infusion should be maintained for 6 to 8 hours and then tapered down to 0.3 IU/min for 12 hours, 0.2 IU/min for 12 hours, 0.1 IU/min for 12 hours, and discontinued if there is no evidence of further GI bleeding. The catheter should be taped to the groin and kept for at least an additional 12 hours with saline infusion.

1.2 Embolization In Gastrointestinal Bleeding

Case 1.2:

Lower GI bleeding from the colon in a 55-year-old male patient with active rectal bleeding.

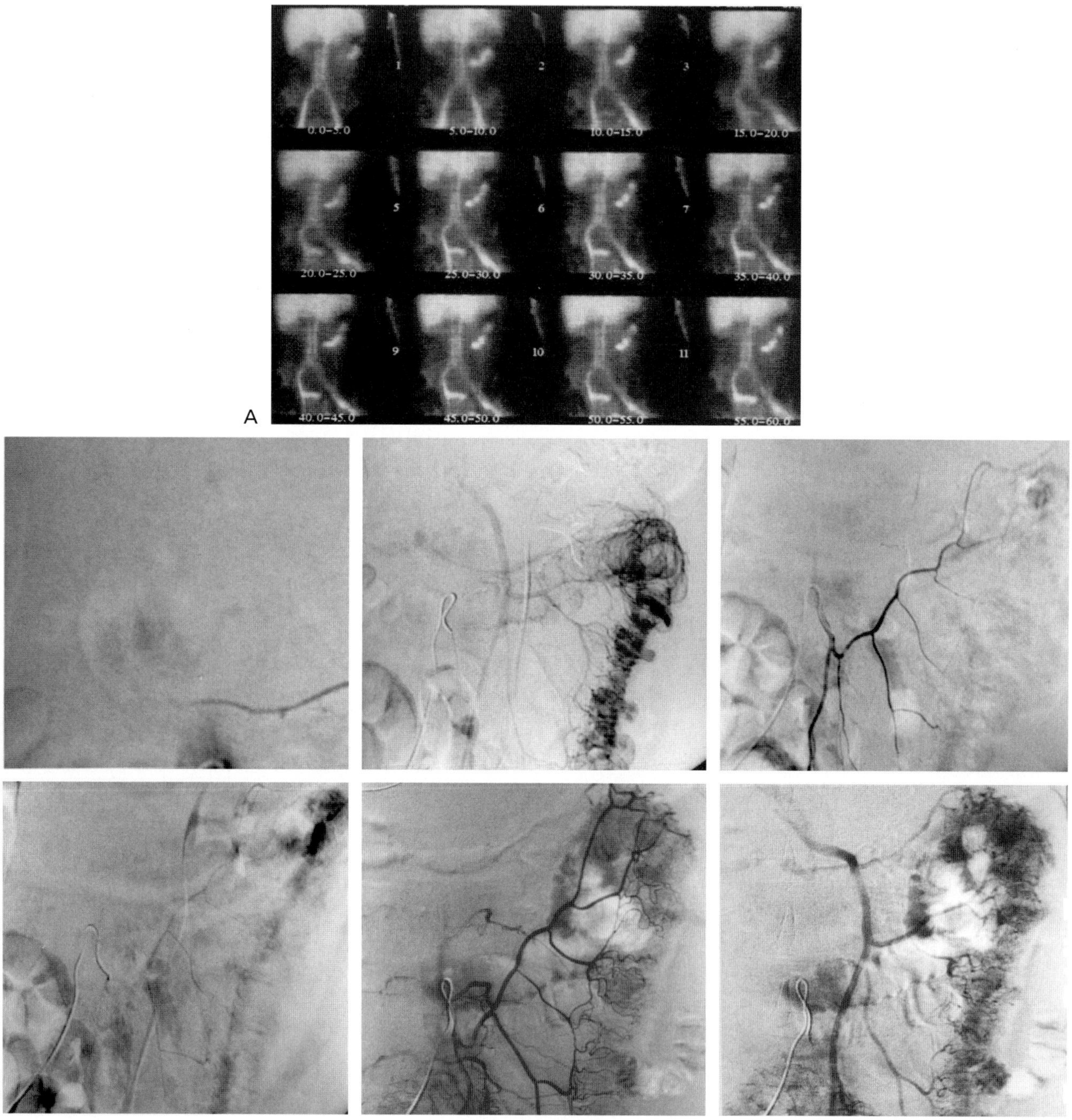

A; B, C; D; E, F; G

Figure 1.2

Bleeding diverticulum of left colon. **A:** Technetium-99m–labeled red blood cell scan. Accumulation of activity in the left side of the abdomen suggests descending colon and moves a relatively short distance in 60 minutes. Bleeding also could be interpreted as coming from the small bowel. **B:** Inferior mesenteric artery (IMA) injection was performed and showed a point of extravasation in the diverticulum in the left colon. **C:** Late-phase IMA angiogram shows some accumulation of contrast in the lumen of the colon. Note spasm of the walls and other diverticula. **D,E:** Arteriogram after infusion into the superior mesenteric artery of vasopressin 0.4 IU/min for 20 minutes shows no extravasation and marked spasm of the arteries. Note absence of venous filling. **F,G:** Follow-up angiogram performed 12 hours after discontinuation of infusion and 36 hours after treatment. Note the excellent blood flow to the left colon and dense venous return.

Comment: Angiography is relatively sensitive for detection of lower GI bleeding. Bleedings as low as 0.5 mL/min are identified. Arteriography is highly specific in localizing bleeding sites and identifying anatomic lesions capable of bleeding, but the overall yield of angiography in localizing the source of lower GI bleeding is 50% to 60%. Patients who continue to pass blood per rectum have a higher positivity rate. Mesenteric arterial infusion of vasopressin controls lower GI bleeding in about 92% of the patients. However, recurrence rates are relatively high, reaching 30% after initial control with vasopressin, within the same admission. Intravenous vasopressin infusion currently is not used to treat arterial bleeding. Highly selective embolization is an alternative to control lower GI bleeding, but it should not be used after vasopressin infusion to reduce risks of infarction in a territory subject to pharmacologic vasospasm.

1.3 Embolization In Gastrointestinal Bleeding

Case 1.3:

Lower GI bleeding from the cecum in a 85-year-old male patient.

A, B

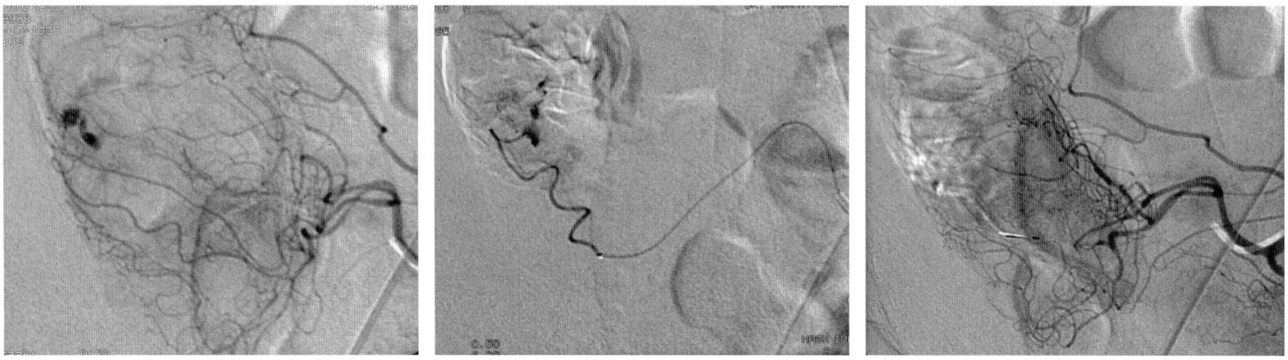

C

Figure 1.3

Bleeding in the cecum after colonoscopic polypectomy. **A:** Superselective angiography of the ileocolic artery shows massive extravasation of contrast in the cecum. **B:** A microcatheter was advanced into the vessel responsible for the bleeding for purpose of embolization. **C:** Angiogram following embolization with one straight microcoil. Note occlusion of the vessel and control of active bleeding; however, there is residual contrast in the lumen of the cecum partially subtracted.

Comment: Embolization is an alternative to vasopressin infusion for controlling lower GI bleeding. There has been great reluctance to use embolization in the colon for bleeding treatment because of the risk of inducing serious ischemic infarction. It has been proved, however, that bowel ischemia is relatively rare, and the technique can be highly effective to control bleeding. Accordingly to some authors, there is an ischemic risk of about 15% to 18%; therefore, monitoring, blood volume replacement, and radiographic assessment of the embolized bowel loop are required. Signs of bowel infarct may present within 24 to 72 hours. Gas in the wall of the bowel loop indicates infarction, and prompt surgery is necessary.

1.4 Embolization In Gastrointestinal Bleeding

Case 1.4:

Lower GI bleeding from the right colon. The 42-year-old patient was a drug user and presented with multiple bleeding colonic ulcerations.

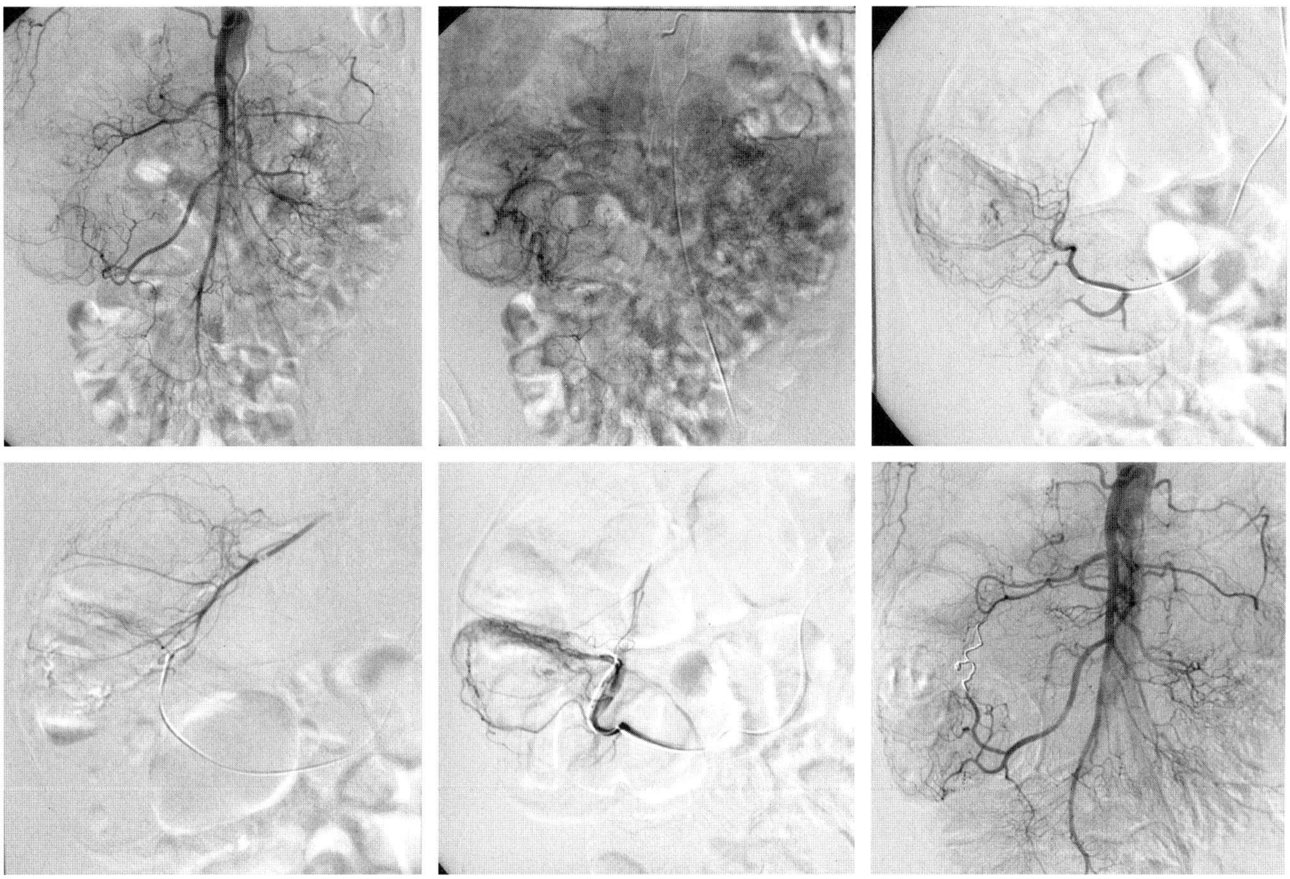

A B, C D E, F

Figure 1.4

A: SMA injection shows an area of extravasation in the middle segment of the right colon supplied by the right colic artery and ileocolic artery. **B:** Late-phase angiogram shows more obvious extravasation of contrast into the bowel lumen. **C:** Superselective catheterization of the ascending branch of the ileocolic artery shows a small extravasation. **D:** Catheterization of the right colic artery beyond the point of bleeding does not show extravasation. **E:** A coil was placed in the distal ascending branch of the ileocolic artery, extending into the right colic artery. **F:** Follow-up arteriogram of the SMA shows control of the bleeding and residual contrast in the lumen of the right colon. Note that the anastomosis between the two systems was embolized with a couple of coils.

Comment: Embolization of anastomotic arcades in the mesenteric circulation is relatively dangerous and should be avoided, if possible. If this patient developed ischemia of the right colon, surgical resection of the colon would be required. No recurrence of bleeding or complications ensued.

1.5 Embolization In Gastrointestinal Bleeding

Case 1.5:

Lower GI bleeding from an angiodysplasia of the ascending colon in an 80-year-old male patient with active rectal bleeding.

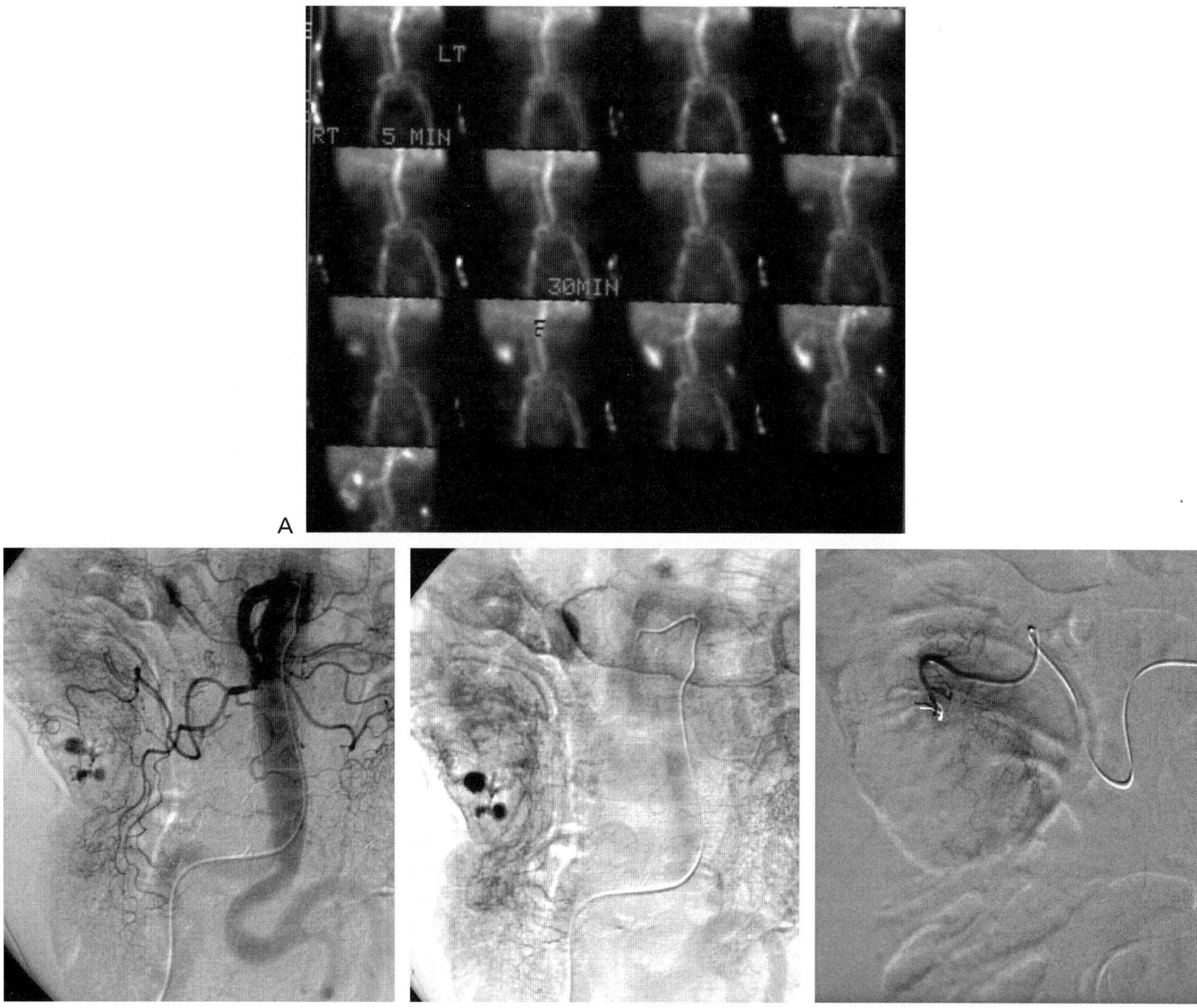

A

B, C

D

Figure 1.5

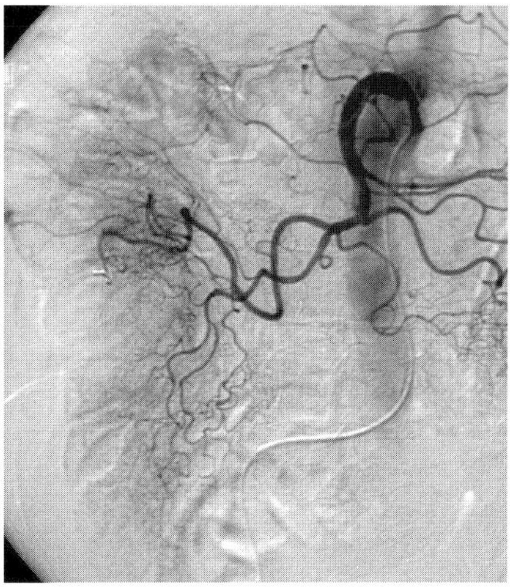

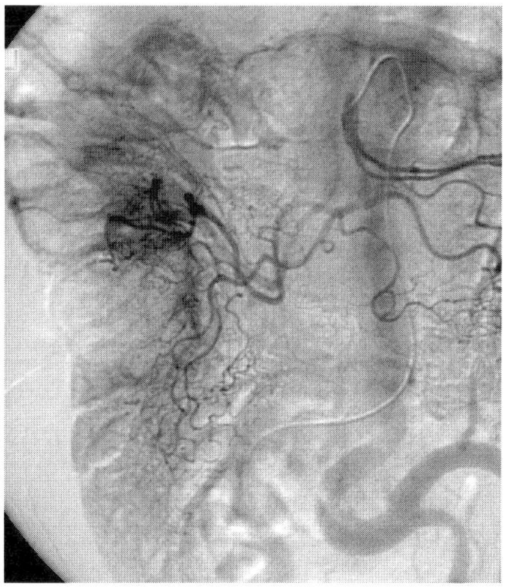

Figure 1.5 *(continued)*

A: Technetium-99m–labeled red blood cell scan shows accumulation of activity in the right side of the abdomen, suggesting right colon bleeding, that moves only a short distance in 65 minutes. **B:** Superior mesenteric angiogram shows active bleeding in the cecum and right colon from an angiodysplasia of the colon. The angiogram shows active extravasation of contrast medium in the lumen of the right colon. **C:** Late-phase angiogram of the SMA shows accumulation of contrast in the bowel lumen. **D:** Superselective catheterization of the ileocecal artery was performed, and the angiogram after embolization with a 2-mm × 2-cm microcoil showed no extravasation. **E,F:** Postembolization SMA angiogram shows bleeding control and patency of the branches of the SMA. Permanent control of the bleeding was achieved without sequelae.

Comment: Identification of acute lower GI bleeding by angiography is limited to about 50% of the cases and is even less frequent in angiodysplasias of the colon. This angiodysplasia was identified by colonoscopy, but the procedure failed to achieve bleeding control. Angiography was not useful for diagnosis of the angiodysplasia in this case, presumably because of the changes in hemodynamics during the active bleeding episode. Cecal or colonic angiodysplasias usually are not identified by active bleeding but by the characteristic angiographic aspects, which include (i) enlarged groups of small arteries on the mesenteric border of the cecum, (ii) accumulation of contrast medium in vascular tufts, (iii) early filling of draining veins, (iv) persistent opacity or late emptying of dilated drainage veins, and (v) occasional contrast extravasation when the study is performed during active bleeding. Superselective catheterization with a microcatheter allows placement of microcoils very close to the point of bleeding. More than one branch may be involved, and multiple selective injections may be necessary. Spasm of the feeding vessel is a problem that may be avoided with careful manipulation and treated with intraarterial nitroglycerin injection. The straight and curved microcoils are not as thrombogenic as the helical and more complex coils, and multiple coils may be necessary for adequate occlusion. The higher the number of coils used, the higher the chances of ischemia in the wall of the bowel. Bleeding was controlled in this patient without complications.

1.6 Embolization In Gastrointestinal Bleeding

Case 1.6:

Lower GI bleeding in a 79-year-old man with previous miocardial infarction and exertional angina. Treatment with vasopressin for 24 hours was attempted in another institution but did not stop the bleeding. Because of the severity of the coronary disease, the infusion was stopped and the patient transferred for possible embolization.

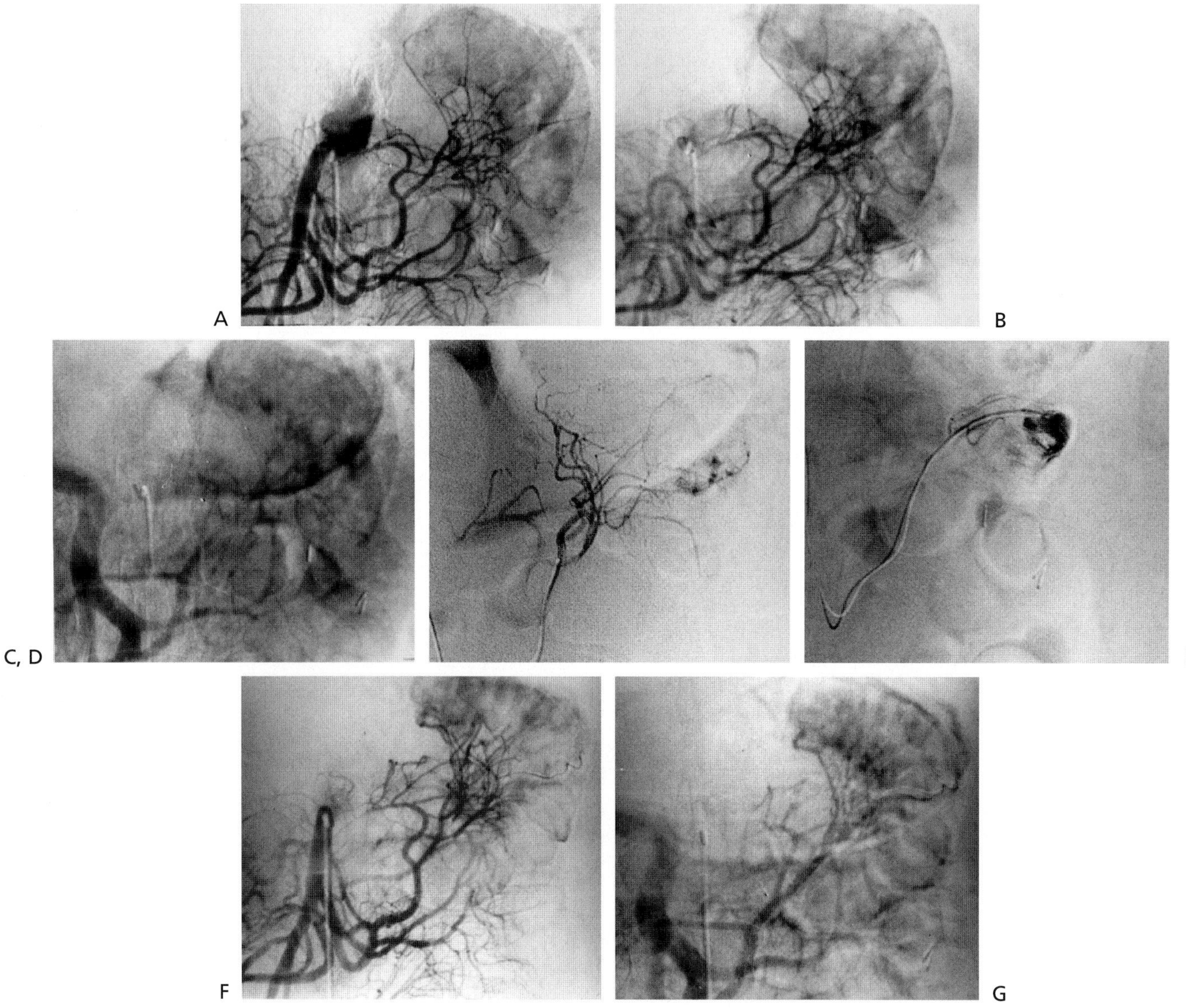

Figure 1.6

A–C: Superior mesenteric angiogram shows small active extravasation of contrast medium in the proximal jejunum. The early-phase angiogram **(A)** suggests a small aneurysm is a peripheral jejunal artery. **D:** More selective catheterization with the microcatheter shows extravasation. **E:** Superselective catheterization and angiogram shows massive extravasation of contrast medium. **F,G:** Embolization with one helical coil occluded the vessel that was involved in the bleeding, and control of the hemorrhage was achieved. Bleeding stopped, and the patient became stable. He was returned to his original hospital, where the surgery service decided to perform a small bowel resection to prevent future bleedings. The coils in the jejunal artery helped in locating the affected small bowel area. The specimen revealed a chronic ulceration in the jejunal mucosa.

Comment: Jejunal bleeding without a predisposing cause is uncommon. There was no explanation for the jejunal ulceration in this patient. Bleeding was massive when it started, and although vasopressin reduced the bleeding rate, it did not stop. The preexisting coronary disease and failure of vasopressin infusion prompted the change of treatment course to embolization. Because the attending surgeon lacked familiarity with mesenteric embolization, it is possible an unnecessary bowel resection was performed. There were no signs of ischemia, and the patient was stable at the time of surgery.

1.7 Embolization In Gastrointestinal Bleeding

Case 1.7:

A 64-year-old woman with active rectal bleeding underwent a nuclear medicine scan that showed bleeding at the 6.5-hour delay film only. This scan was not helpful in locating the site of bleeding. The SMA angiogram was considered negative. Bleeding recurred, and a new angiogram was performed.

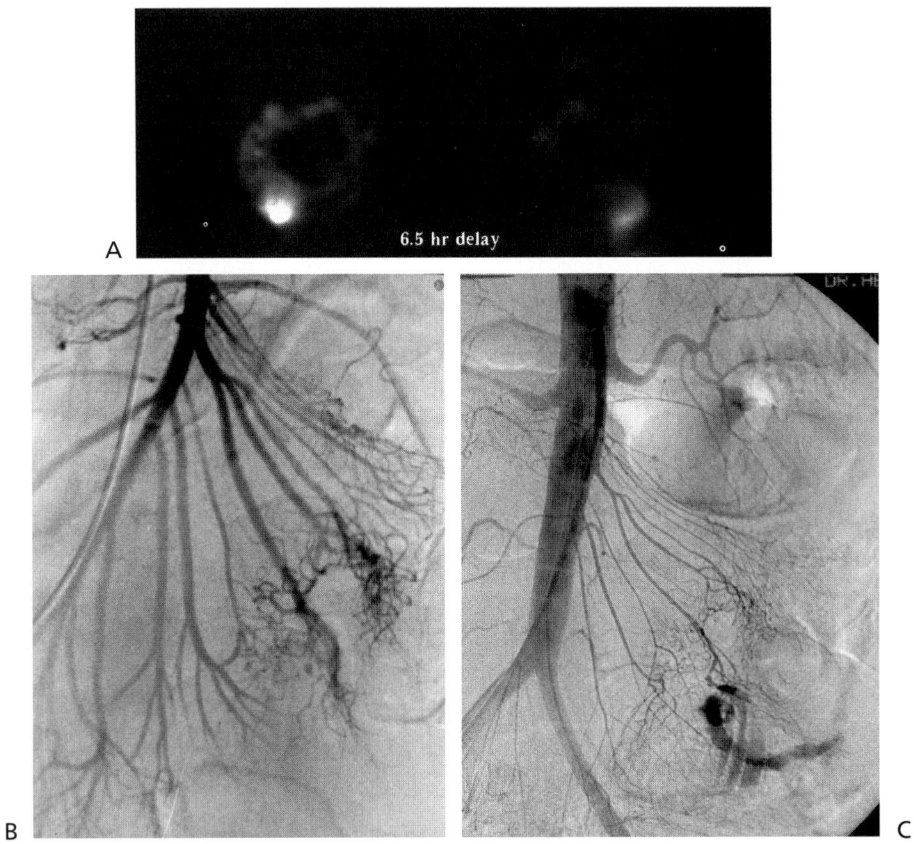

Figure 1.7

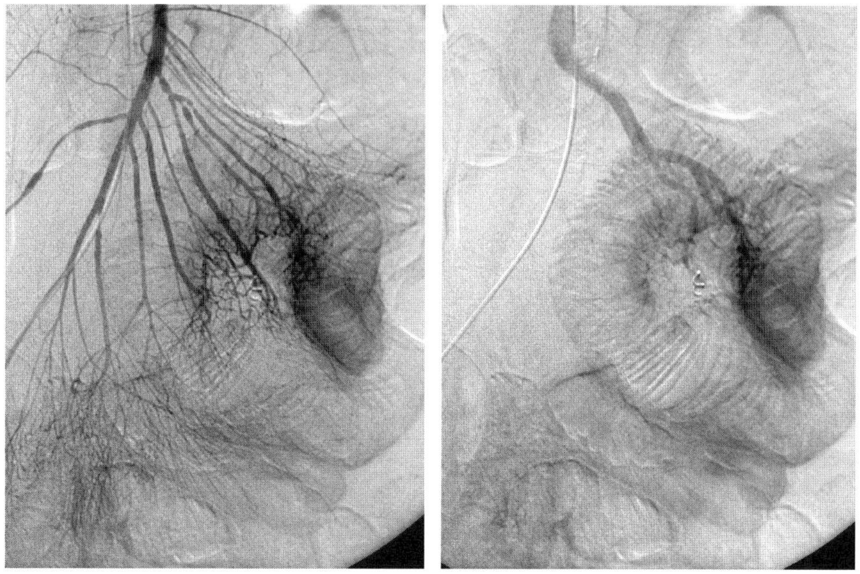

D E

Figure 1.7 *(continued)*

A: Technetium-99m–labeled red blood cell scan performed 6.5 hours after injection shows accumulation of activity in the cecum. **B:** Initial superior mesenteric arteriogram shows no active extravasation of contrast and was considered negative. In retrospect, a small aneurysm was identified in a middle peripheral jejunal artery (fifth branch). **C:** Twelve hours after the initial angiogram, new massive bleeding occurred and prompted a new angiogram. Active extravasation of contrast was identified in the middle jejunal branch with the small aneurysm. Note spasm of the mesenteric branches compared with the previous angiogram in **B**. **D:** Superselective catheterization of the bleeding vessel was performed with a 4F Cobra catheter, and a small 2-mm × 2-cm minicoil was delivered to occlude the bleeding vessel. **E:** Late-phase angiogram shows good venous return and control of bleeding. No further bleeding was observed. The patient did not develop any pain or ischemic symptoms and was discharged 3 days after the procedure.

Comment: In cases of intermittent bleeding, a negative mesenteric arteriographic event is a very frustrating occurrence for the patient and physician. In this specific case, even the technetium-99m–labeled red blood cell scan was not able to show the approximate location of the bleeding. Repeat angiogram during active bleeding showed the actual location of the bleeding. A small aneurysm identified retrospectively in a jejunal branch might have been treated earlier and spared the patient a second procedure and life-threatening bleeding.

1.8 Embolization In Gastrointestinal Bleeding

Case 1.8:

An 82-year-old man with recurrent lower GI bleeding and two negative colonoscopies and one upper endoscopy continued to bleed. Technetium-99m–labeled red blood cell scan was negative. The patient was referred for angiography for diagnosis and possible treatment.

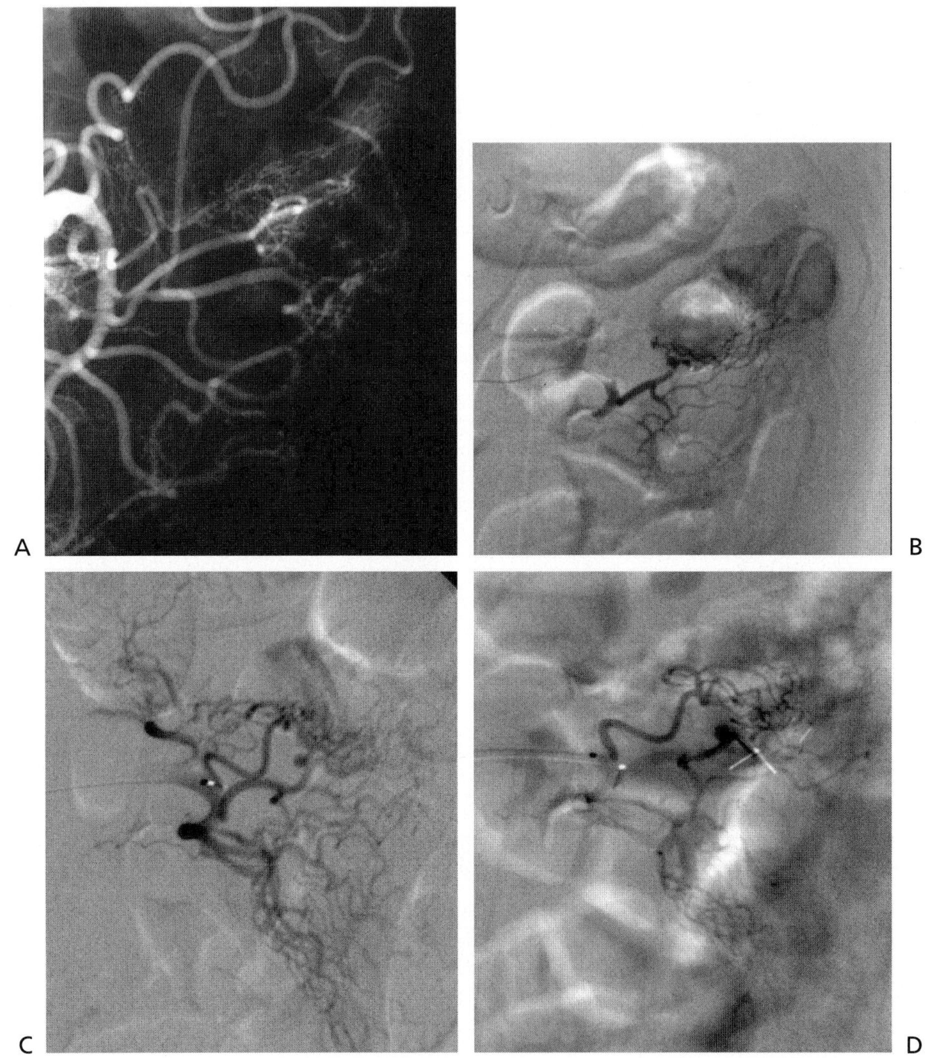

Figure 1.8

A: Initial unsubtracted superior mesenteric arteriogram shows no obvious extravasation or vascular lesion. **B:** More selective injections with a microcatheter shows a small aneurysm at a bifurcation of the third jejunal artery. **C:** Digital arteriogram better demonstrates the lesion, and embolization was performed with two straight microcoils. **D:** Postembolization angiogram shows the artery is still open and filling of the aneurysm. Flow was slower, and occlusion of the aneurysm may have followed the embolization (it was not demonstrated angiographically). The patient did well after the embolization and during 2-year follow-up.

Comment: Due to previous experiences with small mesenteric aneurysms, a decision was made to embolize, even if no active bleeding was identified angiographically. The patient stopped bleeding after the embolization and experienced no recurrence during a relatively long follow-up, which suggests that the treatment may have been adequate. Again, the microcatheter technology was very helpful in achieving embolization.

1.9 Embolization In Gastrointestinal Bleeding

Case 1.9:

A 48-year-old man with lower GI bleeding and a positive nuclear medicine scan presented with active bleeding in the distal ileum seen on angiogram.

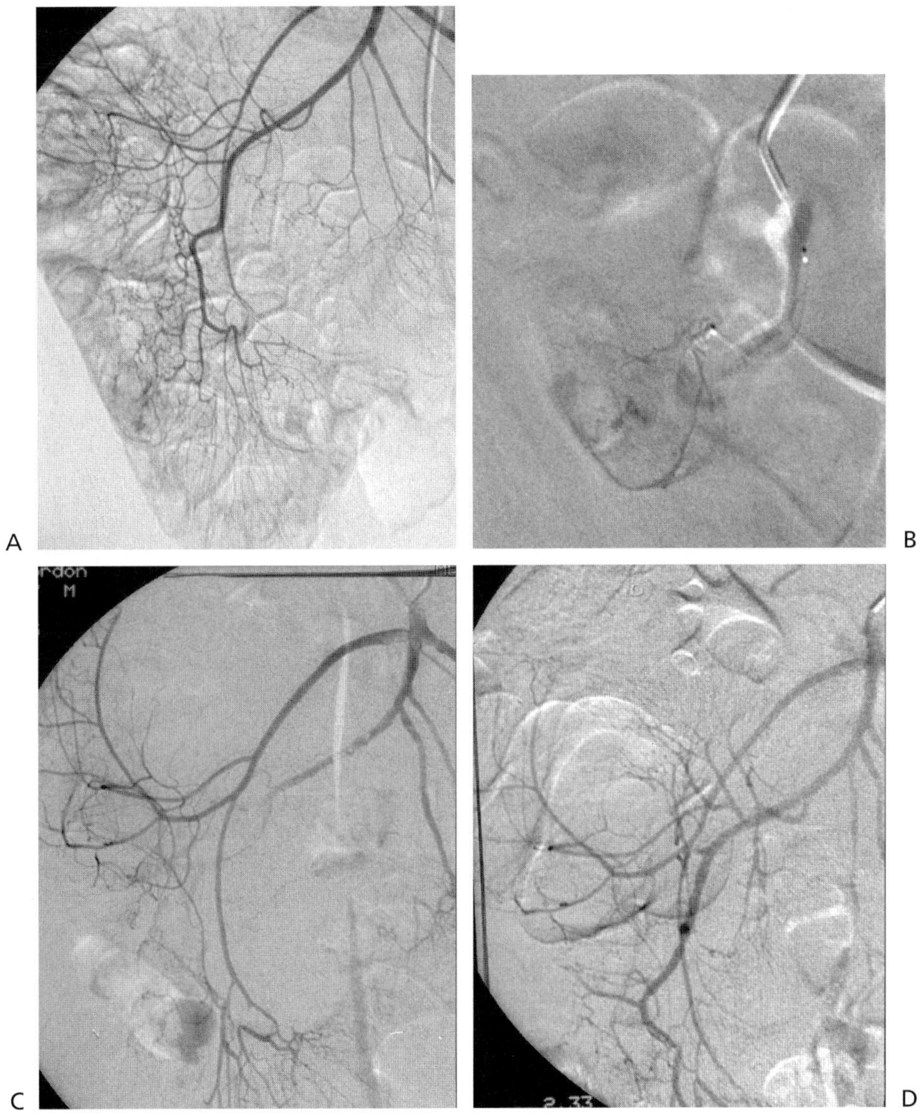

Figure 1.9

A: Selective superior mesenteric arteriogram shows localized bleeding from branches at the distal ileum. **B:** The 5F catheter was advanced into the ileocolic artery, and a microcatheter was advanced into the bleeding vessel. Note extravasation of contrast medium in the dilated bowel loop. **C:** Embolization with one microcoil was performed and the bleeding stopped. The catheter was pulled out, and the ileocolic artery showed extensive thrombosis and spasm. Infusion of urokinase 50,000 IU/h for 2 hours, associated with sublingual vasodilators, was performed and the ileocolic artery recanalized adequately. **D:** Angiogram obtained after urokinase infusion shows patency of the ileocolic artery and no signs of bleeding.

Comment: This was a difficult problem to treat in this patient. The 5F catheter was advanced too far into the ileocolic artery. Only the microcatheter should have been used for peripheral catheterization and embolization. Embolization initially was effective in this patient, but it almost caused a major disaster. Urokinase infusion was a good save of the situation, but there was risk of additional bleeding. Despite initial success, the patient rebled 1 week after the procedure. The distal ileum and the cecum were resected surgically, with good results.

1.10 Embolization In Gastrointestinal Bleeding

Case 1.10:

A 29-year-old man with repeated vomiting and upper GI bleeding was transferred from another hospital after he was transfused with 15 units of blood and underwent surgery that was ineffective in stopping the bleeding. Endoscopy showed Mallory-Weiss tears, with bleeding at the esophagogastric junction. Endoscopic sclerosis did not stop the bleeding, and angiography was requested for possible embolization.

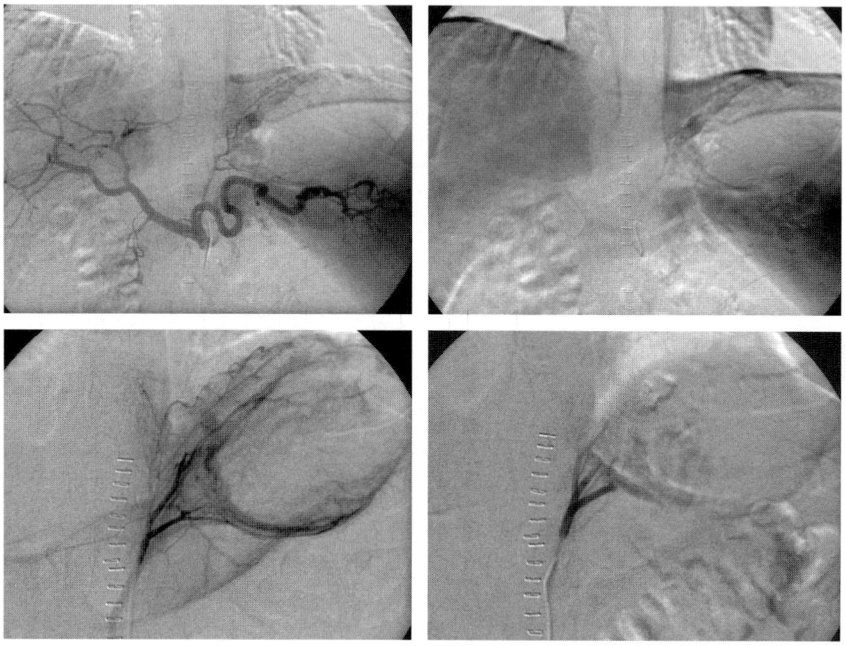

Figure 1.10

A: Celiac arteriogram demonstrates active bleeding at the esophagogastric junction. The liver and spleen are angiographically normal. Note that the gastric fundus and distal esophagus are fed by the left gastric artery, which arises from the celiac artery. **B:** Late-phase angiogram shows collection of contrast in the esophagogastric junction. **C:** The bleeding was not readily visible in the early phase of the selective left gastric artery angiogram. Late-phase arteriogram shows no venous return. A very faint area of bleeding is seen. **D:** Embolization with Gelfoam pledgets attained occlusion of the peripheral branches of the left gastric artery, with control of the bleeding. Note the subtracted shadow of residual contrast in the esophagogastric junction.

Comment: Mallory-Weiss tears as a cause of upper GI bleeding are more common than initially thought, being present in 14% in some series. Tearing of the esophagogastric junction usually is related to severe vomiting and alcohol abuse in the previous 48 hours. Less than half of the patients with Mallory-Weiss tears will require blood transfusion, and a much smaller number of patients may require more aggressive therapy. This type of bleeding usually is intramucosal and can be treated with intraarterial vasopressin infusion or embolization with absorbable particles of Gelfoam, as in this case. More than 90% of cases are controlled by embolization alone. Control of bleeding usually leads to healing of the mucosal tear and recanalization of the left gastric artery if temporary embolizing agents are used. Bleeding recurred 24 hours after embolization; therefore, a new angiogram was obtained, followed by a new embolization of the short gastric arteries. Surgery was performed, but no active bleeding was identified. The tears were sutured, and the patient subsequently did well.

1.11 Embolization In Gastrointestinal Bleeding

Case 1.11:

A 35-year-old woman with unresectable gastric cancer presented with chronic bleeding from superficial tumor erosions that required repeated blood transfusions. Embolization was requested to control or reduce the bleeding.

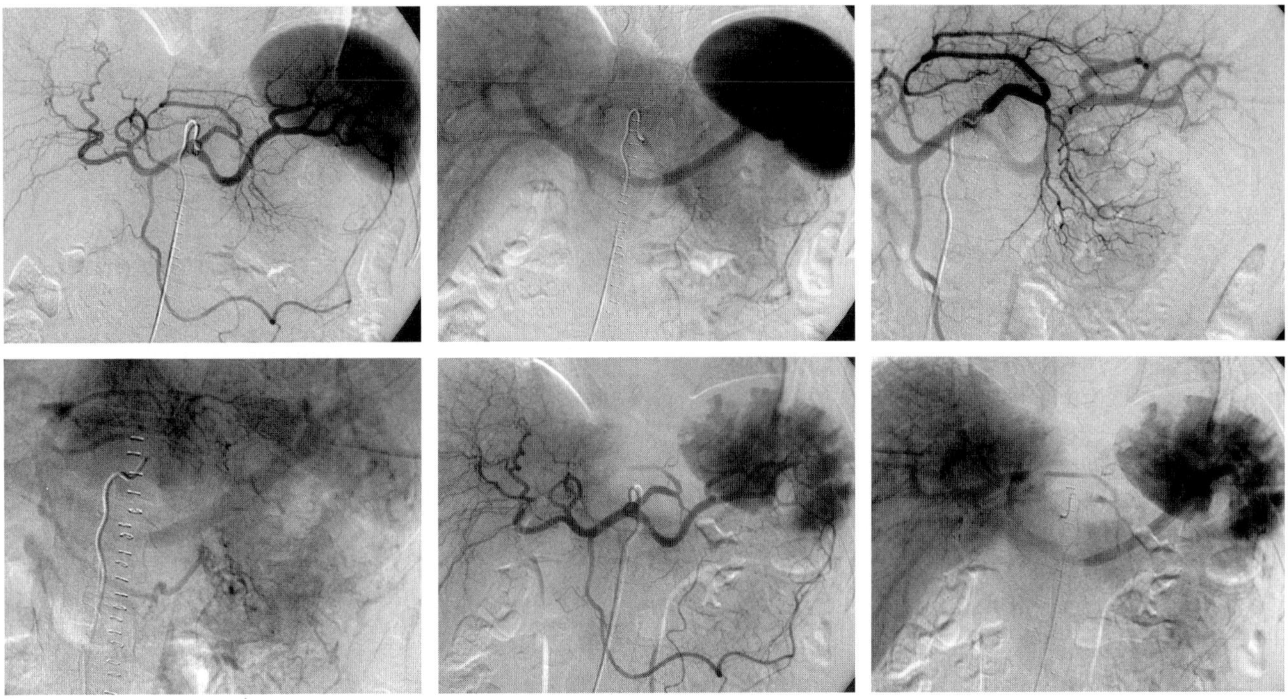

Figure 1.11

A,B: Celiac arteriogram shows normal liver and spleen. The splenic and portal veins were patent. Note the prominent left gastric artery (origin of the left hepatic artery in this case) and hypervascularity in the gastric body, with tumor vessels and some tumor enhancement. **C,D:** Selective angiogram of the left gastric artery shows prominent arteries and hypervascularity in the gastric body at the tumor site. Note the presence of tumor vessel venous lakes and tumor enhancement. A draining vein also was noted. **E,F:** Follow-up celiac arteriogram performed after embolization of the gastric tumor shows total devascularization of the main tumor mass. Ivalon 300 m and Gelfoam pledgets were used for embolization. Splenic artery angiogram also was performed to check for short gastric arteries but demonstrated no filling of the tumor from collaterals. Improvement of bleeding was obtained, which reduced the transfusion needs.

Comment: Tumor vessels are not sensitive to vasoconstrictor infusion because they lack wall musculature; therefore, bleeding in tumors cannot be stopped efficiently by vasopressin infusion. Although larger vessels do contract and may reduce the total blood flow to a tumor with some control of the bleeding, the tumor vessels and the vessels actually involved in the bleeding will not contract. Embolization is the best option in tumoral situations where bleeding control is necessary. However, due to the evolving nature of tumor areas, growth and necrosis will develop, potentially increasing the chances of bleeding. In this case, embolization was palliative and performed to minimize or control bleeding, increase quality of life, and reduce the mortality related to complications. In this patient, improvement of bleeding was achieved in the remaining survival time.

1.12 Embolization In Gastrointestinal Bleeding

Case 1.12:

A 51-year-old female patient with previous partial gastrectomy presented with active upper GI bleeding from the stomach. Endoscopy showed active gastric bleeding from a posterior wall lesion but was not able to stop the bleeding. Initial embolization controlled the bleeding, but rebleeding occurred 1 week after initial treatment and a new arteriogram was performed.

A, B C D, E F G, H I

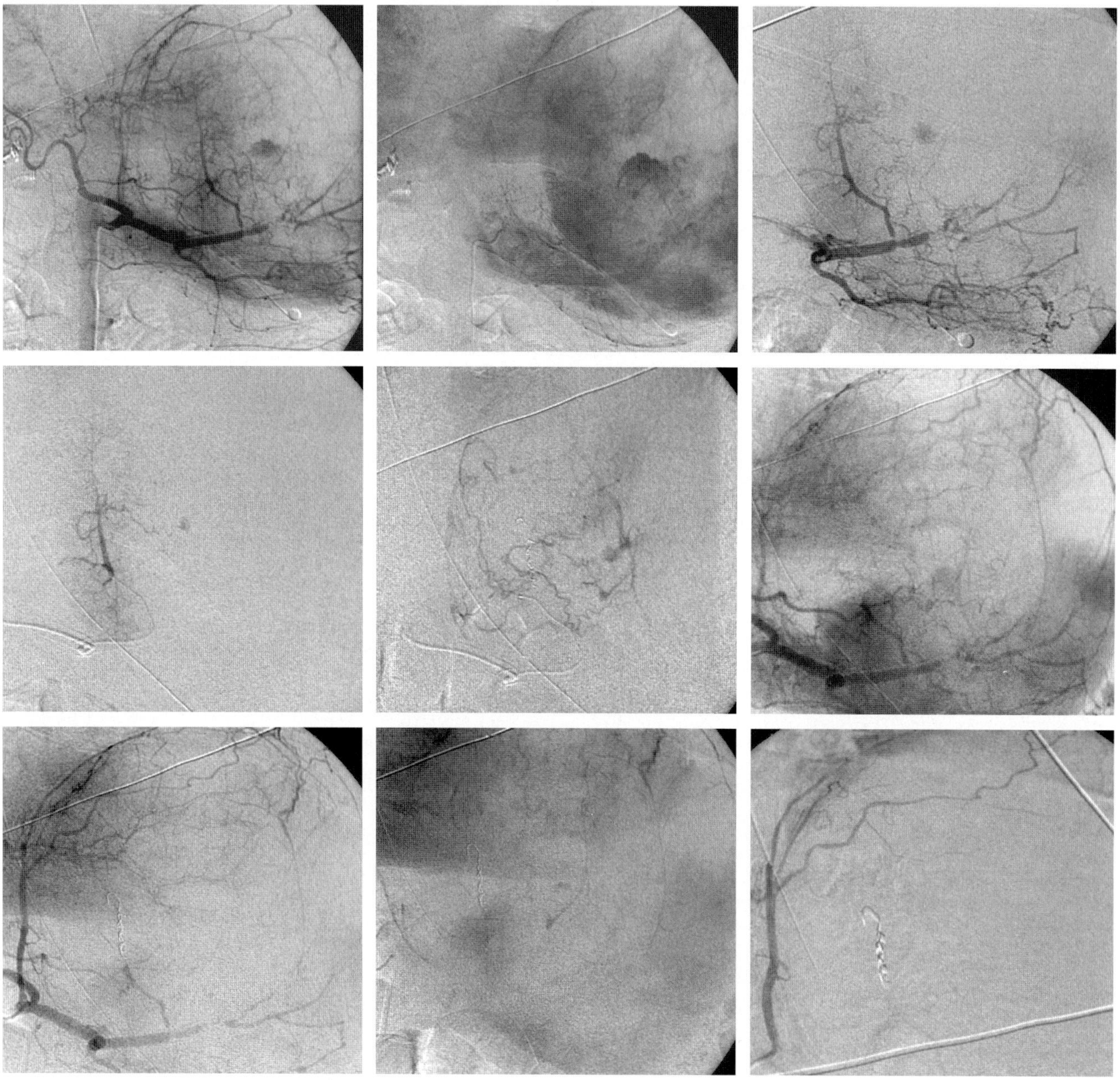

Figure 1.12

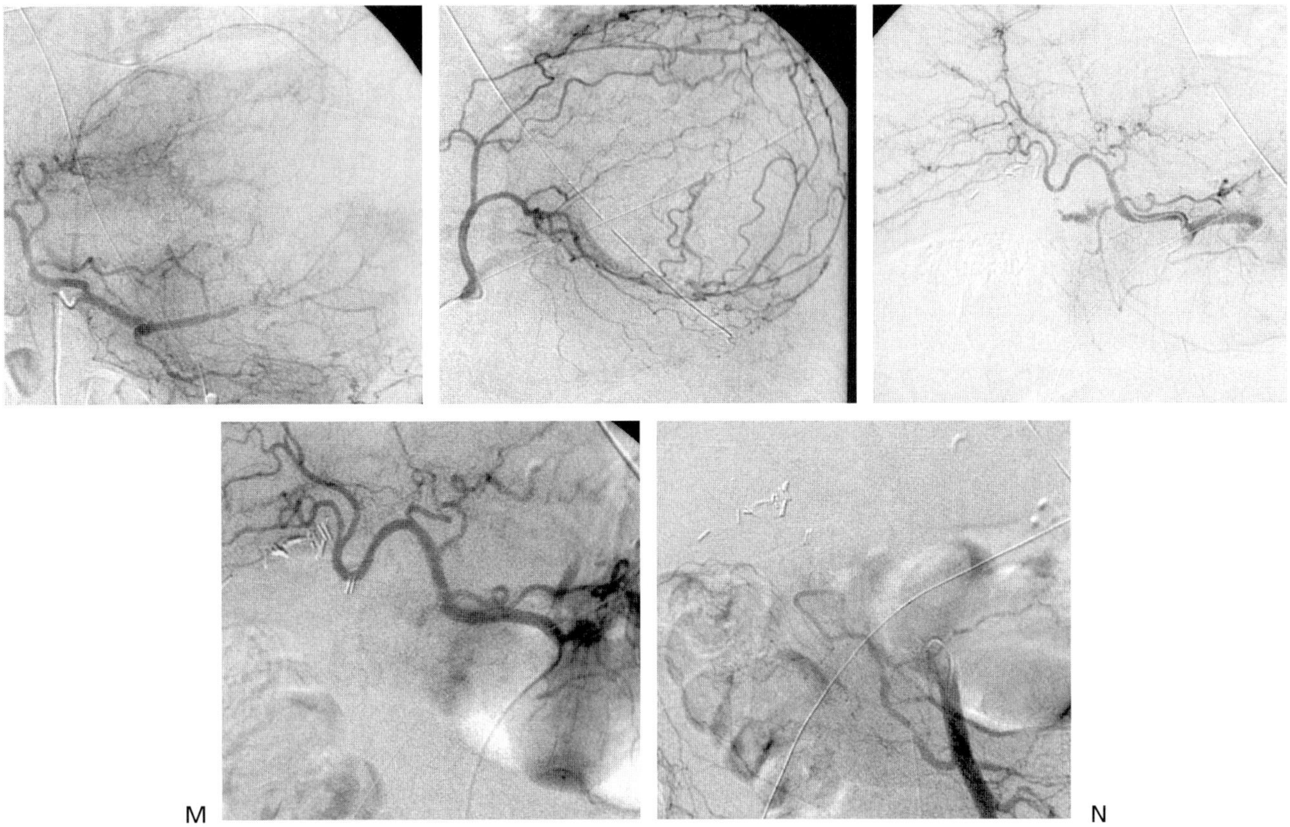

Figure 1.12 *(continued)*

A: Celiac artery injection shows occlusion of the splenic artery due to previous surgery, with reconstitution of distal short gastric branches through the left gastric artery. An area of active bleeding is seen in the center of the stomach. **B:** Late-phase angiogram shows a small arterial aneurysm and spreading of contrast on the mucosa of the stomach. **C:** More selective angiogram of the splenic artery shows active bleeding from the short gastric arteries. **D:** Superselective angiogram of one of the proximal short gastric arteries shows active bleeding. Embolization with a microcoil was performed. **E:** Superselective angiogram performed in another short gastric artery still shows active bleeding. **F:** Celiac arteriogram following embolization shows reduction of bleeding but the aneurysm still is visible. **G:** Left gastric artery shows no extravasation, but there still is filling of the aneurysm. **H:** Distal filling of the aneurysm still is visualized. **I:** Postembolization angiogram of the left gastric artery shows no filling of the aneurysm **J:** Postembolization celiac arteriogram shows faint filling of the aneurysm. Bleeding was controlled. **K:** Arteriogram obtained 10 days after initial treatment because of another episode of upper GI bleeding. Left gastric artery angiogram does not show any active bleeding. **L:** Celiac arteriogram shows active bleeding in the duodenum from a branch of the gastroduodenal artery. **M:** Postembolization arteriogram of the gastroduodenal artery shows control of the bleeding. **N:** Postembolization superior mesenteric arteriogram shows no active bleeding in the gastroduodenal area, from the collateral vessels, originating from the SMA.

Comment: The cause of bleeding in this patient was not well established, but presumably was related to gastritis and duodenitis following surgery. Two separate episodes of bleeding were observed 10 days apart. Initial bleeding was identified in the stomach and the second in the duodenum. Embolization controlled the bleeding and allowed recovery. It was necessary to proceed with a rather extensive embolization that included short gastric arteries and left gastric artery. The second procedure included embolization of the gastroduodenal artery. The left gastric artery was patent on follow-up angiogram. Collateral circulation plays an important role in the embolic management of upper GI bleeding, particularly in the stomach fundus and duodenum, where double circulation is observed. Superselective embolization usually is necessary; however, very distal branches may be difficult to catheterize, as in this case.

1.13 Embolization In Gastrointestinal Bleeding

Case 1.13:

A 54-year-old man with diffuse metastatic disease presented with bleeding from a duodenal ulcer that could not be stopped by endoscopy. An arteriogram and embolization were performed at another institution. Because of recurrence of bleeding, the patient was transferred for treatment.

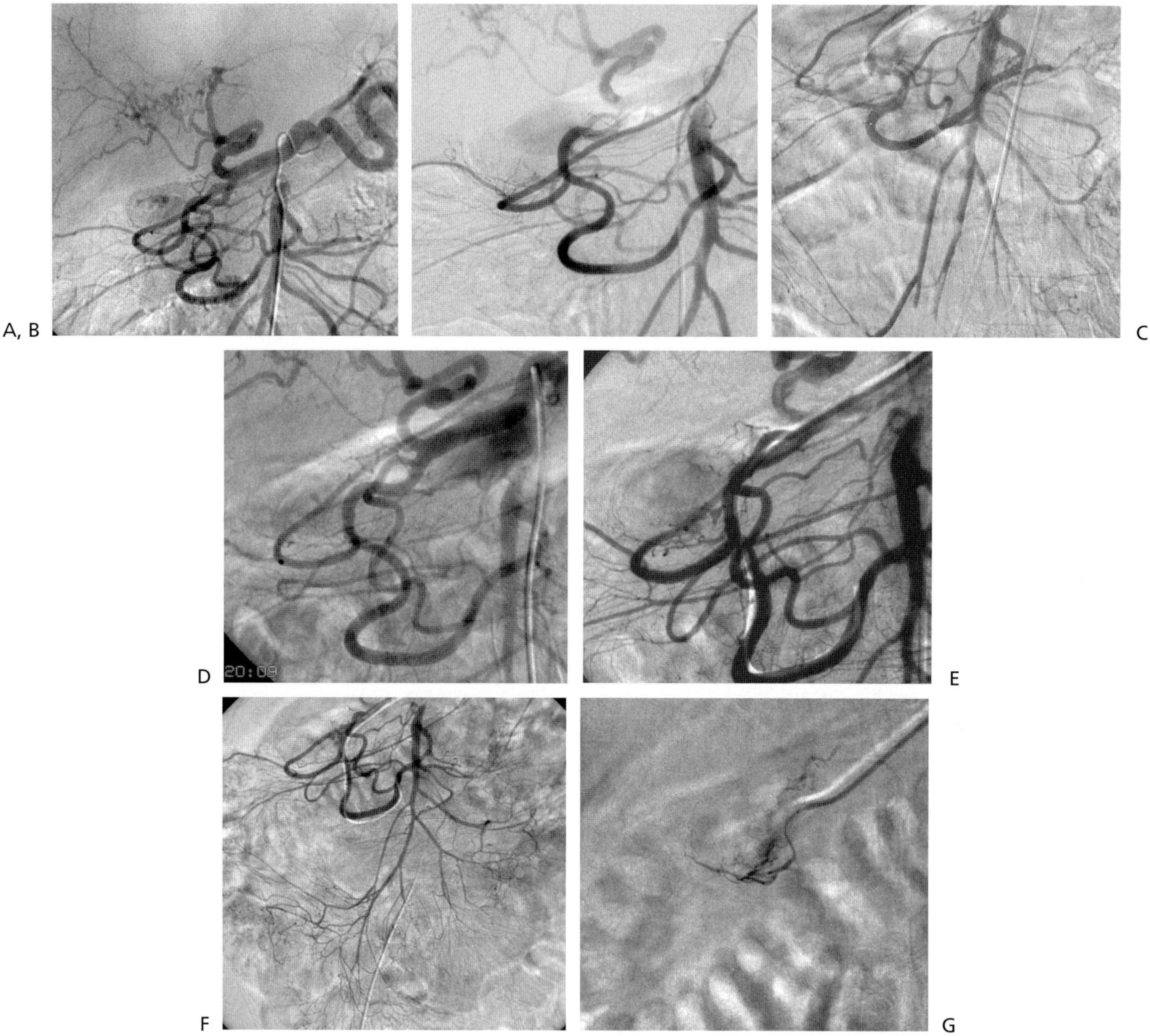

Figure 1.13

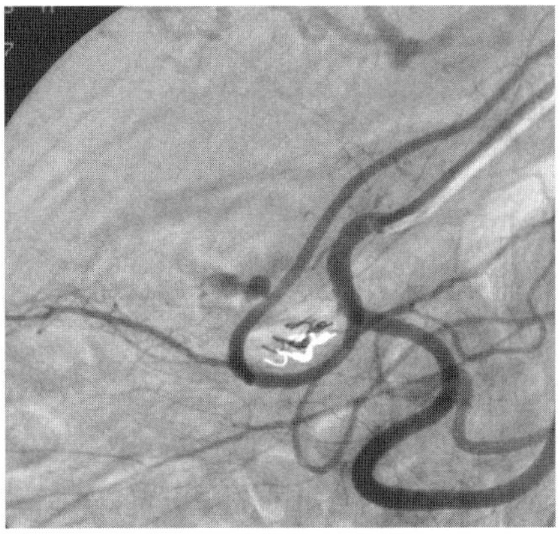

H

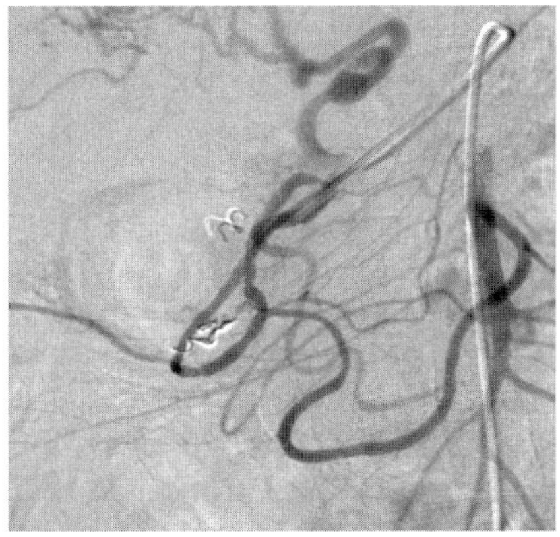

I

Figure 1.13 *(continued)*

A: Outside arteriogram with selective injection in the celiac trunk shows active bleeding from branches of the gastroduodenal artery, into the duodenum. Note development of collaterals that fill the SMA through the pancreaticoduodenal arcades. The SMA presented a stenosis at the orifice. **B:** Selective injection in the gastroduodenal artery shows no bleeding. Note again the direct connection to the SMA. **C:** Despite the large communication between the celiac artery and the SMA, embolization with larger particles of Gelfoam was performed by a less experienced interventionalist. This procedure caused embolism into the distal branches of the SMA, without occlusion of the pancreaticoduodenal arcade. Note occlusion of the distal SMA branches that was not appreciated at the time of embolization. Bleeding improved temporarily but restarted the next morning. The patient was transferred to our institution. **D:** Initial celiac arteriogram does not show active bleeding. **E:** Selective angiography of the gastroduodenal artery shows active bleeding in the duodenal lumen. **F:** SMA injection through the pancreaticoduodenal arcade shows recanalization of the embolized branches of the SMA, with a minor residual occlusion of one branch. Active bleeding is depicted in the duodenum. **G:** Superselective injection with a microcatheter of a branch of the gastroduodenal artery shows active bleeding. Embolization with microcoils occluded the vessel. **H:** More proximal injection shows persistent bleeding. **I:** Multiple other branches were catheterized and embolized with microcoils. The bleeding was controlled; however, the patient could not tolerate the severe blood loss and died of multiorgan failure a couple of days later.

Comment: This case illustrates a common anatomic situation where the gastroduodenal artery is directly connected to the SMA through the inferior pancreatic artery and pancreaticoduodenal arcades. Embolization of the dilated arcades, as in this case, will lead to SMA embolism and ischemia. Unaware of the risks of SMA embolism, improper embolization was performed with Gelfoam particles that went directly into the SMA. No major symptoms of ischemia developed, but persistent bleeding prompted restudy and proper embolization. The patient eventually died due to the severity of clinical problems, but apparently unrelated to the iatrogenic SMA embolism.

1.14 Embolization In Gastrointestinal Bleeding

Case 1.14:

A 41-year-old male prison inmate presented with an actively bleeding ulcer of the duodenum. Endoscopy was performed and the diagnosis was made, but endoscopy could not stop the bleeding.

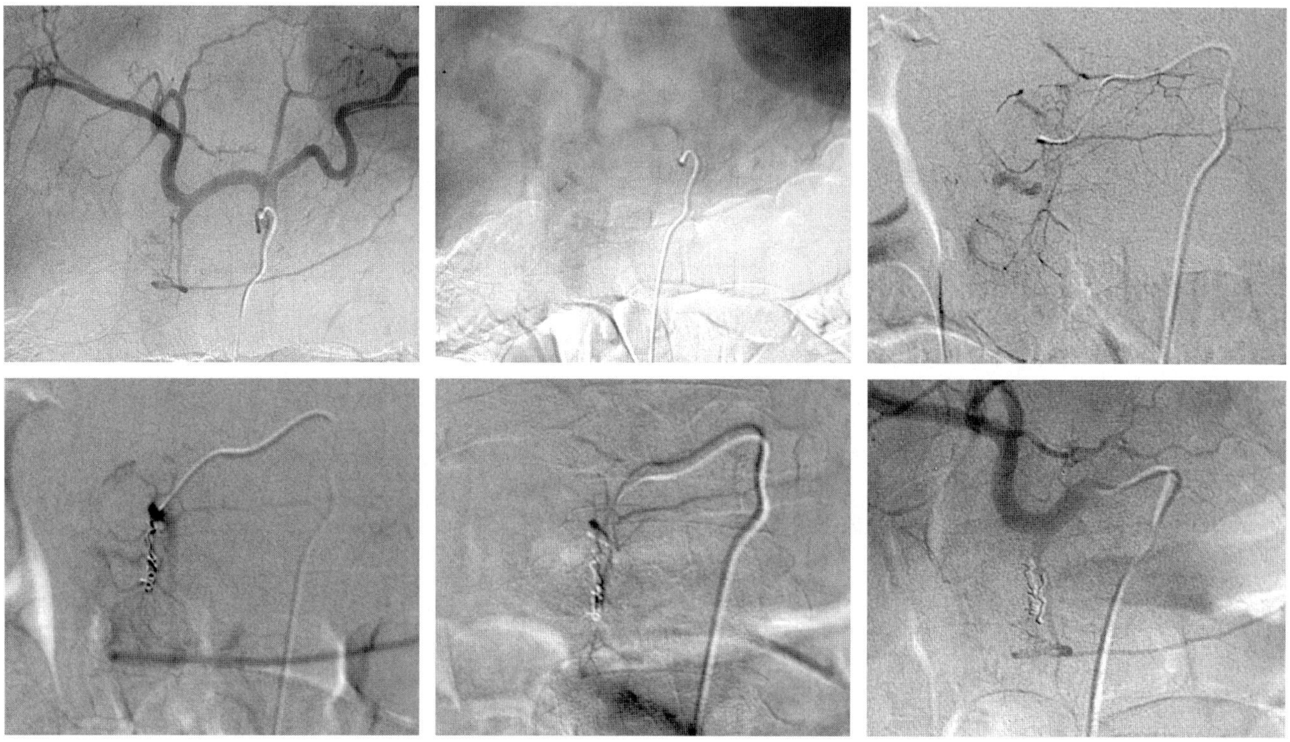

A, B C D, E F

Figure 1.14

A: Celiac arteriogram shows a normal liver and spleen but a small area of extravasation adjacent to the lateral aspect of the gastroduodenal artery. A prominent pancreaticoduodenal arcade is observed. **B:** Late-phase celiac arteriogram shows partial filling of the portal vein and extravasated contrast in the lumen of the duodenum. **C:** Through the 5F Mikaelsson catheter located in the celiac artery, a 1.8F microcatheter was used for superselective catheterization of a branch of the pancreaticoduodenal arcade and demonstrated the extravasation. **D,E:** Embolization with microcoils was performed in a couple of branches to control the bleeding. **F:** A few minutes after embolization, a hepatic artery arteriogram was performed and showed control of the bleeding.

Comment: This case demonstrates well the utilization of the embolization procedure to control upper GI bleeding from an arterial source in the duodenum. With the availability of the new microcatheter technology originally designed and developed for neurointerventional procedures, it became possible to reach bleeding sites never before adequately embolized with particulate matter. In the previous era of microcatheters, embolization of more peripheral arterial branches was possible only with the utilization of fluid materials or very small flow-oriented solid particles. When injected more proximally, a fluid embolic agent may cause occlusion of undesired arterial territories and increase the possibility of necrosis of surrounding healthy tissues. The same risk of necrosis of nontarget tissues is possible with small flow-oriented particles. The availability of microcatheters has allowed the safer use of embolic glues as well as microcoils, as demonstrated in this case. Small embolic particles still are contraindicated for GI bleeding, such as in the presented case.

1.15 Embolization In Gastrointestinal Bleeding

Case 1.15:

A 62-year-old man presented with hypotension due to massive bleeding of duodenal ulcer that could not be controlled by endoscopy. Angiography was requested for possible embolization.

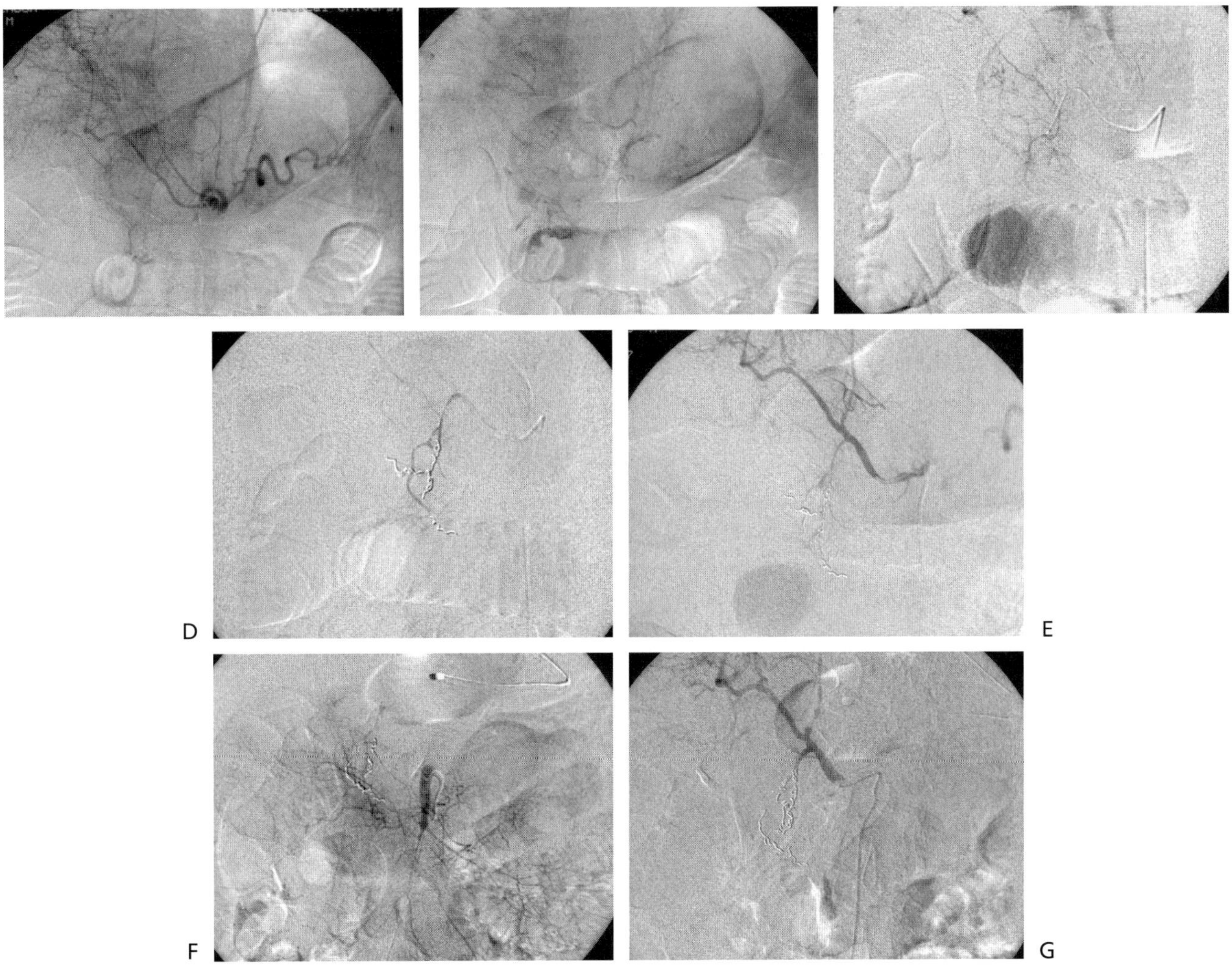

Figure 1.15

A: Celiac arteriogram shows diffuse arterial spasm. An anatomic variation with two independent hepatic arteries arising from the celiac artery is observed. The gastroduodenal artery is barely visible and is connected to the most lateral hepatic artery. **B:** Late-phase celiac arteriogram shows active extravasation in the duodenal lumen from a branch of the gastroduodenal artery. **C:** Superselective injection in one of the pancreaticoduodenal arcades shows filling of the biliary artery (either the 9 or 3 o'clock artery) all the way up to the intrahepatic right hepatic artery. No active bleeding is detected by this injection. **D:** Multiple superselective microcoil embolization in several branches, including one in the area originally visualized as the bleeder artery. **E:** A more proximal selective angiogram shows no active bleeding. **F:** Superior mesenteric angiogram shows diffuse spasm and no bleeding after embolization. **G:** Final arteriogram in the hepatic artery shows improvement of the spasm and control of the bleeding, which was seen as permanent in the follow-up time available.

Comment: GI bleeding and hypotension are accompanied by visceral spasm in an attempt to control shock and exsanguination. Diffuse arterial spasm may make it more difficult to catheterize the artery and even identify the bleeding. Multiple catheterizations and microcoil embolization were necessary to control the bleeding; however, no actual bleeding was detected by the superselective embolizations. One important postembolization angiogram for duodenal bleeding is superior mesenteric angiography, which may show collateral feeding from below that requires additional catheterization if the actual bleeder branch is not embolized.

1.16 Embolization In Gastrointestinal Bleeding

Case 1.16:

A 60-year-old woman with a large duodenal diverticulum that became infected and perforated required percutaneous drainage a couple of weeks after diagnosis and surgical cholecystectomy. About 1 week after drainage, the patient presented with massive bleeding in the diverticulum and hemodynamic instability that prompted diagnostic angiogram and embolization.

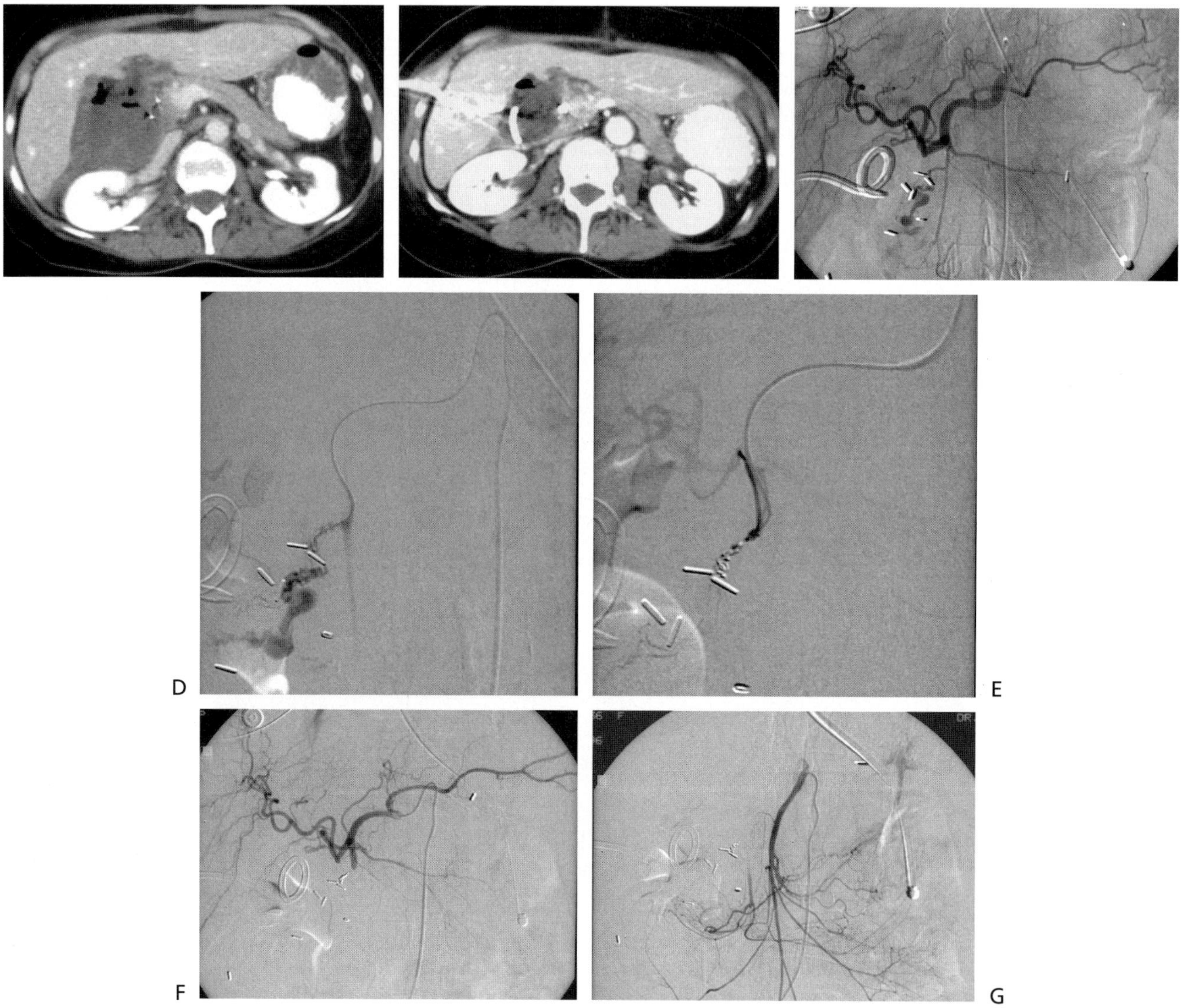

A, B C D E F G

Figure 1.16

A: Computed tomographic scan of the abdomen shows subhepatic fluid collection with air within. Surgery was performed at that time. **B:** Follow-up computed tomographic scan of the abdomen obtained during percutaneous drainage with a 12F catheter for recurrent fluid collection. Note reduction in size of the collection following drainage. **C:** Five days after drainage, the patient presented with massive bleeding inside the duodenal diverticulum. Celiac arteriogram shows active bleeding from the superior posterior pancreaticoduodenal arcade into the diverticulum or peritoneal cavity. **D:** Superselective catheterization with a microcatheter into the pancreaticoduodenal artery and injection shows active extravasation. **E:** Superselective catheterization allowed selective embolization with a single 3-mm × 3-cm microcoil, which arrested the bleeding. Selective angiogram shows no active extravasation of contrast. **F,G:** Postembolization celiac and superior mesenteric angiography show no active bleeding.

Drainage was maintained for several weeks, and eventually the patient was discharged.

Comment: Active massive bleeding in duodenal diverticulum is rare. Infection and arterial erosion certainly played a role in the development of bleeding in this patient. A pseudoaneurysm in the gastroduodenal artery branch most likely was responsible for the bleeding. Pancreatic pseudocysts more commonly cause arterial erosion and bleeding. Angiographic diagnostic was straightforward and bleeding identification was easy. Superselective catheterization with a microcatheter allowed direct embolization of the bleeder artery. One single microcoil was used for the embolization. The modern microcoils are not as thrombogenic as the old Gianturco coils or the minicoils; therefore, a small piece of Gelfoam may be used to precipitate thrombosis around the coil. However, it was not necessary in this procedure.

1.17 Embolization In Gastrointestinal Bleeding

Case 1.17:

A 47-year-old man recovering from a severe myocardial infarction suffered 5 days before developed a bleeding duodenal ulcer that could not be treated surgically or endoscopically due to the high risk of general anesthesia and deep sedation.

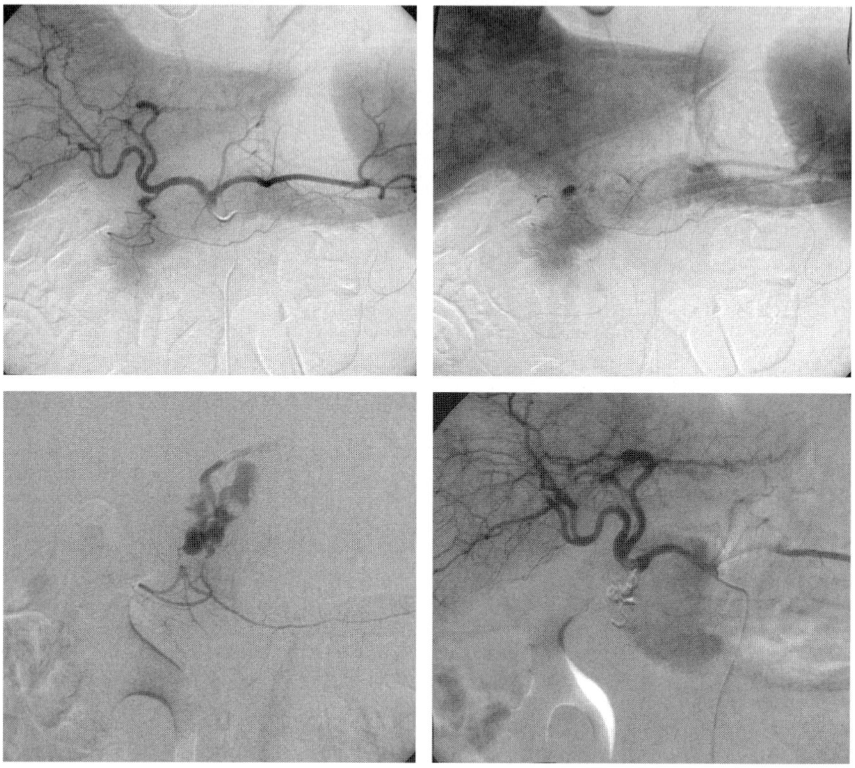

Figure 1.17

A,B: Selective celiac arteriography shows an image suggestive of a pseudoaneurysm of the gastroduodenal artery, which accumulated the contrast in the duodenal lumen, as demonstrated in the late phase. **C:** Superselective catheterization of the gastroduodenal artery and contrast injection shows massive extravasation at the point of bleeding in the duodenum. Superior mesenteric artery injection did not demonstrate retrograde filling of the gastroduodenal artery. **D:** Embolization of the gastroduodenal artery with multiple microcoils and a few particles of Gelfoam was performed, which controlled the bleeding. Common hepatic arteriogram shows total occlusion of the gastroduodenal artery. Note the pseudoaneurysm filled with the coils.

Comment: It is relatively uncommon for duodenal bleedings to be related to direct lesions of the gastroduodenal artery. Erosion of the artery develops at the bottom of the ulceration in the duodenal mucosa, by direct action of the gastric and duodenal juices. A pseudoaneurysm of the gastroduodenal artery was identified in this case. Embolization of the main steam of the gastroduodenal artery must be performed. The embolization must occlude the artery beyond and before the point of the pseudoaneurysm. Coils are the usual best selection for that type of lesion. Because the pseudoaneurysm may be in the bottom lumen of the ulceration, the coils may be placed partially in the lumen of the ulceration. Small particles of Gelfoam were used to promote thrombosis within the mesh created by the coils. A microcatheter was used to deploy the coils and the Gelfoam particles, with the 5F catheter located in the orifice of the gastroduodenal artery.

1.18 Embolization In Gastrointestinal Bleeding

Case 1.18:

A 76-year-old male patient underwent a choledochojejunostomy for pancreatic cancer. The day after surgery, he developed upper GI bleeding from a pseudoaneurysm of the hepatic artery, with severe hemorrhage in the bowel loop used for the choledochojejunostomy. The patient was hypotensive and comatose at the time of the angiogram.

A 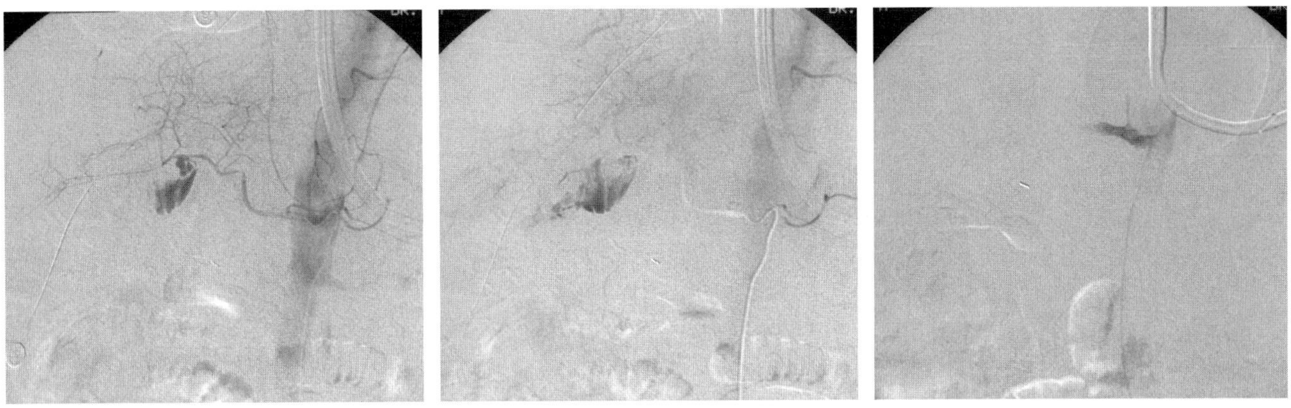 B, C

Figure 1.18

A,B: Selective celiac arteriogram shows marked spasm of the visceral vessels. A pseudoaneurysm of the hepatic artery at the level of the anastomosis is identified, as well as active bleeding into the anastomotic bowel loop. **C:** Embolization was performed with Gelfoam particles. Due to the arterial spasm, total occlusion of the hepatic artery developed and was seen on follow-up angiogram. The patient continued to bleed. He was taken to surgery the next day and died during surgery due to cardiac and respiratory complications.

Comment: This very high-risk patient developed a severe complication of surgery with massive GI hemorrhage. Angiography demonstrated the cause of bleeding, which was related to a pseudoaneurysm in the anastomotic site. In this case, embolization was done with Gelfoam, from a more proximally located catheter, which caused total occlusion of the hepatic artery. The best technique in this case would be the use of a microcatheter and coils to ensure total and permanent occlusion of the hepatic artery at the level of the pseudoaneurysm. The use of Gelfoam in this case may have caused the recurrent bleeding due to recanalization of the artery, requiring further surgery.

1.19 Embolization In Gastrointestinal Bleeding

Case 1.19:

A 45-year-old man presented with recurrent upper GI bleeding with repeated normal endoscopies. Endoscopic ultrasound showed periduodenal varices. An angiographic study was requested for diagnosis and possible treatment.

A, B

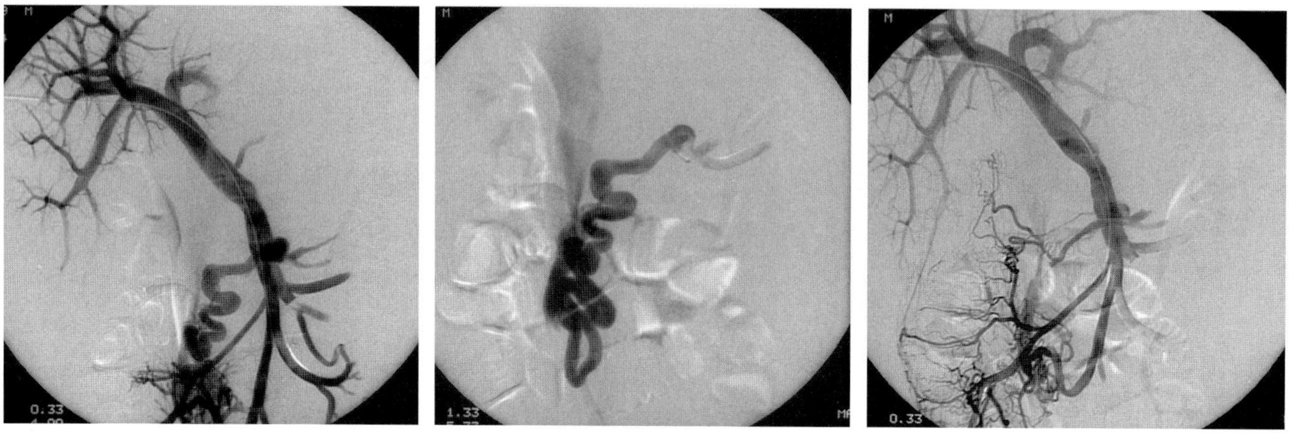

C

Figure 1.19

A: Percutaneous transhepatic portogram shows a large varicose vein with hepatofugal flow, draining in the inferior vena cava and coursing along the duodenal wall. **B:** Selective catheterization of the varix was performed for embolization with coils. **C:** Transhepatic portogram after embolization with coils shows total occlusion of the varix. The recurrent bleeding was controlled permanently. Pressures were recorded and showed no evidence of portal hypertension.

Comment: Percutaneous transhepatic portogram with varices embolization is a time-honored procedure with a relatively high success in controlling acute variceal bleeding, but with a high rate of recurrence within 3 to 6 months. It is unusual for a small varix in the wall of a bowel structure without portal hypertension to cause clinically significant bleeding. The transhepatic approach is a very adequate technique to deal with the portal system and for selective embolization of varices related to the portal system. Access usually is made with a Lunderquist needle, and the selective catheterization usually requires a curved tip catheter. The liver tract is embolized with a large Gelfoam torpedo to reduce the possibility of intraperitoneal bleeding.

1.20 Embolization In Gastrointestinal Bleeding

Case 1.20:

A 49-year-old man presented with recurrent upper GI bleeding with esophageal varices identified by endoscopy.

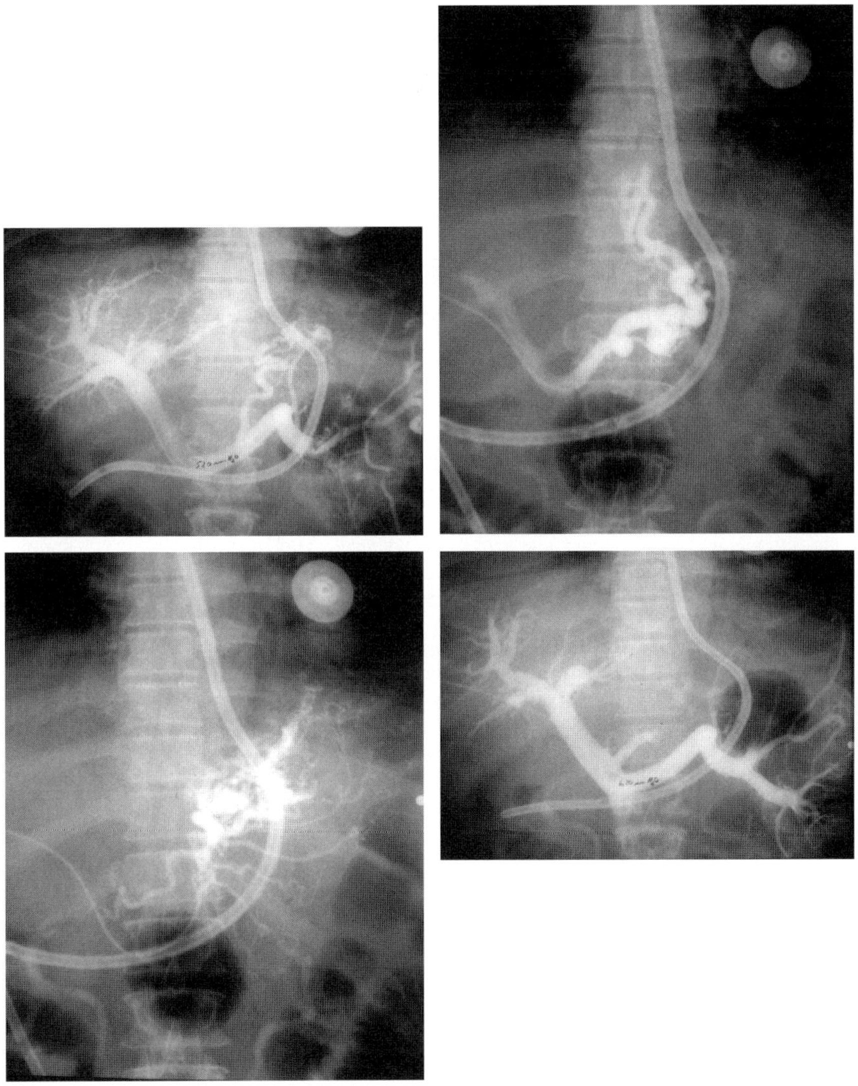

A B C D

Figure 1.20

A: Transhepatic portography shows patency of the splenic and portal vein, with a short gastric vein coming off the splenic vein and filling of varices in the stomach. **B:** Selective injection at the left gastric vein shows filling of gastric veins and distal esophageal varices. **C:** Selective injection in the short gastric vein shows gastric varices. Selective embolization performed with Gelfoam pledgets and absolute alcohol, achieved occlusion of the gastroesophageal varices, with control of the bleeding. **D:** Postembolization transhepatic portogram shows occlusion of the varices.

Comment: About 10% of patients with upper GI bleeding bleed from esophageal varices. Among the population with proven esophageal varices, less than 50% bleed from these varices during an episode of upper GI bleeding. Initial diagnostic tool is endoscopy followed by endoscopic sclerosis. The transhepatic approach for variceal embolization was popular in the late 1970s and early 1980s. The widespread availability of endoscopic sclerosing techniques and, more recently, banding changed the management of the patients with bleeding esophageal varices. Transhepatic esophageal varices embolization is able to stop active bleeding in more than 80% of the patients. However, there is recanalization or development of new varices in about half of the patients within 3 months, with a high chance of rebleeding. This case showed good occlusion of varices, and bleeding was controlled. The point of entrance into the portal vein was too low and carried a risk of intraperitoneal bleeding. No complications developed following the procedure.

1.21 Embolization In Gastrointestinal Bleeding

Case 1.21:

A 50-year-old man presented with acute upper GI bleeding. Alcoholic cirrhosis was the diagnosis. An angiographic study was requested for diagnosis and possible treatment.

A 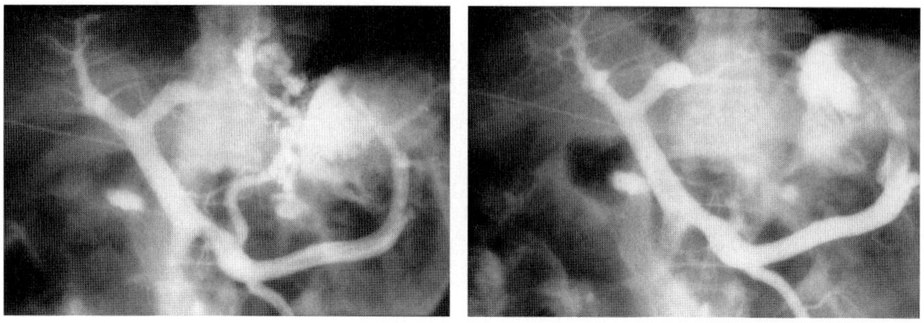 B

Figure 1.21

A: Transhepatic portogram was performed under fluoroscopic guidance. Note the low position of the puncture in the portal vein, which carries a risk of bleeding, and the gastroesophageal varices. There is residual barium in the stomach from the day before. **B:** Selective catheterization of the left gastric vein was followed by occlusion with absolute alcohol. Bleeding stopped, and the patient remained stable for the next 3 weeks. The patient's clinical status progressively deteriorated, with development of encephalopathy and coma.

Comment: The results of variceal embolization are worse in Child's C class patients. Percutaneous transhepatic catheterization and embolization of variceal varices may be performed during the acute phase of bleeding, as in this case. The procedure is performed through transhepatic puncture, under fluoroscopic guidance. The puncture site is the right middle axillary line at the level of the ninth and tenth intercostal spaces. A peripheral portal branch should be selected for access into the portal vein. Puncture of the main portal vein may be extrahepatic and cause bleeding. Various embolization materials are used, including Gelfoam, metallic coils, and sclerosing agents. Absolute alcohol is an efficient substance to achieve thrombosis of the varices and may occlude more distal, esophageal varices. Coils are proximal occluders and should not be used alone.

1.22 Embolization In Gastrointestinal Bleeding

Case 1.22:

A 54-year-old woman presented with acute upper GI bleeding due to esophageal varices and portal hypertension caused by postnecrotic cirrhosis.

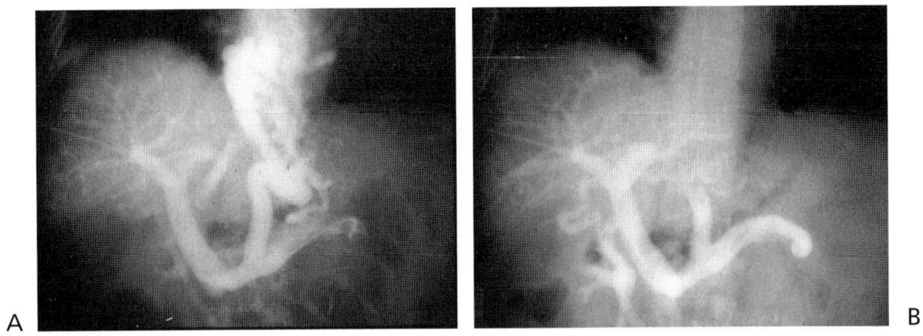

Figure 1.22

A: Transhepatic portogram shows massive gastroesophageal varices from the left gastric vein arising from the splenic vein. **B:** After selective catheterization, embolization with metal coils, absolute alcohol, and Gelfoam pledgets and complete occlusion of the large varices were achieved.

Comment: Catheterization of the portal vein through the liver parenchyma in patients with chronic liver disease and coagulopathy carries a significant risk of bleeding. During removal of the catheter, its pathway through the liver parenchyma is embolized to prevent intraperitoneal bleeding. The catheter is pulled, and several "torpedoes" of Gelfoam are carefully introduced through the catheter and deposited in the parenchyma to seal off the tract. Care should be exercised to avoid introducing the Gelfoam into the portal system to minimize risks of acute thrombosis. The trauma of portal vein catheterization associated with the stagnation that may follow embolization and preexisting hepatofugal flow may cause acute thrombosis of the portal vein with disastrous consequences, acute liver failure, and death.

1.23 Embolization In Gastrointestinal Bleeding

Case 1.23:

A 60-year-old male patient presented with acute upper GI bleeding due to esophageal varices and portal hypertension caused by alcoholic cirrhosis. Encephalopathy was difficult to control.

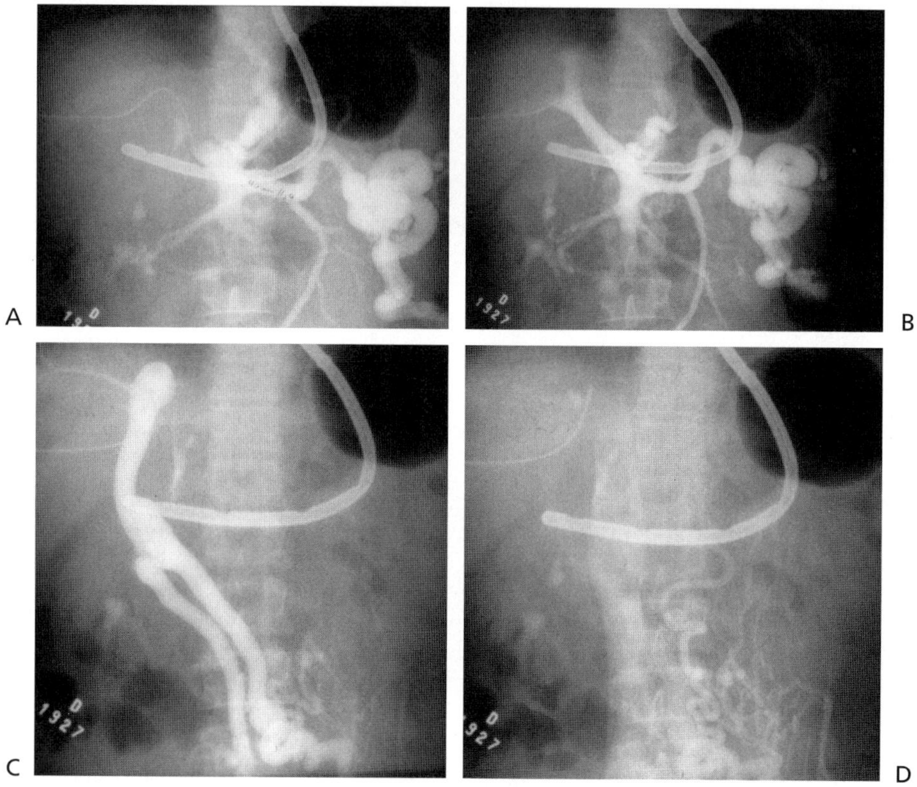

Figure 1.23

A: Percutaneous transhepatic portogram shows hepatofugal flow with filling of a large perisplenic varix, most likely connected to the systemic circulation. **B:** Embolization of the esophagogastric varices improved portal flow in hepatopetal direction. **C:** After pulling the catheter back into the main portal vein, a large paraumbilical vein was identified draining the portal system into the caput medusae. **D:** Later-phase angiogram shows filling of the inferior vena cava and multiple collaterals.

Comment: Percutaneous puncture of the portal system is ideally made at the level of a branch of the right portal vein. Hepatofugal flow as demonstrated in this case may be due to increased resistance at the sinusoidal level, arterioportal shunting, and development of portosystemic shunts in the periphery of the portal circulation. Hepatofugal flow may be temporary and reversible. Improvement in hepatic function and resolution of lesions, such as acute alcoholic hepatitis, may reverse direction of the portal flow. Embolization of esophageal varices may cause disturbance of portal flow, and in occasional cases the stagnation provoked by embolization may trigger acute thrombosis in the portal vein. The presence of large portosystemic shunts usually prevents thrombosis. Spontaneous portosystemic shunts are not able to decompress adequately the portal system, but may cause changes in flow direction.

1.24 Embolization In Gastrointestinal Bleeding

Case 1.24:

A 64-year-old man had schistosomiasis combined with chronic encephalopathy for 7 years and three recent episodes of coma despite intensive clinical treatment with a low-protein diet. Splenectomy was performed 2 years earlier in an attempt to reduce portal hypertension. A massive portosystemic shunt was identified.

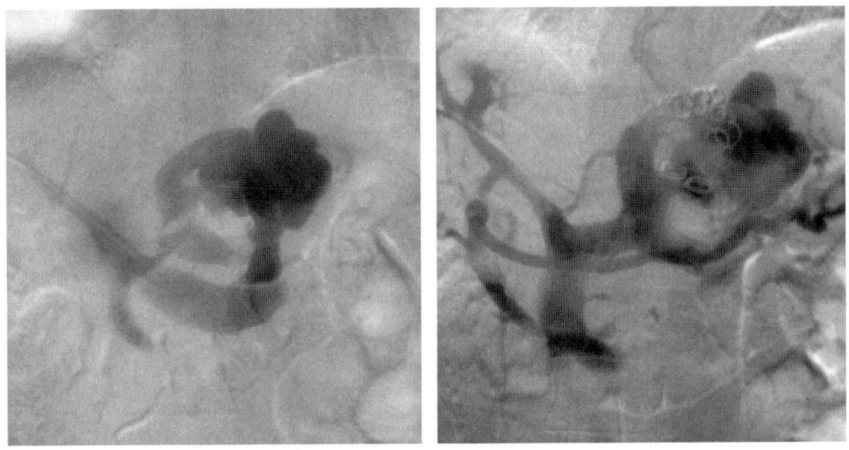

Figure 1.24

A: Percutaneous transhepatic portogram shows hepatofugal flow and total blood drain through the left gastric vein into the splenorenal shunt. **B:** Partial occlusion of the spontaneous shunt was performed with multiple Gianturco coils. There was improvement of portal flow with reversal of flow to a hepatopetal direction. Marked increase in portal pressure developed, and about 1 week after embolization the patient developed bleeding in the gallbladder fossa, which was treated surgically, but the patient died of uncontrollable bleeding.

Comment: Massive splenorenal shunts may cause encephalopathy that is difficult to control clinically. Hepatic encephalopathy can be characterized as the occurrence of mental confusion or episodes of disorientation detected by a patients' family or the attending physician. Permanent mental confusion and coma are more advanced stages that usually precede death from hepatic failure. Massive shunting usually is not amenable to clinical treatment, and invasive treatment is necessary. Occlusion of the spontaneous portosystemic shunt may effectively reduce the blood shunting with clinical improvement, but it may cause an acute increase in portal hypertension that increases the risk of intraperitoneal bleeding.

1.25 Embolization In Gastrointestinal Bleeding

Case 1.25:

A 54-year-old male patient with cirrhosis presented with chronic encephalopathy from spontaneous portosystemic shunt and upper GI bleeding from gastric varices after endoscopic sclerosis.

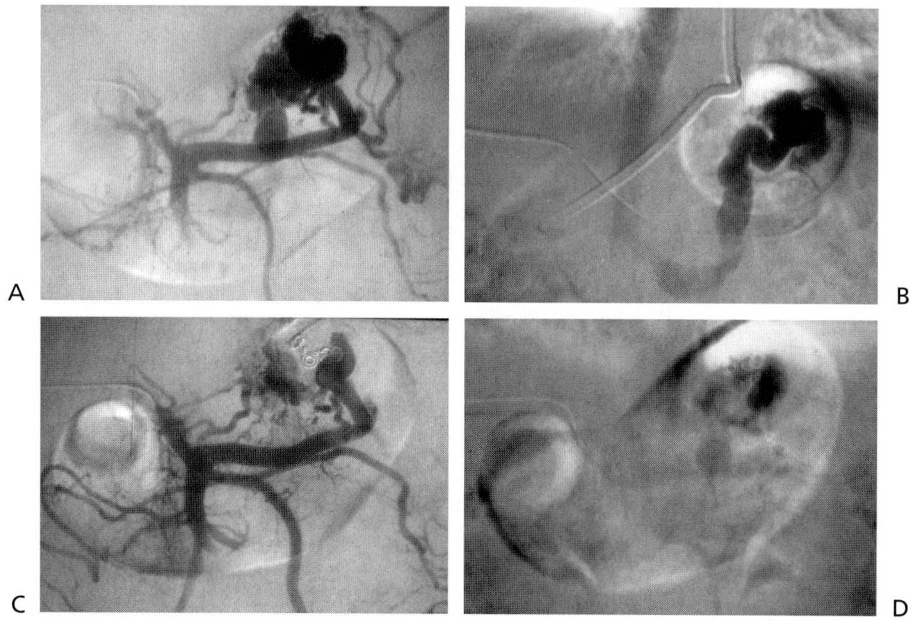

Figure 1.25

A: Transhepatic portogram shows hepatofugal flow and filling of large varices in the gastric fundus and a spontaneous splenorenal shunt originating from a short gastric vein. **B:** Later-phase angiogram shows the shunt communicating with the left renal vein and filling the inferior vena cava. **C:** Embolization with Gianturco coils was performed. Bleeding did not recur and encephalopathy was controlled. **D:** Late phase of the injection shows significant occlusion of the shunt.

Comment: The embolization procedure effectively occluded the shunt in this patient. Endoscopic sclerosis treated only the bleeding related to the esophageal varices and did not touch the gastric fundus varices involved in the shunt. A short gastric vein was the main source of flow into the shunt. Note that the flow was hepatofugal in the portal vein and persisted hepatofugally after embolization of the shunt. The shunt involved large veins that created a potential threat of systemic embolism when the embolization coils were deployed. In this case, large 8-mm coils were used but became trapped inside the venous network. Progressive thrombosis of the shunt is desirable as opposed to acute thrombosis, which may cause a severe increase in portal pressure and variceal bleeding. When the shunt is the cause or the main component of the hepatic encephalopathy, the response is good and improvement is observed over the next several days following the embolization procedure. Improvement is not so good if there is established brain damage or reduced liver function is responsible for the encephalopathy.

Suggested Reading

Bradley EL, Goldman M. Gastric infarction after therapeutic embolization. *Surgery* 1976;79:421–424.

Brucharth F. Percutaneous transhepatic portography: I. Technique and application. *AJR* 1979;132:177–182.

Chandler JG, Fechner RE. Hepatopetal flow restoration in patients intolerant of total portal diversion. *Ann Surg* 1983;197:574–583.

Chung JW, Park JH, Han JK, et al. Perforation of the gastroduodenal artery induced by steerable guidewires in two cases: treatment of haemorrhage by embolization. *Cardiovasc Intervent Radiol* 1994;17:41–43.

Gordon BM, Herlong J, Uflacker R, et al. Recurrent lower gastrointestinal hemorrhage: ileal neoplasm diagnosed by scintigraphy with Tc 99m red blood cells and angiography. *South Med J* 1996;89:1204–1207.

Guy GE, Shetty PC, Sharma RP, et al. Acute lower gastrointestinal hemorrhage: treatment by superselective embolization with polyvinyl alcohol particles. *AJR* 1992;159:521–526.

Hashizume M, Tsugawa K, Migo S, et al. Eradication of large gastric varices by sclerotherapy combined with percutaneous transhepatic obliteration. *Hepatogastroenterology* 1997;44:221–226.

Hoevells J, Lunderquist A, Tylen U. Percutaneous transhepatic portography. *Acta Radiol* 1977;19:643–658.

Kawanaka H, Ohta M, Hashizume M, et al. Portosystemic encephalopathy treated with balloon occluded retrograde transvenous obliteration. *Am J Gastroenterol* 1995;90:508–510.

Keller FS, Dotter CT, Rosch J. Percutaneous transhepatic obliteration of gastroesophageal varices: some technical aspects. *Radiology* 1978;129:327–332.

Lang EV. Transcatheter embolization in management of hemorrhage from duodenal ulcer: long-term results and complications. *Radiology* 1992;182:703–708.

Lunderquist A, Vang J. Transhepatic catheterization and obliteration of the coronary vein in patients with portal hypertension and esophageal varices. *N Engl J Med* 1974;646–649.

Okazaki M, Ono H, Higashihara H, et al. Angiographic management of massive hemobilia due to iatrogenic trauma. *Gastrointest Radiol* 1991;16:205–211.

Uflacker R, Amaral NM, Lima S, et al. Angiography in primary myomas of the alimentary tract. *Radiology* 1981;139:361–369.

Uflacker R, d'Albuquerque LA, de Oliveira e Silva A, et al. Embolization to reverse severe recurrent hepatic encephalopathy. *Arq Gastroenterol* 1988;25:21–25.

Uflacker R, Lima S. Percutaneous transhepatic portography for obliteration of gastroesophageal varices in partial and total portal vein occlusion. *Radiology* 1980;137:325–330.

Uflacker R, Silva AO, Albuquerque LAC, et al. Chronic portosystemic encephalopathy: embolization of portosystemic shunts. *Radiology* 1987;165:721–725.

Uflacker R. Percutaneous transhepatic obliteration of gastroesophageal varices using absolute alcohol. *Radiology* 1983; 146:621–625.

Uflacker R. Transcatheter embolization for treatment of acute lower gastrointestinal bleeding. *Acta Radiol* 1987;28:425–430.

Waltman AC, Fourey WR, Athanasoulis CA, et al. Technique for left gastric catheterization. *Radiology* 1973;109:732–734.

Winick AB, Malloy PC, Lund GB. Retained contrast after embolization of a right gastric artery pseudoaneurysm. *Cardiovasc Intervent Radiol* 1996;19:110–112.

CHAPTER 2

Chemoembolization In The Liver

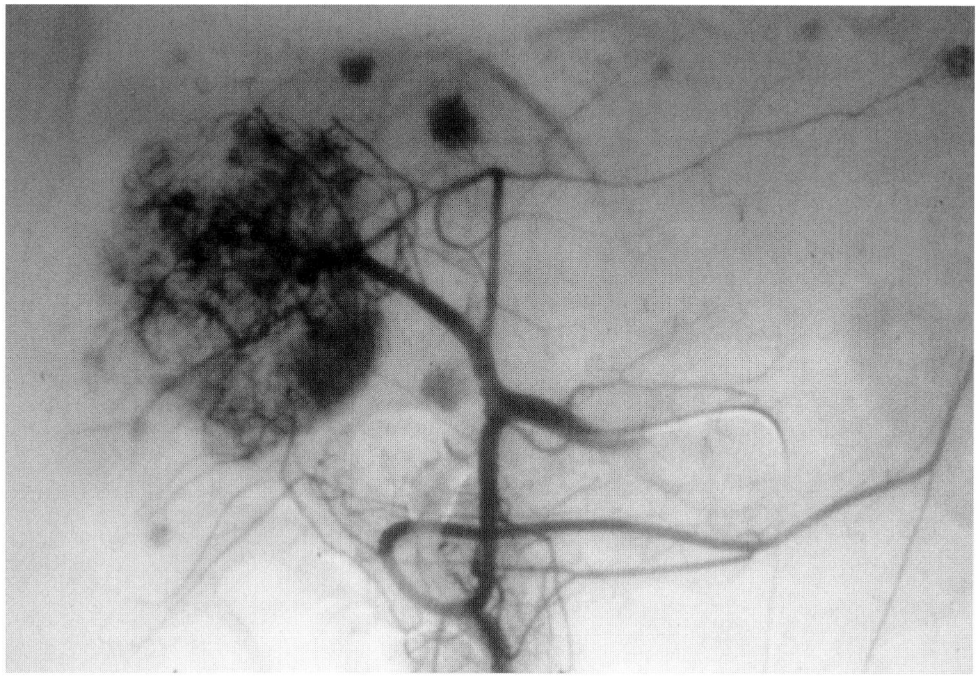

2.1 Chemoembolization In The Liver

Case 2.1:

A 59-year-old female patient presented with painful metastatic liver disease and weight loss due to a breast cancer resected 5 years earlier. Initial treatment with two cycles of intravenous (IV) chemotherapy produced no response. The patient was referred for transcatheter chemoembolization of the liver.

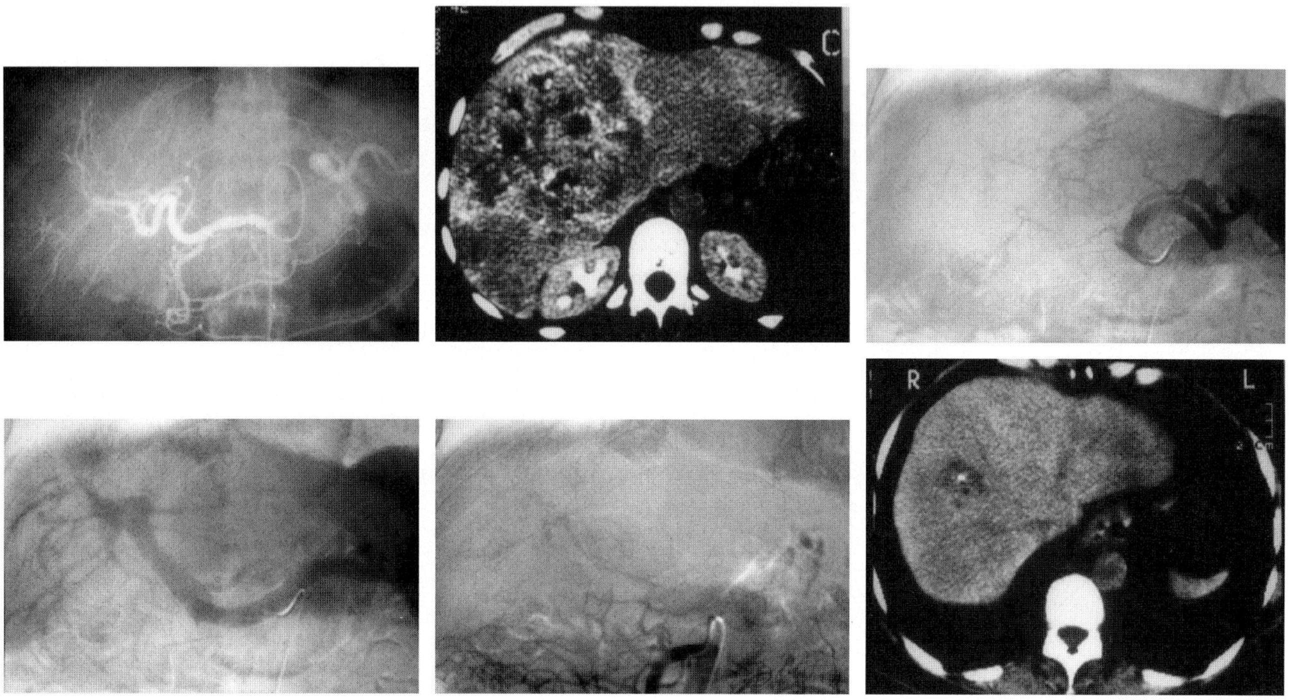

A, B — C — D, E — F

Figure 2.1

A: Initial unsubtracted celiac arteriogram shows displacement of arteries of the right lobe of the liver, but no significant hypervascularity, although the capillary phase shows some tumoral stain (not shown). **B:** Computed tomographic (CT) scan of the liver shows a large confluent metastatic liver mass with areas of enhancement around hypovascular nodules. Six chemoembolization procedures using mitomycin C, lipiodol, and Gelfoam particles were performed every 6 to 8 weeks for 10 months. Pain improved progressively and disappeared 3 weeks after the first procedure. **C:** Celiac arteriogram 1 year after the chemoembolization treatment shows occlusion of the main hepatic artery and collateral circulation through the phrenic arteries and extrahepatic biliary vascular plexus. **D:** Late-phase arteriogram shows patent splenic and portal vein. **E:** Selective superior mesenteric artery angiogram shows partial reconstitution of the intrahepatic artery through the biliary vascular plexus. **F:** Follow-up CT scan 2 years after the chemoembolization treatment shows a remarkable response of the tumor to the treatment. A small low-density liver lesion is still identified in the right liver lobe, with a small drop of lipiodol in the center. A needle biopsy was performed and showed nonviable cells. Follow-up of this patient is now 10 years, without change in clinical status or lesion size.

Comment: This case demonstrates a remarkable response of liver metastatic breast cancer to chemoembolization treatment. About 72% of our patients with metastatic breast cancer to the liver responded well to chemoembolization using mitomycin C, lipiodol/Ethiodol, and embolic particles, showing up to 90% clinical improvement. Mean survival time of the patients in our series was 18.3 months.

2.2 Chemoembolization In The Liver

Case 2.2:

A 65-year-old male patient presented with metastatic liver disease from colon cancer and subsequently underwent a left colectomy for primary tumor resection. IV chemotherapy did not arrest the growth of the liver metastasis. A 12-kg weight loss and severe liver pain developed in the 5-month period after surgery. The patient eventually was referred for chemoembolization.

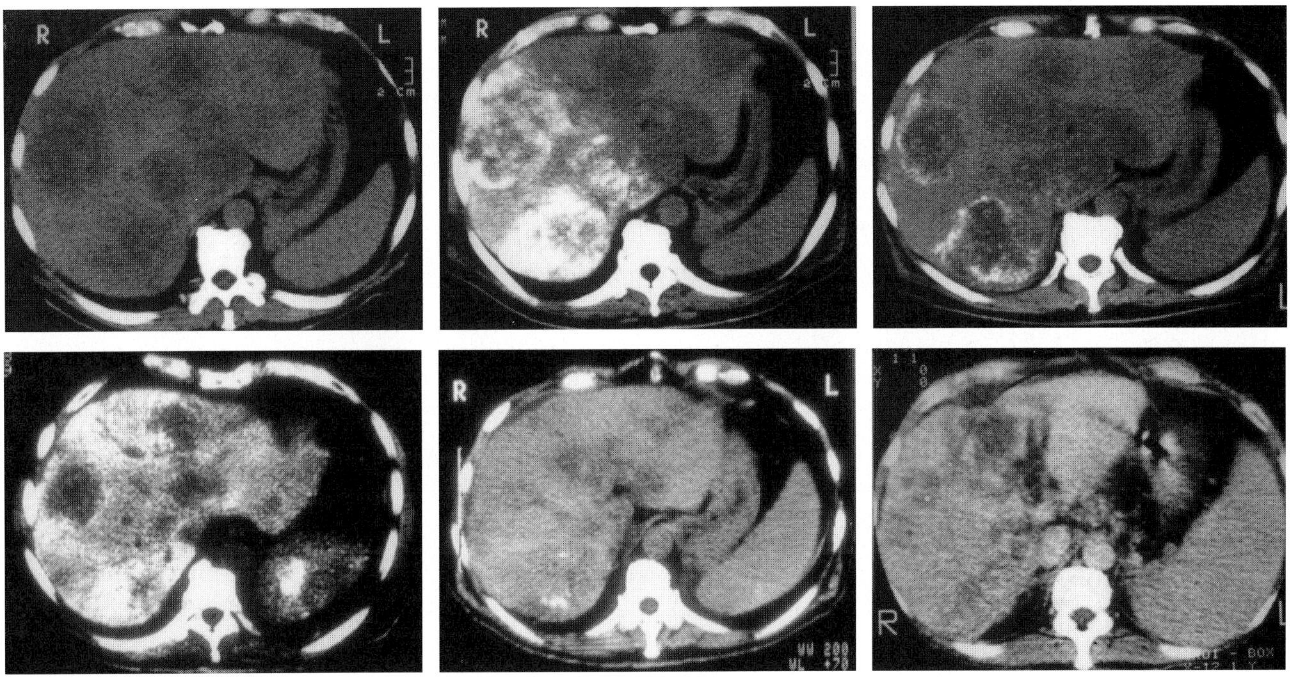

Figure 2.2

A: Initial liver CT scan shows multiple hypodense lesions throughout the organ and marked enlargement in liver size. **B:** Postchemoembolization CT scan of the liver. Due to the extension of the disease and the existence of a replaced left hepatic artery from the left gastric artery supplying the left lobe of the liver, only the right hepatic artery was selectively catheterized for treatment. Chemoembolization with mitomycin C, lipiodol, and Ivalon particles was performed. Note enhancement of the lesions in the right lobe of the liver. **C:** CT scan of the liver 6 weeks after chemoembolization shows some response of the targeted lesions and growth of the left lobe tumors. **D:** CT scan follow-up after the fifth chemoembolization shows significant response to treatment. **E:** CT scan of the liver 6 weeks after the final procedure, at the seventh chemoembolization, 10 months after the initial treatment, shows marked response of the liver metastasis. **F:** Follow-up CT scan of the liver 17 months after beginning treatment shows some recurrence of a lesion in the medial segment of the left lobe and a small amount of ascites. The patient rapidly deteriorated and died 1 month later. Total survival time for this patient was 18 months from the first chemoembolization, but he had good quality of life.

Comment: Alternate chemoembolization of the right and left lobes of the liver was performed every 6 weeks in the first four rounds of treatment. The whole liver was chemoembolized in the remaining three rounds, for a total of seven chemoembolization procedures. There was remarkable clinical improvement that allowed the patient to return to his full-time job as an engineer for the full course of the treatment. The patient was extremely resilient. All chemoembolization procedures were performed on an outpatient basis, and the patient returned to work the next day. Note the time interval enlargement of the spleen. Mean survival time of patients with metastatic colon cancer is 10.6 months in our initial series of 16 patients treated with chemoembolization. Clinical improvement was observed in all patients, but tumor response was identified in only 57.2% of patients.

2.3 Chemoembolization In The Liver

Case 2.3:

A 72-year-old Japanese male patient, who was positive for B virus and had a history of hepatitis, presented with weight loss and a palpable epigastric mass related to the liver. CT scan with biopsy diagnosed a hepatocellular carcinoma (HCC) in the left hepatic lobe.

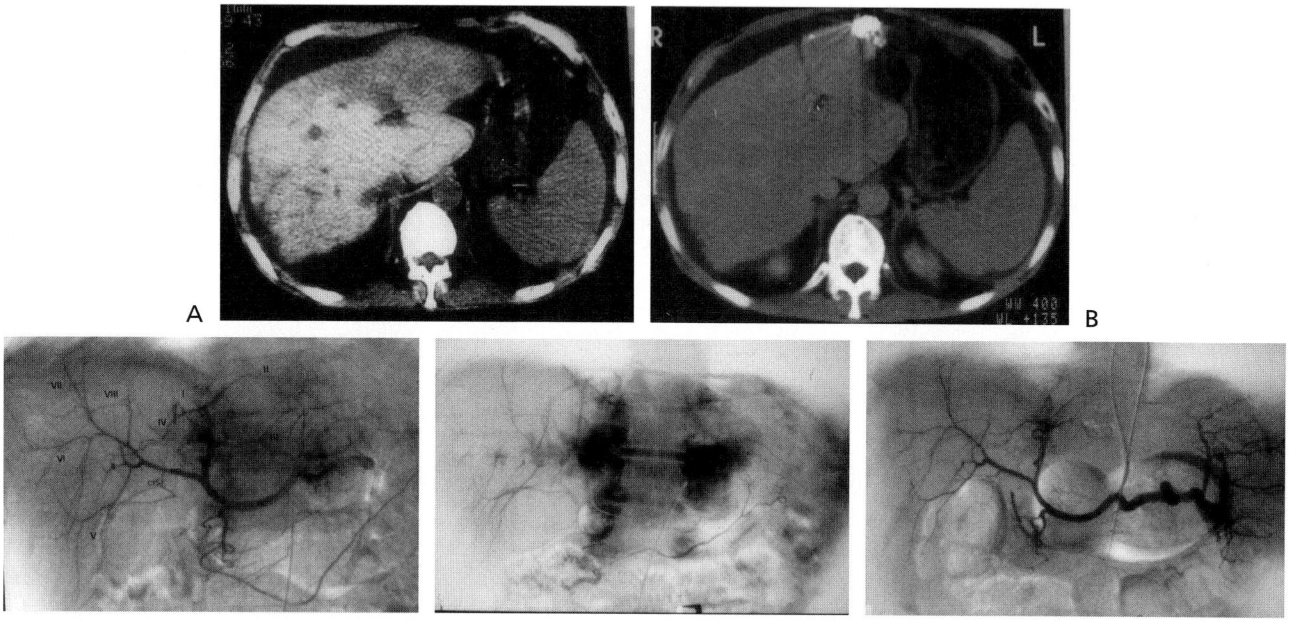

Figure 2.3

A: CT scan shows a large tumoral mass occupying the left hepatic lobe. Note the difference in contrast enhancement. **B:** Postchemoembolization CT scan obtained after two procedures shows marked response of the tumor. Note a high-density nodule (stained by lipiodol) resulting from tumor shrinkage after chemoembolization. **C:** Prechemoembolization hepatic arteriogram shows a large hypervascular HCC in segments IV, II, and III of the left lobe. Note the segment numbers in the picture. **D:** Late-phase arteriogram shows tumor enhancement and extension of the tumor to the right lobe, which contraindicate resection. **E:** Follow-up arteriogram after two chemoembolization procedures shows total regression of the mass. Note the small hyperdense nodule at the tip of the left hepatic lobe. Survival of this patient was almost 3 years.

Comment: This case illustrates the marked response of an HCC after chemoembolization. The more hypervascular the lesion, the better the response. Chemoembolization includes administration of mitomycin C, lipiodol, and Ivalon. In our initial series of 33 patients, there was clinical improvement in 74% of cases and tumoral response in 74% of patients. Mean survival of patients with HCC was 13.2 months.

2.4 Chemoembolization In The Liver

Case 2.4:

A 45-year-old male patient of Japanese extraction, who had a history of hepatitis and was B virus positive, presented with some pain in the right upper quadrant. Ultrasound study showed a tumoral lesion in the right lobe extending from the liver hilum. Chemoembolization was requested.

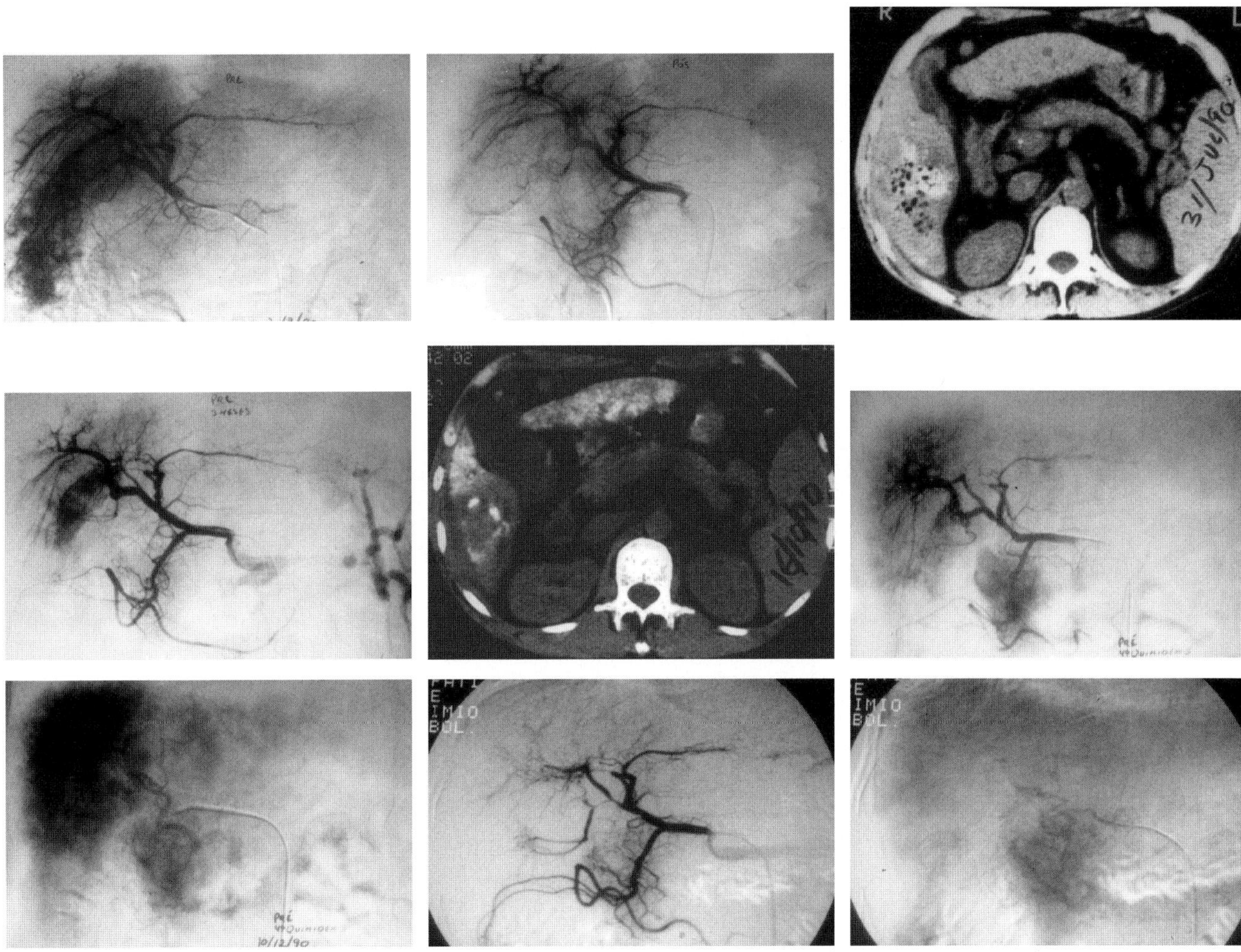

Figure 2.4

A: Selective hepatic arteriogram shows a large, hypervascular HCC in the right hepatic lobe extending from the liver hilum. **B:** Postchemoembolization arteriogram shows total ablation of the tumor. **C:** Postembolization CT scan obtained 24 hours after the procedure shows tumor staining by lipiodol and areas of gas in the tumor. **D:** Three-month follow-up angiogram shows a smaller but still hypervascular tumor in the right lobe of the liver. Another chemoembolization was performed. **E:** Postchemoembolization CT scan shows significant response with tumor reduction. Note enhancement of the left lobe. **F,G:** Five-month follow-up angiogram shows absence of tumor vessels. Another chemoembolization was performed at that time. **H,I:** Follow-up arteriogram shows total devascularization of the HCC. Note significant reduction in liver size. Four procedures were performed in this patient, with excellent response. Survival was more than 3 years.

Comment: This is a relatively atypical HCC located in the right hepatic lobe. Chemoembolization was effective in producing tumoral response and clinical improvement; survival was good. The liver was reduced in size and the spleen enlarged, which suggest development of portal hypertension. Metastatic disease developed in the chest and was the cause of the patient's death. Chemoembolization of the liver for metastatic disease or HCC improves quality of life. Increased survival is not always achieved. In patients with significantly increased survival, metastatic deposits usually develop in different areas of the body, which is not seen in untreated patients with average survival time.

2.5 Chemoembolization In The Liver

Case 2.5:

A 55-year-old man from the Amazon region presented with palpable enlargement of the liver and pain in the right upper quadrant. He was positive for B virus and delta virus. Multiple hepatic masses and nodules were identified in the liver. Hepatic arteriogram and chemoembolization were undertaken.

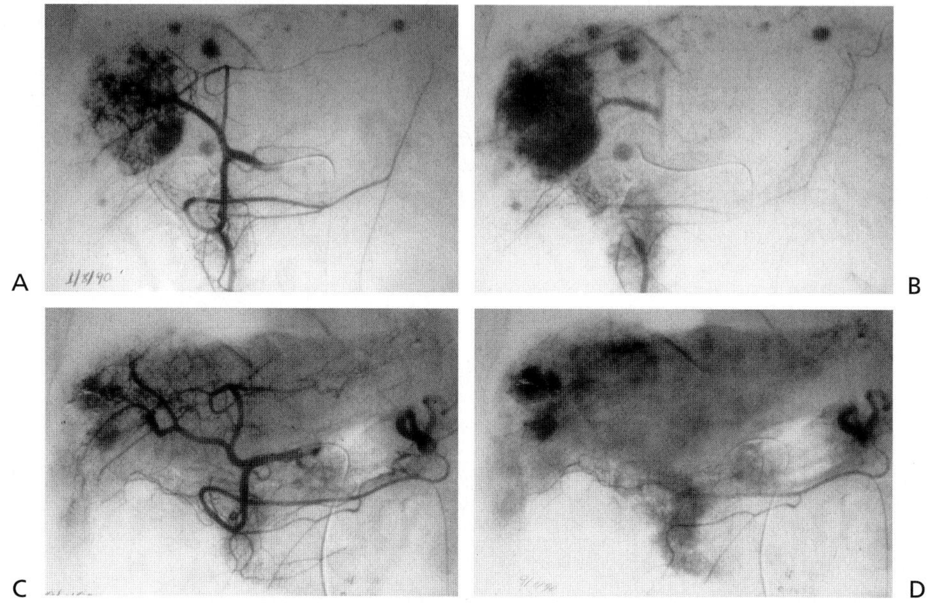

Figure 2.5

A: Hepatic arteriogram shows a large hypervascular mass in the right lobe of the liver and multiple hypervascular nodules throughout the liver, including the left lobe, consistent with HCC. **B:** Late-phase arteriogram shows multiple hypervascular lesions with dense uptake of contrast. Early venous return into the cava is seen from the larger mass. Chemoembolization was performed with mitomycin C, lipiodol, and Ivalon particles. **C,D:** Follow-up angiogram 3 months after the first treatment shows adequate response of the tumor lesions, with reduction in size of the right lobe of the liver. The smaller nodules are not visible or are less prominent. A second chemoembolization was performed. Significant clinical improvement was observed. The patient was lost to follow-up and did not return for further chemoembolization procedures. To our knowledge, his total survival was 12 months.

Comment: The delta agent is encountered all over the world, but there are endemic areas, such as some Mediterranean countries, Sweden, the Amazon basin, and Asia. The delta virus is a "symbiont" of the B virus. A significant number of patients (18%) with hepatitis B and delta virus develop a fulminant hepatitis, which is associated with high mortality. A number of patients develop chronic active hepatitis, cirrhosis, and HCC. These patients have limited survival. HCC has a mean survival time of about 6 months. Although improvement in survival can be obtained using chemoembolization and a relatively good response was achieved with the treatment in this patient, the total survival time was not increased to a great extent.

2.6 Chemoembolization In The Liver

Case 2.6:

A 35-year-old male patient with chronic active hepatitis and cirrhosis presented with a large liver mass and excruciating pain. Hepatic biopsy showed HCC. Hepatic arteriogram and chemoembolization were undertaken.

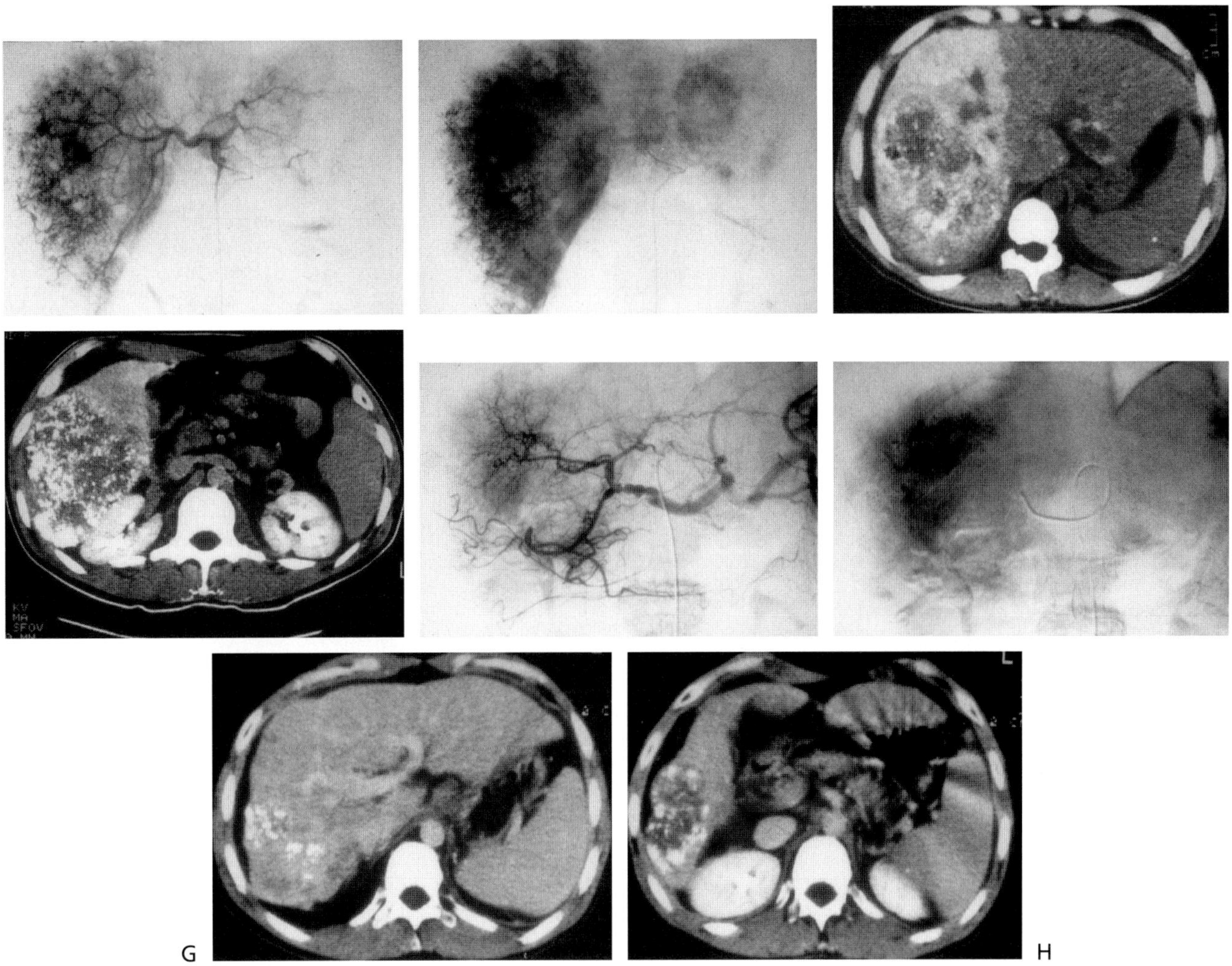

Figure 2.6

A: Hepatic arteriogram shows a large hypervascular mass with tumor vessels and blood pooling. Two other lesions were noted in the left liver lobe. **B:** Late-phase liver arteriogram shows dense tumor stain, with demonstration of the right liver lobe lesion and two smaller lesions in the left lobe. Chemoembolization was performed with mitomycin C, lipiodol, and Ivalon particles. **C,D:** Postchemoembolization CT scan shows dense enhancement of the larger tumor and mild enhancement of a rim in one of the lesions in the left liver lobe. **E,F:** Follow-up liver arteriogram shows significant response, with reduced hypervascularity and size. **G,H:** Follow-up CT scan after four chemoembolization procedures shows significant reduction in liver tumor size. Four procedures were performed in this patient.

Comment: HCC is the cancer most related to environmental factors. It has a variety of geographic distributions, with areas of higher incidence in Africa and Asia, and a growing presence worldwide. The incidence of HCC in the United States doubled in the last 5 years. Hepatitis B virus has been considered the most important etiologic factor and is one of the few cancers that is preventable through vaccination. The areas with the highest incidence of HCC are also the areas with the highest incidence of hepatitis B virus. Males are predominantly affected, and they are younger in areas of higher incidence and older in areas of lower incidence. From 40% to 90% of patients with HCC present with concomitant cirrhosis. Other etiologic factors also are important for the growth of HCC around the world, including contamination of food with aflatoxins, abuse of alcohol, use of steroids, and growing presence of other viruses (such as hepatitis C virus).

2.7 Chemoembolization In The Liver

Case 2.7:

A 53-year-old female patient presented with a large liver mass and severe abdominal pain. Hepatic biopsy showed HCC. B virus serology was positive. Hepatic arteriogram and chemoembolization were requested.

A, B C

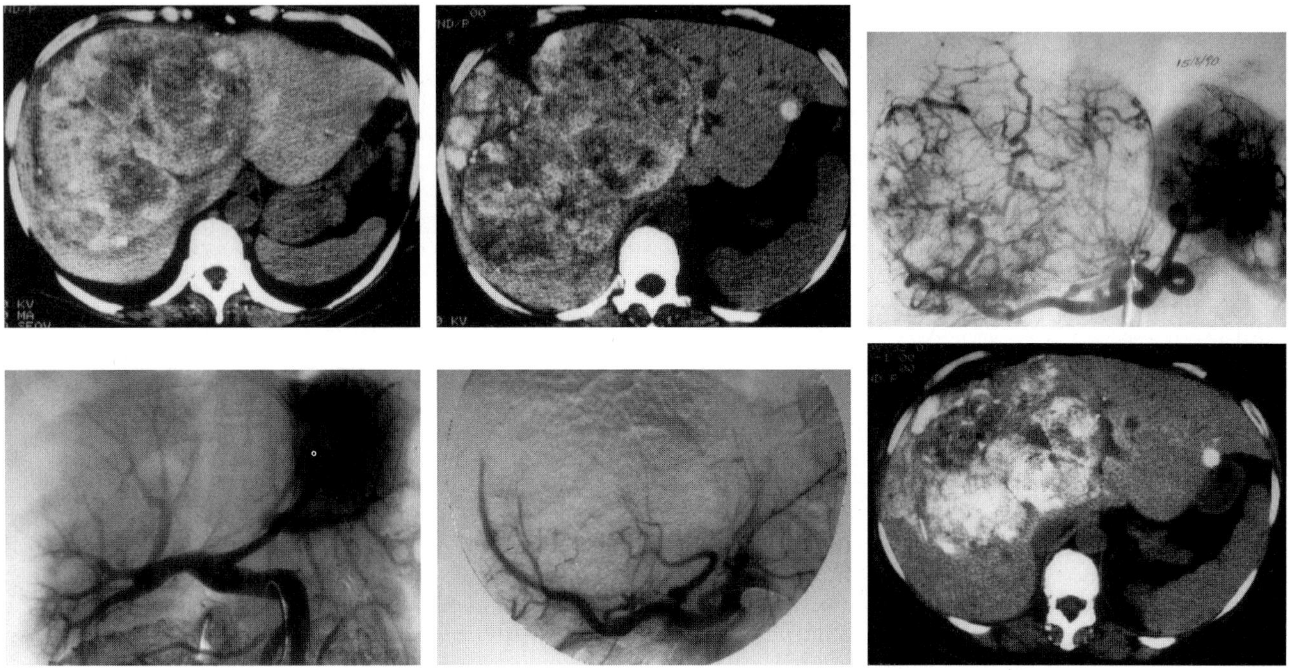

D, E F

Figure 2.7

A: IV contrast-enhanced CT scan of the liver shows a large hepatic mass with heterogenous areas of enhancement and areas of low density occupying the right lobe of the liver and laterally displacing the left lobe. **B:** Postchemoembolization CT scan of the liver shows lipiodol enhancement of the large mass, with an additional small nodule in the periphery of the left lobe, which was not visible before lipiodol injection. **C:** Hepatic arteriogram shows a large hypervascular mass in the right lobe of the liver with tumor vessels and enlarged hepatic artery. **D:** Late-phase arteriogram of the superior mesenteric artery shows a patent portal vein with bowed and displaced intrahepatic portal branches. The left lobe is massively displaced. **E:** Postchemoembolization hepatic arteriogram after treatment. **F:** Follow-up CT scan 4 months after initial treatment shows significant response in tumor size. There was clinical improvement as well. The patient decided to discontinue chemoembolization treatment and received IV chemotherapy only. Survival was 18 months.

Comment: Large HCCs are not very common in younger patients. Larger liver masses tend to be more symptomatic due to displacement of adjacent structures and distention of the liver capsule. Liver tumors with greater hypervascularity respond better to chemoembolization; however, advanced tumors are associated with shorter survival. This case demonstrates the need to document portal vein patency. If the portal vein is occluded, superselective chemoembolization should be performed in an attempt to spare the remaining normal liver parenchyma. In this case, selective chemoembolization was performed in the tumor area. Only a small amount of treatment was delivered to the left lobe. When large portions of the liver are substituted by tumor, care should be taken to perform partial chemoembolization in multiple procedures and to alternate the areas of treatment.

Suggested Reading

Berger DH, Carrasco CH, Hohn DC, et al. Hepatic artery chemoembolization or embolization for primary and metastatic liver tumors: posttreatment management and complications. *J Surg Oncol* 1995;60:116–121.

Cascinu S, Wadler S. Chemoembolization in the treatment of liver metastases from colorectal cancer. *Cancer Treat Rev* 1996;22:355–363.

Chung JW, Park JH, Han JK, et al. Hepatic tumors: predisposing factors for complication of transcatheter oily chemoembolization. *Radiology* 1996;198:33–40.

Clouse ME, Perry L, Stuart K, et al. Hepatic arterial chemoembolization for metastatic neuroendocrine tumors. *Digestion* 1994;55:92–97.

Farinati F, De Maria N, Marafin C, et al. Unresectable hepatocellular carcinoma in cirrhosis: survival, prognostic factors, and unexpected side effects after transcatheter arterial chemoembolization. *Dig Dis Sci* 1996;41:2332–2339.

Ferguson JM, Flinn J. Intracranial meningioma with hepatic metastases and hypoglycaemia treated by selective hepatic arterial chemoembolization. *Australas Radiol* 1995;39:97–99.

Portolani N, Tiberio AM, Bonardelli S, et al. Arterial chemoembolization in hepatocellular carcinoma suitable for resective surgery. *Hepatogastroenterology* 1996;43:1566–1574.

Recchia F, Passalacqua G. Role of polychemoembolization in the treatment of a primitive and secondary liver tumor. *Clin Ter* 1995;146:117–122.

Uflacker R, Mourao GS, Piske RL. Lipiodol retention within hepatic cavernous hemangioma. *Cardiovasc Intervent Radiol* 1989;12:76–79.

Wangberg B, Westberg G, Tylen U, et al. Survival of patients with disseminated midgut carcinoid tumors after aggressive tumor reduction. *World J Surg* 1996;20:892–899.

CHAPTER 3

Embolization In The Liver

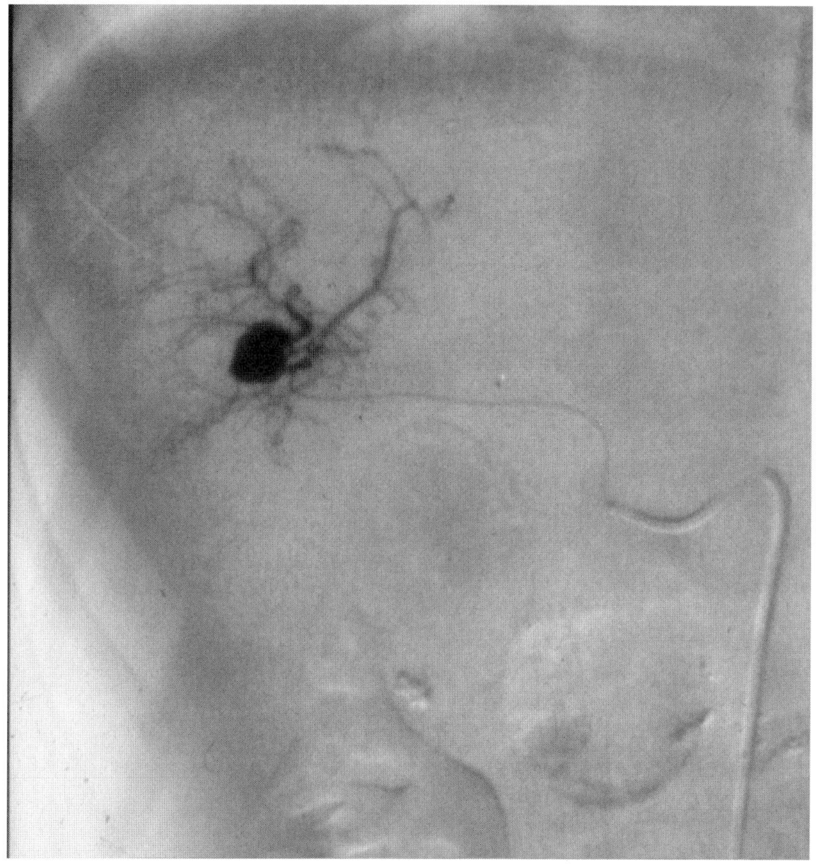

3.1 Embolization In The Liver

Case 3.1:

A 3-year-old male patient who presented with fever and diarrhea and a heart murmur had an arterioportal fistula. An outside abdominal ultrasound (US) and computed tomographic (CT) scan showed a "liver mass" and ascites.

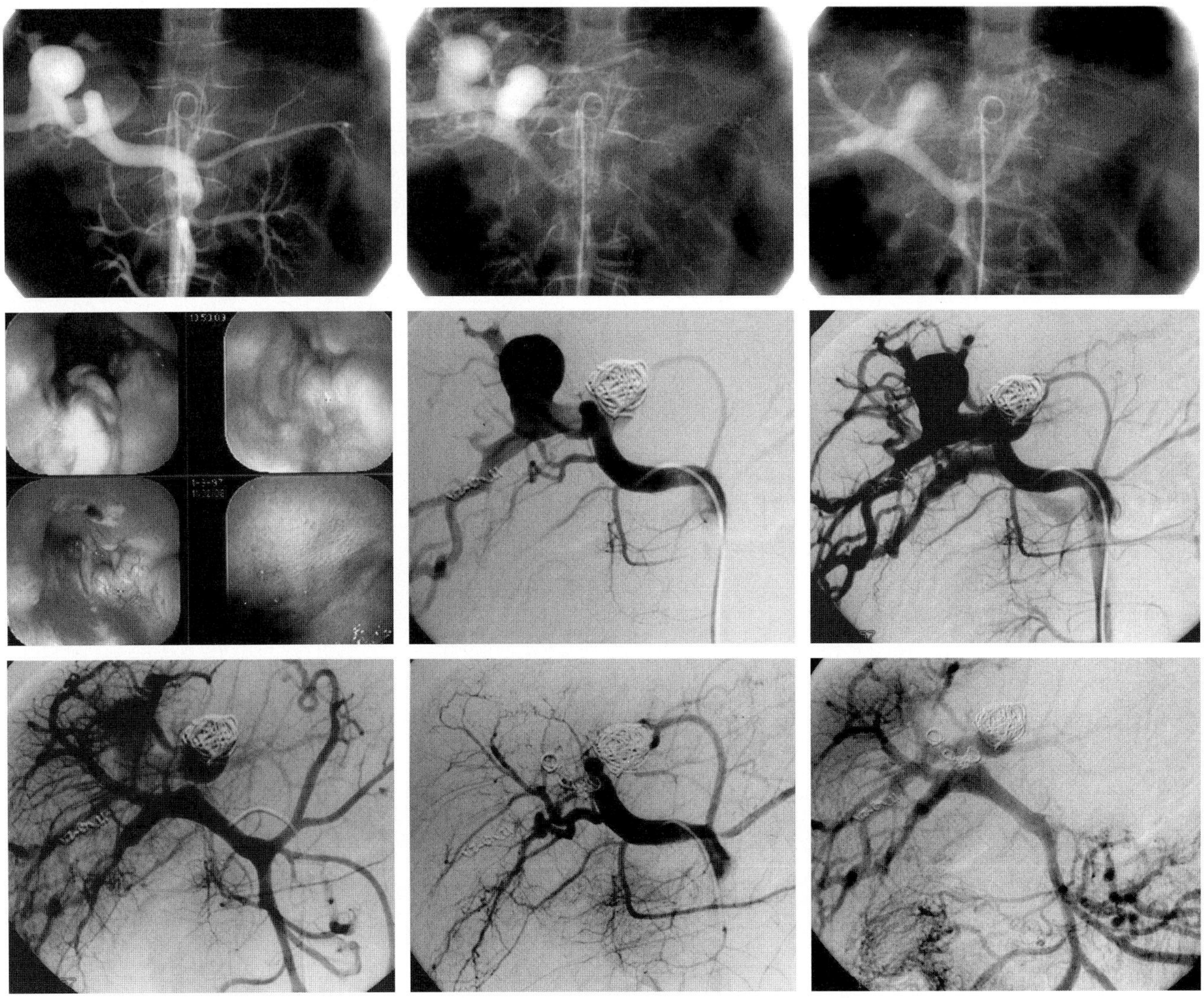

A, B C

D, E F

G, H I

Figure 3.1

A–C: Cine film of the abdominal aorta. During cardiac catheterization, a large arterioportal fistula having direct communication with an enlarged hepatic artery (segment VIII) to the left branch of the portal vein was observed on the cine film. Portal vein pressure was elevated to 30 mm Hg. Note hepatofugal flow in the portal system and an enlarged left gastric vein. The cardiologist failed to recognize the real location of the rent of the arteriovenous (A-V) fistula between the artery to segment VIII and the venous aneurysm. Embolization of the outlet of the A-V fistula into the left portal vein was performed with coils, which increased the pressure into the anomalous segment of portal vein, the hepatofugal flow, and the size of the varices. A small patent ductus arteriosus also was embolized during the same procedure. **D:** Endoscopic view of the esophageal varices. At that point, the patient developed gastrointestinal (GI) bleeding that required blood replacement. **E–G:** Selective hepatic arteriogram shows persistence of the A-V fistula despite embolization with coils performed by the cardiology department. **H:** Adequate embolization of the A-V fistula using coils performed by the interventional radiology department resulted in total occlusion of the A-V communication. Note enlargement of the left hepatic artery after embolization and resolution of the A-V fistula. **I:** Postembolization arteriogram with papaverine shows hepatopetal flow of the superior mesenteric vein and portal vein in the late phase. Note that the left gastric vein is not opacified. A later arteriogram showed occlusion of the left branch of the portal vein and further enlargement of the left hepatic artery. Follow-up Doppler US 6 months after treatment showed no evidence of A-V fistula. The patient improved remarkably, gained weight, and remained feeling well more than 1 year after treatment.

Comment: Embolization of a liver A-V fistula is the treatment of choice. Extensive surgical procedures are avoided when embolization is used, and the outcomes are excellent. However, this case demonstrates the need to understand the disease process, anatomy, and treatment alternatives for adequate interventional correction. The actual A-V fistula was not embolized correctly, and the small patient continued to have portal hypertension with recurrent variceal bleeding. General anesthesia was used for the procedures, and the inadequacy of the initial procedures exposed the small patient to additional risks. The type of fistula between the hepatic artery and portal vein can be treated best by coil embolization or detachable balloon embolization. Immediate correction of the fistula was achieved once the real fistula was identified and the proper technique used. Superselective catheterization is necessary; when the tract is tortuous, a microcatheter may be necessary. Immediate resolution of the portal hypertension follows occlusion of the A-V fistula. In cases of prolonged exposure of the liver to portal hypertension related to increased flow, changes in the liver may develop and create a situation of irreversible chronic liver disease

3.2 Embolization In The Liver

Case 3.2:

A 16-year-old girl was unrestrained in the back seat of a car during a head-on motor vehicle accident. She suffered severe abdominal contusion with spleen and liver lacerations, probably grade 2, which were treated surgically by splenectomy and suture of the liver lesion. Upper GI bleeding developed 2 months after surgery. Endoscopy confirmed hemobilia.

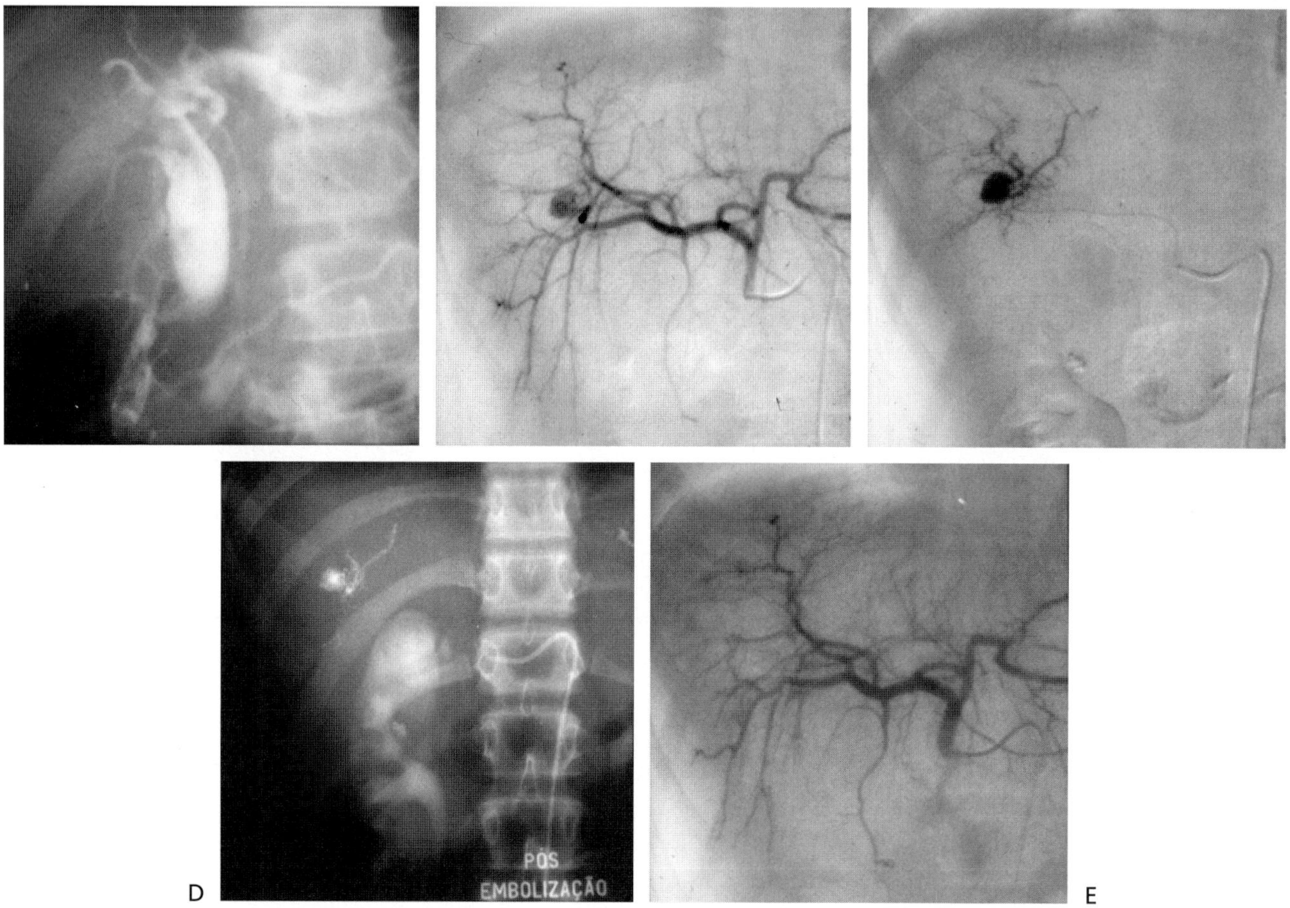

A, B C D E

Figure 3.2

A: Endoscopic retrograde cholangiopancreatography demonstrates a dilated common bile duct with a filling defect inside that extended into the right bile duct, which was occluded. **B:** Celiac arteriogram shows a pseudoaneurysm in a branch of segment VIII of the right hepatic artery that supposedly was responsible for the bleeding. **C:** A microcatheter was used to catheterize the pseudoaneurysm and perform embolization with cyanoacrylate. **D:** Embolization with cyanoacrylate was performed and occluded the lumen of the pseudoaneurysm and two adjacent branches. **E:** Postembolization angiogram shows total occlusion of the pseudoaneurysm that permanently controlled the bleeding during several years of follow-up.

Comment: Trauma to the liver may cause acute bleeding just after the trauma, or the liver may develop a pseudoaneurysm or A-V fistula related to hemobilia during evolution of the lesion. Pseudoaneurysms are usually located deep in the liver parenchyma and result from trauma to a relatively large artery. Embolization is the most efficient method to treat a traumatic pseudoaneurysm and has the greatest chance of success. Cyanoacrylate, although not readily available in the United States, is a good alternative that allows superselective occlusion of the mouth of the pseudoaneurysm with minimal ablation of normal adjacent parenchyma.

3.3 Embolization In The Liver

Case 3.3:

A patient with sepsis and mycotic hepatic aneurysm following heart valve surgery presented with right upper quadrant pain and at least one episode of hemobilia.

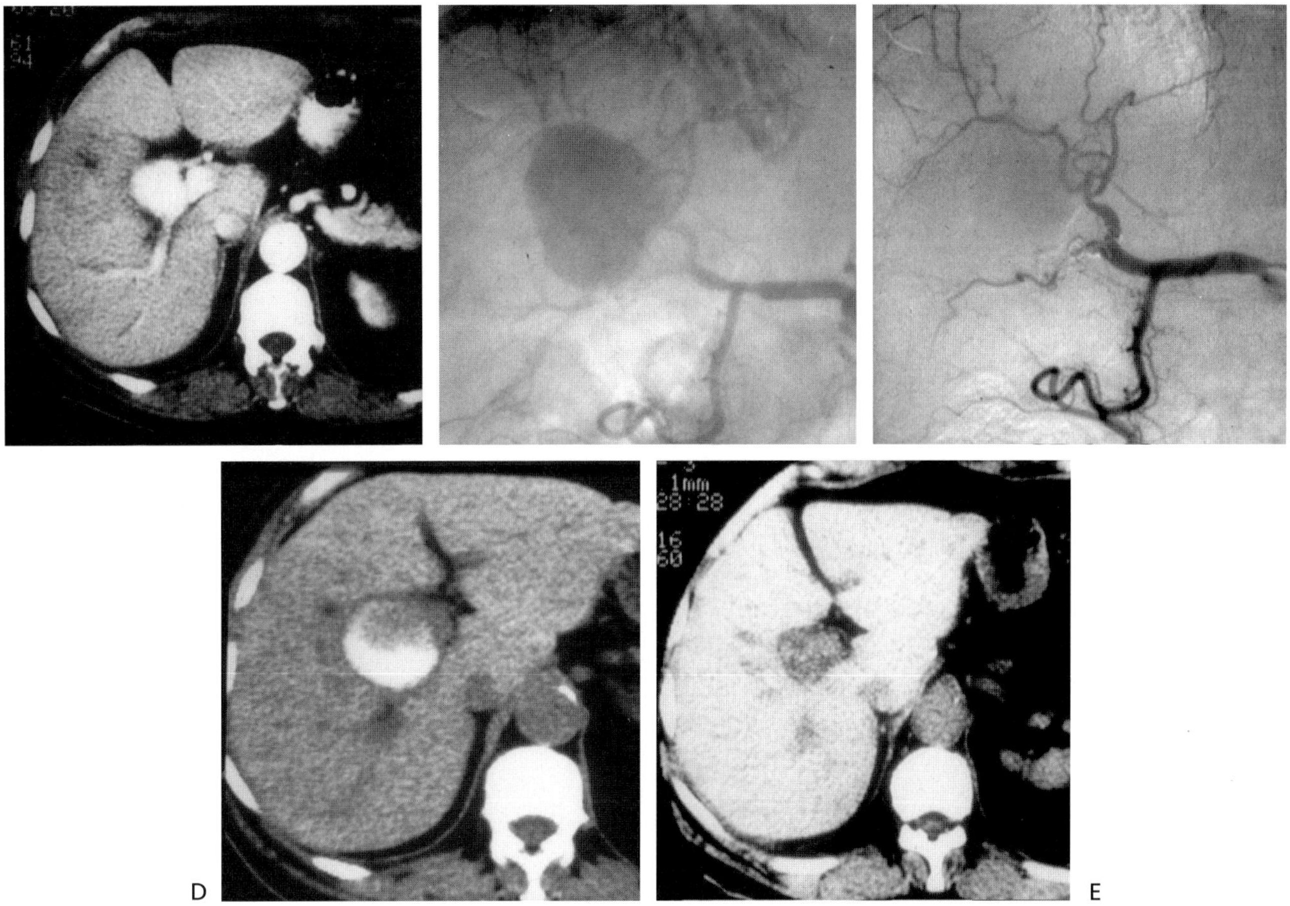

A B, C D E

Figure 3.3 *(continued)*

A: Dynamic CT scan of the liver shows the aneurysm and the connection with a peripheral arterial branch. **B:** Hepatic arteriogram shows the mycotic aneurysm cavity connected with the right hepatic artery. The portal vein was patent but is not shown. **C:** Postembolization arteriography shows occlusion of the aneurysm by the two coils used in this case. **D:** CT scan without intravenous (IV) contrast 4 days after the embolization shows the partially thrombosed mycotic aneurysm with residual angiographic contrast inside. **E:** Follow-up CT scan 4 months after the embolization shows resolution of the mycotic aneurysm.

Comment: Mycotic hepatic artery aneurysms are uncommon. Despite the infectious etiology of such a lesion, embolization is still the best way to treat an obviously large aneurysm in the middle of the liver substance. Surgical treatment would require extrahepatic hepatic artery ligation, which may not be effective, or right hepatic resection, which would expose the patient to major surgery. Coils are a good alternative for embolization, as long as the catheter can be advanced beyond the entrance of the aneurysm and the coils can be deployed beyond and before the aneurysm to reduce chances of recanalization.

3.4 Embolization In The Liver

Case 3.4:

A 76-year-old man presented with a hepatic artery aneurysm and active bleeding following left hepatectomy for metastatic colon carcinoma.

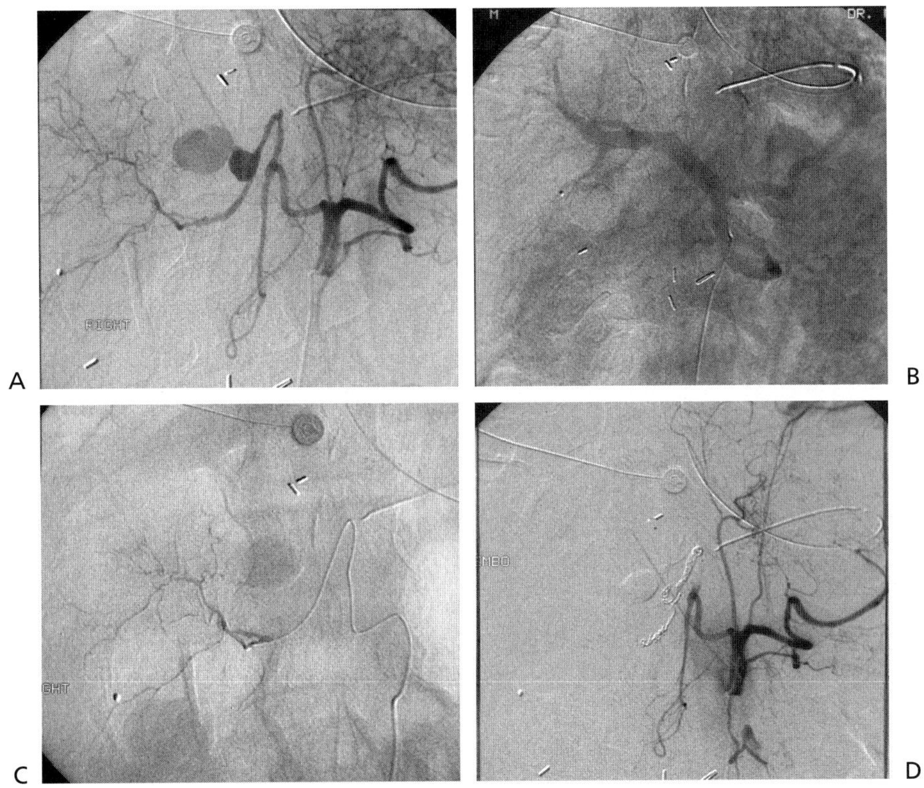

Figure 3.4

A: Selective celiac arteriogram shows diffuse spasm of the hepatic artery and a focal pseudoaneurysm of the right hepatic aneurysm with active bleeding during the arteriogram. Note occlusion of the left hepatic artery by surgical ligation. **B:** Superior mesenteric arteriogram shows patency of the main and right portal vein. **C:** Superselective catheterization of the right hepatic artery beyond the pseudoaneurysm with the 2.8F microcatheter used to deploy the microcoils. **D:** Postembolization angiogram shows occlusion of the right hepatic artery and thrombosis of the pseudoaneurysm. Note the shadow of residual contrast media in the lumen of the pseudoaneurysm.

Comment: It is important to note that, in this case, the lesion was traumatic/iatrogenic and related to a surgical vascular lesion that developed into a pseudoaneurysm in a very sick patient the day after he underwent a left hepatectomy. The initial clinical presentation was GI bleeding, and emergency arteriogram was performed to locate a surgery-related lesion in the hepatic artery. Microcatheter technology provided the means to reach the tortuous right hepatic artery at the level of the pseudoaneurysm and safely embolize the parent artery, thus occluding the lesion and controlling the bleeding.

3.5 Embolization In The Liver

Case 3.5:

A 23-year-old man who was unrestrained at the time of a motor vehicle accident suffered a major liver laceration, grade 3 to 4. He presented with unstable blood pressure, required blood replacement, and underwent CT and angiographic evaluation.

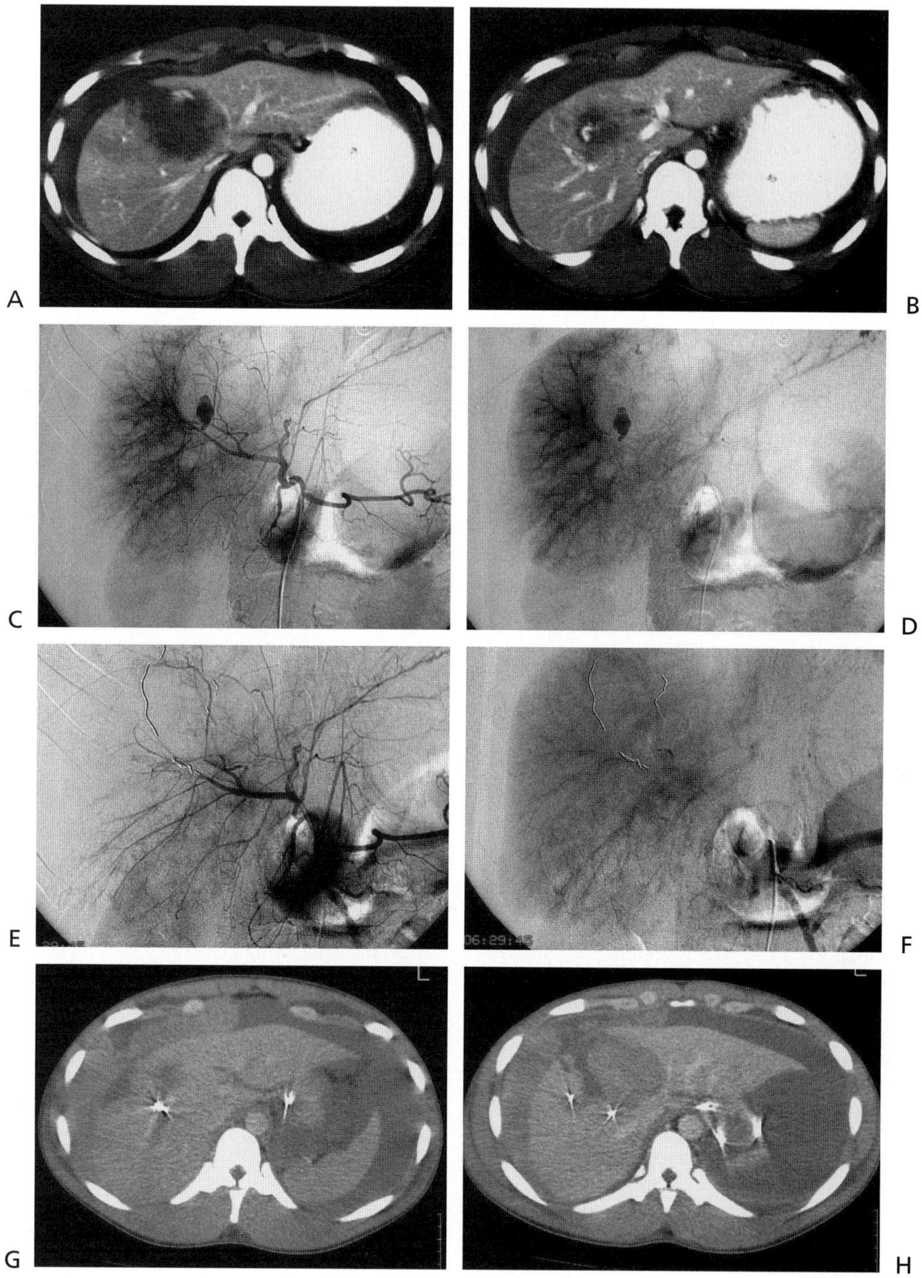

Figure 3.5

A,B: Dynamic CT scan of the liver at two levels shows a large laceration of the liver, with areas of active bleeding and a large amount of fluid around the liver and inside the peritoneal cavity. **C:** Hepatic artery arteriogram shows the large intrahepatic hematoma displacing the surrounding vessels, an area of active extravasation of contrast arising from the right hepatic artery, and a small area of bleeding from a peripheral branch on the edge of the hematoma. **D:** Late-phase angiogram shows the large intrahepatic hematoma, extravasation from at least two points, a large subcapsular hematoma, and intraperitoneal blood collection. **E,F:** Embolization with a microcatheter and microcoils was performed to control the bleeding. Postembolization angiogram shows occlusion of the pseudoaneurysm and control of the bleeding. **G,H:** Follow-up CT scan shows control of the bleeding without enhancement of the pseudoaneurysms. Note the radiopaque coils. The patient recovered and was discharged without further interventions 2 weeks later.

Comment: Most liver traumas do not require immediate treatment for bleeding. Traditional treatment includes surgical ligation of the hepatic artery, suture of the hepatic wound with drainage of the hematoma, lobectomy, or surgical packing with Gelfoam. When the patient is stable, observation only may be the best approach. Acute or continuous intraperitoneal bleeding will require treatment, either surgical or transcatheter. Embolization is very effective when performed appropriately and expeditiously. This case demonstrates the utilization of embolization to treat an acute liver trauma. Intraperitoneal blood collection may be treated conservatively. Peritoneal cavity evacuation may be necessary if fever or infection develops. It is not uncommon to develop a biloma in the cavity created by the hematoma that requires percutaneous drainage and/or surgical evacuation.

3.6 Embolization In The Liver

Case 3.6:

The 27-year-old female patient, who was unrestrained at the time of a motor vehicle accident, was admitted with multiple injuries. The patient was hemodynamically unstable on arrival. A grade 3 liver laceration and extensive hemoperitoneum were diagnosed. During observation in the intensive care unit, multiple other problems in addition to the liver lesion presented, including pulmonary contusion with development of adult respiratory distress syndrome and a closed head injury. Fever and jaundice developed associated, with elevated liver function tests. US demonstrated a biloma. Laparoscopy was performed and revealed free bile in the peritoneal cavity. A cholecystectomy was performed, and intraoperative cholangiography demonstrated injury to the left main duct. The lateral segment of the left lobe of the liver was found to be necrotic and was removed, followed by drainage for 3 weeks. The patient was discharged approximately 5 weeks after initial admission. About 3 months later, the patient presented with hematemesis and hemobilia. CT and angiography were performed.

A, B

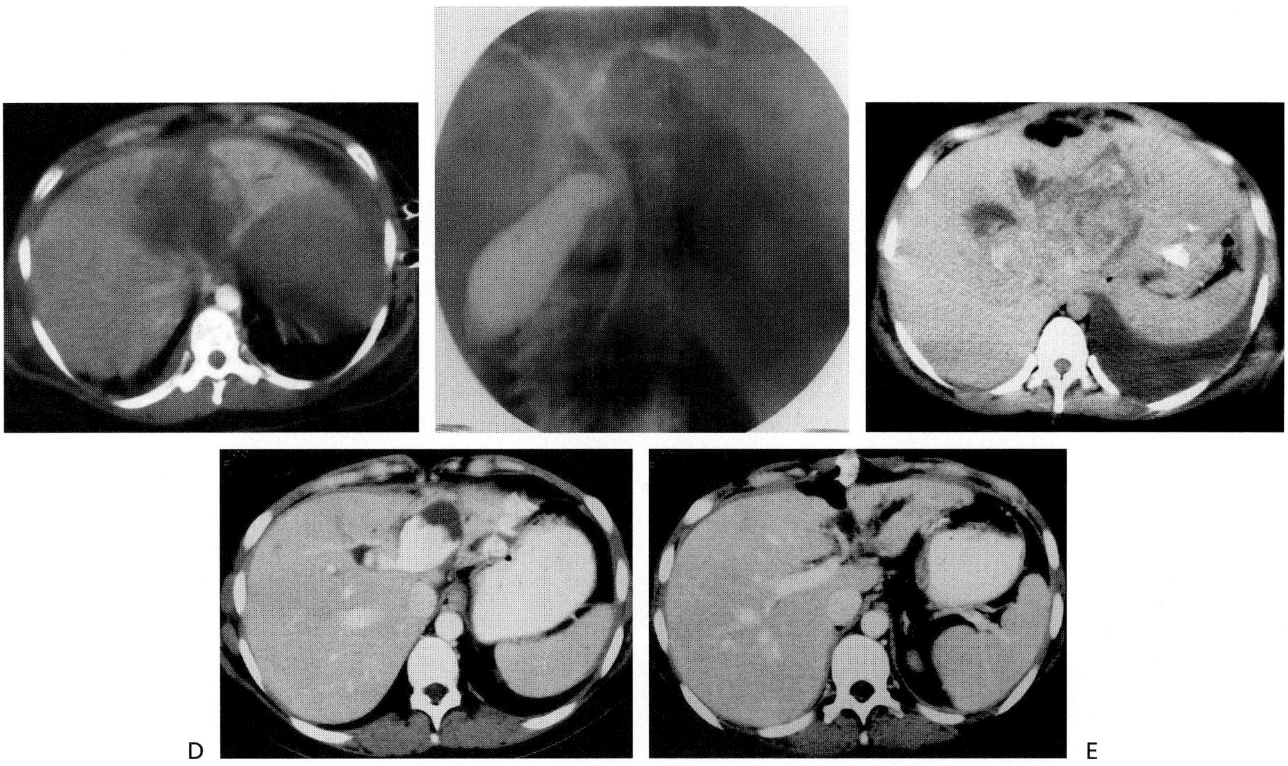

C

D

E

Figure 3.6

A: Admission CT scan shows laceration of the liver without active extravasation of contrast. Note the perihepatic blood. **B:** Intraoperative cholangiogram shows lesion of the left bile duct. **C:** Predischarge CT scan shows partial resolution of the liver laceration with organized hematomas in the parenchyma. **D,E:** Readmission CT scan, with IV contrast, after upper GI bleeding due to hemobilia shows a large pseudoaneurysm in the corresponding area of the hematoma and the laceration below the level of the pseudoaneurysm. **F:** Hepatic artery angiography shows a large pseudoaneurysm related to the left hepatic artery and an A-V fistula with the hepatic vein. **G:** Late-phase hepatic arteriogram shows the A-V fistula and the right hepatic draining vein. Note the large venous pseudoaneurysm. **H:** The catheter was advanced into the left hepatic artery and embolization with one Gianturco coil was performed. The angiogram shows immediate occlusion of the A-V fistula. **I,J:** Later-phase hepatic angiogram shows hyperemia in the right liver lobe, probably caused by the previous hypertension in the venous territory, suddenly released by the embolization. Note total occlusion of the A-V fistula. **K,L:** Follow-up CT scan shows the high-density coil and the "resolved" pseudoaneurysm. Note that there is no contrast enhancement of the pseudoaneurysm and A-V fistula. **M:** Fever

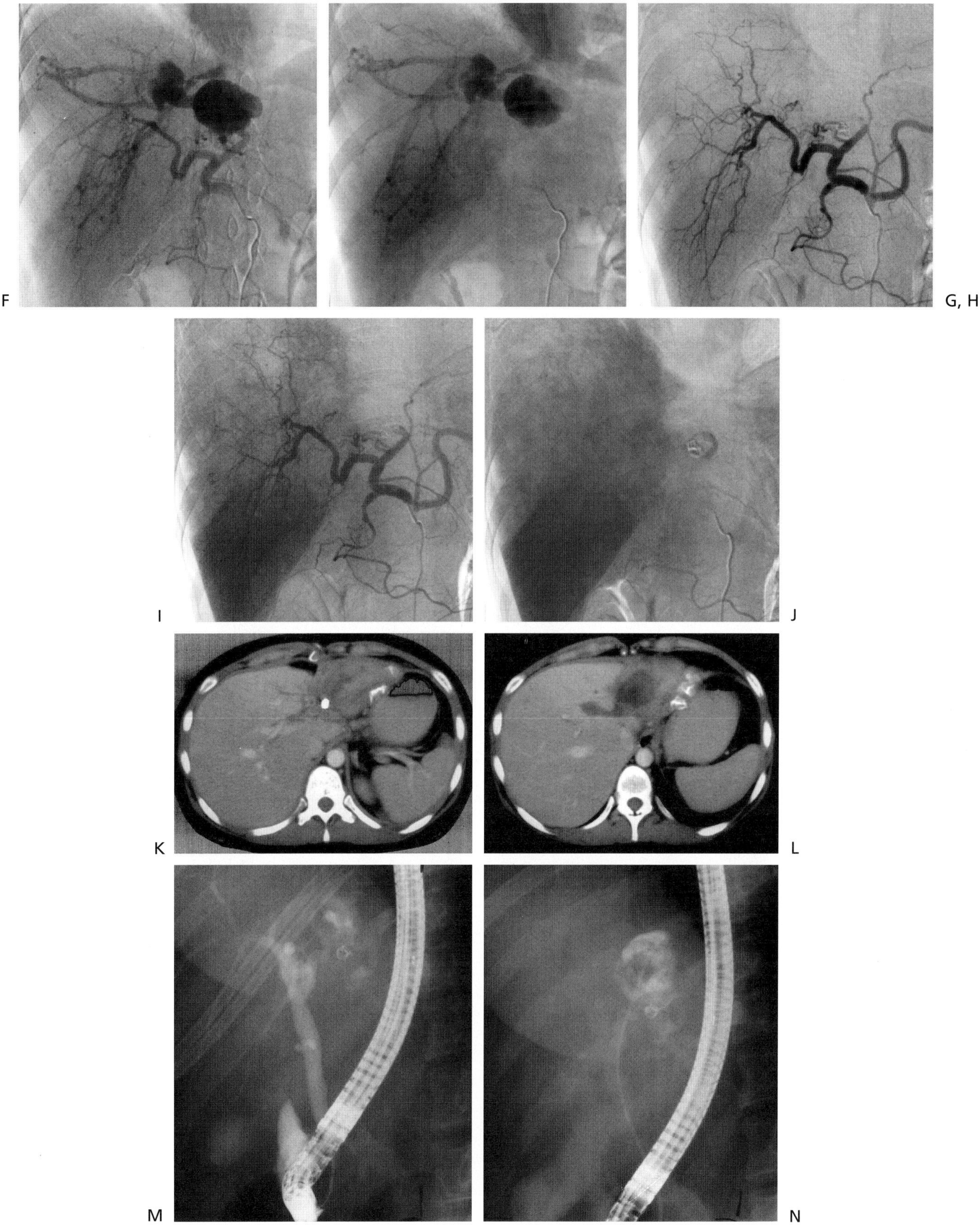

Figure 3.6 *(continued)*

recurred, and a small biloma was identified by endoscopic retrograde cholangiopancreatography. **N:** Injection of contrast demonstrated the cavity, and a stent was placed. The stent was removed after 4 weeks. Follow-up is now more than 3 years, and the patient is doing well.

Comment: Massive lacerations of the liver may develop large fractures of the liver parenchyma, with hematoma formation. When a through-and-through laceration is observed, a large bile duct also may be lacerated, creating a biloma. Endoscopic stent placement usually is necessary to reestablish the continuity of the bile duct and control the bile leak; however, the biloma may need percutaneous drainage. Hematomas may cavitate and result in pseudoaneurysms with or without A-V fistulas. Massive A-V fistulas may cause hemobilia and severe hemodynamic changes in liver circulation. Surgical correction of such a lesion would require left hepatectomy and voluminous blood reposition, with high morbidity and mortality. Transcatheter embolotherapy, as in this case, provided fast and safe control of the bleeding. Coils and detachable balloons are the techniques of choice for massive lesions in the liver. Recovery was uneventful and required only biliary stent exchanges.

3.7 Embolization In The Liver

Case 3.7:

A 68-year-old man suffered hepatic trauma in a motor vehicle accident and experienced intraperitoneal bleeding and drop in hematocrit. CT scans showed active bleeding. Angiography was performed.

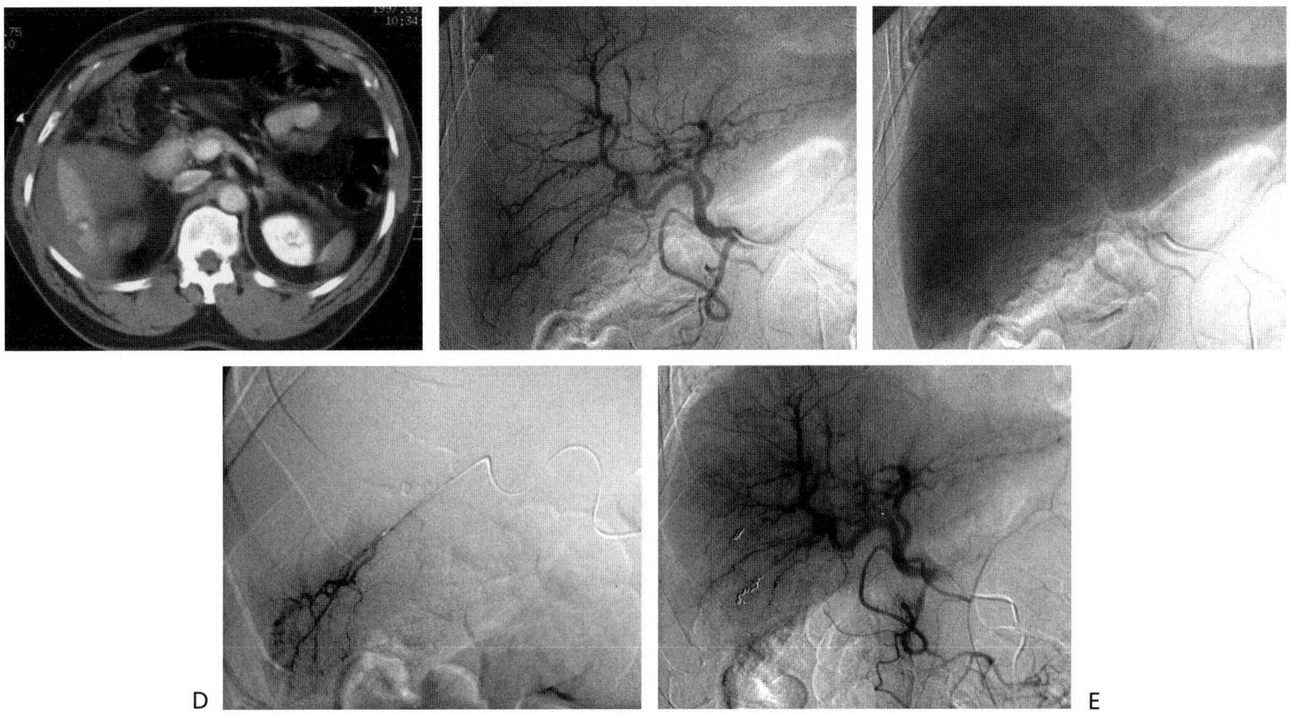

A B, C D E

Figure 3.7

A: CT scan of the liver shows a small area of laceration and extravasation of contrast in segment VI. Large amounts of blood are visible around the liver. **B:** Selective hepatic arteriogram shows area of hyperemia in segment VI but no active extravasation of contrast. **C:** Late-phase arteriogram shows hyperemia in the trauma area and punctuated areas of contrast accumulation. **D:** Superselective injection shows limited areas of contrast accumulation. **E:** Embolization of arterial branches in segment VI occluded the vessels involved and there was no further bleeding. Three 2-mm × 2-cm microcoils were used for embolization.

Comment: CT scan shows active bleeding and free blood in the peritoneal cavity. The angiographic image was less dramatic than expected, but showed areas of contusion and questionable extravasation. Due to the CT finding, embolization was performed, which permanently controlled the bleeding.

3.8 Embolization In The Liver

Case 3.8:

A 1-year-old male patient who was diagnosed with advanced neuroblastoma, coagulopathy, and liver nodular lesions underwent US-guided biopsy of the liver. The patient suffered three episodes of cardiac arrest in the last 48 hours before the biopsy. He was intubated and comatose at the time of the biopsy. After biopsy, the patient developed clinical and US signs of intraperitoneal bleeding associated with acute drop in hematocrit.

A, B

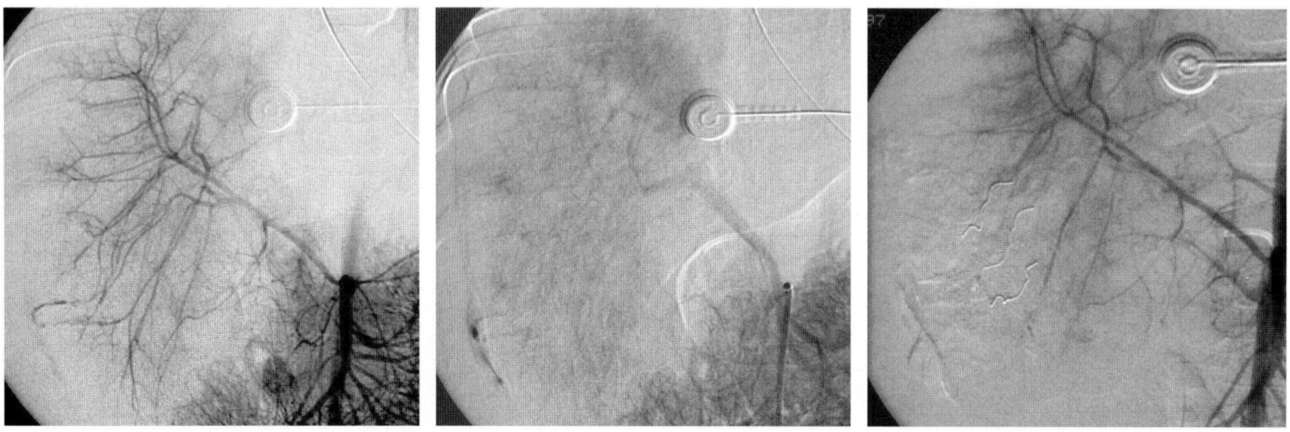

C

Figure 3.8

A: Replaced right hepatic artery angiography shows two linear liver lacerations with active extravasation of contrast in the peritoneal cavity. **B:** Late-phase hepatic artery arteriogram shows contrast accumulation in the subcapsular area and peritoneal cavity. **C:** Superselective catheterization was difficult because of the patient's size, but in 25 minutes the embolization of three hepatic artery branches of segments V and VI was performed with three microcoils. At the end of the procedure, the patient arrested again but recovered. Note occlusion of the involved arteries with successful control of the bleeding. Despite hemodynamic stability achieved after embolization, the patient died about 12 hours after the procedure.

Comment: This very unstable young patient underwent a liver biopsy that resulted in a serious complication. He was treated successfully by embolization alone. Superselective catheterization technique was the only choice to occlude the bleeding vessels without a major intervention. Despite the immediate adequate result of embolization, the patient was not clinically stable and did not survive long. It is relatively unusual to identify hepatic bleeding from biopsy tracts without an A-V fistula or pseudoaneurysm. Coagulopathy is certainly a cause for that atypical situation. However, the embolic technique showed efficacy for the presented problem. Cyanoacrylate glue probably would be an effective alternative for treatment of such a lesion.

3.9 Embolization In The Liver

Case 3.9:

A 41-year-old male patient with alcohol-related chronic liver disease underwent a blind liver biopsy with a 16-gauge needle and developed massive intraperitoneal bleeding. Coagulopathy certainly played a role in the development of the complication. Profuse intraperitoneal bleeding was observed by US.

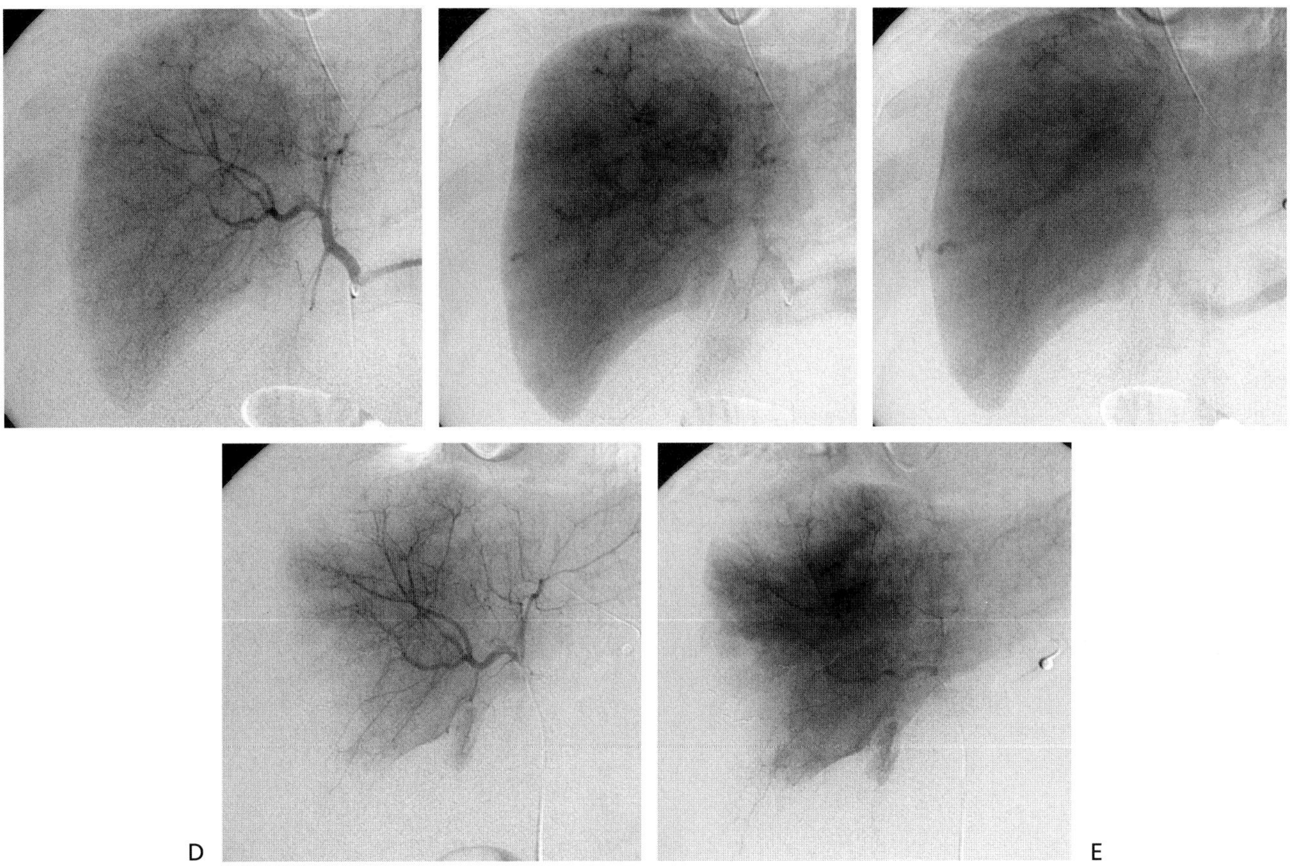

Figure 3.9

A: Hepatic arteriogram shows medial displacement of the liver by the intraperitoneal and subcapsular hematoma. A very subtle extravasation started to be observed. **B,C:** Later phase of the hepatic arteriogram shows the tract of the biopsy and extravasation of contrast into the hematoma. **D,E:** Postembolization angiogram shows occlusion of the arteries involved in the bleeding and control of the hemorrhage. Microcoils deployed through a microcatheter were used for embolization.

Comment: Unusual demonstration of the biopsy tract with active bleeding into the peritoneum. Note that there is no pseudoaneurysm formation. It was difficult to find the arterial branch and no definite bleeding was identified upon superselective injections. Embolization of several branches was performed and eventually the bleeding was stopped.

3.10 Embolization In The Liver

Case 3.10:

A 42-year-old male patient presented with a gunshot wound to the right upper quadrant of the abdomen and a penetrant wound in the liver. The large caliber of the bullet opened a large tunnel in the upper part of the liver and caused abundant bleeding. A compressive expansive latex tube was used for hemostasis inside the tunnel in the liver. Upon retrieval of the compression device, copious bleeding ensued, which required reinflation of the device and referral for arteriography and embolization.

A

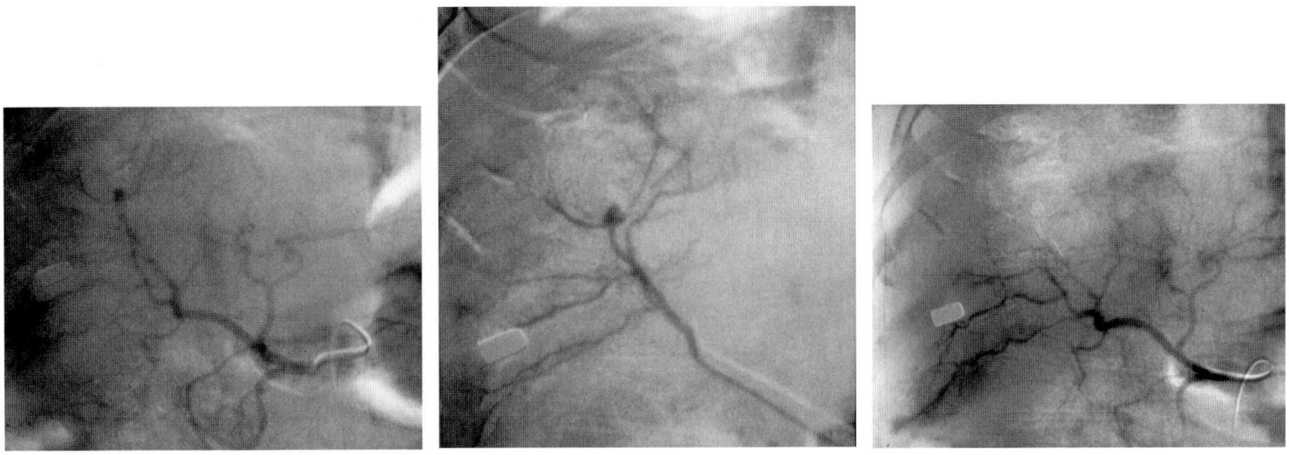

B, C

Figure 3.10

A: Selective hepatic arteriogram shows displacement and bowing of the peripheral hepatic artery branches around the tunnel created by the bullet wound. A pseudoaneurysm is visible at the top of it. Note the bullet on the right side of the liver. **B:** A more selective hepatic artery angiogram shows the pseudoaneurysm in detail. **C:** Embolization with cyanoacrylate was performed using a microcatheter. Total occlusion of the pseudoaneurysm resulted in permanent control of the bleeding and allowed removal of the compression device. Occlusion of some adjacent arteries branches also was performed. Note the good patency of the remaining branches. The portal vein was patent but did not participate in the bleeding.

Comment: Penetrating liver gunshot wounds are devastating because of the size of the channel created in the liver parenchyma by cavitation and laceration. Chances for development of a vascular trauma and laceration are high, and pseudoaneurysm formation is likely. Massive bleeding and rebleeding are common. Despite surgical measures and compression inside the tubular channel created by the bullet, angiography is very helpful for assessment and endovascular treatment. Embolization may be performed with coils, if very selective, or with cyanoacrylate glue, through a microcatheter. Embolization with absorbable particles is not generally advisable, but it may be effective. Risks of rebleeding are higher with Gelfoam than with coils or glue. Superselective embolization occludes the lesion with maximal preservation of the surrounding normal circulation, as seen in this case and in case 3.2.

3.11 Embolization In The Liver

Case 3.11:

A 60-year-old female patient developed acute pain in the right upper quadrant and a palpable and painful liver edge. CT scan showed an intrahepatic hematoma with an image suggesting an aneurysm. Angiography and embolization were requested.

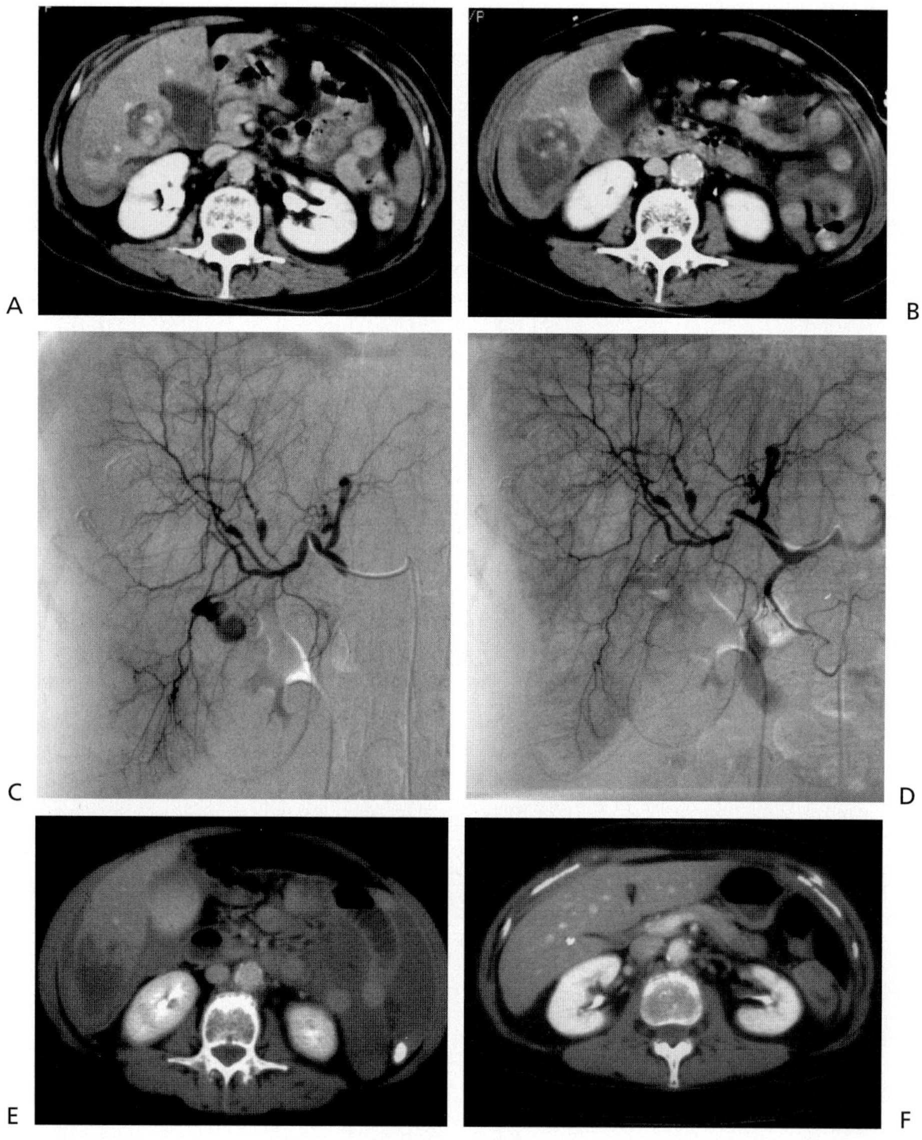

Figure 3.11

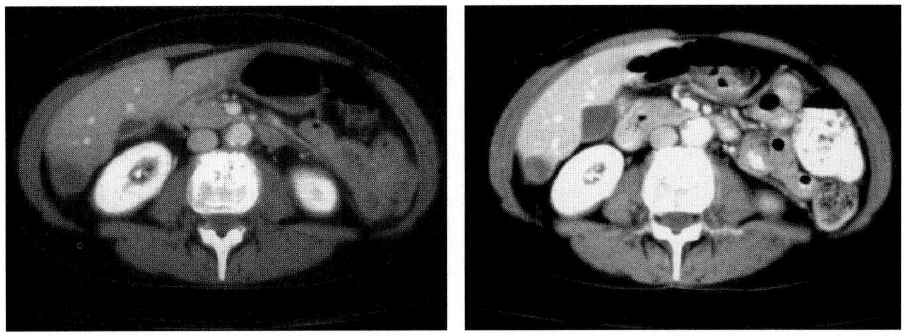
G H

Figure 3.11 *(continued)*

A: CT scan of the liver shows a hyperdense area of contrast accumulation surrounded by a hematoma located in segment VI. **B:** CT scan of the liver at a lower level shows a larger hematoma with areas of high density inside. **C:** Selective arteriogram of the common hepatic artery shows fusiform aneurysms in proximal segmental hepatic artery branches, a large saccular aneurysm of the artery in segment VI, and an area of extravasation inside the large hematoma in the right lobe of the liver. Note displacement of the branches in the right lobe of the liver. **D:** Superselective catheterization and embolization of the segmental artery of segment VI were performed, and embolization with a 2-mm × 2-cm minicoil was performed through a 5F Cobra catheter. Occlusion of the arterial branch, the aneurysm, and the pseudoaneurysm was achieved. Bleeding was controlled and the patient's pain improved. **E:** CT scan follow-up 1 week after embolization shows partial resolution of the intrahepatic hematoma and disappearance of the vessels inside the lesion. **F:** Follow-up CT scan 5 months after embolization shows marked resolution of the hepatic hematoma. **G,H:** Three-year follow-up CT scan shows a residual cavitary lesion at the tip of the right lobe of the liver. No further bleeding has occurred since the embolization.

Comment: This case raises many questions about the etiology of the bleeding. Several attempts to confirm the diagnosis of vasculitis were unsuccessful. The possibility of atherosclerotic aneurysms should be considered, but vasculitis is still an alternative diagnosis. The differential diagnosis should include segmental arterial mediolysis (formerly called segmental mediolytic arteritis), which is a nonatherosclerotic, noninflammatory vascular disease of unknown cause. It is characterized by necrosis of the outer tunica media vasorum of the arterial wall, with fibrous deposits at the medial adventitial junction and replacement of the lysed muscle fibers by fibrin, erythrocytes, and granulation tissue. The gaps in the vascular wall structure allow the dissecting hematomas and aneurysms. Involvement of visceral arteries is rare but has been reported in elderly patients, usually with simultaneous involvement of other abdominal arteries. The segmental arterial mediolysis is believed to be a precursor to, or variant of, fibromuscular dysplasia. There was no clinical evidence suggesting infection, trauma, or chemical etiology. Embolization was easy to perform and was a less invasive solution. A microcatheter was not available at the time of this procedure, but a 5F catheter could be advanced into the affected artery and deploy the coil, thus permanently occluding the aneurysm. Long follow-up available in this patient showed resolution of the hematoma, but there was a persistent small area of residual collection. Longer follow-up will be necessary in this patient, because other aneurysms may evolve and rupture in the future.

3.12 Embolization In The Liver

Case 3.12:

A 53-year-old woman had pain in the right upper quadrant and an aneurysm identified by CT scan of the upper abdomen and confirmed by angiography.

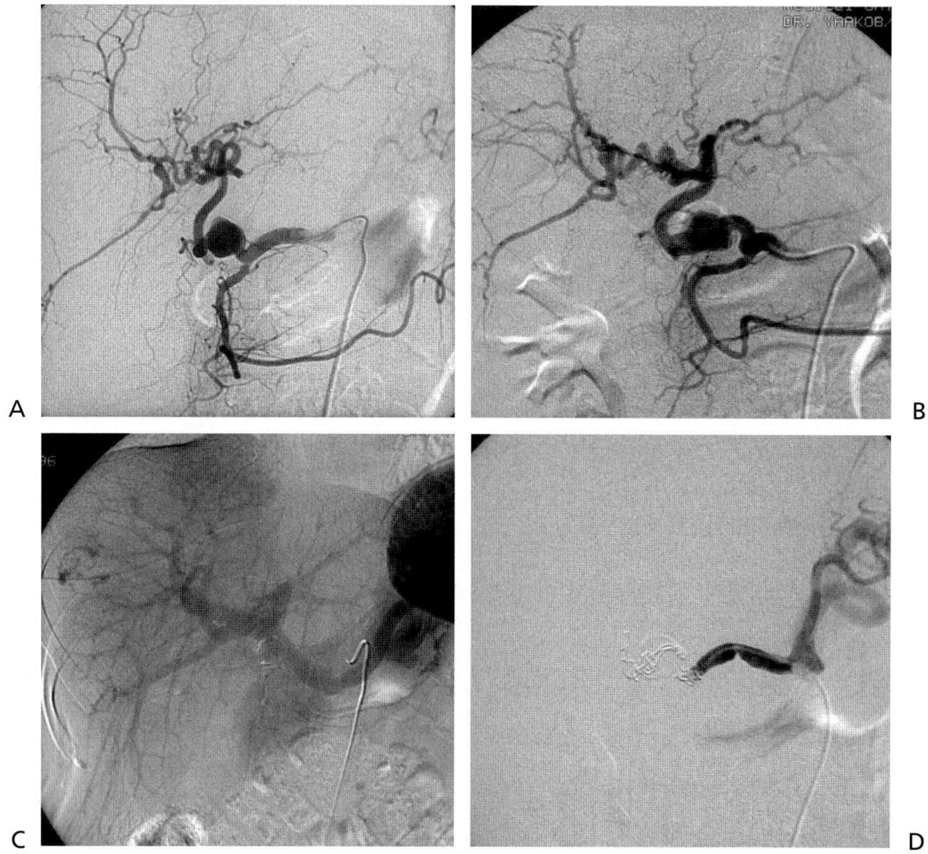

Figure 3.12

A: Selective common hepatic arteriogram shows a saccular aneurysm of the proper hepatic artery and excessive tortuosity of the intrahepatic arteries, associated with fusiform aneurysmatic dilation of at least one intrahepatic branch. **B:** Hepatic angiogram in the oblique view shows that the aneurysm is not as saccular as viewed in the anteroposterior projection. Intrahepatic aneurysmatic changes are confirmed in this view. **C:** Late-phase celiac angiogram shows patency of the splenic and portal veins. Note the calcifications in the wall of the aneurysm and a small hemangioma of the right lobe of the liver. **D:** Embolization was performed with multiple microcoils, which bridged the aneurysm location and resulted in total occlusion of the common hepatic artery and proper hepatic artery.

Comment: Aneurysms of the hepatic artery might be detected as masses or by bleeding into the bile ducts. Severe and massive intraperitoneal bleeding may be the first sign of an extrahepatic aneurysm or pseudoaneurysm. Most common causes include trauma, infection, atherosclerosis, and collagenous diseases with vascular involvement. In the past, the most common cause was infection; currently the most frequent cause of hepatic artery pseudoaneurysm is trauma. As the population gets holder, atherosclerotic disease becomes more common. Hepatic artery aneurysms may rupture into the peritoneal cavity (44%), biliary tract (41%), GI tract (11%), or portal vein (5%). Traditional treatment has been surgical ligation or reconstruction of the artery, but this is associated with a high 75% presurgical and postsurgical morbidity/mortality. After utilization of transcatheter embolization, the morbidity/mortality decreased to around 30%. Unruptured hepatic artery aneurysms may cause pain and jaundice. Ideal embolization technique requires filling the aneurysm cavity and preserving the parent artery, if possible. Fusiform aneurysms, if embolized, will require occlusion of the parent artery. A covered stent may be an option, but experience with such a device for that purpose is not yet available despite a case report showing successful treatment.

3.13 Embolization In The Liver

Case 3.13:

A 63-year-old male patient with a known large cholangiocarcinoma developed acute massive bleeding during endoscopy and exchange of plastic stents. Pulsatile hemobilia was observed as the patient's blood pressure dropped and he complained of abdominal pain in the right upper quadrant. Emergency angiography was undertaken.

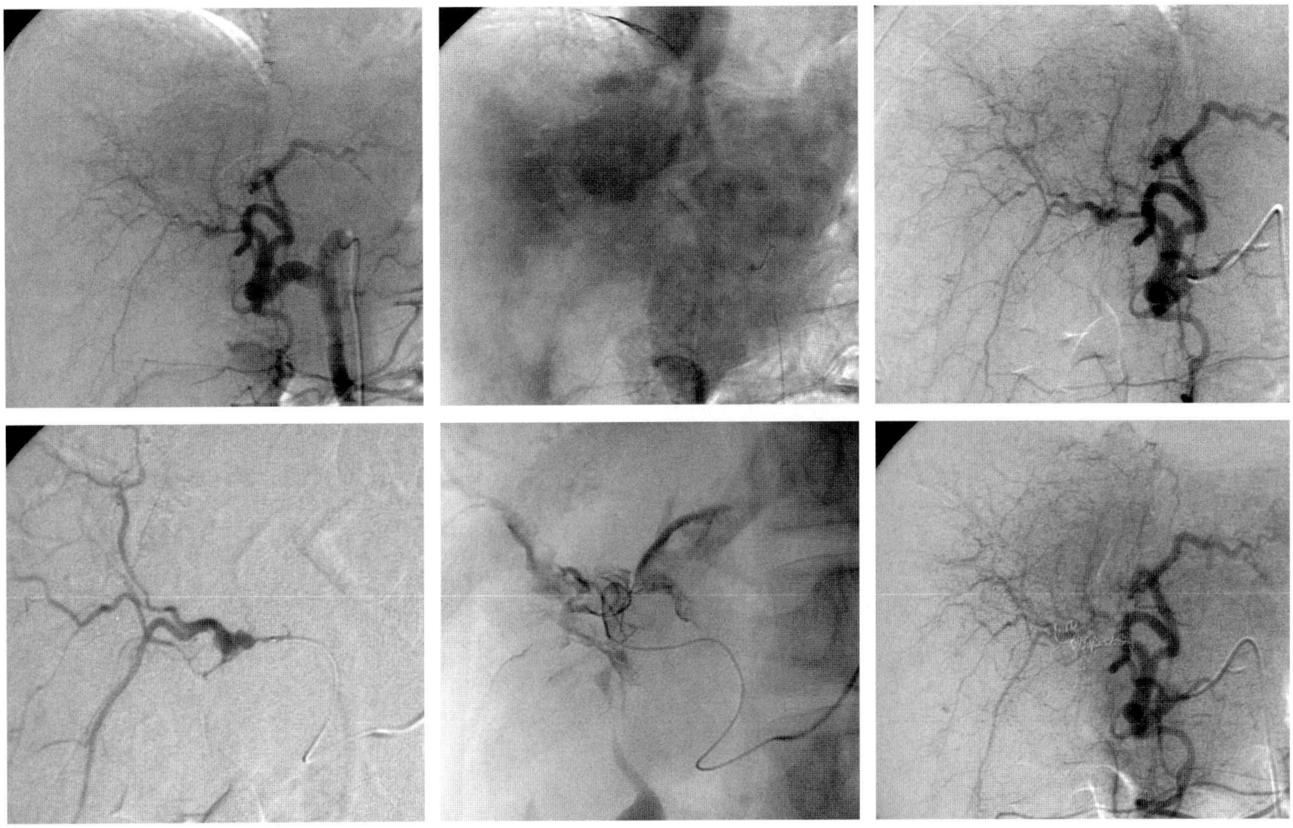

Figure 3.13

A: Selective angiography demonstrates total replaced common hepatic artery from the superior mesenteric artery, a pseudoaneurysm in the proximal right hepatic artery, and an adjacent tumoral mass with tumoral vessels. No active extravasation is observed. **B:** Late-phase hepatic arteriogram shows tumor enhancement in the right and left lobes of the liver. **C:** More selective arteriogram of the common hepatic artery shows the pseudoaneurysm and the tumor mass in greater detail. **D:** Superselective catheterization of the right hepatic artery with a 2.8F microcatheter demonstrates the bilobular pseudoaneurysm. **E:** A more wedged injection with the microcatheter beyond the pseudoaneurysm shows extravasation of dye into the bile ducts and demonstrates the communication of the lesion with the bile ducts. **F:** Embolization with fourteen 2-mm × 2-cm microcoils filling the aneurysm cavity and the proximal right hepatic artery. Note persistent patency of the left hepatic artery and the segment IV artery, with reconstitution of peripheral branches of the right hepatic artery. The bleeding was controlled permanently and the bile ducts were drained percutaneously. Metal stents were placed at a later date.

Comment: In this case, it is impossible to know for certain if the pseudoaneurysm was created by tumoral invasion or erosion/trauma by the biliary stent. It is more likely, however, that the pseudoaneurysm was created by tumoral growth and invasion. The actual bleeding may have been started by stent manipulation inside the bile duct. Hepatic carcinoma growth inside the liver most frequently causes arterioportal fistulas rather than arterial invasion and pseudoaneurysm formation. Embolization is the most adequate treatment for this kind of arterial lesion and, as demonstrated in this case, usually is successful.

3.14 Embolization In The Liver

Case 3.14:

A 65-year-old male patient presented with acute intraperitoneal bleeding, severe pain in the upper abdomen, and a ruptured liver tumor (hepatocellular carcinoma), identified by a CT scan of the abdomen. He was treated by surgical "scooping" of the necrotic tumor and wide surgical suture of the bleeding liver. Despite the surgical procedure, the patient continued to bleed. After 14 units of blood replacement, he was flown to our institution for treatment. Cirrhosis and coagulopathy played a role in the bleeding. Emergency angiography was performed.

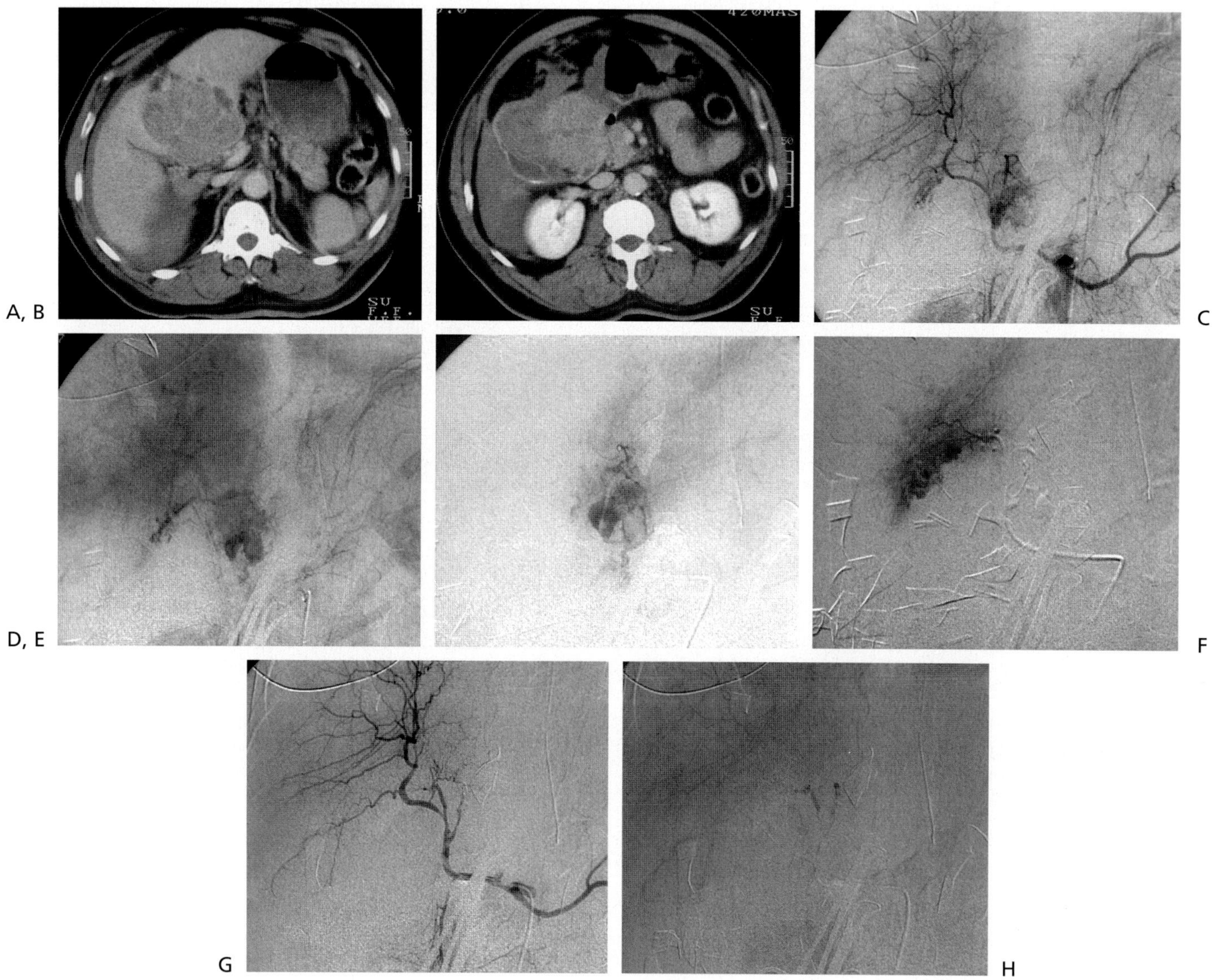

Figure 3.14

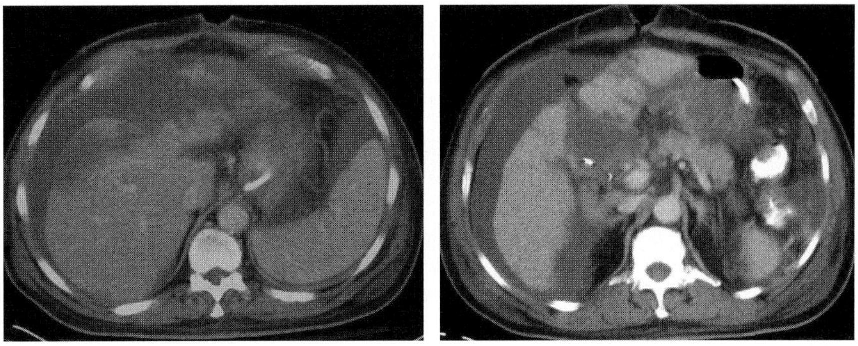

I J

Figure 3.14 *(continued)*

A,B: CT scan of the liver shows the mass in the left lobe of the liver ruptured in the anterior aspect. Note the free fluid in the abdomen and necrotic areas within the liver mass. **C:** Liver arteriogram shows areas of active bleeding in the lateral aspects of the residual mass. Note the multiple metal clamps used to close the abdominal wound for patient transportation. **D:** Later-phase arteriogram shows two active areas of contrast accumulation. **E:** Superselective arteriogram with a microcatheter in the lateral arteriogram of segment IV shows active bleeding. **F:** Superselective arteriogram in the medial arteriogram of segment IV and some branches toward the right lobe shows active areas of bleeding on the surface of the residual tumor. **G:** Embolization with distally placed Gelfoam and more proximal 2-mm × 2-cm microcoils occluded both bleeding arteries. Postembolization arteriogram shows control of the bleeding. **H:** Late-phase angiogram shows contrast medium retained in the embolized arteries. The bleeding was permanently controlled. **I,J:** CT scan of the liver 2 weeks after embolization shows a large volume of residual blood in the peritoneal cavity with subcapsular hematoma and a cavity at the tumor location filled with old blood. Note the metal coils and metal clips in **H.** Despite control of bleeding, this patient never left the hospital. He experienced progressive clinical deterioration and died of multiple organ failure about 4 weeks after the embolization.

Comment: Spontaneous rupture of hepatocellular carcinoma is a rare cause (7.5%) of intraperitoneal bleeding but is associated with high morbidity and mortality. Thirty-day mortality is elevated. Traditional surgical treatment includes emergency hepatectomy, hepatic packing with Gelfoam, and hepatic artery ligation, with hepatic artery ligation being the most successful. Hepatic artery embolization has been used in relatively few cases, based on literature reports, but it is the most effective and obvious treatment. Embolization with smaller particles placed distally and microcoils to seal off the bleeding vessel is the treatment of choice. Proximal embolization of the hepatic artery should be avoided at all costs because it may not stop the bleeding and will preclude further endovascular treatment, if necessary.

3.15 Embolization In The Liver

Case 3.15:

A 31-year-old female patient with hepatic hemangiosarcoma presented with spontaneous rupture and intraperitoneal bleeding, following a cesarean section, which had been treated by coil embolization at another institution. Recurrence of bleeding prompted transfer of the patient to our institution, and an angiogram was performed for possible embolization.

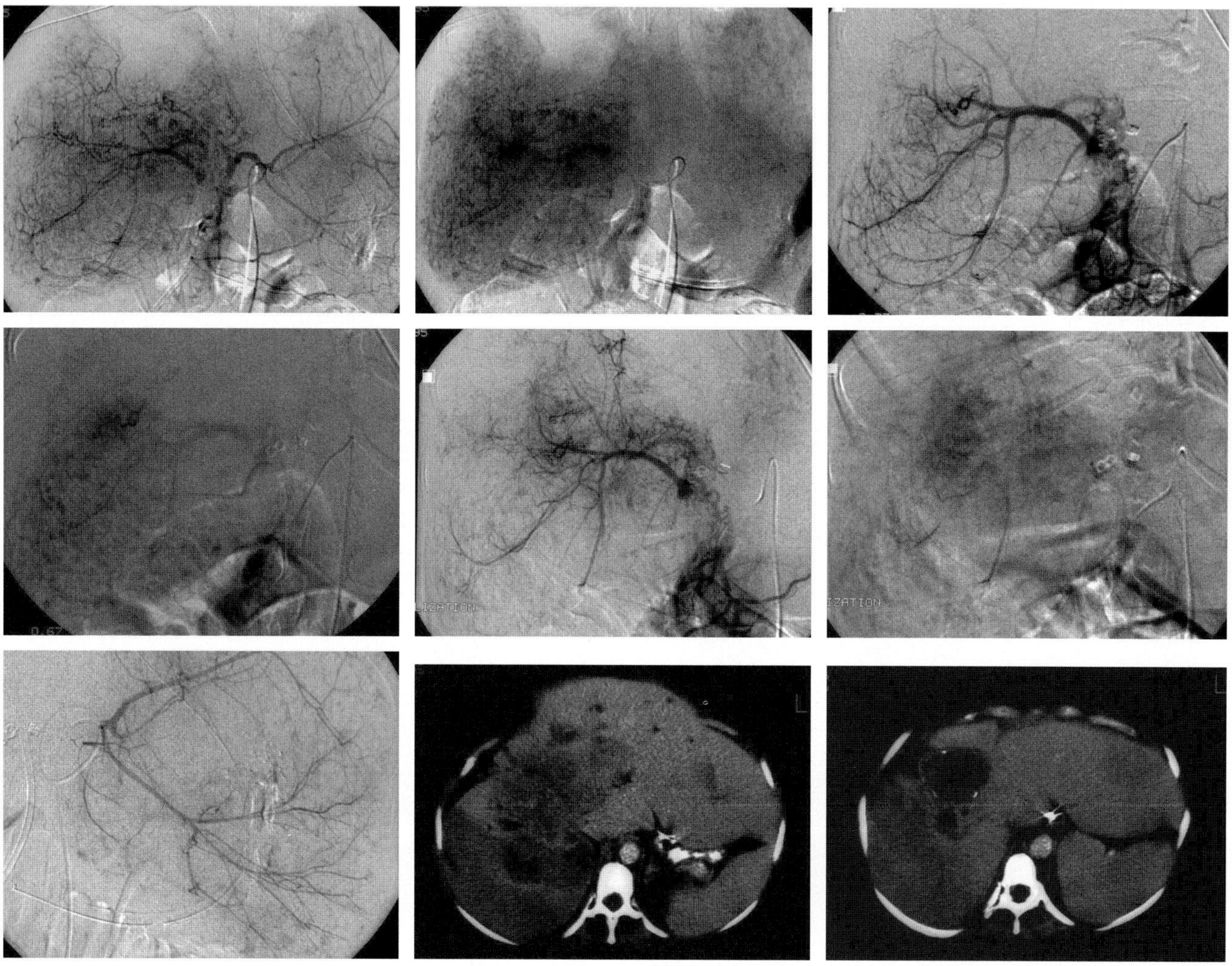

A, B C

D, E F

G, H I

Figure 3.15

A: Hepatic arteriogram shows the right hepatic artery occluded by coils placed quite proximally, beyond the origin of the gastroduodenal artery. Note hypervascularity and tumor vessels within the right hepatic lobe feeding from the reconstituted right hepatic artery through collaterals originating from the gastroduodenal artery and left hepatic artery. The peripheral branches are bowed and displaced by the mass. The left hepatic lobe is enlarged. A plastic, endoscopically placed, biliary stent also is seen. **B:** Capillary phase angiogram shows tumor stain and abnormal and patchy hepatogram with small punctate collections consistent with the diagnosis of peliosis hepatis. **C:** Superselective gastroduodenal artery angiogram shows abundant collaterals reconstituting the right hepatic artery beyond the occlusive coils. **D:** Superselective catheterization of the right hepatic artery with a Tracker microcatheter to allow access for smaller particles embolization (100 to 200 μm). **E,F:** Postembolization angiogram shows significantly reduced tumor vascularity. **G:** Selective angiogram of the left hepatic artery shows some degree of peripheral peliosis hepatis. **H,I:** CT scan of the liver 3 days after the angiogram and embolization shows a large hepatic mass with aspect suggesting rupture of the periphery of the lesion and a large hypodense nodule.

Comment: Hemangiosarcoma is a rare malignancy of the liver that has been linked to exposure to several substances in approximately 40% of the cases. Vinyl chloride, Thorotrast, arsenicals, and radium are the most common related exposures reported. Hepatic arteriography shows normal-sized hepatic arteries, tumoral staining and puddling, and central areas of hypovascularity. Peliosis hepatis is a relatively rare hepatic abnormality with a characteristic appearance that includes blood-filled cystic spaces of various sizes, which may or may not be lined by endothelium. This abnormality has been associated with use of anabolic steroids, estrogens, oral contraceptives, and azathioprine; exposure to vinyl chloride; angiosarcoma; and hepatoma. Hemangiosarcoma may develop spontaneous rupture, as well as peliosis hepatis, and intraperitoneal bleeding may be the first symptom. Peripheral embolization with particles should be the preferred technique. Metal coils can be used to seal off the arteries but not placed as proximal as initially used in this case.

3.16 Embolization In The Liver

Case 3.16:

A 40-year-old female patient using contraceptives presented with liver cell adenoma with spontaneous rupture and intraperitoneal bleeding.

A, B

C

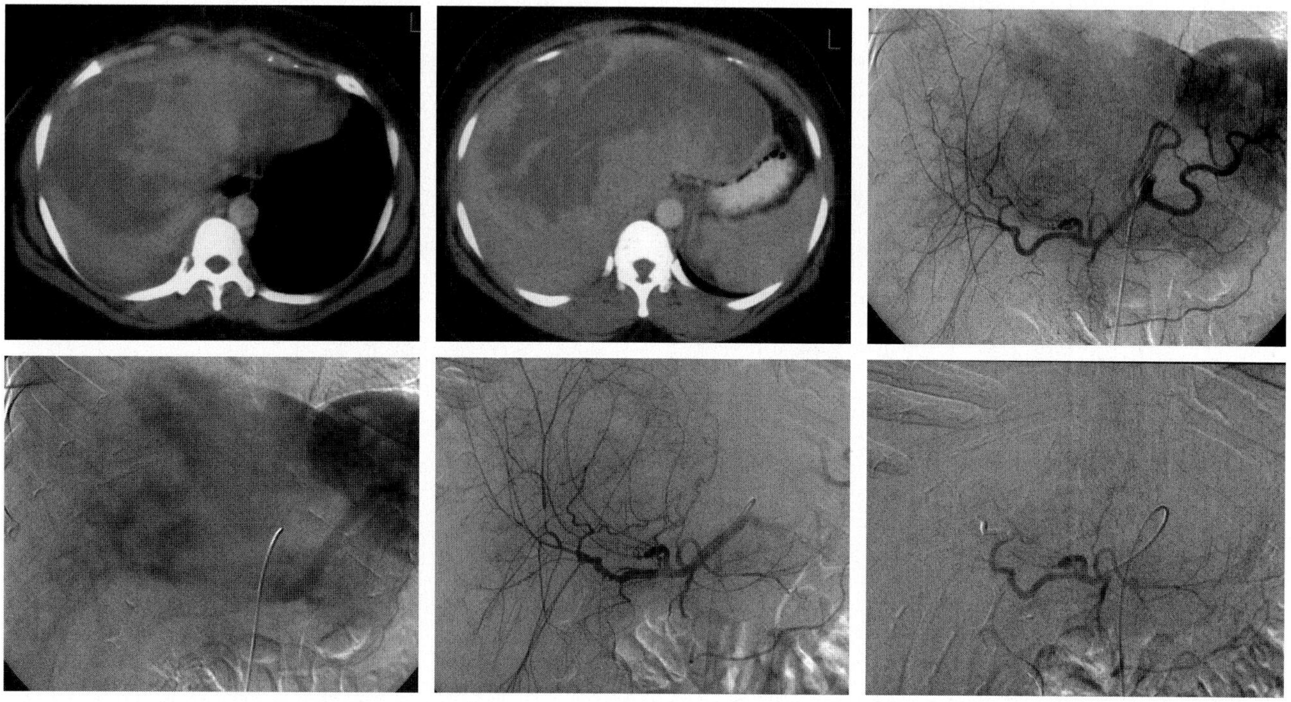

D, E

F

Figure 3.16

A,B: CT scan with IV contrast shows a large liver mass with areas of hypodensity and intrahepatic areas of hemorrhage. **C:** Celiac arteriogram shows a large left lobe liver mass displacing the hepatic arteries with neovascularity and moderate tumor stain. **D:** The portal vein is patent but is displaced by the tumor. **E:** Superselective hepatic arteriogram shows partial filling of the lesion from the right hepatic artery. No active extravasation is observed. **F:** Embolization with Gelfoam particles was performed to control the bleeding. Surgical resection was performed electively a few weeks later.

Comment: Hepatic adenomas are benign tumors consisting of hepatocytes without biliary elements. There is a higher incidence in females, mainly associated with oral contraceptive use. There is a propensity for spontaneous hemorrhage that can be life threatening. There is a small chance of malignant degeneration. There is support in the literature for resolution of hepatic adenomas after cessation of oral contraceptive intake. Angiographically, hepatic adenomas show a spectrum from hypovascular to hypervascular, and A-V shunting does not occur in a usually well-circumscribed homogeneous mass in the capillary phase. Surgical resection is indicated because of the small risk of malignant degeneration and the possibility of bleeding. Embolization may be the initial treatment to control spontaneous bleeding and save the patient's life during the acute phase. Small-sized (200 to 500 μm) particles (Ivalon or Gelfoam) should be used for embolization. Proximal embolization with coils is not indicated.

Suggested Reading

Althaus S, Ashdown B, Coldwell D, et al. Transcatheter arterial embolization of two symptomatic giant cavernous hemangiomas of the liver. *Cardiovasc Intervent Radiol* 1996;19:364–367.

Aso N, Matsunaga N, Fukuda T, et al. Multiple intrahepatic aneurysms following transcatheter arterial embolization. *Radiology* 1994;193:743–746.

Ault GT, Wren SM, Ralls PW, et al. Selective management of hepatic adenomas. *Am Surg* 1996;62:825–829.

Bakker J, Robben SGF, Hazerbroek F, et al. Congenital arterioportal fistula of the liver with reversal of flow in the superior mesenteric vein. *Pediatr Radiol* 1994;24:198–199.

Blue JM, Burney DP. Current trends in the diagnosis and treatment of hepatic artery aneurysms. *South Med J* 1990;83:966–969.

Cacho G, Abreu L, Calleja J, et al. Arterioportal fistula and hemobilia with associated acute cholecystitis: a complication of percutaneous liver biopsy. *Hepatogastroenterology* 1996;34:1020–1023.

Cascinu S, Wadler S. Chemo-embolization in the treatment of liver metastases from colorectal cancer. *Cancer Treat Rev* 1996;22:355–363.

de Baere T, Roche A, Amenabar JM. Liver abscess formation after local treatment of liver tumors. *Hepatology* 1996;23:1436–1440.

Demachi H, Matsui O, Kawamori Y, et al. The protective effect of portoarterial shunts after experimental hepatic artery embolization in rats with liver cirrhosis. *Cardiovasc Intervent Radiol* 1995;18:97–101.

Doppman JL, Girton M, Kahn R. Proximal versus peripheral hepatic artery embolization experimental study in monkeys. *Radiology* 1978;128:577–588.

Fellows K, Hoffer F, Markowitz R, et al. Multiple collateral to hepatic infantile hemangioendothelioma and arteriovenous malformation: effect on embolization. *Radiology* 1991;181:813–818.

Gibril F, Doppman J, Jensen R. Recent advances in the treatment of metastatic pancreatic endocrine tumors. *Semin Gastrointest Dis* 1995;6:114–121.

Gorenflo M, Waldschmidt J, Bein G, et al. Arterioportal fistula in infancy. *J Pediatr Gastroenterol Nutr* 1993;16:87–89.

Gryboski J, Clemett A. Congenital hepatic artery aneurysm with superior mesenteric artery insufficiency: a steal syndrome. *Pediatrics* 1967;39:344–347.

Hazerbroek F, Tibboel D, Robben S, et al. Hepatic artery ligation for hepatic vascular tumors with arteriovenous and arterioportal venous shunts in the newborn: successful management of two cases and review of the literature. *J Pediatr Surg* 1995;30:1127–1130.

Heaton N, Davenport M, Karani J, et al. Congenital hepatoportal arteriovenous fistula. *Surgery* 1995;117:170–174.

Helikson MA, Shapiro DL, Seashore JH. Hepatoportal arteriovenous fistula and portal hypertension in an infant. *Pediatrics* 1977;60:921–924.

Inon A, D'Agostino D. Portal hypertension secondary to congenital arterioportal fistula. *J Pediatr Gastroenterol Nutr* 1987;6:471–473.

Jeans WD, Leven HO. A new technique for nonsurgical repair of peripheral pseudoaneurysm. *Acta Radiol* 1995;36:100–101.

Khan KN, Nakata K, Shima M, et al. Pancreatic tissue damage by transcatheter arterial embolization for hepatoma. *Dig Dis Sci* 1993;38:65–70.

Kishimoto W, Nakao A, Takagi H, et al. Acute pancreatitis after transcatheter arterial embolization (TAE) for hepatocellular carcinoma. *Am J Gastroenterol* 1989;84:1396–1399.

Kitahara S, Makuuchi M, Ishizone S, et al. Successful left trisegmentectomy for ruptured hepatoblastoma using intraoperative transarterial embolization. *J Pediatr Surg* 1995;30:1709–1712.

Lee SI, Chew FS. Splanchnic segmental arterial mediolysis. *AJR* 1998;170:122.

Lina JR, Jaques P, Mandell V. Aneurysm rupture secondary to transcatheter embolization. *AJR* 1979;132:553–556.

Liou TC, Ling CC, Pang KK. Liver abscess concomitant with hemobilia due to rupture of hepatic artery aneurysm: a case report. *Hepatogastroenterology* 1996;43:241–244.

Livraghi T, Giorgio A, Marin G, et al. Hepatocellular carcinoma and cirrhosis in 746 patients: long term results of percutaneous ethanol injection. *Radiology* 1995;197:101–108.

Marchand V, Uflacker R, Baker SS, et al. Congenital hepatic arterioportal fistula in a 3-year-old child. *J Pediatr Gastroenterol Nutr* 1999;28:435–441.

Meunier C, Dabadie A, Darnault P, et al. Fistule arterioporte intrahepatique congenitale: aspects diagnostiques et therapeutiques. *Pediatrie* 1993;48:211–216.

Miyagawa S, Makuuchi M, Kawasaki S, et al. Outcome of major hepatectomy with pancreatoduodenectomy for advanced biliary malignancies. *World J Surg* 1996;20:77–80.

Mounedji Boudiaf L, Rougier P, Culine S, et al. Treatment of metastatic malignant insulinomas 2 cases. *Presse Med* 1995;24:894–896.

Pavcnik D, Saxon RR, Kubota Y, et al. Attempted induction of chronic portal venous hypertension with polyvinyl alcohol particles in swine. *J Vasc Interv Radiol* 1997;8:123–128.

Routh WD, Keller FS, Cain WS, et al. Transcatheter embolization of a high flow congenital intrahepatic arterial portal venous malformation in an infant. *J Pediatr Surg* 1992;27:511–514.

Samuel M, Spitz L. Infantile hepatic hemangioendothelioma: the role of surgery. *J Pediatr Surg* 1995;30:1425–1429.

Shapiro AM, Lakey JR, Rajotte RV, et al. Portal vein thrombosis after transplantation of partially purified pancreatic islets in a combined human liver/islet allograft. *Transplantation* 1995;7:1060–1063.

Slavin RE, Seki K, Bhagavan B, et al. Segmental arterial mediolysis: a precursor to fibromuscular dysplasia? *Mod Pathol* 1995;8:287–294.

Sonomura T, Yamada R, Kishi K, et al. Dependency of tissue necrosis on gelatin sponge particle size after canine hepatic artery embolization. *Cardiovasc Intervent Radiol* 1997;20:50–53.

Stain SC, Woodburn DA, Stephens AL, et al. Spontaneous hepatic hemorrhage associated with pregnancy. Treatment by hepatic arterial interruption. *Ann Surg* 1996;224:72–78.

Suzuki H, Nimura Y, Kamiya J, et al. Preoperative transcatheter arterial embolization for giant cavernous hemangioma of the liver with consumption coagulopathy. *Am J Gastroenterol* 1997;92:688–691.

Tharp R, Fillmore D. Multiple hepatic hemorrhagic mycotic pseudoaneurysms treated with embolization. *J Vasc Interv Radiol* 1995;6:876–878.

Thibodeaux LC, Deshmukh RM, Hearn AT, et al. Management options for hepatic artery aneurysms. *Ann Vasc Surg* 1995;9:285–288.

Uflacker R, Mourao GS, Piske RL, et al. Hemobilia: transcatheter occlusive therapy and long-term follow-up. *Cardiovasc Intervent Radiol* 1989;12:136–141.

Uflacker R, Paolini RM, Nobrega M. Ablation of tumor and inflammatory tissue with absolute ethanol. *Acta Radiol* 1986;27:131–138.

Walker WJ. Case report: successful internal iliac artery embolisation with glue in a case of massive obstetric haemorrhage. *Clin Radiol* 1996;51:442–444.

Wangberg B, Westberg G, Tylen U, et al. Survival of patients with disseminated midgut carcinoid tumors after aggressive tumor reduction. *World J Surg* 1996;20:892–899.

Zepeda HO. Treatment of hepatic metastasis provenient of endocrine tumors of the pancreas. *Rev Gastroenterol Mex* 1997;62:50–56.

CHAPTER 4

Embolization In The Spleen

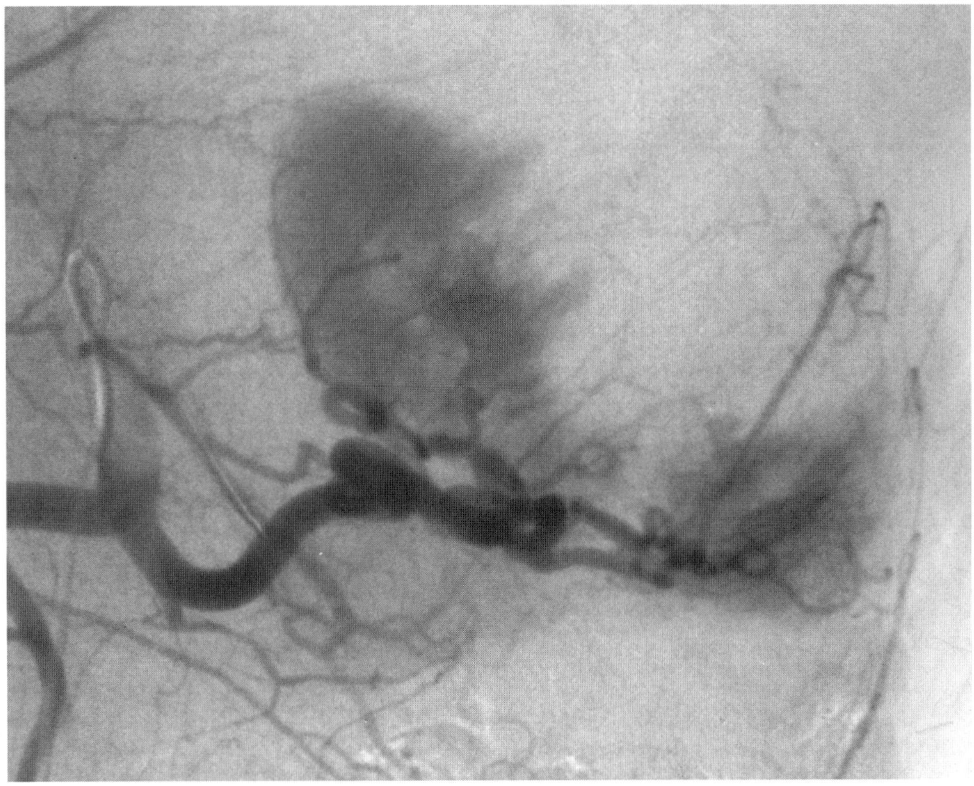

4.1 Embolization In The Spleen

Case 4.1:

A 66-year-old male patient presented with repeated gastric and esophageal varices bleeding. Several attempts at treatment with endoscopic sclerosis did not result in improvement. Ultrasound and computed tomographic (CT) scan demonstrated occlusion of the splenic and portal veins, which was causing extrahepatic portal hypertension. No liver disease or cause of portal vein thrombosis was identified. Arteriography and embolization of the splenic artery were requested to reduce the splenic component of the portal hypertension.

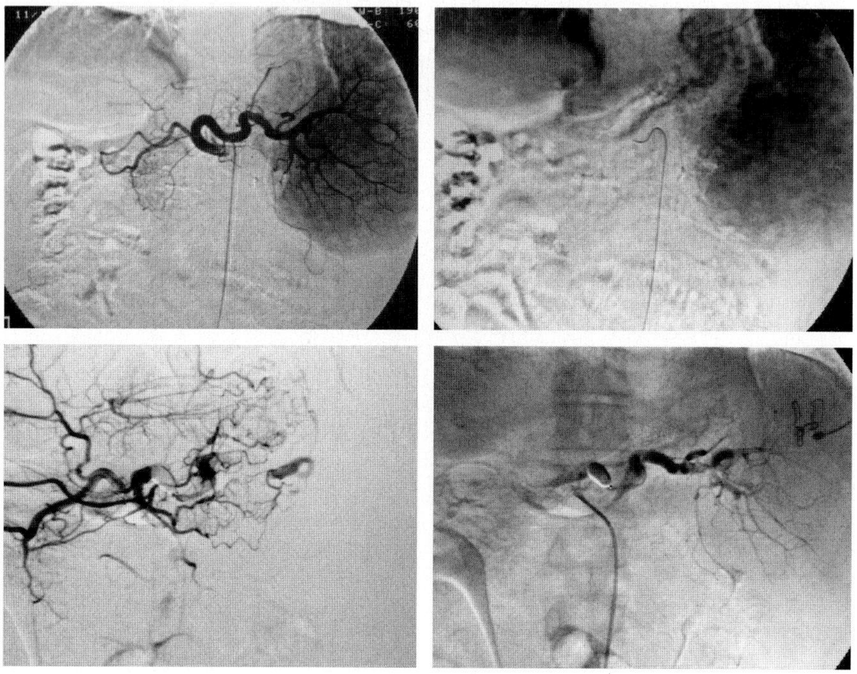

A B C D

Figure 4.1

A: Celiac arteriogram shows a large spleen supplied by an enlarged splenic artery. Note that there is no main hepatic artery, which is replaced to the superior mesenteric artery. Only a small hepatic artery branch is observed. **B:** Late-phase celiac arteriogram shows no filling of the splenic and portal veins. Note enhancement of gastric fundus varices. A decision was made to occlude the splenic artery using a detachable balloon, to reduce flow and pressure into the spleen and hopefully reduce pressure in the venous system, which would allow reconstitution of the distal splenic artery and maintain splenic perfusion. **C:** Early-phase arteriogram of the celiac trunk, which is occluded by the balloon, shows development of collateral circulation and reconstitution of the distal splenic artery. **D:** Late-phase celiac injection shows perfusion of the splenic substance with a much slower flow.

Comment: Extrahepatic portal hypertension most commonly is due to portal and/or splenic vein thrombosis. Occlusion of the splenic vein caused development of venous collateral circulation through the short gastric veins and perisplenic venous circulation and possible draining into the portal vein through the left gastric vein. If the portal vein also is occluded, the hypertension extends into the superior mesenteric vein and the mesenteric circulation, and there is no drainage of the gastric fundus in the portal vein through the left gastric vein. Varices in the esophagus also develop due to regional hypertension and reversal of flow in the lower esophageal veins. The contribution of the splenic flow is very significant, mainly when the spleen enlarges. In patients with cirrhosis, the contribution by the spleen to portal hypertension is about 20%. In patients with hepatosplenic schistosomiasis due to hypersplenism, the contribution is greater, close to 40%. The outcome in this patient was good, and bleeding was controlled during follow-up of more than 8 months.

4.2 Embolization In The Spleen

Case 4.2:

A 56-year-old male patient with chronic liver disease due to posthepatitic cirrhosis presented with hypersplenism and untreatable hepatic encephalopathy.

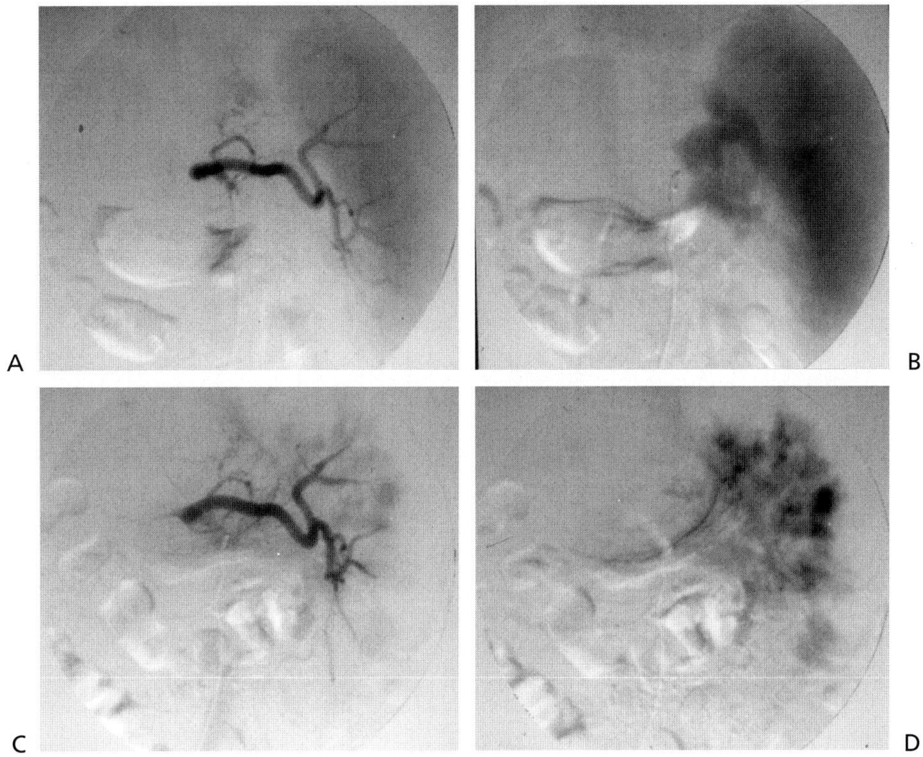

Figure 4.2

A: Selective injection into the splenic artery shows a large spleen. **B:** Late-phase angiogram shows opacification of the splenic vein and splenorenal shunt. **C:** After partial embolization of the splenic circulation with Gelfoam, reduction of the splenic perfusion was obtained. Note reduced filling of peripheral arterial branches. **D:** Late-phase postembolization angiogram shows mottled appearance of the splenic substance and no filling of the shunt. Encephalopathy was controlled for more than 1 year following embolization.

Comment: Diversion of splanchnic blood from the hepatic circulation is the major element in encephalopathy caused by a portosystemic shunt. When splenic flow is increased in situations of hypersplenism, spontaneous portosystemic shunts may develop, creating localized shunts between the splenic vein and the systemic circulation. Hyperflow through the splenic vein draining into a collateral may cause a sump situation, diverting splenic vein flow and sucking blood from the portal system into the systemic circulation. Reduction of arterial splenic flow reduces venous flow, diminishes the sump through the shunt, and reduces flow into the systemic circulation. The possibility to control encephalopathy is achieved by reducing spleen perfusion. In general, there is no need for dietary control, or only a minimal reduction in protein intake is required. Reduction of portal venous pressure also is a probable factor that reduces the shunting and diversion of blood flow from the liver.

4.3 Embolization In The Spleen

Case 4.3:

A 50-year-old female patient with chronic liver disease due to alcoholic cirrhosis presented with hypersplenism and untreatable low platelet count.

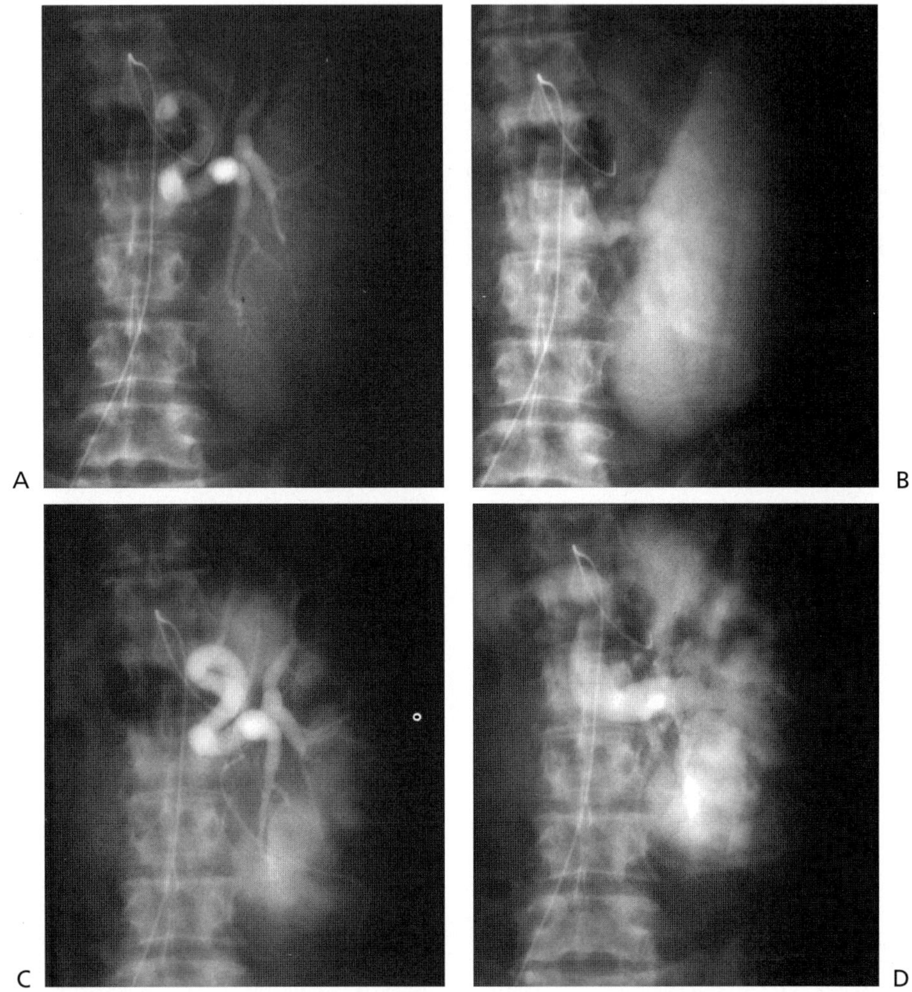

Figure 4.3

A: Selective splenic arteriogram shows a large spleen with increased arterial flow. **B:** Late-phase arteriogram shows parenchymatous enhancement of the large spleen. **C:** Angiogram after partial embolization performed with Gelfoam shows reduced flow and irregular staining of the splenic parenchyma. **D:** Late-phase arteriogram shows highly irregular enhancement and increased density during filling of the splenic vein.

Comment: Embolization of the spleen for control of hypersplenism is an efficient way to reduce platelet consumption. However, embolization must be partial and preserve splenic function, but it also must reduce the volume of parenchyma available and the total organ flow. Splenic blood supply is complex, and there is evidence of a microcirculatory open bed, with some shunting. Partial embolization was established to be effective in 1979. The procedure then was standardized, with a dramatic reduction of complications initially related to the procedure. Today, partial embolization of the spleen is a reliable technique to treat hypersplenism related to immunosuppressive states, portal hypertension, and chronic liver disease. In cases of large splenomegaly, partial embolization can be used to improve patient comfort and reduce abdominal pain. Hypersplenism is characterized by sequestration of formed blood elements inside the spleen. The aim of embolization is to reduce perfusion of the enlarged spleen by blood and thus reduce the level of sequestration. Infection was the most threatening complication of partial splenic embolization. Intravenous antibiotic coverage is required 6 to 12 hours before the procedure, should be maintained during the procedure, and given for 7 to 10 days following the procedure. Postembolization syndrome is tolerated by most patients, but pain may require morphine and sedation for effective control. It is also important that hydration be available to the patient. The spleen may enlarge initially and will reduce progressively in size after day 30. Leukocytosis is common following embolization, returning to normal levels after 2 or 3 days.

4.4 Embolization In The Spleen

Case 4.4:

A 40-year-old female patient with a history of chronic pancreatitis was admitted to the hospital with signs of intraabdominal bleeding, initially thought to be related to the pancreatitis process. CT scan of the abdomen showed splenic laceration with active bleeding. Angiography was requested. At the time of the angiogram, the patient presented with bruises on the face and abdomen, which suggested previous physical aggression and probably were related to the splenic trauma. The splenic injury was considered class III according to the Buntain classification.

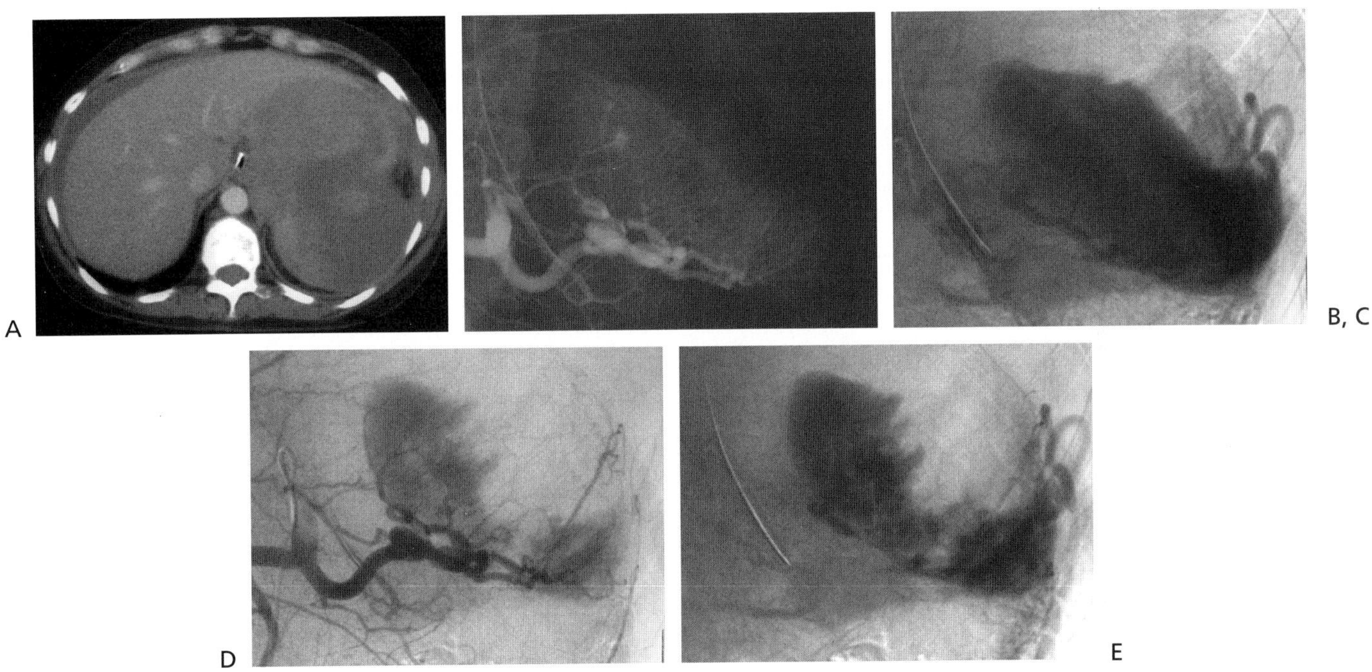

Figure 4.4

A: CT scan shows splenic laceration and active contrast extravasation. **B,C:** Selective arteriogram of the celiac artery shows splenic laceration with a subcapsular hematoma and active bleeding within the splenic substance. **D,E:** A Tracker microcatheter was used for superselective catheterization of the splenic artery. Partial splenic embolization was performed with Ivalon 100 to 200 μm and Gelfoam 1 × 1 mm. The arteriogram shows reduced perfusion of the spleen and control of active bleeding.

Comment: Following embolization, the patient improved hemodynamically and was discharged from the intensive care unit. Three days after the improvement, the patient deteriorated again. Free air in the peritoneal cavity due to rupture of the stomach was identified. Surgery was performed, after which the patient slowly improved.

Splenic injuries are classified according to Buntain (1988), in ranked and nominal variable scales.

The ranked variable scale is as follows:

Class I: Localized capsular disruption or subcapsular hematoma, without significant parenchymal injury

Class II: Single or multiple capsular and parenchymal disruptions, transverse or longitudinal, that do not extend into the hilum or involve major vessels; intraparenchymal hematoma may or may not coexist.

Class III: Deep fractures, single or multiple, transverse or longitudinal, extending into the hilum and involving major blood vessels

Class IV: Completely shattered or fragmented spleen, or spleen separated from its normal blood supply at the pedicle

Absence of extravasation on arteriography is a reliable indicator of successful nonoperative therapy, but most of patients present with persistent or recurrent hemorrhage or require delayed laparotomy. Indications for exploratory laparotomy after CT scan or angiography are hemodynamic instability, ongoing blood loss, peritonitis, pancreatic, diaphragmatic or bowel injury, and failure to complete embolization successfully.

Embolization should be performed when active extravasation is seen by celiac or splenic arteriography. Embolization can be performed proximally with coils or, according to other authors, with flow-directed particles. Focal and superselective embolization with smaller pledgets of Gelfoam or other particles may be performed when the extravasation extends outside the capsule into the peritoneum. At that point, embolization of other structures, such as the liver, kidney, or pelvic vessels, may be performed as well. Angiography usually refines the CT characterization of the splenic injury. In patients with active extravasation but who are hemodynamically stable, embolization is successful and can increase the number of patients who can be managed nonoperatively.

Complications of the procedure are infection and pain. The overall percentage of patients treated nonoperatively is about 88%, with a salvage rate of 97%. Embolization may be the sole treatment in about 30% of the cases, whereas observation only may be the main form of treatment in about 60% of the patients with splenic trauma.

Suggested Reading

Arias Diaz J, Gomez Gutierrez M, Torres Melero J, et al. Embolization of the gastroduodenal artery for the treatment of massive haemorrhage in a patient with chronic pancreatitis. *Eur J Surg* 1994;160:393–395.

Hagiwara A, Yudioka T, Ohta S, et al. Nonsurgical management of patients with blunt splenic injury: efficacy of transcatheter arterial embolization. *AJR* 1996;167:159–166.

Mukaiya M, Hirata K, Yamashiro K, et al. Changes in portal hemodynamics and hepatic function after partial splenic embolization (PSE) and percutaneous transhepatic obliteration (PTO). *Cancer Chemother Pharmacol* 1994;33:S37–S41.

Murata K, Shiraki K, Takase K, et al. Long term follow up for patients with liver cirrhosis after partial splenic embolization. *Hepatogastroenterology* 1996;43:1212–1217.

Noguchi H, Hirai K, Aoki Y, et al. Changes in platelet kinetics after a partial splenic arterial embolization in cirrhotic patients with hypersplenism. *Hepatology* 1995;22:1682–1688.

Rutledge R. The increasing frequency of nonoperative management of patients with liver and spleen injury. *Adv Surg* 1996;30:385–415.

Sakata K, Hirai K, Tanikawa K. A long term investigation of transcatheter splenic arterial embolization for hypersplenism. *Hepatogastroenterology* 1996;43:309–318.

Sclafani SJA, Shaftan GW, Scalea TM, et al. Nonoperative salvage of computed tomography-diagnosed splenic injuries: utilization of angiography for triage and embolization for hemostasis. *J Trauma* 1989;39:818–825.

Sclafani SJA, Weisberg A, Scalea TM, et al. Blunt splenic injuries: nonsurgical treatment with CT, arteriography, and transcatheter arterial embolization of the splenic artery. *Radiology* 1991;181:189–196.

Spigos DG, Jonasson O, Mozes M, et al. Partial splenic embolization in the treatment of hypersplenism. *AJR* 1979;132:777–782.

Umlas S-L, Cronan JJ. Splenic trauma: can CT grading systems enable prediction of successful nonsurgical treatment. *Radiology* 1991;178:481–487.

CHAPTER 5

Embolization In The Pancreas

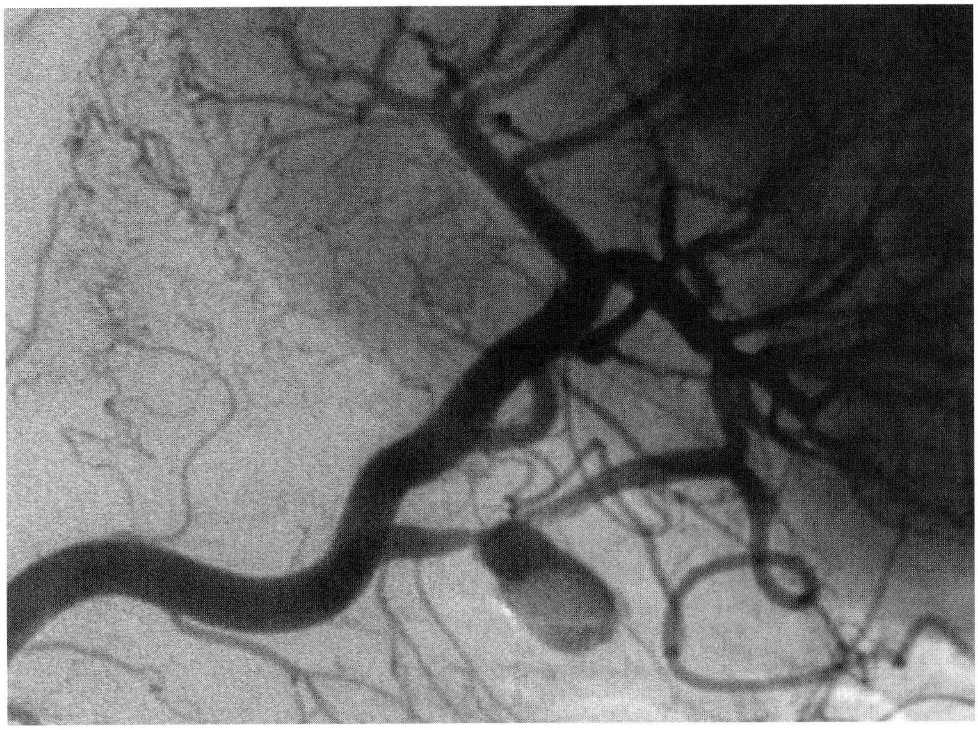

5.1 Embolization In The Pancreas

Case 5.1:

A 54-year-old man with acute pancreatitis developed a pancreatic pseudocyst, which became painful and did not respond to clinical treatment. Drainage guide by computed tomography (CT) was performed, but acute bleeding occurred later.

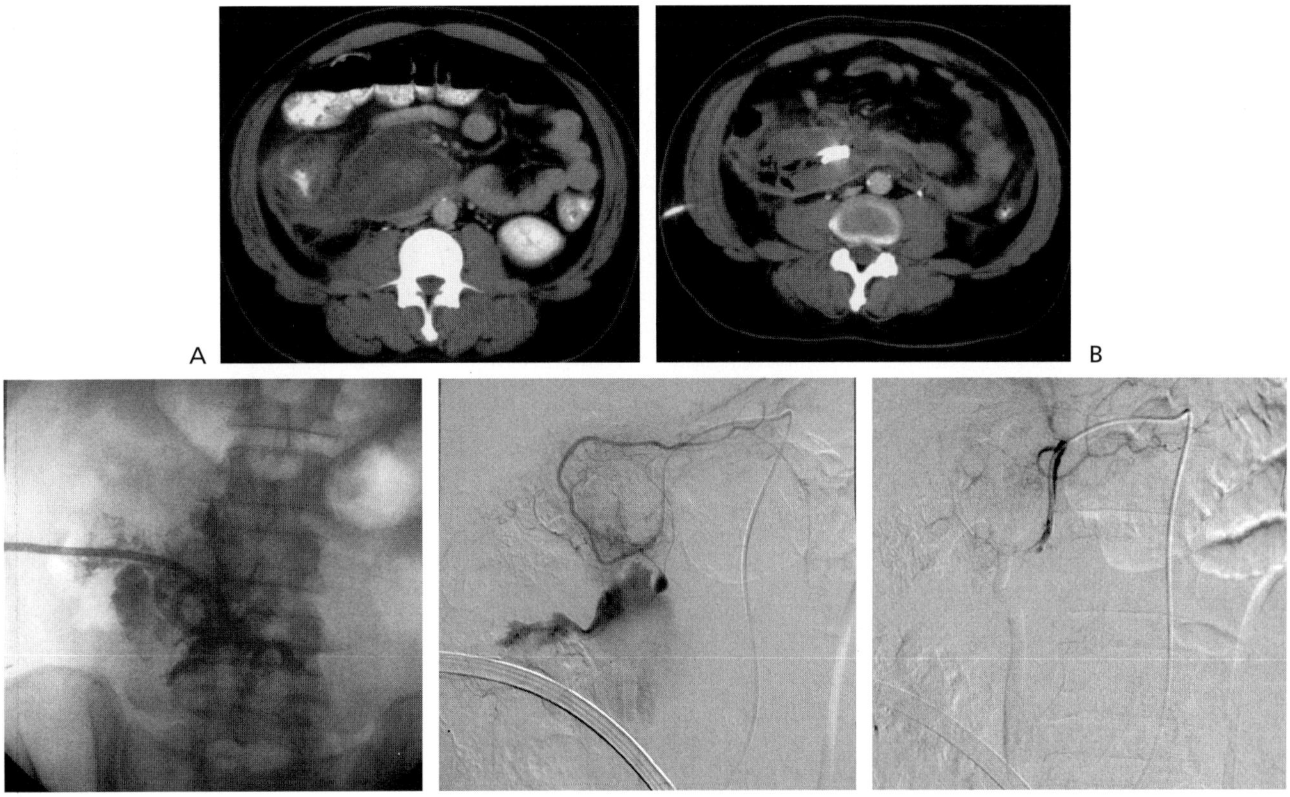

Figure 5.1

A: CT scan shows a large pancreatic pseudocyst with signs of recent bleeding inside. **B:** Two weeks after clinical treatment, there was no resolution of the pseudocyst, and the patient continued to experience pain and discomfort. Drainage with a 12F catheter was performed under CT guidance. **C:** Film of the abdomen after catheter injection shows a highly irregular cavity well drained by the catheter. **D:** Three days after percutaneous drainage, acute bleeding developed, which required emergency arteriogram and embolization. Selective gastroduodenal arteriogram shows a pseudoaneurysm of a pancreaticoduodenal arcade just on the wall of the pseudocyst, with active extravasation of contrast in the cyst lumen. Note the drainage catheter in the lumen of the cyst. **E:** Postembolization angiogram shows complete control of the bleeding with occlusion of the gastroduodenal artery and pseudoaneurysm. Note the microcoils in the lumen of the gastroduodenal artery.

Comment: This case illustrates the complexity of the management of patients with pancreatitis and serious related complications. Pancreatic pseudocysts may develop and regress in a matter of a few weeks, and they may be asymptomatic. However, when the cysts do not regress or the patient develops complications such as infection or bleeding, the lesions may become very symptomatic, cause severe pain, and be life threatening.

Bleeding is one of the most severe complications of pancreatic pseudocysts. When moderate and self limited, bleedings inside pseudocysts may resolve spontaneously. The cyst may follow its natural course, perhaps with an increased possibility of infection. Abrupt enlargement of the pseudocyst caused by intracystic bleeding may cause pain and, in some cases, rupture. Larger, massive acute bleedings inside pseudocysts are life threatening, and blood replacement may be necessary to stabilize patient hemodynamics. Angiography is a safe and reliable technique for diagnosis and treatment of acute pancreatic bleeding.

5.2 Embolization In The Pancreas

Case 5.2:

A 48-year-old man with acute pancreatitis required percutaneous biliary drainage for main common bile duct obstruction. Surgical drainage and scooping of the pancreatic bed had been performed previously. The patient developed pancreatic pseudocysts, recurrent gastrointestinal (GI) bleeding, and abdominal pain. Emergency CT and angiography were performed.

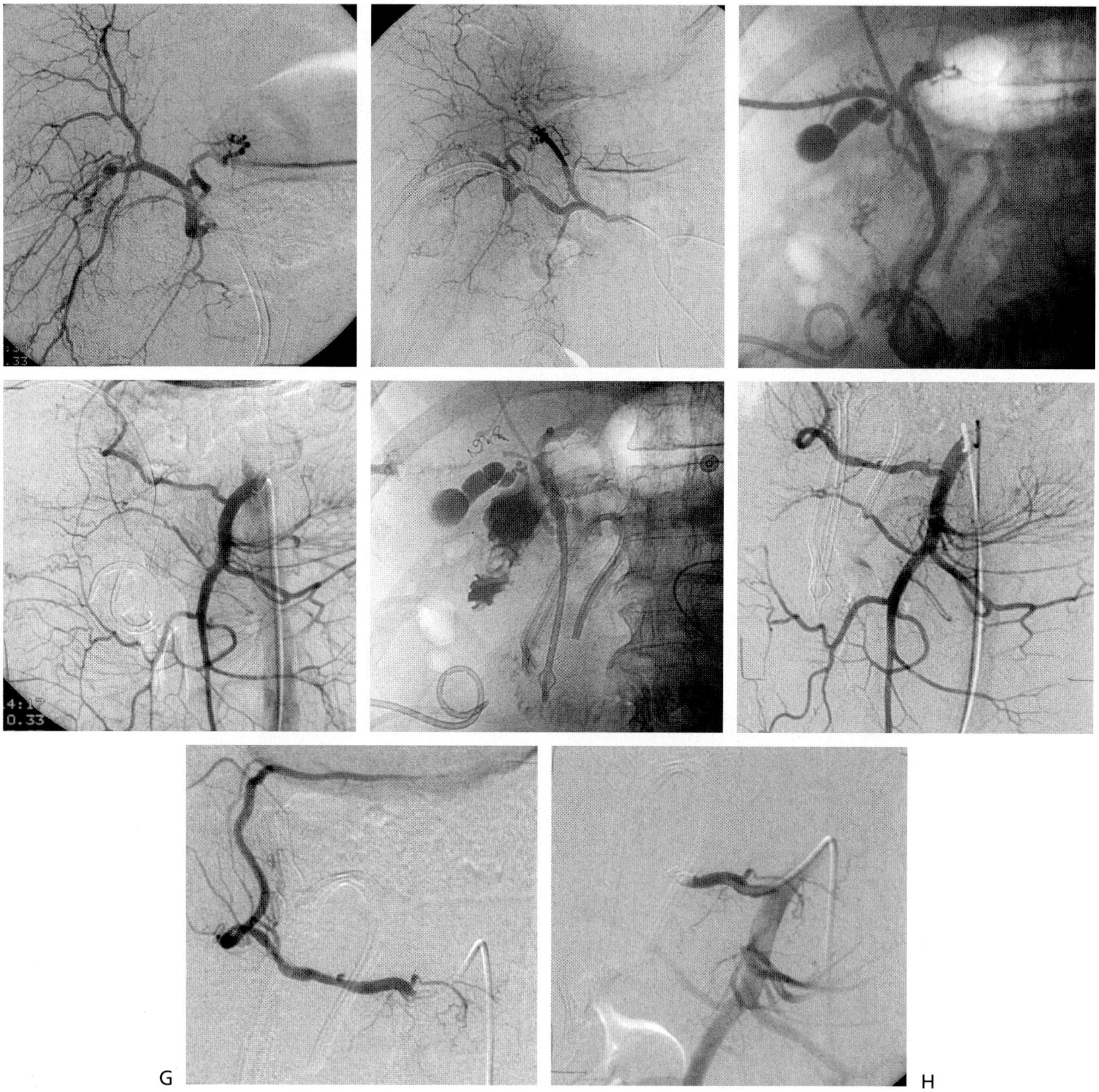

A, B C D, E F G H

Figure 5.2

A: Initial angiogram shows a pseudoaneurysm in a branch of the right hepatic artery, related to the biliary drainage. **B:** Transcatheter coil embolization was used to occlude the pseudoaneurysm. **C:** Cholangiogram through the catheter shows improvement of biliary drainage and the coils in the hepatic artery branch. Note the percutaneous drainage and the surgical drain around the duodenum. **D:** Superior mesenteric artery (SMA) angiogram at this time did not show any abnormalities. **E:** An internal biliary stent was placed for internal drainage. **F:** Twelve days after the first embolization, a new episode of GI bleeding developed. Celiac arteriogram shows no abnormalities, except for the embolized hepatic artery. Injection at the SMA shows a small pseudoaneurysm in the inferior pancreatic artery just at the edge of one of the surgical drains. **G:** Superselective injection in the inferior pancreatic artery shows the lesion was larger than previously thought and the artery provided access for treatment. **H:** Embolization performed with three microcoils beyond and before the pseudoaneurysm resulted in total occlusion of the lesion. Permanent control of the bleeding was achieved. Biliary drainage was maintained for several weeks, and eventually the stent was endoscopically removed.

Comment: Visceral artery aneurysms occur in up to 10% of patients with pancreatitis, most commonly in the region of the splenic artery and less frequently in the pancreatic head region. When complicated by bleeding, the mortality rate is high and therapeutic intervention is necessary. Surgical ligation of the bleeding pseudoaneurysm has been the usual treatment. However, some of the involved arteries are located very deep in the inflamed pancreatic tissues, and surgical exposure of the vessel for ligation may be impossible. Due to the relatively easy reach capability of the angiographic catheter, visceral peripancreatic pseudoaneurysms can be treated safely.

Rupture of visceral artery pseudoaneurysms occurs in about 50% of the cases, causing bleeding into the gastrointestinal tract, retroperitoneal space, pseudocyst, pancreatic duct, or peritoneal cavity. Often, however, bleeding occurs as self-limited brisk episodes, which may represent vessel rupture with rapid bleeding stopped by thrombus formation and temporary hemostasis. Subsequent lysis may cause further episodic hemorrhages that may recur over days, weeks, or months. Embolization is a safe and reliable treatment for pancreatic-related bleedings.

5.3 Embolization In The Pancreas

Case 5.3:

A 67-year-old man with alcoholic necrotizing pancreatitis developed a retroperitoneal pseudocyst with a pseudoaneurysm in the vicinity of the pancreatic head, visualized on CT scan. He was transferred to our institution for treatment. Clinical evidence of bleeding was present for several days, and the patient's health was progressively deteriorating. Arteriography was requested for possible embolization.

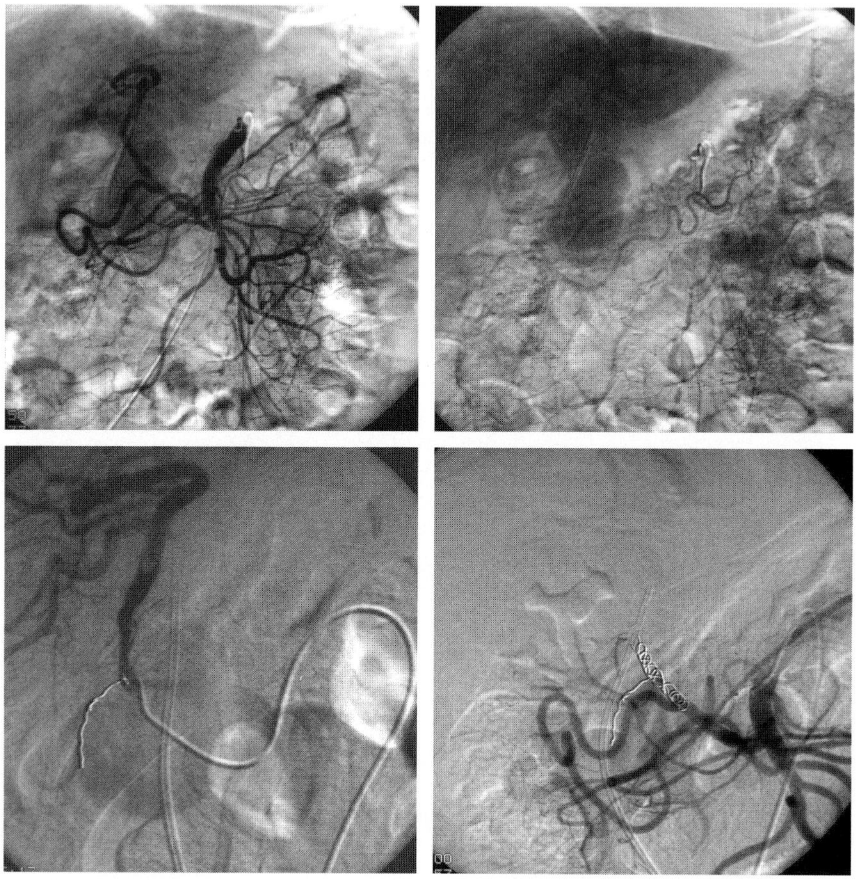

A B C D

Figure 5.3

A: Superior mesenteric artery angiogram shows a large pseudoaneurysm filling with contrast medium during the arterial phase of the angiogram. **B:** Late-phase angiogram shows the large pseudoaneurysm just behind the replaced right hepatic artery but no evidence of arterial opening. The communication with the pseudoaneurysm was not visualized, even during superselective injections of the gastroduodenal artery or replaced hepatic artery. The patient continued to bleed, and a new arteriogram was performed 2 days after the first procedure. **C:** During the second arteriogram, the gastroduodenal artery was prophylactically embolized, and only then was the jet into the pseudoaneurysm visualized coming out of the replaced right hepatic artery. **D:** Embolization of the replaced hepatic artery with microcoils located beyond and before the level of the pseudoaneurysm permanently occluded the lesion and controlled the bleeding. Bleeding was permanently controlled, and eventually the patient recovered and was discharged.

Comment: Pancreatic enzymes released by recurrent or persistent pancreatic inflammation weakens the walls of the peripancreatic vasculature. Angiographically, the vessel wall lesion may appear as an aneurysmatic dilation or as a free extravasation or perforation with a jet into the cavity of the pseudocyst (or pseudoaneurysm). In selected cases, during brisk bleeding, angiography may show extravasation into the bowel lumen. Conventional treatment has been surgery with arterial ligation, but even more radical duodenopancreatectomy procedures may became necessary. Vasopressin infusion may reduce or stop the bleeding, but the effect will not last. Embolotherapy with nonabsorbable particles is the current indicated treatment. Embolization of the splenic artery initially raised concerns of splenic infarction and abscess formation, but more recent cases proved that this is not a cause for major concern. Temporary balloon occlusion of the hepatic artery may be used to control splenic artery/vein flow when the bleeding is related to splenic vein occlusion or rupture. Balloon control of splenic flow also can be utilized in preparation for splenectomy to control left-sided portal hypertension secondary to portal vein thrombosis, which would significantly reduce perioperative bleeding.

Accordingly to a recent published series of 180 patients, arterial complications may occur in about 7% of patients with pancreatic pseudocysts. The clinical presentation of bleeding was variable, and sudden onset of abdominal pain was the most frequent symptom. Upper GI bleeding and signs suggesting hypovolemia were observed less frequently. In that series, the most useful diagnostic technique for diagnosis of the bleeding lesion was CT scan and angiography. In cases reported after 1980, embolization was the most successful technique used, whereas surgery was the most frequently used treatment in previous years.

5.4 Embolization In The Pancreas

Case 5.4:

A 55-year-old male patient developed acute duodenal bleeding due to alcohol abuse and pancreatitis.

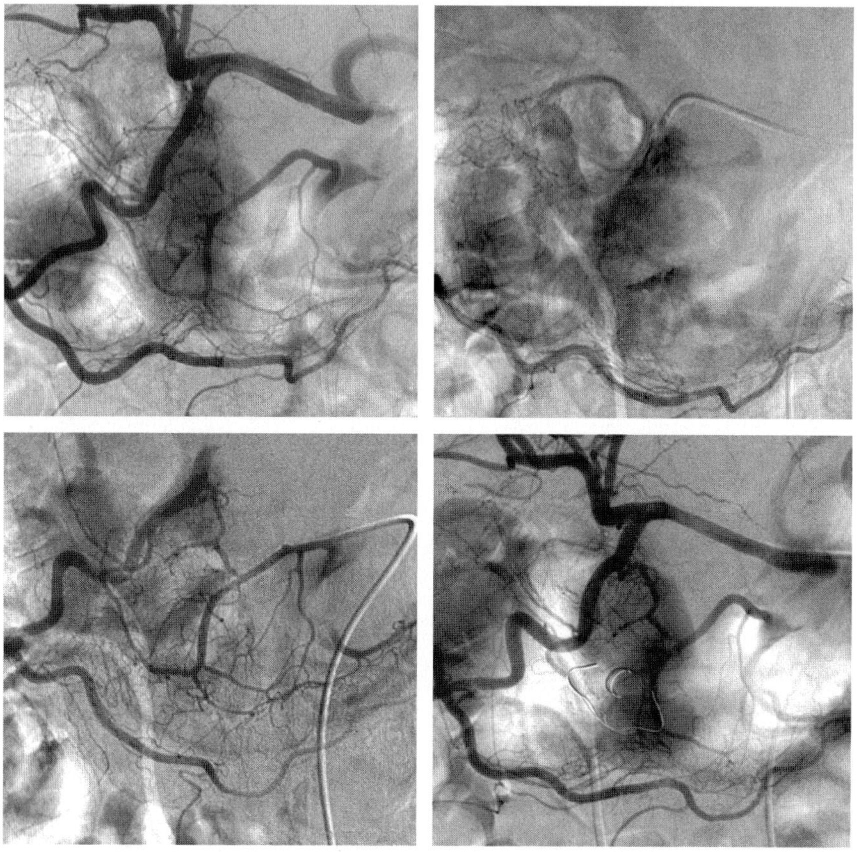

Figure 5.4

A: Selective gastroduodenal artery angiogram shows an area of active bleeding originating from a small pseudoaneurysm of the posterosuperior pancreaticoduodenal arcade. Note filling of the inferior pancreatic artery. **B:** Late-phase angiogram shows active bleeding spreading inside a "cavity" delineated by the bowing of the surrounding arteries. **C:** Injection into the inferior pancreatic artery did not show the bleeding. **D:** Postembolization angiogram with the microcoils placed in branches of the anterior and posterior pancreaticoduodenal arcades shows complete cessation of the bleeding. Permanent control of the bleeding was achieved.

Comment: Because the cause of pancreatitis is alcohol related in the majority of patients, other sources of bleeding may be encountered. Angiography in association with endoscopy is the best way to differentiate among the several possible etiologies of bleeding. Prompt diagnosis of pancreatic pseudoaneurysm remains a challenge, and bleeding related to cirrhosis may lead to a faulty diagnosis. Chronic bleeding due to pancreatic inflammation also is difficult to recognize because of the subtle presentation. Very small pseudoaneurysms remain a special problem, because their size is beyond the spatial resolution of noninvasive imaging. In these circumstances, angiography is the only diagnostic tool capable of determining the source of bleeding. Many authors reported the reliability of embolization for treatment of the arterial complications of pancreatitis. Pseudoaneurysms associated with pseudocysts are more difficult to treat surgically. Transcatheter embolization has proved to be effective and reliable in both elective and emergency treatment of arterial complications of pancreatitis, such as simple pseudoaneurysms, regardless of the location.

5.5 Embolization In The Pancreas

Case 5.5:

A 33-year-old man with acute pancreatitis developed pancreatic pseudocysts, recurrent GI bleeding, and abdominal pain. Emergency CT and angiography were performed.

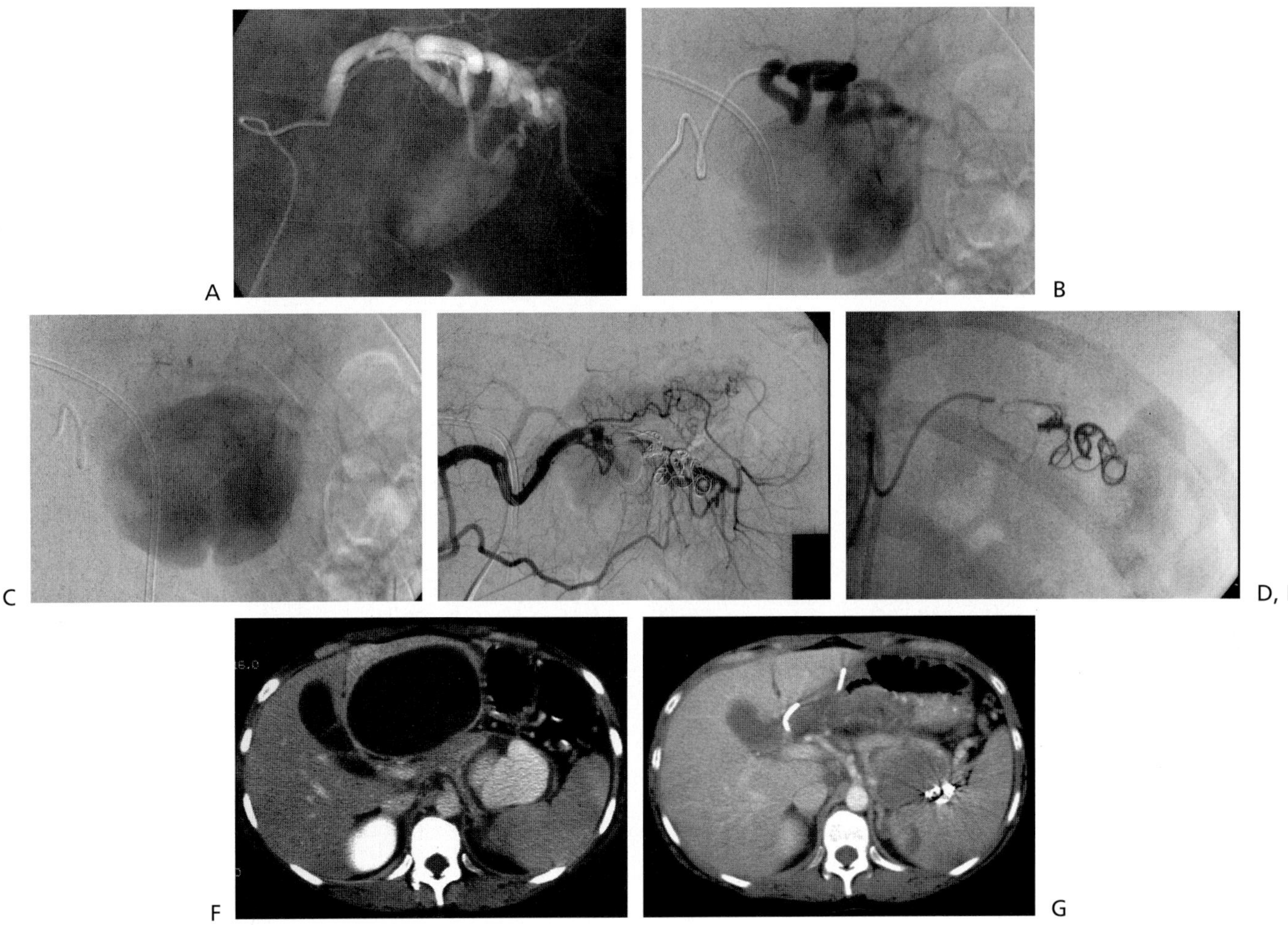

Figure 5.5

A: Selective splenic arteriogram shows a perforation in the distal artery, close to the splenic hilus, and a large pseudoaneurysm. Note the jet of contrast in the pseudoaneurysm. **B,C:** Later-phase angiogram shows filling of the pseudoaneurysm, with septate lumen. **D:** Embolization with microcoils resulted in total occlusion of the splenic artery and mouth of the pseudoaneurysm. **E:** Coils are seen inside the splenic artery and the microcatheter delivering the coils is still in place. Superselective catheterization was facilitated by the microcatheter. **F:** CT scan before treatment shows a large pancreatic pseudocyst and the massive pseudoaneurysm enhanced by contrast medium in front of the pancreatic tail. CT-guided drainage of the pseudocyst was performed at that time. **G:** Follow-up CT scan shows total occlusion of the pseudoaneurysm by the coils (high-density metal at the posterior wall of the pseudoaneurysm) and resolution of the pseudocyst drained using a 10F catheter.

Comment: Bleeding caused by pancreatitis is related to digestion of the arterial wall by pancreatic juices. Intimate contact of the pseudocyst with the artery may cause acute rupture of the artery. Bleeding may be massive and may be directly in the pancreatic duct, inside the peritoneal cavity, into a pancreatic pseudocyst, or less frequently in the bowel lumen. In general, the pseudoaneurysm ruptures in the posterior wall, inside a pseudocyst. In general, surgical treatment of this condition is difficult. In some cases it is impossible to locate the source of the bleeding. A less invasive treatment is advisable, as demonstrated in this case. Control of bleeding is immediate and, in most cases, definitive.

5.6 Embolization In The Pancreas

Case 5.6:

A 35-year-old male patient with pancreatitis presented with chronic GI bleeding for 2 months and developed acute upper GI bleeding that required 15 units of blood replacement.

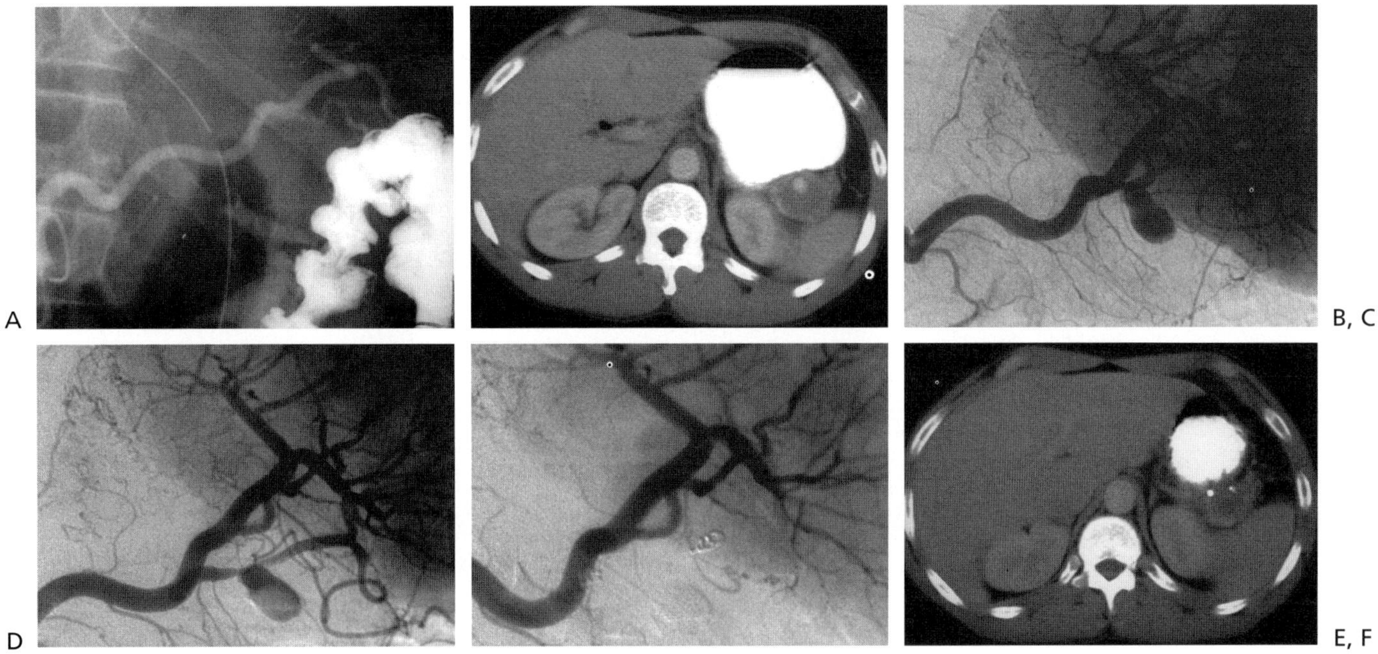

Figure 5.6

A: Celiac arteriogram during the previous investigation for recurrent GI bleeding did not show abnormalities of the arterial system. **B:** Two months later, CT scan performed at the time of acute bleeding shows a pseudoaneurysm in the region of the pancreatic tail. Note the enhanced lumen of the lesion. **C:** Anteroposterior view of the splenic artery angiogram shows a pseudoaneurysm that seems to arise from the splenic artery. **D:** Oblique view of the splenic artery shows the lesion is related to the left gastroepiploic artery and does not arise from the main splenic artery, as initially thought. **E:** After selective catheterization of the gastroepiploic artery beyond and before the level of the pseudoaneurysm, coil embolization resulted in total occlusion of the lesion. Note the coils, which are visible close to the splenic artery. The splenic vein was patent (not shown). **F:** Follow-up CT scan 14 days after embolization and control of the bleeding shows reduction in pseudoaneurysm size and absence of enhancement in the lumen. The patient was discharged shortly afterward.

Comment: Embolization of peripancreatic arteries is a safe and effective procedure. It has a success rate of approximately 80% and compares favorably with surgery. Steel coils are preferred to achieve permanent arterial occlusion, but smaller pseudoaneurysms can be treated effectively with gelatin sponge. The risk of rupturing the pseudoaneurysm during embolization with high-pressure injectable material must be borne in mind. Coils are delivered through low-pressure systems, whereas Gelfoam is delivered through a high-pressure system by injection using a syringe. The newer microcoils are delivered through microcatheters either by flushing with a syringe (generating pressure) or with a metallic pusher (without significant increase in pressure). In pancreatic embolization, the pusher technique is preferred to reduce the pressure during coil delivery. When rupture of the pseudoaneurysm results from embolization, continuing with embolization can stop the bleeding in most cases.

Recurrence of hemorrhage after embolization is seen occasionally and usually is related to incomplete arterial blockage, feeding arteries, or development of collaterals that feed a branch related to the lumen of the artery involved in the pseudoaneurysm.

5.7 Embolization In The Pancreas

Case 5.7:

A 47-year-old male patient with chronic pancreatitis, chronic pain, and recurrent pseudocyst formation was treated with a Whipple procedure (choledochojejunostomy). Twenty-seven days after surgery, the patient developed acute massive bleeding from the gastroduodenal artery stump.

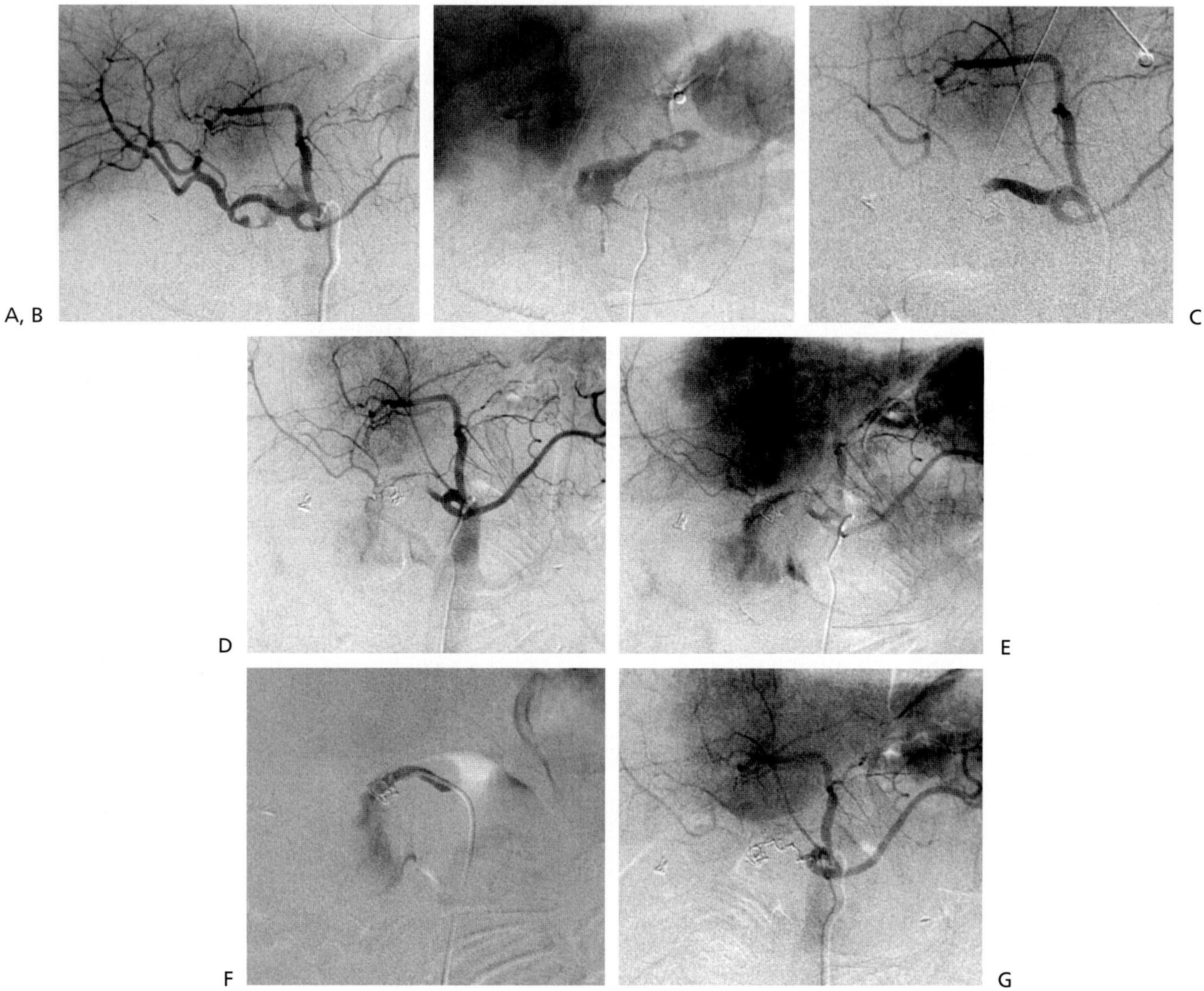

Figure 5.7

A: Selective celiac artery angiogram shows massive bleeding from the gastroduodenal artery stump. **B:** Late-phase angiogram shows contrast medium spread around the bowel anastomosis. **C:** Embolization of the gastroduodenal stump was performed with coils, and immediate control of the bleeding was achieved. Note that the hepatic artery was occluded proximally, with reconstitution of the intrahepatic segment. **D,E:** Four days after the embolization, bleeding recurred and a new arteriogram was performed. Celiac injection demonstrated occlusion of the hepatic artery and distal reconstitution with active bleeding from the gastroduodenal stump, best seen on the late-phase angiogram **(E)**. **F:** Selective injection in the gastroduodenal artery stump shows active bleeding. **G:** New embolization was performed with a couple more coils and pieces of Gelfoam, and total occlusion with permanent control of the bleeding was achieved.

Comment: Surgery frequently is performed to treat chronic recurrent pain in patients with chronic pancreatitis for decompression of the pancreatic duct or resection of the diseased pancreas. Sphincteroplasty, which is used infrequently today, is effective when the sphincter of Oddi is the only point of obstruction. Caudal pancreaticojejunostomy (Du Val procedure) may be performed when there is a single point of obstruction in the middle of the pancreas with distal duct dilation and when only the distal segment needs to be removed or decompressed. Longitudinal pancreaticojejunostomy (Puestow procedure) is performed when the pancreatic duct has alternating segments of narrowing and dilation, also known as "chain of lakes appearance." In this situation, the Puestow procedure is the most effective drainage method. The entire main pancreatic duct is opened longitudinally and the stones are extracted. A defunctionalized jejunal segment is opened and sewn over the opened duct. The drainage procedure relieves pain in 75% of cases. Pancreatectomy of 95% of the pancreas with preservation of a small rim of tissue near the duodenum is the most commonly used resection procedure. Total pancreatectomy and pancreaticoduodenectomy (Whipple procedure) are performed less frequently because of their greater morbidity and mortality. Relief of pain with resection is achieved in about 80% of cases.

One of the complications of the Whipple procedure is bleeding from the gastroduodenal stump or other paraduodenal artery. Reoperation carries a high morbidity/mortality risk, and noninvasive procedures such as embolization are the preferred means of treatment. Although recurrence of bleeding may occur, it is possible, as demonstrated in the reported case, to reintervene and control the bleeding.

5.8 Embolization In The Pancreas

Case 5.8:

A 35-year-old man with pancreatitis due to obstruction of the ampulla and factor VIII deficiency hemophilia developed upper GI bleeding after endoscopic papillotomy. His status became unstable, despite blood replacement.

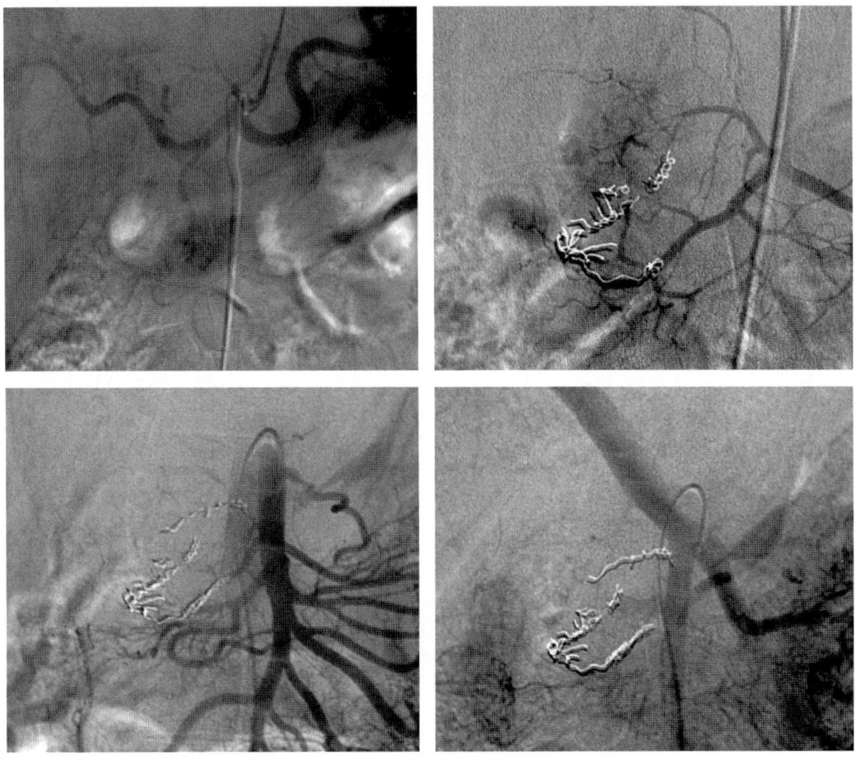

A B C D

Figure 5.8

A: Selective celiac arteriogram demonstrates active bleeding in the duodenum. **B:** Inferior pancreatic artery injection, at a branch of the SMA, after partial embolization still shows a small area of extravasation of contrast originating from a more proximal arterial branch. **C:** Follow-up angiogram with injection at the main SMA shows control of the bleeding. **D:** Late-phase angiogram shows the portal vein has no active bleeding. Note the small amount of residual contrast in the duodenum.

Comment: Although related to pancreatitis, the cause of bleeding in this patient was not vessel wall digestion. Papillotomy damaged an artery, a branch of the gastroduodenal artery, at the cranial aspect of the papilla; coagulopathy created the conditions for bleeding. Embolization in this case had to be superselective, but due to the diffuse arterial spasm a single vessel source of the bleeding could not be identified at once. Embolization of the gastroduodenal artery and branches was not effective. Only catheterization of the branch originating from the inferior pancreatic artery allowed control of the bleeding. Minicoils were used in this case, but Gelfoam pledgets probably would have been as useful.

5.9 Embolization In The Pancreas

Case 5.9:

A 50-year-old woman presented with chronic pancreatitis, pain, and pancreatic duct obstruction. A longitudinal pancreaticojejunostomy (Puestow procedure) was performed to drain the pancreatic duct. Acute bleeding occurred 2 weeks after surgery.

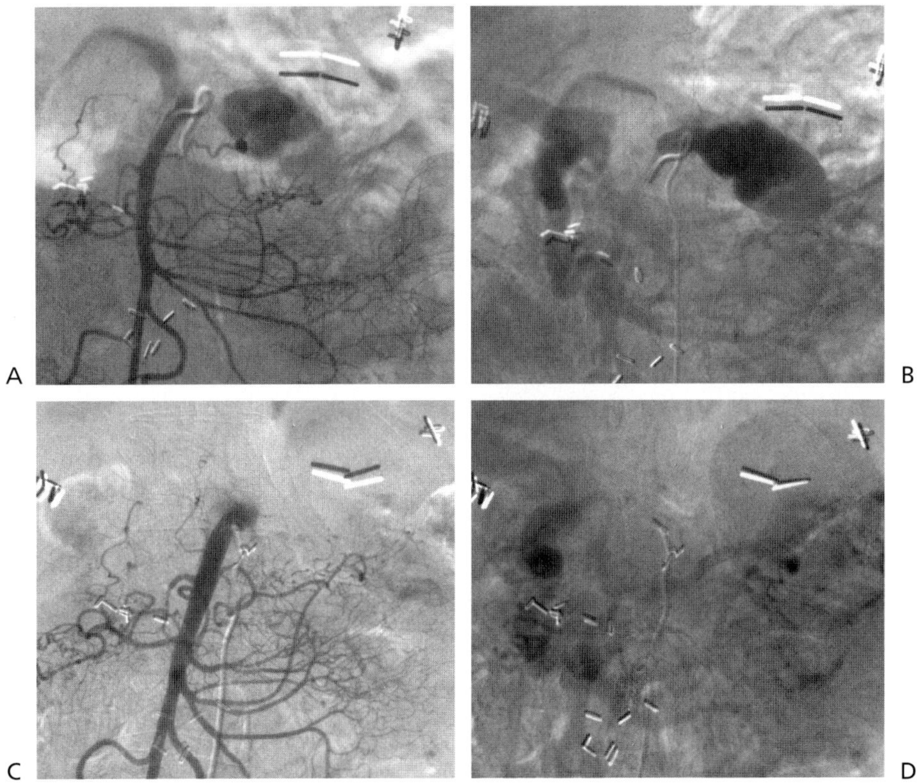

Figure 5.9

A: Selective SMA arteriogram shows a small pseudoaneurysm in a proximal jejunal artery branch. Note large active contrast extravasation originating from the pseudoaneurysm into the bowel lumen. **B:** Late-phase SMA angiogram shows the large extravasation of contrast into the bowel lumen and occlusion of the superior mesenteric vein. Note the collateral circulation bypassing the obstruction of the superior mesenteric vein. **C:** Embolization of the first jejunal artery performed with one minicoil delivered via a microcatheter resulted in immediate control of the bleeding. **D:** Postembolization late-phase angiogram shows control of the bleeding and occlusion of the superior mesenteric vein. The splenic vein also is occluded.

Comment: Surgical drainage procedures relieve pain in 75% of cases when properly selected. Morbidity and mortality are low, but bleeding at the anastomosis and dehiscence of the suture may be encountered. The bowel wall and vessels are in close contact with the pancreatic juice and enzymes, and vessel wall digestion is a very real possibility. The development of pseudoaneurysms in the bowel vessels may cause massive bleeding. Superselective embolization, as performed in this case, allows for precise and safe embolization of the small bowel artery related to the bleeding. No ischemia is expected when only the artery involved in the bleeding is embolized. The patient must be monitored carefully following embolization. In cases of pancreatitis-related pseudoaneurysms, vasopressin infusion is not effective but may reduce the bleeding rate. Embolization following vasoconstrictor infusion is not advisable, because it can cause ischemia of the bowel wall and perforation.

5.10 Embolization In The Pancreas

Case 5.10:

A 70-year-old man with acute pancreatitis, pain, and active bleeding was referred for angiography and possible embolization. No cause for the bout of pancreatitis was identified.

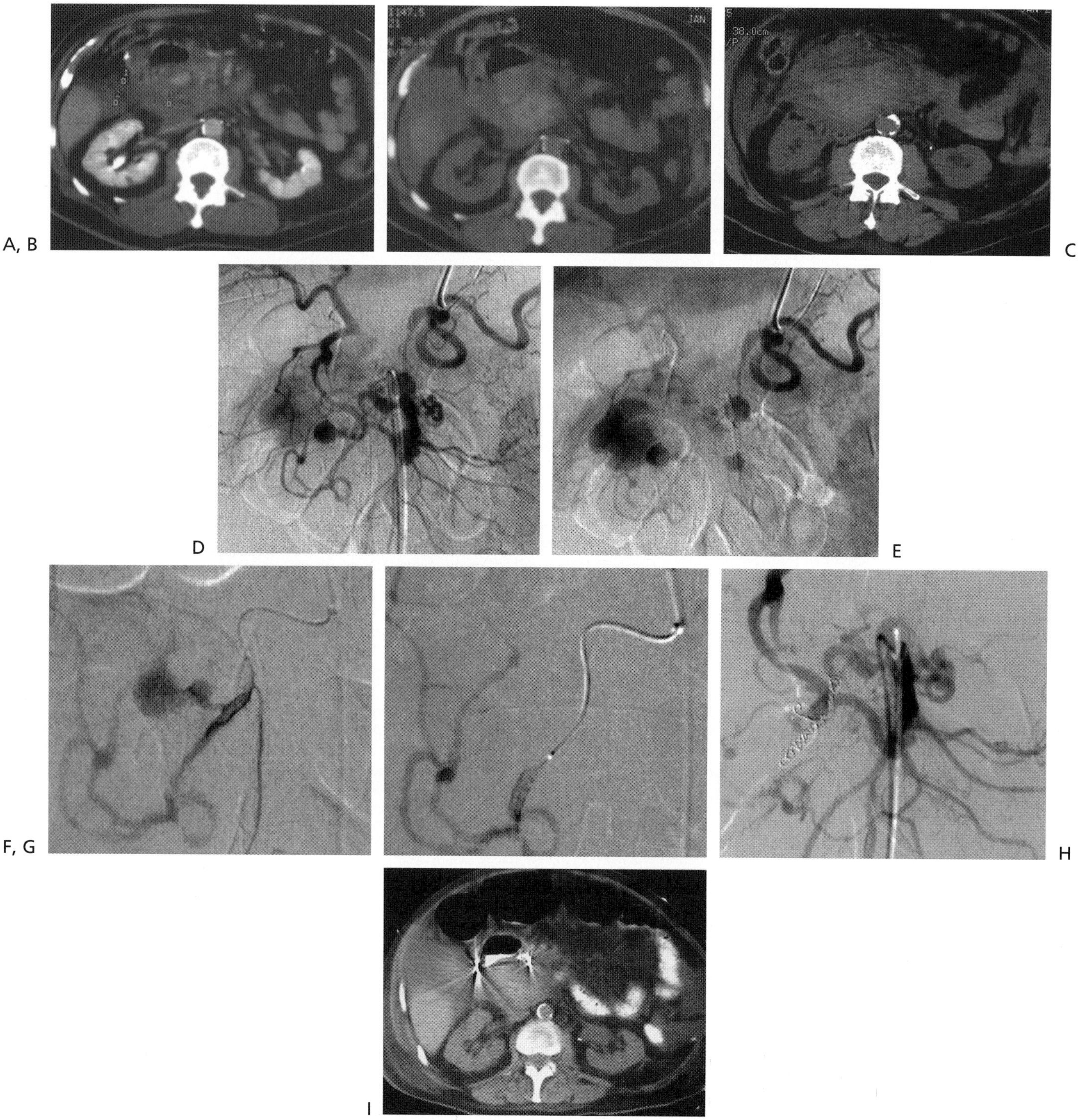

Figure 5.10

A: CT scan of the pancreas shows changes consistent with pancreatitis and a retroperitoneal hematoma, with signs of recent bleeding. **B,C:** Follow-up CT scan 3 days after the initial CT scan, with clinical indications of active bleeding, shows signs of hematoma expansion and active bleeding. **D:** SMA arteriogram shows dilation of the proximal SMA and spasm of the distal artery. At least three round pseudoaneurysms and focal dilation of the proximal inferior pancreatic artery were identified. One of the pseudoaneurysms was bleeding actively at the time of angiography, as demonstrated by massive extravasation of contrast medium. Note filling of the hepatic and splenic arteries due to stenosis of the celiac artery. **E:** Late-phase angiogram shows persistent filling of the round pseudoaneurysm from the inferior pancreatic artery and a large amount of extravasated contrast. **F,G:** A microcatheter was used to selectively catheterize the inferior pancreatic artery. An injection was performed before and beyond the level of the pseudoaneurysm. Embolization with ten 3-mm × 3-cm microcoils was performed to occlude the parent vessels and the pseudoaneurysm. **H:** Postembolization angiogram shows total occlusion of the artery and pseudoaneurysm, with permanent control of the bleeding. **I:** Follow-up CT scan at 5 days shows actual reduction in size of the lesion and the coils. Follow-up at 25 days shows the lesion is stable. In the interim, the patient underwent surgery for treatment of pseudocysts and was septic at the time of follow-up CT scan. The patient remained in the hospital for the following 2 months.

Comment: Severe damage to the pancreas and surrounding structures can result from necrotizing pancreatitis. In this case, the SMA and main branches were affected, and massive bleeding developed. This is a high-risk lesion; the prognosis of the disease is very reserved and low survival is anticipated due to the very high morbidity and mortality. The development of several pseudoaneurysms is unusual and, due to their location, it was not possible to embolize all of them. A decision was made to embolize only the complicated lesion and to observe the evolving disease. The patient eventually was discharged 3 months after initial embolization.

5.11 Embolization In The Pancreas

Case 5.11:

A 49-year-old man who was admitted for severe hypoglycemia had a 1-year history of fainting episodes, consistent with an insulinoma in the pancreas. While in the hospital for workup, the patient developed uncorrectable hypoglycemia, with glucose levels as low as 17 mg/dL despite intravenous administration of 50% glucose solution. Emergency arteriography and embolization of the tumor were requested, because the patient refused surgery and the condition was life threatening.

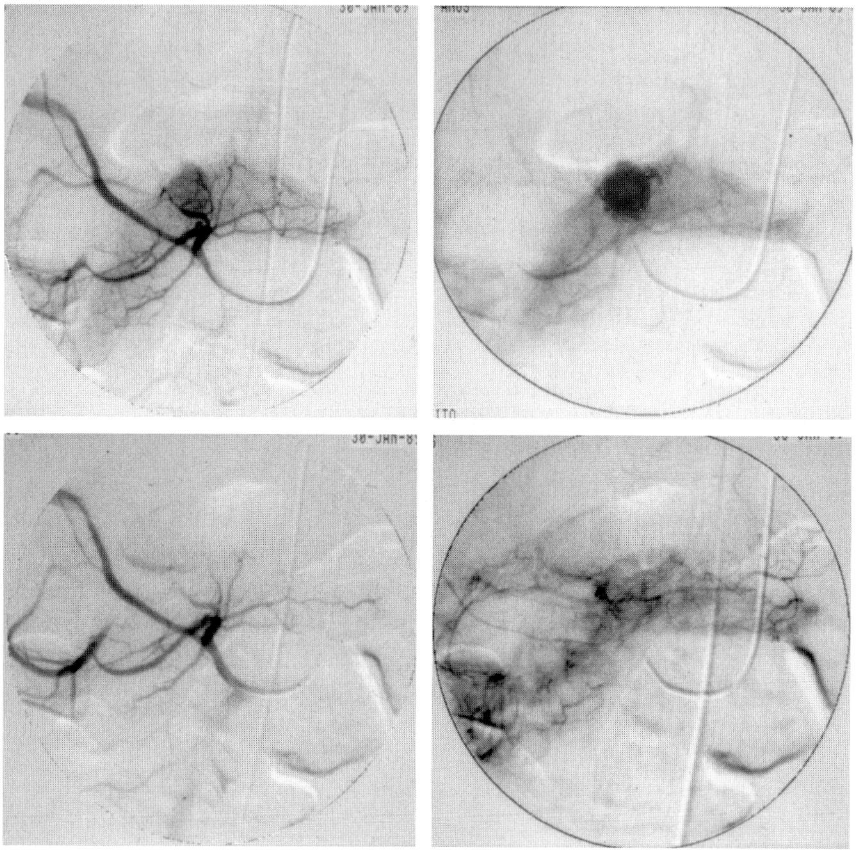

A B C D

Figure 5.11

A: Selective angiogram of the dorsal pancreatic artery arising from the superior mesenteric artery with a 5F Cobra catheter in a Waltman loop configuration was performed. Note the tumor blush at the early arterial phase. **B:** Late arterial phase shows dense tumor staining of the insulinoma in the body of the pancreas. **C:** After embolization with polyvinyl alcohol particles (150 to 300 μm), the lesion was devascularized. **D:** Late arterial phase shows no tumor staining. The patient has been free of symptoms for more than 5 years.

Comment: Therapeutic embolization is a standard method for palliative treatment of malignant tumors, particularly hormone-producing endocrine tumors, in selected patients. In some cases, the tumor responds by reducing in size, which then allows surgical resection. Although the liver has been the most common target for palliative embolization, other organs with endocrine tumors also benefit from the technique. Insulinomas are relatively rare benign pancreatic tumors, and the diagnosis is still a challenge, requiring several imaging modalities for adequate localization and diagnosis. There are only a few reports of insulinomas treated by embolization. Small particles should be used to shut down insulinoma circulation, which may cause pancreatitis, while avoiding nontarget vessels, as described in the literature. Surgical enucleation and partial pancreatic resection have been the traditional and time-honored treatments for insulinomas in the pancreas; recurrence is about 8% at 20 years. Embolization of insulinomas has been used in only a few cases but has proved to be effective in mid- to long-term follow-up, with control of hypoglycemia. Transcatheter embolization proved to be a lifesaver for this patient. However, embolization should be limited to patients who are poor candidates for surgery or who refuse surgery entirely.

Suggested Reading

Abbott G, McDermott V, Smith TP. Successful endovascular treatment of a celiac artery pseudoaneurysm complicating pancreatitis. *J Vasc Interv Radiol* 1996;7:103–106.

Adams DB, Mauterer Dj, Vujic I, et al. Preoperative control of splenic artery inflow in patients with pancreatitis and splenic vein thrombosis. *South Med J* 1984;77:390–394.

Adams DB, Zellner JL, Anderson MC. Arterial hemorrhage complicating pancreatic pseudocysts: role of angiography. *J Surg Res* 1993;54:150–156.

Agarwal P, Phadke RV, Baijal SS, et al. Calcific pancreatic-induced gastroduodenal artery pseudoaneurysms: non-surgical management. *Pediatr Radiol* 1994;24:539–540.

Boudghène F, L'Hermine C, Bigot JM. Arterial complications of pancreatitis: diagnostic and therapeutic aspects in 104 cases. *J Vasc Interv Radiol* 1993;4:551–558.

Bretagne JF, Heresbach D, Darnault P, et al. Pseudoaneurysms and bleeding pseudocysts in chronic pancreatitis: radiological findings and contribution to diagnosis in 8 cases. *Gastrointest Radiol* 1990;15:916–918.

Cahow CE, Gusberg RJ, Gottlieb LJ. Gastrointestinal hemorrhage from pseudoaneurysms in pancreatic pseudocysts. *Am J Surg* 1983;145:534–540.

Capek P, Rocco M, McGahan J, et al. Direct aneurysm puncture and coil occlusion: a new approach to peripancreatic arterial pseudoaneurysms. *J Vasc Interv Radiol* 1992;3:653–656.

De Filippi VJ, Vargish T, Block GE. Massive gastrointestinal hemorrhage in pancreatitis secondary to visceral artery aneurysms. *Am Surg* 1992;58:618–621.

Golzarian J, Braude P, Bank WO, et al. Case report: color Doppler demonstration of pseudoaneurysms complicating pancreatic pseudocysts. *Br J Radiol* 1994;67:91–93.

Golzarian J, Nicaise N, Devière, et al. Transcatheter embolization of pseudoaneurysms complicating pancreatitis. *Cardiovasc Intervent Radiol* 1997;20:435–440.

Heathon DI, Reid AW, Murray WR. Bleeding pseudocysts and pseudoaneurysms in chronic pancreatitis. *Br J Surg* 1992;79:281–284.

Knight RW, Kadir S, White RI. Embolization of bleeding trans verse pancreatic artery aneurysms. *Cardiov Invervent Radiol* 1982;5:37–39.

Lina JR, Jaques P, Mandell V. Aneurysm rupture secondary to transcatheter embolization. *AJR* 1979;132:553–556.

Lossing AG, Grosman H, Mustard RA, et al. Emergency embolization of a ruptured aneurysm of the pancreaticoduodenal arcade. *Can J Surg* 1995;38:363–365.

Mandel SR, Jaques PF, Sanofsky S, et al. Nonoperative management of peripancreatic arterial aneurysms. *Ann Surg* 1987;205:126–128.

Mauro MA, Jaques P. Transcatheter management of pseudoaneurysms complicating pancreatitis. *J Vasc Interv Radiol* 1991;2:527–532.

Modlin IM, Lewis JJ, Ahlman H, et al. Management of unresectable malignant endocrine tumors of the pancreas. *Surg Gynecol Obstet* 1993;176:507–518.

Morita R, Muto N, Konagaya M, et al. Successful transcatheter embolization of pseudoaneurysm associated with pancreatic pseudocyst. *Am J Gastroenterol* 1991;86:1264–1267.

Salam TA, Lumsden AB, Martin LG, et al. Nonoperative management of visceral aneurysms and pseudoaneurysms. *Am J Surg* 1992;164:215–219.

Sand JA, Seppanen SK, Nordback IH. Intracystic hemorrhage in pancreatic pseudocysts: initial experiences of a treatment protocol. *Pancreas* 1997;14:187–191.

Steckman ML, Doodley MC, Jaques PF, et al. Major gastrointestinal hemorrhage from peripancreatic blood vessels in pancreatitis. Treatment by embolotherapy. *Dig Dis Sci* 1984;29:486–497.

Suter M, Doenz F, Chapuis G, et al. Haemorrhage into the pancreatic duct (Hemosuccus pancreaticus): recognition and management. *Eur J Surg* 1995;161:887–892.

Uflacker R, Diehl JC. Successful embolization of a bleeding splenic artery pseudoaneurysm secondary to necrotizing pancreatitis. *Gastrointest Radiol* 1982;7:379–382.

Uflacker R. Arterial embolization as definitive treatment for benign insulinoma of the pancreas. *J Vasc Interv Radiol* 1992;3:639-644; discussion 644–646.

Uflacker R. Interventional management of visceral arterial aneurysms. In: Strandness DE, Van Breda A, eds. *Vascular diseases: surgical and interventional therapy.* New York: Churchill Livingstone, 1994: 823–844.

Valette PJ, Souquet JC, Chayvialle JA. Arterial chemoinfusion and embolization of iliac metastasis from pancreatic islet cell carcinoma. *AJR* 1989;153:13–18.

Vujic I, Andersen BL, Stanley JH, et al. Pancreatic and peripancreatic vessels: embolization for control of bleeding in pancreatitis. *Radiology* 1984;150:51–55.

Vujic I, Anderson MC, Meredith HC, et al. Successful embolization of the dorsal pancreatic artery to control massive upper gastrointestinal hemorrhage. *Am Surg* 1980;46:184–186.

Vujic I. Vascular complications of pancreatitis. *Radiol Clin North Am* 1989;27:81–91.

Wagner WH, Cossman DV, Treiman RL, et al. Hemosuccus pancreaticus for intraductal rupture of a primary splenic artery aneurysm. *J Vasc Surg* 1994;19:158–164.

Waltman AC, Luers PR, Athanasoulis CA, et al. Massive arterial hemorrhage in patients with pancreatitis. *Arch Surg* 1986;121:439–443.

Winick AB, Malloy PC, Lund GB. Retained contrast after embolization of a right gastric artery pseudoaneurysm. *Cardiovasc Intervent Radiol* 1996;19:110–112.

Woods MS, Traverso LW, Kozarek RA, et al. Successful treatment of bleeding pseudoaneurysms of chronic pancreatitis. *Pancreas* 1995;10:22–30.

Yamagishi S, Yamashita H, Sasaki M, et al. Control of a massive bleeding of a pancreatic pseudoaneurysm penetrating into the colon by transcatheter arterial embolization. *Am J Gastroenterol* 1994; 89:1268–1269.

CHAPTER 6

Embolization In The Kidneys

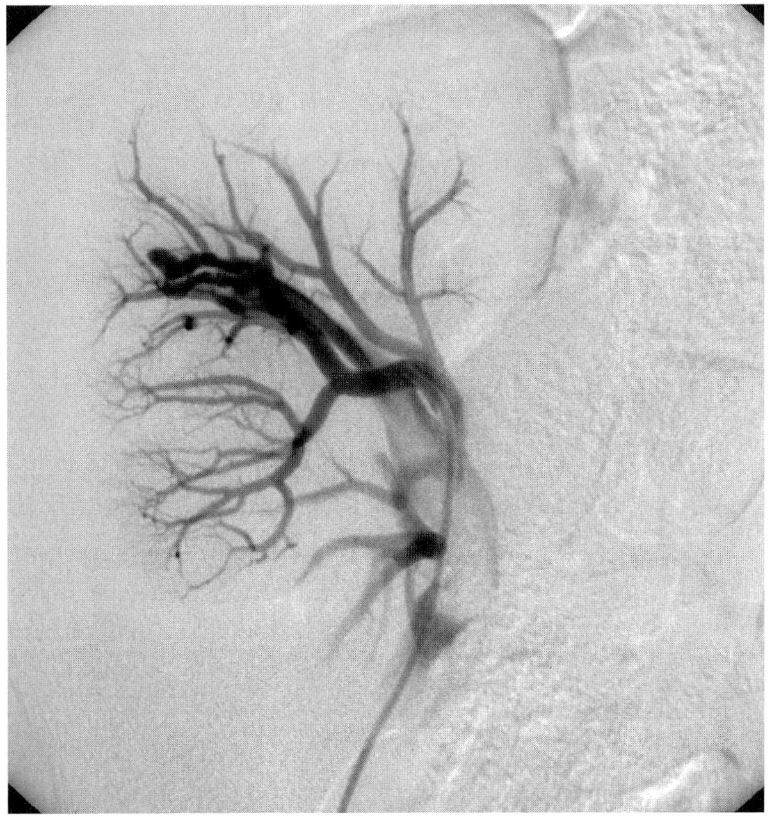

6.1 Embolization In The Kidneys

Case 6.1:

A 62-year-old man presented with massive hematuria following surgical biopsy of a transplanted kidney in the right pelvis. Embolization of an iatrogenic lesion in the transplanted kidney was performed.

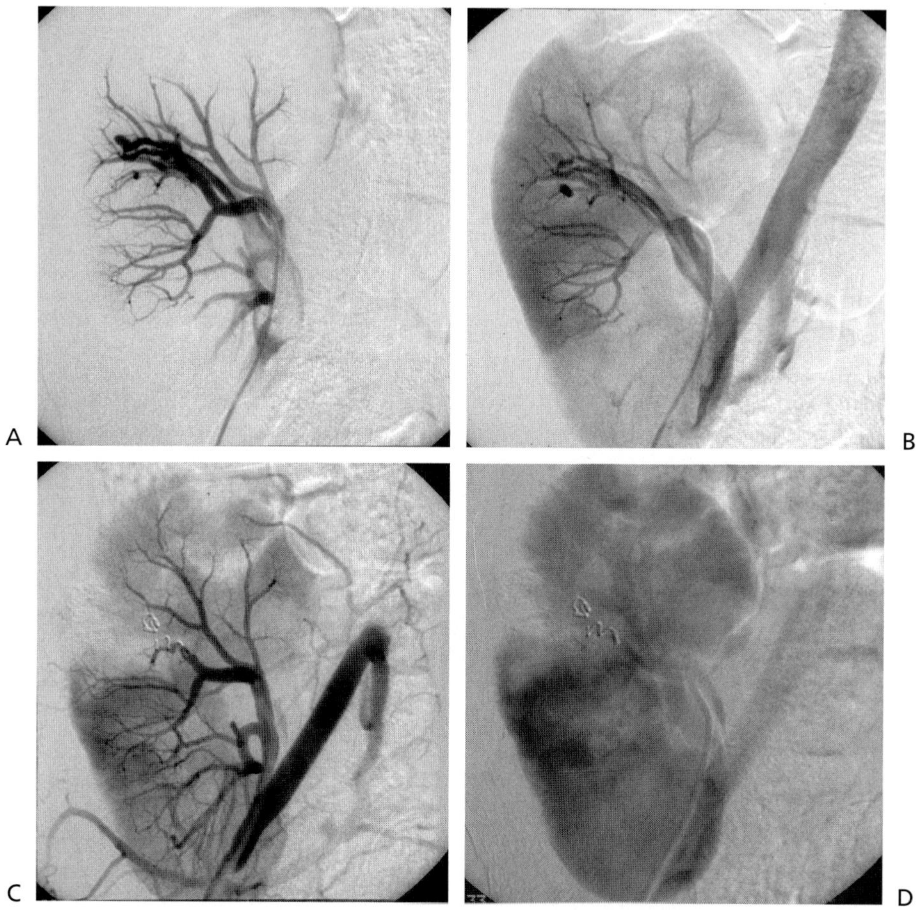

Figure 6.1

A: Selective transplanted kidney arteriogram through an ipsilateral femoral puncture was performed. Note the presence of two small pseudoaneurysms and massive arteriovenous (A-V) fistula in the periphery of the kidney. The renal artery was anastomosed end to side with the iliac artery. **B:** Later-phase angiogram shows massive venous return, with filling of the renal and right iliac veins. The pseudoaneurysms still were filled with contrast. **C:** Embolization was performed. Renal arteriogram after embolization with two 3-mm Gianturco metal coils shows occlusion of the arteries involved in the bleeding. **D:** Late-phase angiogram shows the wedged peripheral filling defect after embolization. There was permanent control of bleeding and no changes in renal function.

Comment: Traumatic hematuria may be secondary to blunt or penetrating trauma, diagnostic needle biopsy, or surgical procedures. In the past, trauma with A-V fistula and massive hematuria required total or partial nephrectomy to control bleeding. Superselective embolization now allows conservation of more renal parenchyma and function. Immediate control of hemorrhage by embolization alone is achieved in 94% of cases. There may be recurrence in up to 23% of patients. Additional embolization of small adjacent branches usually resolves the recurrent bleeding permanently. The final clinical success rate is more than 82%. The most effective embolic material is the Gianturco coil, followed by an absorbable gelatin sponge pledget to enhance clotting around the coil. Blood clots and small particles should be avoided, especially with pseudoaneurysms, due to rupture potential by pressure injection.

6.2 Embolization In The Kidneys

Case 6.2:

Embolization of a traumatic lesion in the kidney of an 18-year-old man was performed. A stab wound to the back caused the renal lesion, followed by massive hematuria with a drop in hematocrit and hypotension.

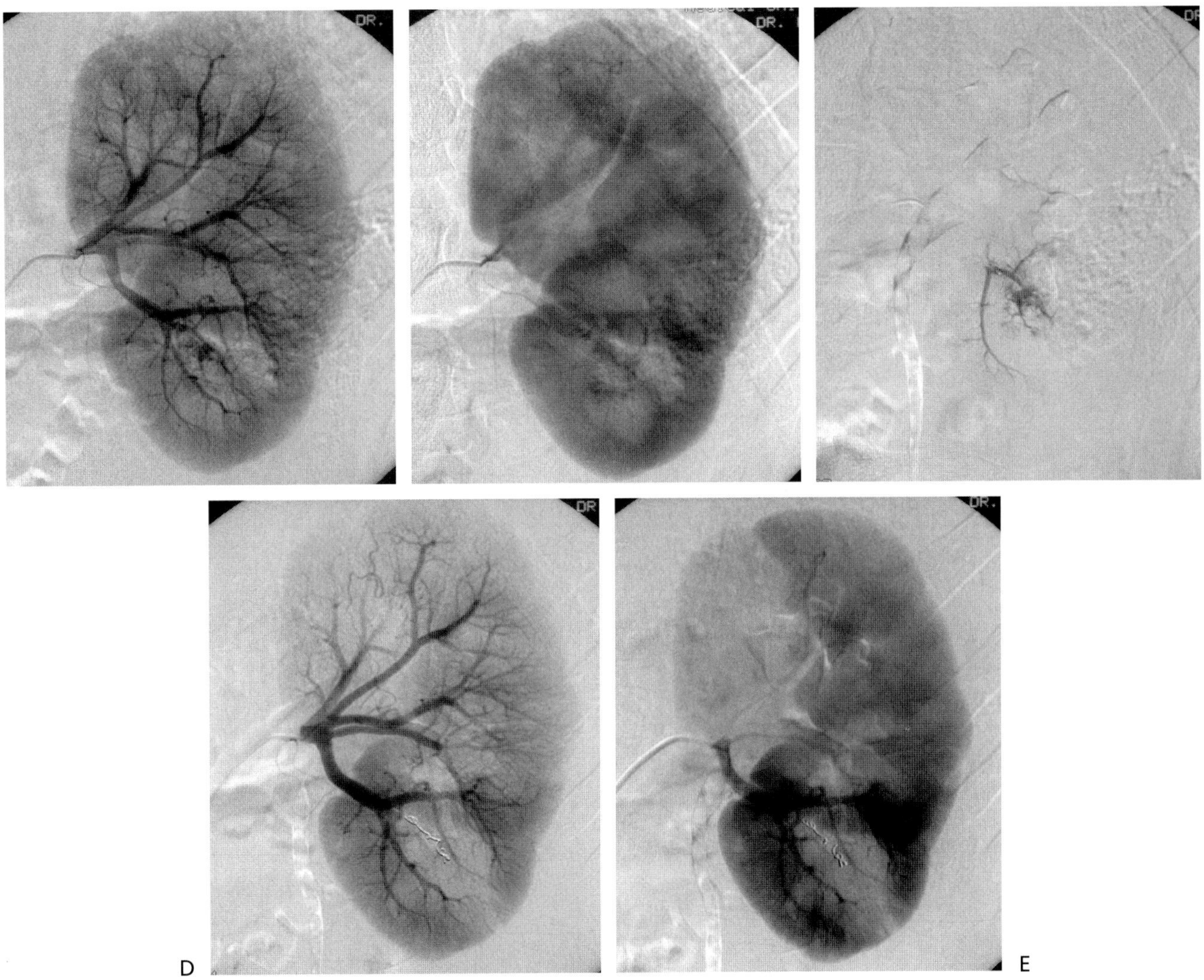

A B, C D E

Figure 6.2

A: Selective left renal artery angiogram shows a pseudoaneurysm of a segmental branch of the lower pole of the kidney. Note the hematoma surrounding the vascular lesion causing displacement of vessels. **B:** Late-phase angiogram shows an enhancement defect in the area of the pseudoaneurysm. **C:** Superselective angiogram with a 2.8F microcatheter in the artery related to the traumatic lesion. Note the small pseudoaneurysm. **D:** Two 2-mm × 2-cm microcoils were used to embolize the pseudoaneurysm, with total occlusion of the artery leading to the lesion. **E:** Late capillary phase of the angiogram shows devascularization of the embolized area. Complete control of the bleeding was obtained, and there was no recurrence. The patient was discharged 2 days after the embolization with unchanged renal function and stable hemodynamic status.

Comment: In the past, renal trauma with pseudoaneurysm and A-V fistula often required total or partial nephrectomy to achieve control of bleeding. More recently, several attempts have been made to conserve more renal parenchyma and function using local or segmental surgical procedures, including excision of the fistula, endofistulorrhaphy, renal artery branch ligation, and venous channel occlusion. However, results have been mixed, and some form of kidney resection often has been required. Maximal preservation of renal parenchyma is obtained with superselective embolization of the involved artery, sparing the adjacent parenchyma of ischemia. Development of microcatheter technology has allowed maximum preservation of renal function.

6.3 Embolization In The Kidneys

Case 6.3:

A 47-year-old male patient with chronic renal failure underwent renal transplant in the right pelvis. Due to a progressive increase in creatinine level, surgical revision of the arterial anastomosis was performed based on an ultrasound Doppler examination suggestive renal artery flow reduction. As the artery was revised for a lower branch stenosis, a transoperative biopsy was performed. Surgical biopsy was followed by massive hematuria and hypotension. Arteriography was requested for possible embolization.

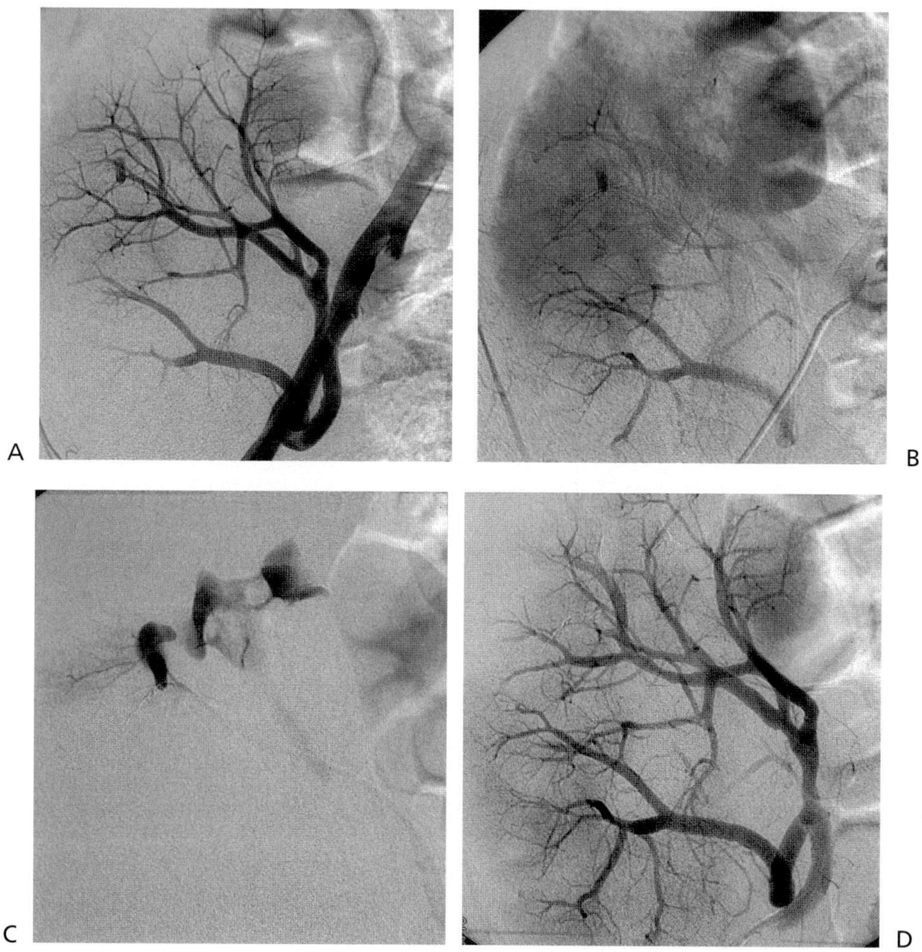

Figure 6.3

A: Right iliac artery angiography shows surgical ligature of the right internal iliac artery and direct end-to-side anastomosis of the graft renal artery to the external iliac artery. Peripherally, a small pseudoaneurysm is observed in a midsegmental renal artery. **B:** Late capillary phase shows stagnant contrast into the pseudoaneurysm and sluggish flow into the lower pole arterial branch. **C:** A 4F catheter was advanced into the branch containing the pseudoaneurysm, and a gentle test injection ruptured the pseudoaneurysm with extravasation into the upper calix. Embolization was performed with one metal coil. **D:** Postembolization renal arteriogram shows occlusion of the pseudoaneurysm and the damaged branch. The coil was barely noted in the subtracted angiogram. Bleeding was controlled and renal function fully recovered.

Comment: Surgical needle biopsy caused massive bleeding in the kidney of this patient. Surgical control of the bleeding was impossible without causing loss of renal function and parenchyma. Superselective catheterization and embolization is the best method to treat this type of kidney lesion. A 4F catheter was used to catheterize the branch involved in the bleeding. This usually is a poor option, because it frequently triggers spasms that may preclude embolization. Microcatheter technology allows access to very peripheral cortical arterial branches and embolization with microcoils. Fortunately, in this case it was possible to deliver the one coil into the proper position. Complications related to this type of embolization procedure are rare, and mortality associated with the procedure has not been reported. Hemodynamic instability is rapidly controlled by embolization in most patients. However, bleeding may recur in up to 23% of patients, and a second embolization may be necessary. Nephrectomy may be necessary in some cases. Failure of embolization is related more frequently to inadequate materials, such as Gelfoam and blood clots. Fragmentation of the embolic material is the major cause of failure and recurrence of hematuria. Even patients with massive fracture of the kidney will stop bleeding after effective adequate embolization.

6.4 Embolization In The Kidneys

Case 6.4:

A 36-year-old male patient with a horseshoe kidney underwent percutaneous nephrolithotripsy at another institution, followed by placement of a ureteral stent and 14F nephrostomy catheter for temporary external drainage. Hypotension and hematuria developed shortly after surgery, and the patient was transferred to our institution for further treatment. A diagnostic arteriogram was requested for possible embolization.

A

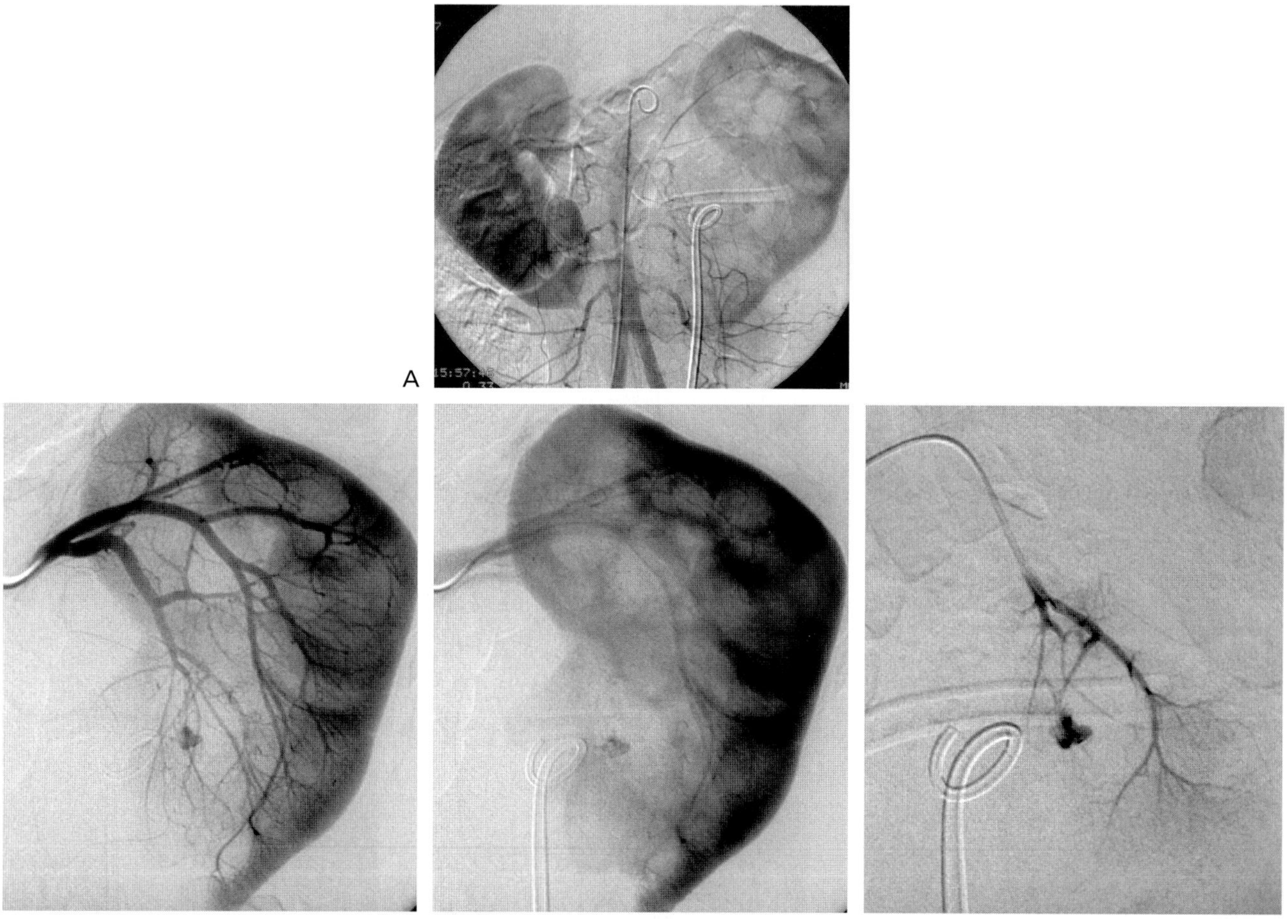

B, C

D

Figure 6.4

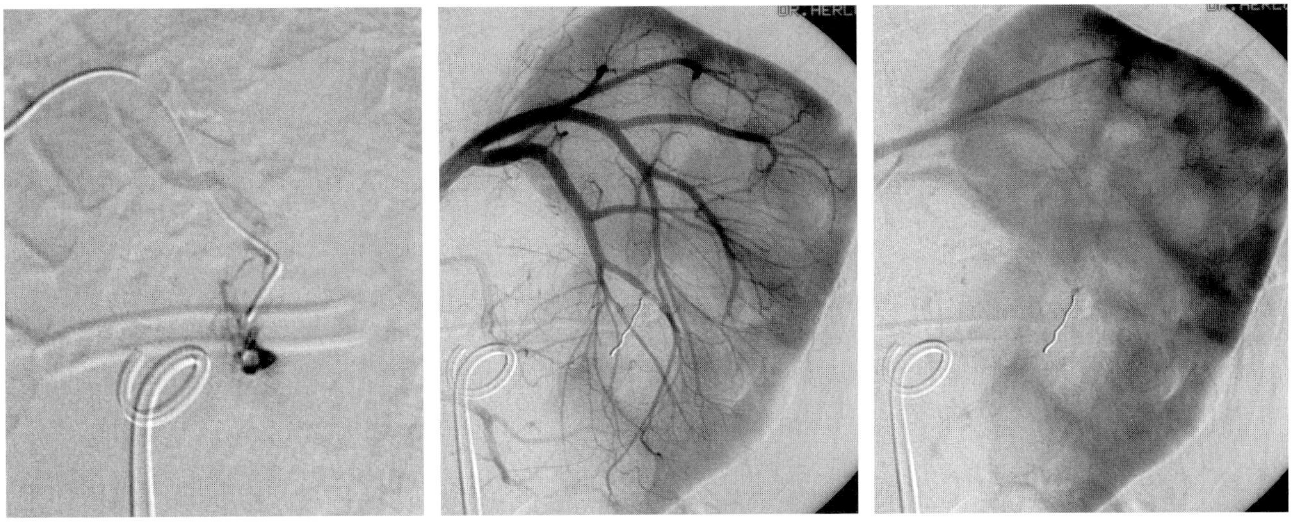

E F, G

Figure 6.4 *(continued)*

A: Late-phase abdominal aortogram shows the large horseshoe kidney with a dilated pelvis, by clots (not readily visible), the nephrostomy catheter, and the ureteral stent. A relatively small pseudoaneurysm was noted, adjacent to the shaft of the nephrostomy catheter. **B:** Main left renal artery angiogram shows a pseudoaneurysm in a lower branch of the renal artery. **C:** Late-phase arteriogram shows the pseudoaneurysm and a hypovascular area around the lesion. **D:** A more selective arteriogram was performed using a microcatheter in an attempt to locate the compromised arterial branch. **E:** The microcatheter was advanced into the artery containing the tear. Note a small A-V fistula related to the pseudoaneurysm. **F:** Embolization with one microcoil was performed. Postembolization renal arteriogram shows total occlusion of the pseudoaneurysm and damaged artery. A single 2-mm × 2-cm microcoil was placed into the damaged artery for embolization. **G:** Late-phase left renal arteriogram shows occlusion of the lesion.

Comment: Percutaneous kidney stones lithotripsy requires transparenchymal access. If the puncture is medial and closer to the infundibular or segmental arterial branches, a major artery may be struck and a puncture-related complication may develop. Multiple punctures with larger needles increase the possibility of arterial trauma and bleeding. As the percutaneous endourologic procedures became more popular 10 to 15 years ago, an increased number of vascular traumas to the kidney have been seen. A horseshoe kidney is naturally more prone to vascular trauma due to its rotation and unusual anatomy. As the number of cases increased, the role of transcatheter intravascular procedures became more important in controlling acute/massive bleeding in the kidney. Microcatheter technology has allowed very precise catheterization and embolization. Renal segments are isolated and no arterial collaterals communicate between the segments. Proximal occlusion of the feeder artery to the pseudoaneurysm usually is sufficient to occlude the lesion permanently. It may be necessary to embolize the whole segment, because some intrasegmental collaterals may develop distal to the occlusion. It is wise to perform the embolization as selectively as possible, with occlusion of the rent in the artery.

6.5 Embolization In The Kidneys

Case 6.5:

A 27-year-old male patient had advanced right renal cell carcinoma, with retroperitoneal lymph node metastasis, pain, and hematuria. An arteriogram and embolization were requested to boost immunologic response against the tumor and control the hematuria.

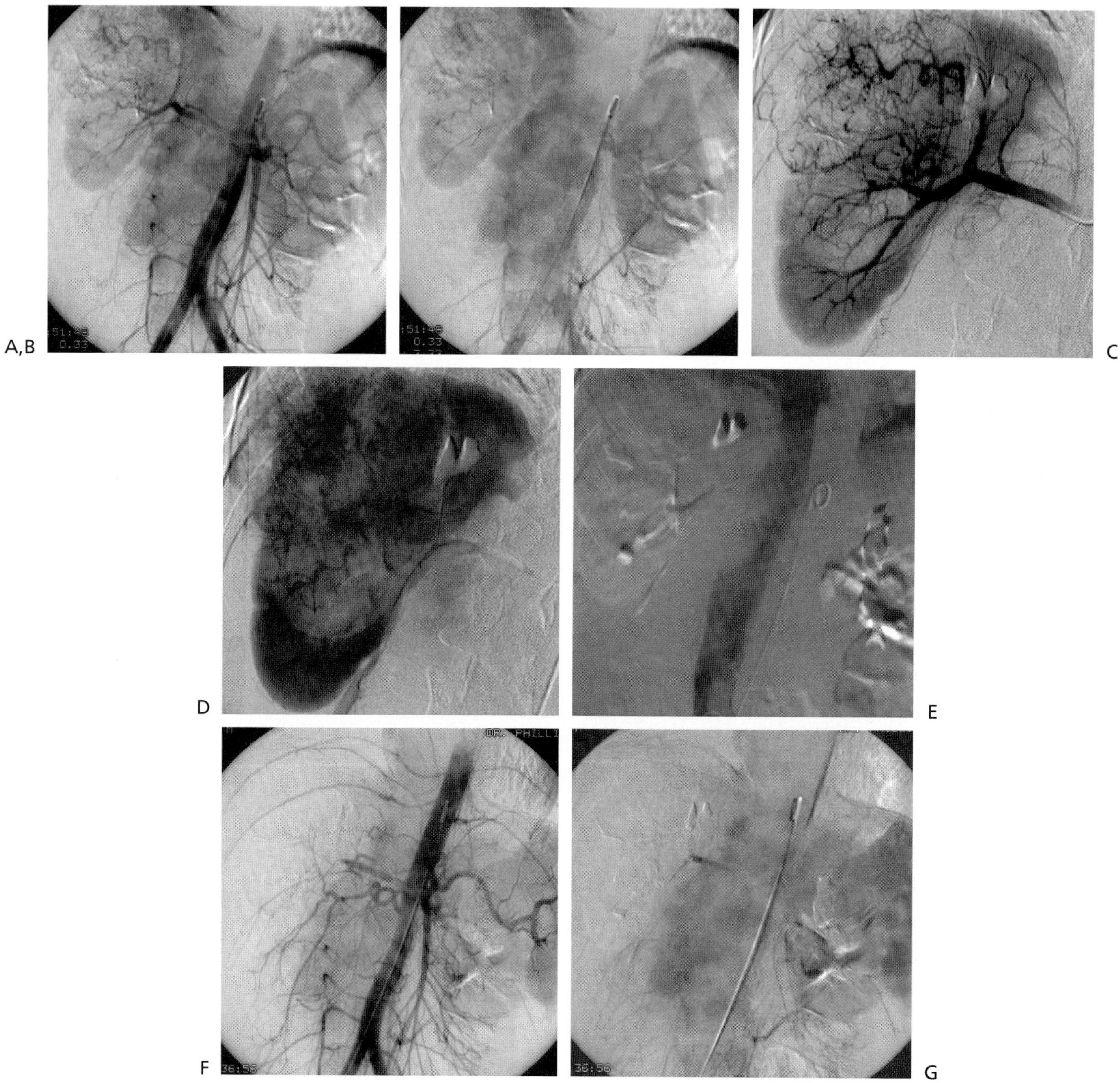

Figure 6.5

A: Abdominal aortogram shows a large hypervascular tumor in the middle and upper half of the right kidney and a paraaortic mass on the right. **B:** Late-phase aortogram shows enhancement of the paraaortic mass. **C,D:** Selective arteriogram of the right kidney shows the hypervascular mass breaking through the renal capsule and displacing the collecting system. **E:** Inferior cavogram shows compression and invasion of the inferior vena cava by the paraaortic tumor. **F,G:** Postembolization aortogram shows total devascularization of the kidney but persistent enhancement of the paraaortic mass. Embolization was performed with Ivalon particles and microcoils.

Comment: Renal cell carcinomas are hypervascular tumors that respond well to embolization. The diagnostic angiographic protocol should include aortogram, bilateral selective renal arteriogram, cavogram, and renal vein visualization for assessment of metastatic disease. Embolization of malignant renal tumors is performed as a preoperative procedure, for palliation of unresectable tumors, and perhaps to boost immunologic response against the tumor. A variety of embolic materials are used for renal tumor embolization, including Gelfoam sponge, polyvinyl alcohol particles, Gianturco coils, and absolute ethanol. Ethanol should be used carefully. The renal artery should be catheterized with a balloon catheter to reduce the risks of intraaortic reflux. Absolute ethanol floats in the aortic blood, and anterior laminar flow will enter the inferior mesenteric circulation if allowed to reflux into the aorta. The balloon used for occlusion may not prevent nontarget organ embolization. Special care should be exercised to prevent left colon ischemia. When embolizing the left renal artery by balloon occlusion, the alcohol can reach the bowel arteries through parasitic circulation between the tumor and the left colon. The maximum usable dose of absolute ethanol is 0.5 mL/kg; this dose reduces the risks of alcohol intoxication and coma. Association of multiple embolic materials frequently is necessary, especially when high-flow A-V fistulas are present. Coils or other devices are always necessary to occlude larger vessels.

Suggested Reading

Avolio L, Savasta S, Matteotti C, Fusillo M, Bragheri R. Symptomatic unilateral renal angiomyolipoma in a child with tuberous sclerosis. *Urol Int* 2001;67:249–251.

Bookstein JJ, Goldstein HM. Successful management of postbiopsy arteriovenous fistula with selective arterial embolization. *Radiology* 1973;109:535–537.

Ekelund L. Transcatheter embolization in the management of neoplastic and benign diseases of the kidney. In Lang EK (ed). *Percutaneous and interventional urology and radiology.* New York; Springer-Verlag 1986;177–187.

Fisher RG, Ben-Menachen V, Whigham C. Stab wounds of the renal artery branches: angiographic diagnosis and treatment by embolization. *AJR* 1989;152:1231–1235.

Hamaguchi T, Kasahara K, Shuin T, Kataoka S. Spontaneous rupture of renal aniomyolipoma with tuberous sclerosis during long-term follow-up: A case report. *Hinyokika Kiyo* 2001;47:645–648.

Hora M, Hes O, Michal M. Histoligic classification of kidney tumors for clinical practice in adults. *Cas Lek Cesk* 2001;140:362–369.

Jimenez RE, Eble JN, Reuter VE, et al. Concurrent angiomyolipoma and renal cell neoplasia: a study of 36 cases. *Mod Pathol* 2001;14:157–163.

Moudouni SM, En-Nia I, Patard JJ, Lobel B, Guille F. Arterial embolization in hemorrhagic renal angiomyolipoma. *Prog Urol* 2001:11: 235–238.

Radin R, Ma Y. Malignant epithelioid renal angiomyolipoma in a patient with tuberous sclerosis. *J Comput Assist Tomogr* 2001;25:873–875.

Sampaio FJ, Aragao AH. Anatomical relationship between the intrarenal arteries and the kidney collecting system. *J Urol* 1990;143: 679–681.

Tanaka M, Kyo S, Inoue M, Kojima T. Conservative management and vaginal delivery following ruptured renal angiomylolipoma. *Obstet Gynecol* 2001;98:932–933.

Tazelaar HD, Batts KP, Srigley JR. Primary extrapulmonary sugar tumor (PEST): a report of four cases. *Mod Pathol* 2001;14:615–622.

Uflacker R, Paolini RM, Lima S. Management of traumatic hematuria by selective renal artery embolization. *J Urology* 1984;132:662–667.

Uflacker R, Paolini RM, Nobrega M. Ablation of tumor and inflammatory tissue with absolute ethanol. *Acta Radiol Diagn* 1986;27:131–138.

Young A, Tadavarthy M, Coleman CC, et al. Embolotherapy: agents, equipment and techniques. In: Castaneda-Zuniga WR, Tadavarthy SM, eds. *Interventional radiology.* Baltimore: Williams & Wilkins, 1988;13–76.

CHAPTER 7

Embolization In The Chest And Lungs

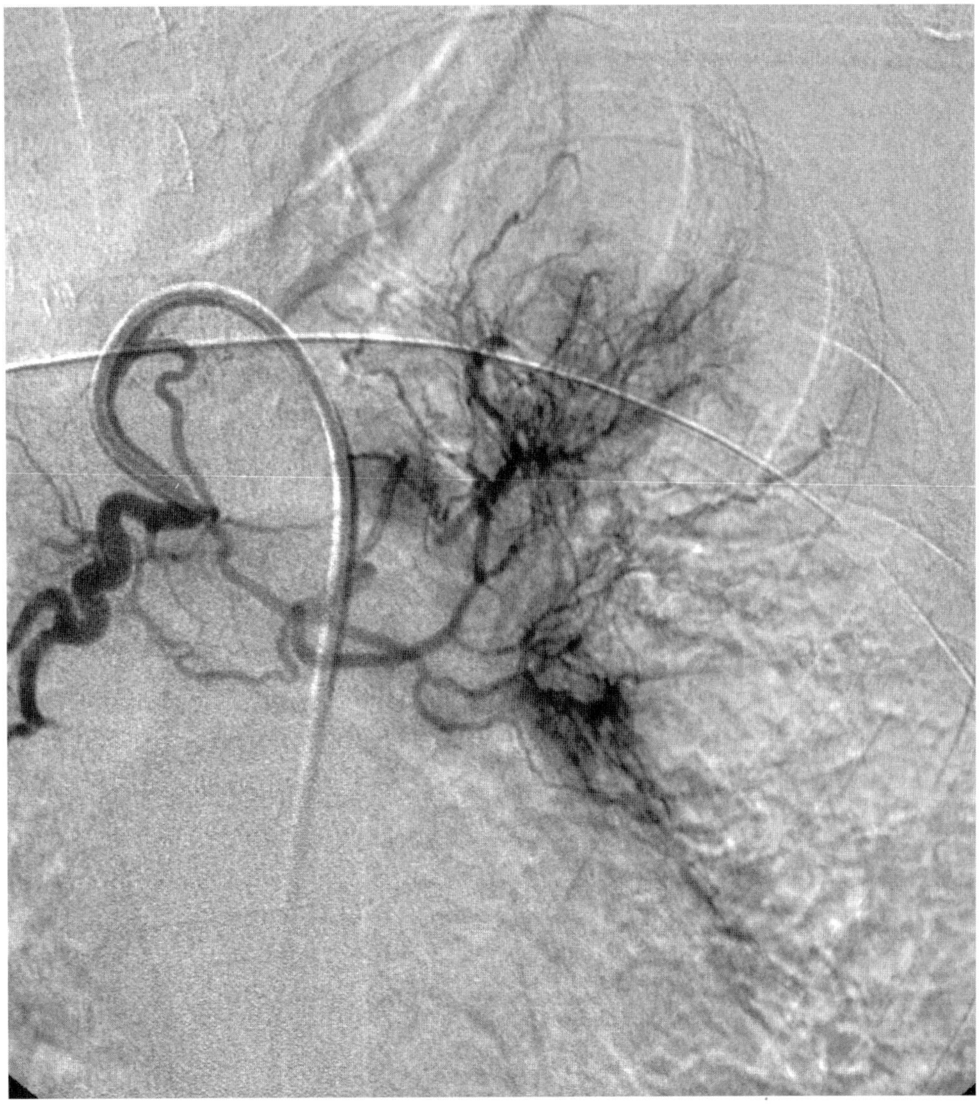

7.1 Embolization In The Chest And Lungs

Case 7.1:

A 3-year-old boy with a history of recurrent pulmonary infections presented with infected bronchiectasis and massive hemoptysis. Bronchial artery angiography and embolization were requested.

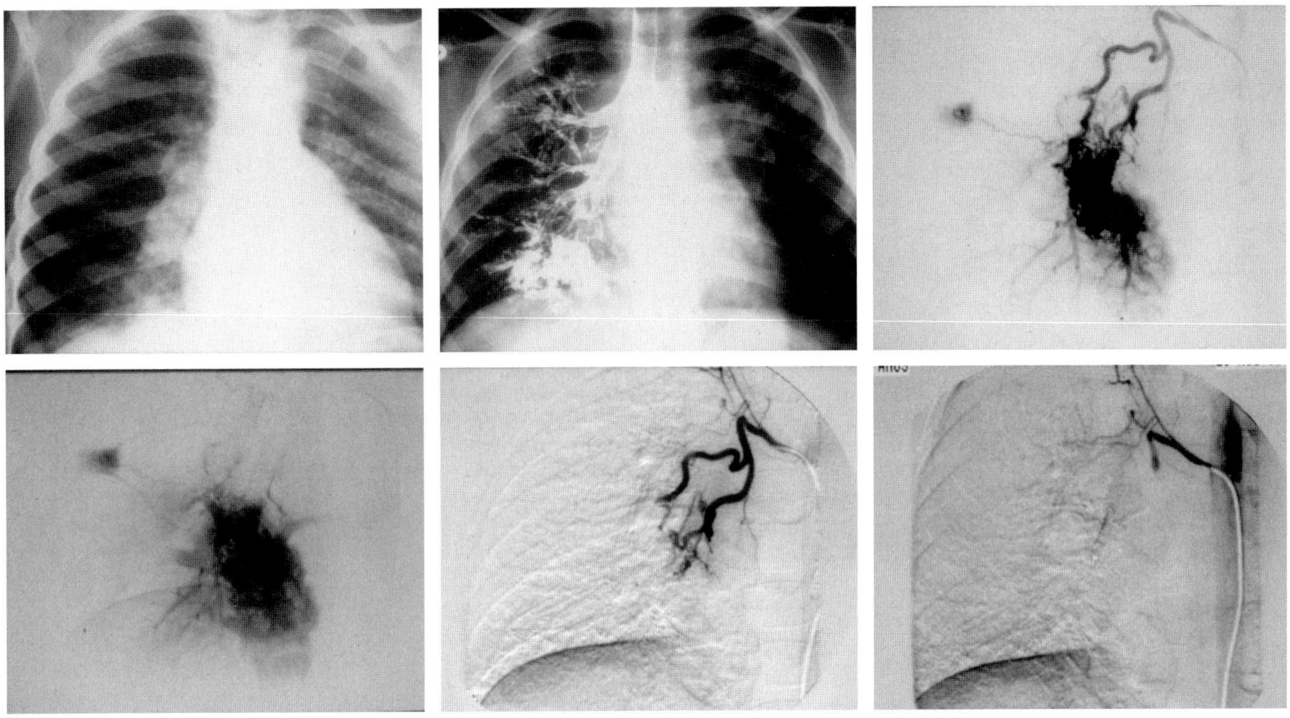

A B, C D E, F

Figure 7.1

A: Previous chest radiograph shows a mass in the middle and right lower lobes. **B:** Bronchography shows massive lower lobe bronchiectasis. **C:** Bronchial artery angiography with injection in the right intercostobronchial trunk shows a massive area of hypervascularity in the right lower lobe, with a nodular area of hypervascularity possibly in the middle lobe. Note the large size of the bronchial arteries branches of the intercostobronchial trunk. **D:** Late-phase arteriogram shows dense enhancement of the inflammatory lesion and massive shunting with the pulmonary artery of the lower lobe. **E:** Angiogram following partial embolization with Ivalon shows marked reduction of the vascularity in the inflammatory lesion. **F:** Following embolization of the more proximal artery with Gelfoam, there was total occlusion of the bronchial arteries branching off the intercostobronchial trunk. Total control of the bleeding was achieved, and the patient was later treated by surgery.

Comment: Massive hemoptysis is a highly significant clinical and surgical problem that is associated with a mortality rate of 50% to 100%. Death in these cases is related more to asphyxia than hypovolemia. The most frequent cause of massive hemoptysis is active or residual tuberculosis. In 10% to 20% of patients, chronic lung disease with residual inflammatory process develops, and a significant number of those patients experience massive hemoptysis. Other major causes of massive hemoptysis are bronchiectasis, pneumoconiosis, aspergilloma, carcinoma, cystic fibrosis, and abscess.

Surgery is a definitive treatment for massive hemoptysis; however, it is viable only for patients with unilateral and localized disease. Diffuse disease is a contraindication for surgery, and some lesions, such as cystic fibrosis, are not amenable to surgical treatment. The case presented is typical: a patient with an infectious unilateral disease, who is amenable to surgical treatment but first requires clinical and hemodynamic stabilization. Embolization of the bronchial arteries controlled the bleeding and allowed the patient to be treated surgically when convenient.

7.2 Embolization In The Chest And Lungs

Case 7.2:

A 10-year-old girl with cystic fibrosis presented with massive hemoptysis. Bronchial artery angiography and treatment by embolization were requested. Despite embolization, recurrence of bleeding necessitated additional embolization.

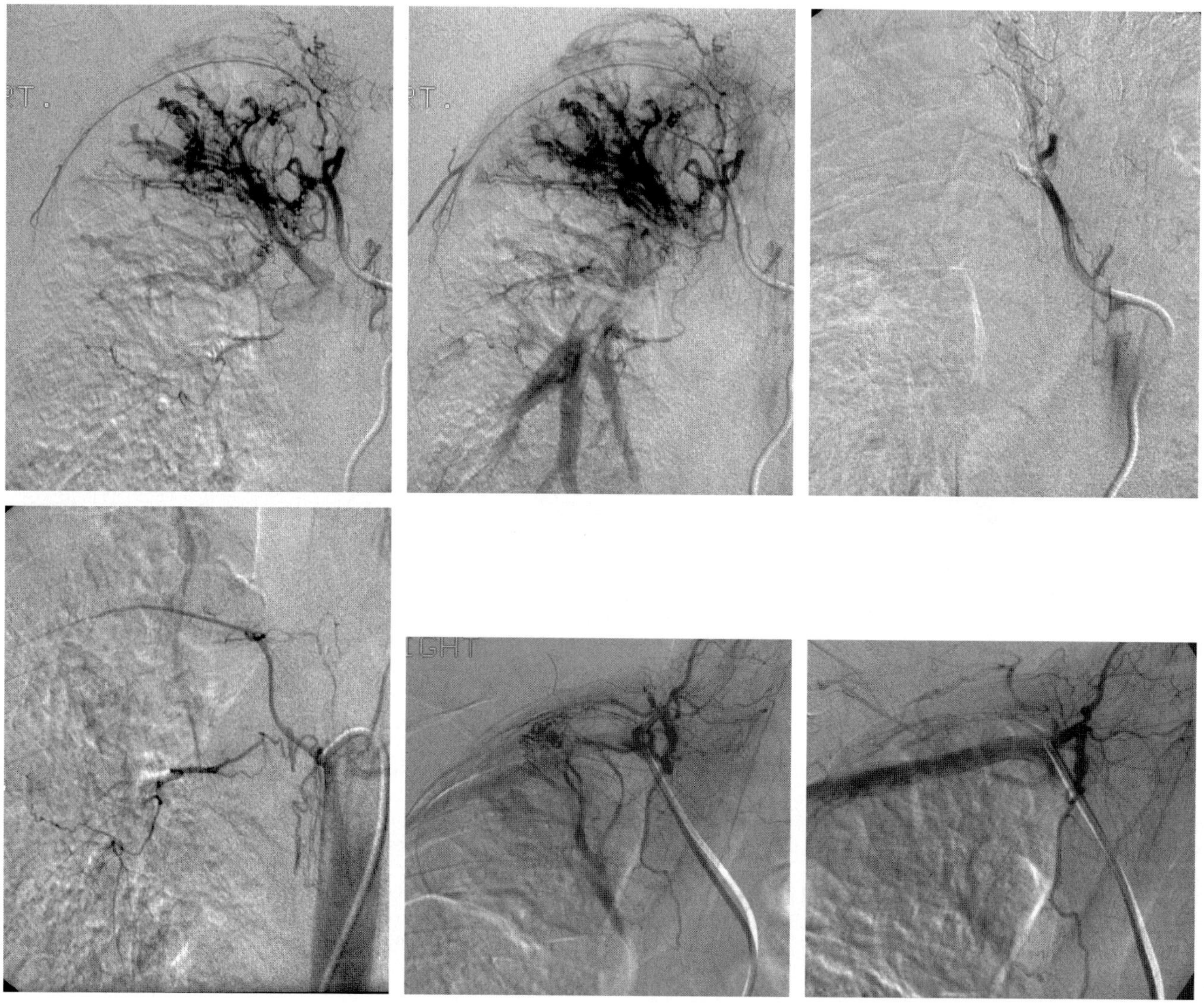

A, B C D, E F

Figure 7.2

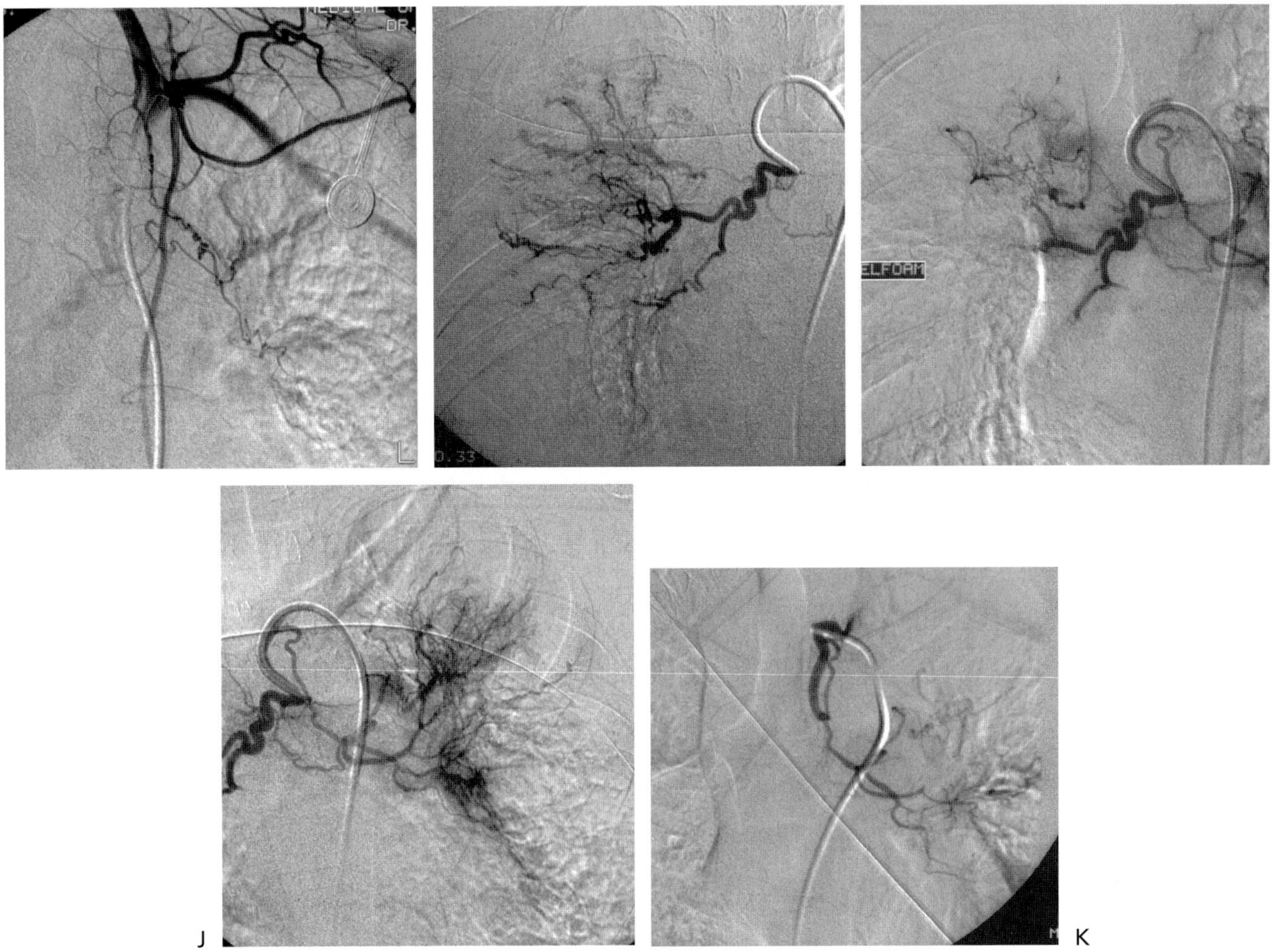

G H, I J K

Figure 7.2 *(continued)*

A: Selective arteriogram in the intercostobronchial trunk shows massive inflammatory lesions in the right upper lobe. Note massive shunting to the peripheral branches of the pulmonary artery. **B:** Later phase shows filling of the pulmonary artery, also in the right lower lobe. **C:** Embolization with Ivalon and Gelfoam produced occlusion of the intercostobronchial trunk branches. **D:** Catheterization of a more inferior intercostal artery reveals connection with the right lower lobe bronchial artery. **E:** Selective injection into the right thyrocervical trunk shows development of collateral vessels from the thoracic wall into the inflammatory lesion in the lung. Note the anterior spinal artery connected to the thyrocervical trunk medially. **F:** Embolization with Gelfoam was performed, which spared the anterior spinal artery. **G:** Selective injection into the left thyrocervical trunk shows a small tortuous connection with the left bronchial artery. **H:** Selective injection in the common bronchial trunk reveals a main right bronchial artery supplying the right upper lobe bronchus. **I:** Embolization was performed with Ivalon and Gelfoam. Note occlusion of the main terminal branches. **J:** After embolization of the dominant right branch, the left artery became more visible, as did the inflammatory lesion in the left lung, upper and lower lobes. Embolization was performed. **K:** Bleeding recurred 2 days later, and an unusual variation was discovered. There was a left bronchial artery connection arising from the origin of the left subclavian artery that descended into the mediastinum and connected to the left bronchial artery circulation. Embolization was performed, and the bleeding was controlled.

Comment: As massive hemoptysis has such a high morbidity and mortality rate, recognition of the event causing the bleeding and definition of alternative treatments should be rapid. Immediate interventional treatment should be available to all patients, as surgery has a high mortality rate. In cases of uncontrollable bleeding, endotracheal intubation and assisted ventilation may be required to avoid asphyxiation. A double-lumen endotracheal tube (Carlens tube) should be available to confine the bleeding to one lung while the normal lung is being ventilated. Bronchoscopy is important in the management of patients with massive hemoptysis. It can establish the origin of bleeding in about 86% of patients, although it may be difficult to perform bronchoscopy during a massive bleeding episode. Some endobronchial procedures, such as endobronchial balloon tamponade, are useful for control of hemoptysis. Irrigation with adrenaline also is useful to control the bleeding. Immediate control of acute, massive bronchial bleeding (hemoptysis) can be achieved by bronchial artery embolization in more than 85% of cases with tuberculosis. However, bleeding recurrence may occur in up to 21% of patients, with 9% mortality. Although the embolic materials are thrombogenic, patency of the vessel may be restored by either lysis or recanalization of thrombosed arteries.

7.3 Embolization In The Chest And Lungs

Case 7.3:

A 35-year-old woman with sarcoidosis and aspergillosis presented with massive hemoptysis. Bronchial artery angiography and embolization were requested.

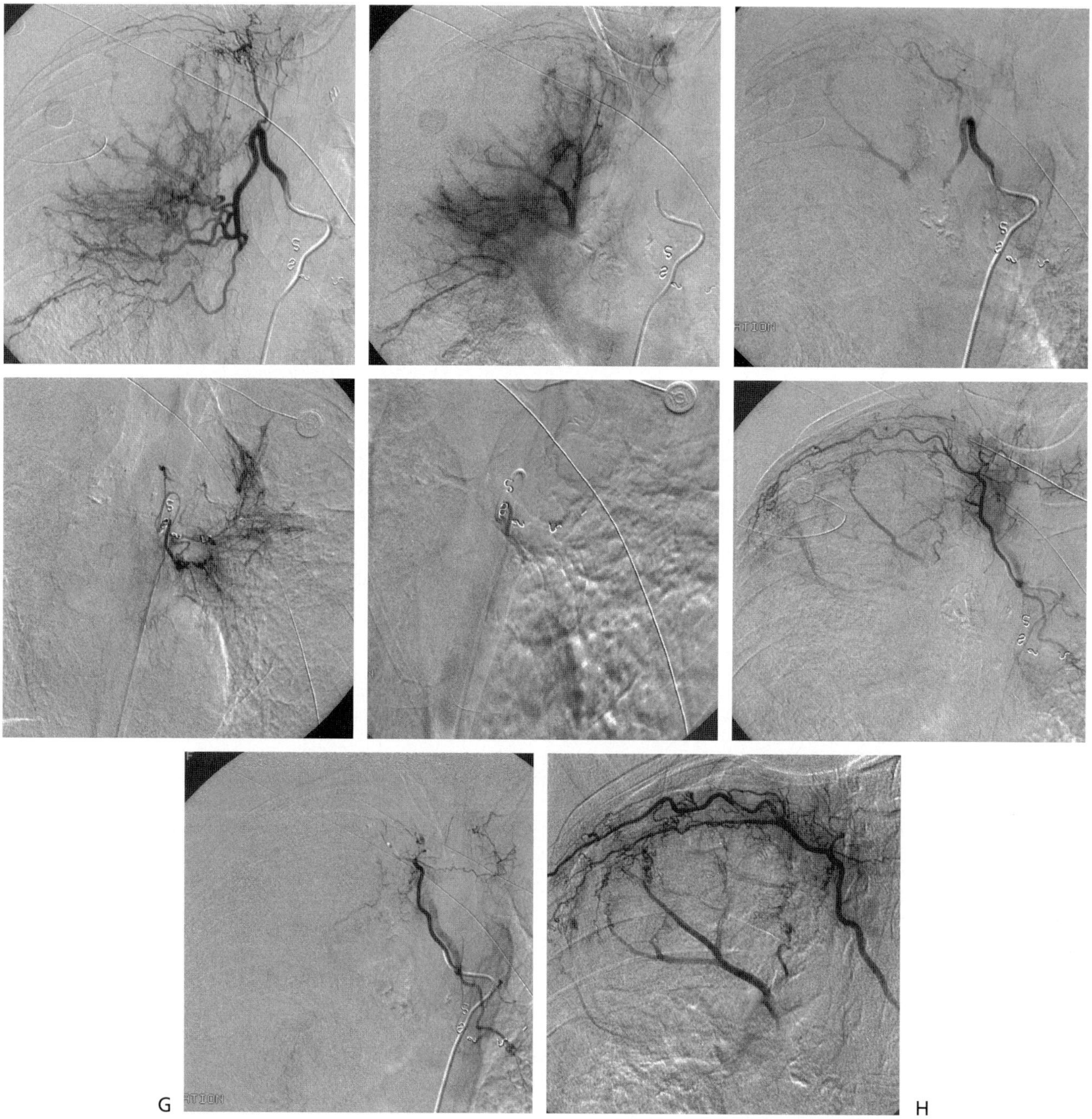

A, B C D, E F G H

Figure 7.3

A: Selective arteriogram of the intercostobronchial trunk shows massive hypervascularity of the right lung in more prominent areas with the chronic inflammatory process. **B:** Late-phase angiography shows shunts into the right pulmonary artery. **C:** Embolization of the intercostobronchial trunk was performed with Ivalon and Gelfoam. Total occlusion was achieved. **D:** Selective injection into the left bronchial artery shows hypervascularity in the left lung. **E:** Embolization was performed with Ivalon and Gelfoam, and total occlusion was achieved. **F–H:** Multiple intercostal arteries were injected. Communications with the intrapulmonary inflammatory hypervascularity and shunts with branches of the pulmonary artery are shown. Embolization with Gelfoam produced further occlusion of the shunts.

Comment: The bronchial arteries anatomy is now well established. There usually are two to four main bronchial arteries but there is a variable anatomic presentation. There are at least ten possible combinations, but the most common findings are either one right and one left artery with an upper lobe and a lower lobe bronchus branch; one right and two left arteries; or two right and two left arteries. In 33% to 43% of cases, there is a common trunk giving origin to right and left bronchial arteries. The anterior spinal artery rarely or never arises from a bronchial artery or trunk. The anterior spinal artery may arise from intercostal arteries or thyrocervical trunk. If the anterior spinal artery is visualized, there is a contraindication for embolization. Advancement of the catheter beyond the origin of the anterior spinal artery is a useful method to prevent accidental occlusion of that vessel. The presence of the posterior spinal artery and spinal artery radicles arising from the bronchial arteries or other feeders is not a total contraindication to the embolic procedure. Chronic inflammatory conditions cause enlargement of the bronchial arteries and development of bronchopulmonary anastomoses. Other systemic arteries, such as the subclavian, axillary, phrenic, and intercostal arteries, also contribute to the systemic supply to the lungs under conditions of chronic inflammation or infection. Embolization of the other blood sources also should be performed. Embolization of the bronchial arteries is indicated in a patient with life-threatening hemoptysis who is unsuitable for surgery. Usually the patients are treated by embolization during active bleeding or in the intervals lasting a few hours between bleeding episodes.

7.4 Embolization In The Chest And Lungs

Case 7.4:

A 4-year-old boy with tetralogy of Fallot and pulmonary artery atresia presented with excessive systemic-to-pulmonary collateral vessels causing congestive heart failure and low oxygenation due to massive arteriopulmonary shunting. Diagnostic angiography and possible embolization were requested before undertaking corrective surgery.

A, B

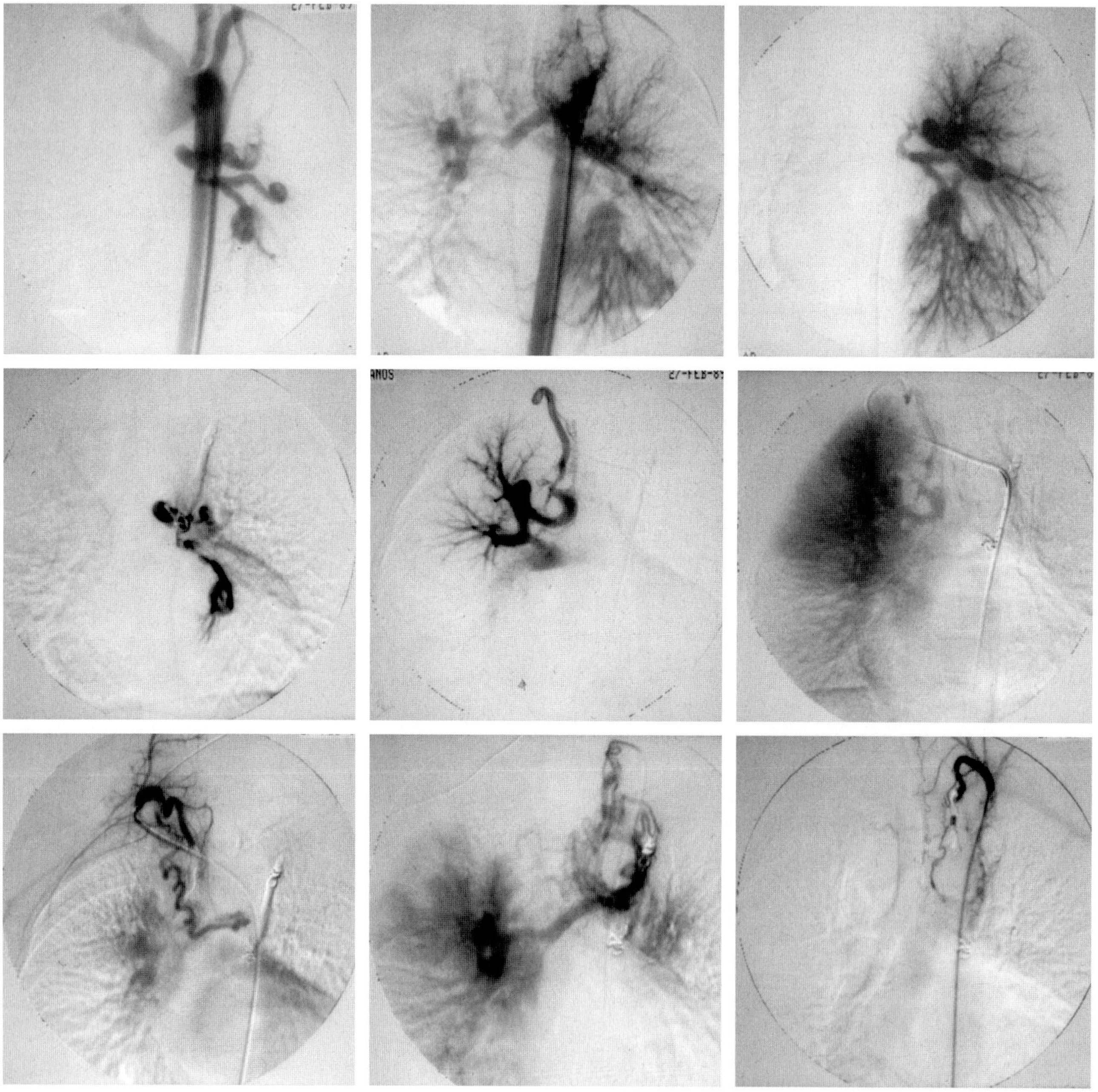

C

D, E

F

G, H

I

Figure 7.4

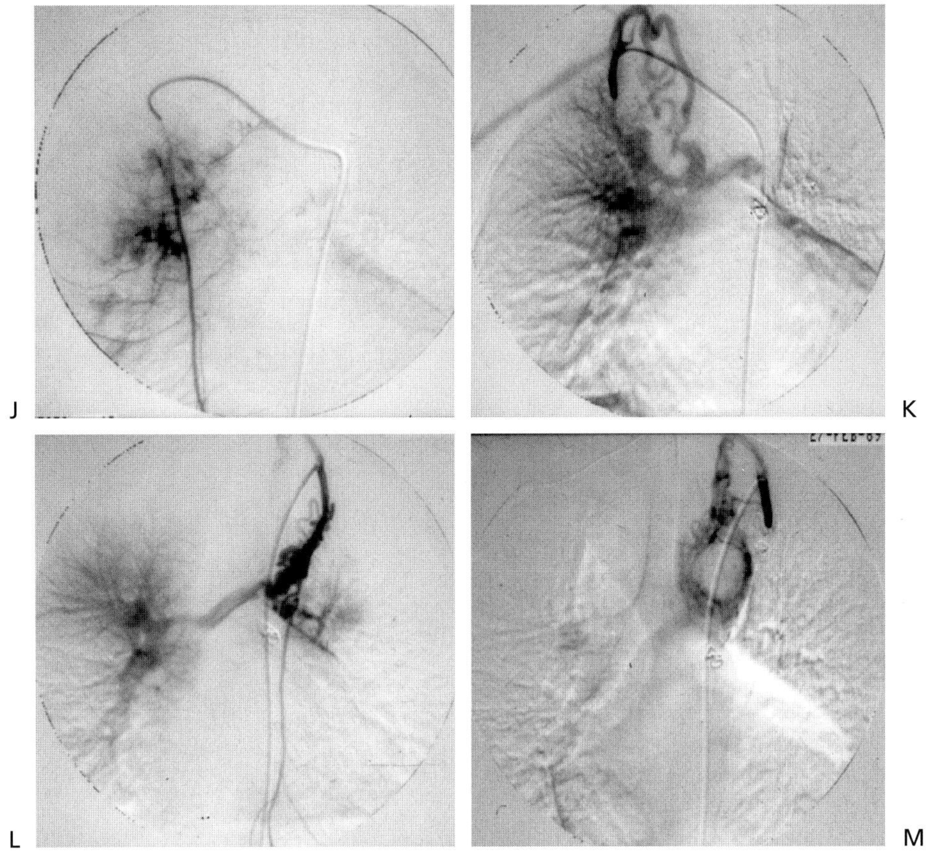

Figure 7.4 *(continued)*

A,B: Early and late phases of the thoracic aortogram show markedly enlarged branches arising from the descending thoracic aorta and cervical branches. Note the size of the bronchial arteries and perfusion of the peripheral pulmonary branches. **C:** Selective injection in the left bronchial artery shows filling of the peripheral branches of the left pulmonary artery. **D:** Proximal embolization of the left bronchial artery performed with Gianturco coils resulted in significant reduction in perfusion. **E:** Selective injection into a descending branch of the right thyrocervical trunk anastomosed to an anomalous mediastinal artery, which is connected with the peripheral branches of the right pulmonary artery. **F:** Late phase shows pulmonary perfusion. **G:** Following embolization of the anomalous artery with coils, there was marked reduction in flow to the right lung. **H:** Injection in the left thyrocervical trunk shows anastomotic vessels to the pulmonary branches connected to the right lower lobe. **I:** Embolization was performed and reduction of flow was obtained. **J,K:** Pre- and postembolization angiograms of the right internal mammary arteries show partial perfusion of the pulmonary arteries of the right lung. Following embolization, significant reduction in flow was obtained. **L:** Injection into the left internal mammary artery (IMA) shows anastomosis with the pulmonary artery of the right lower lobe. **M:** Embolization was performed and reduction of flow was obtained. Note the vasa vasorum around the aortic arch.

Comment: Patients with congenital heart disease, especially right ventricular outflow tract or pulmonary artery obstruction, develop large systemic-to-pulmonary collateral vessels. The enlarged vessels usually arise from the aorta or its branches and anastomose with the pulmonary artery at various levels. The collateral vessels may be the only source of blood flow to portions of the lungs in which no pulmonary artery is connected to the main pulmonary artery. Excessive systemic-to-pulmonary shunts through these collaterals may cause heart failure, low arterial oxygen saturation from the excessive flow, or even pulmonary hemorrhage from rupture of these thin-walled vessels, with clinical deterioration. There are three types of collateral arteries, each having a distinctive anastomosis with the pulmonary artery: (i) bronchial artery collaterals, which are anastomosed to more peripheral segments of the pulmonary artery through developed collaterals; (ii) direct aortic collateral vessels, which originate from the descending aorta and usually supply a lobe or segment of lung and anastomose with segmental pulmonary arteries; and (iii) indirect aortic collateral vessels, which arise from major branches of the aorta and usually anastomose with central pulmonary arteries outside the lungs. These vessels frequently develop stenoses. Surgical ligation is an accepted form of treatment to eliminate the shunts, following correction of the congenital heart disease. Identification and ligation of these anomalous vessels may prolong surgical time and add to its difficulty. Occasionally, a separate surgical procedure may be necessary to achieve adequate treatment. Embolization has been used to occlude the shunts to the pulmonary arteries, either before or after surgical correction of the heart disease. When there is hemoptysis, the embolization procedure is highly successful in controlling the bleeding. There is improvement of heart failure and oxygen saturation in 80% to 90% of patients with previous surgical correction of the congenital heart disease. The success rate may be even higher when the embolization procedure is performed before the heart surgery. Possible complications are related to pulmonary infarction and infection. Embolization should be performed with coils or detachable balloons, usually in the arterial side of the shunt, avoiding the distal pulmonary circulation. Small particles or fluid materials are contraindicated and may be the cause of complications reported in the literature, mostly related to pulmonary infarction.

7.5 Embolization In The Chest And Lungs

Case 7.5:

A 56-year-old man with previously undiagnosed hereditary hemorrhagic telangiectasia (HHT), chronic hypoxia, and adynamia presented with a pulmonary nodule detected on chest x-ray film and was referred for biopsy. Revision of the chest x-ray film taken at the other institution showed a nodule in continuity with a vascular structure, which prompted the diagnosis of a pulmonary arteriovenous (A-V) fistula. Inspection of the patient's face showed multiple telangiectasia, and the history included recurrent nose bleeds since youth.

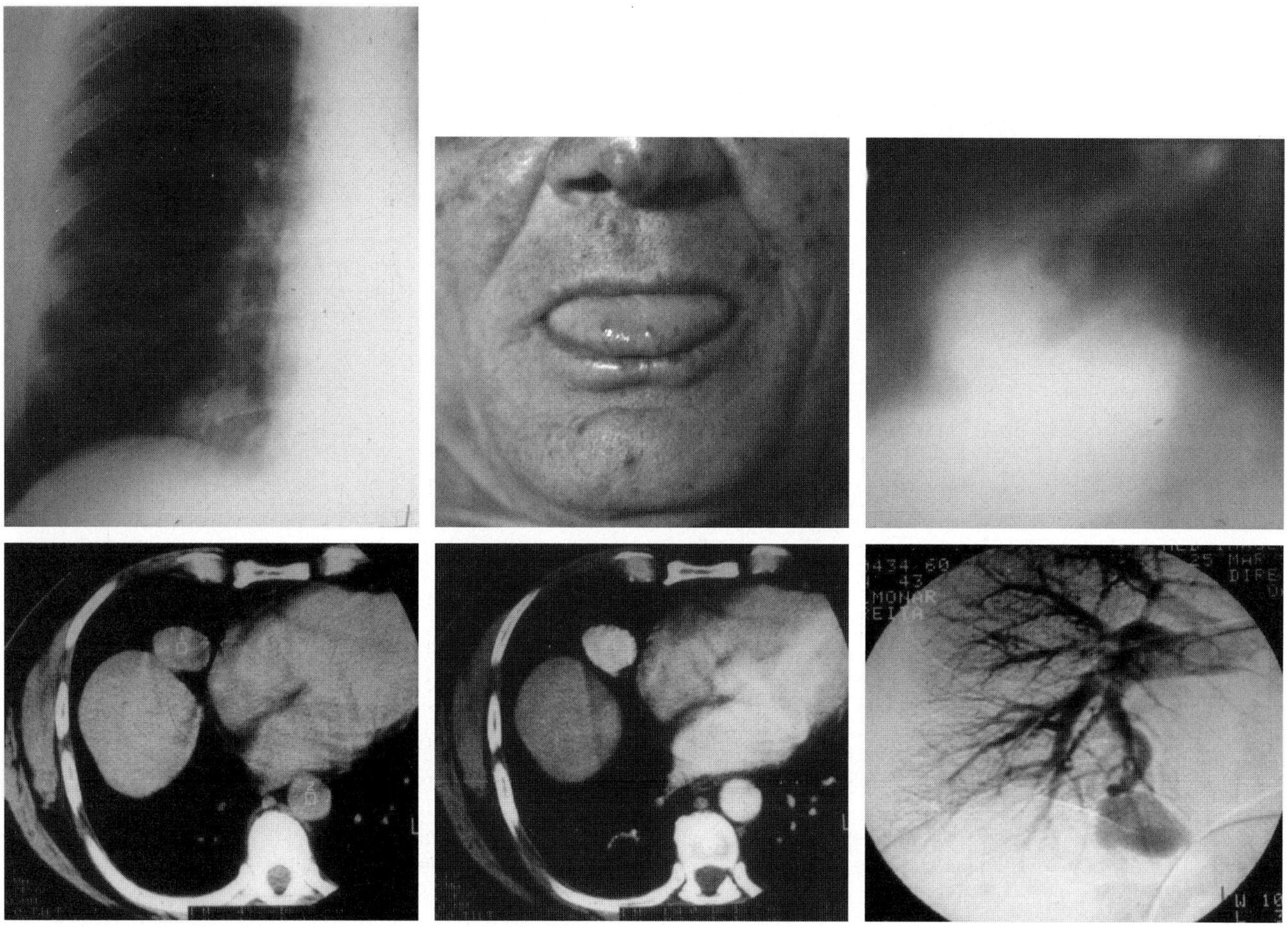

A, B C

D, E F

Figure 7.5

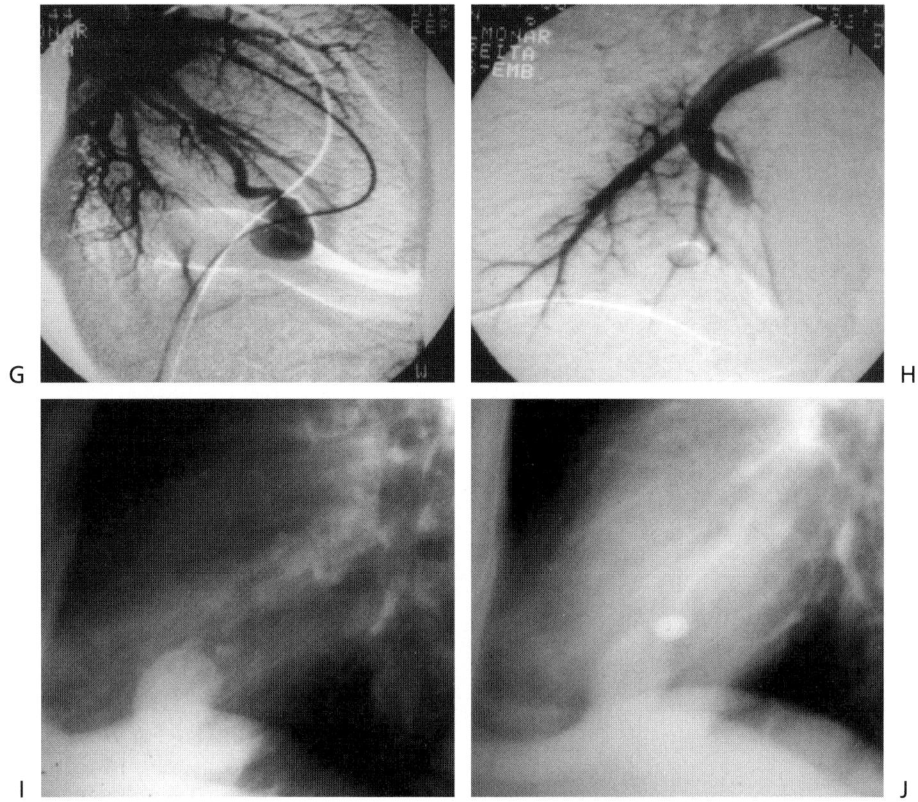

Figure 7.5 *(continued)*

A: Anteroposterior view of the chest shows the nodule near the right cardiophrenic angle. **B:** The face of the patient presented multiple telangiectasia in the tongue, lips, and face, which is consistent with the diagnosis of HHT. **C:** Conventional planigram shows the vascular aneurysm connected to efferent and afferent vessels. **D,E:** Pre- and postcontrast computed tomographic (CT) scans show the nodule enhanced with intravenous contrast injection. **F:** Anterior view of the pulmonary arteriogram demonstrates the (simple type) A-V fistula with a large aneurysm in the medial part of the middle lobe. **G:** Lateral view of the A-V fistula shows only one pulmonary feeding artery communicating through the aneurysm to a single draining vein in the later phase (not shown). **H:** Embolization performed with one detachable balloon in the single feeding artery resulted in total occlusion of the flow through the fistula. **I,J:** Lateral view of the chest shows the aneurysm before and after embolization. Note the balloon in **J**. Progressive reduction in aneurysm size was observed.

Comment: Pulmonary A-V malformations are uncommon lesions that can be treated by surgery or embolization. They are most commonly multiple but may be isolated. Clinical presentation is variable. Tiredness and shortness of breath are frequently the main symptoms and may result from chronic hypoxia or cardiac overload when there is a systemic shunt, or be of neurologic origin when there is paradoxic embolization. Pulmonary A-V fistulas are classified as simple or complex. The simple type has one feeding vessel and occurs in 79% of cases. The complex type has multiple feeding arteries and draining veins and occurs in 21% of cases. When the shunt is large, cyanosis develops, with digital clubbing, dyspnea, and polycythemia; however, there are no cardiac hemodynamic changes as seen in peripheral A-V fistulas.

The prognosis of untreated patients is poor, particularly when the condition is associated with HHT. Repeated epistaxis, hematuria, and hematemesis are relatively common among patients with HHT due to multiple telangiectasia. Pulmonary arterio-venous fistula (PAVF) may cause hemoptysis, pulmonary hematoma, hemothorax, and shock. Brain abscess and paradoxic embolism may be present in 33% to 41% of the patients with HHT and in 18% of patients without HHT.

Embolization with detachable balloons or Gianturco coils are equally efficient in controlling the shunts, with maximum preservation of the functional lung parenchyma. A selective and careful embolization procedure is necessary to minimize risks and complications. Complications include systemic coil embolization, premature balloon deflation, transient stroke, and myocardial puncture during procedure. Less common complications include persistent pneumothorax related to use of the occlusive spider and severe pulmonary hypertension related to coexistent hepatic A-V shunts. All symptomatic patients should undergo embolization or surgical treatment. All PAVFs over 3 mm in diameter also should be embolized, even if the patient is asymptomatic, to prevent strokes and brain abscesses.

7.6 Embolization In The Chest And Lungs

Case 7.6:

A 32-year-old woman with previously undiagnosed hereditary hemorrhagic telangectasia (HHT), chronic hypoxia, and adynamia presented with heart failure and a bruit over the liver and was referred for hepatic angiogram. Revision of a chest x-ray film taken at the other institution for examination of a postpartum hemothorax showed a large peripheral pulmonary nodule, which prompted the diagnosis of a pulmonary A-V fistula. Inspection of the patient's face showed multiple telangiectasia, and the history included recurrent nose bleeds since an earlier age.

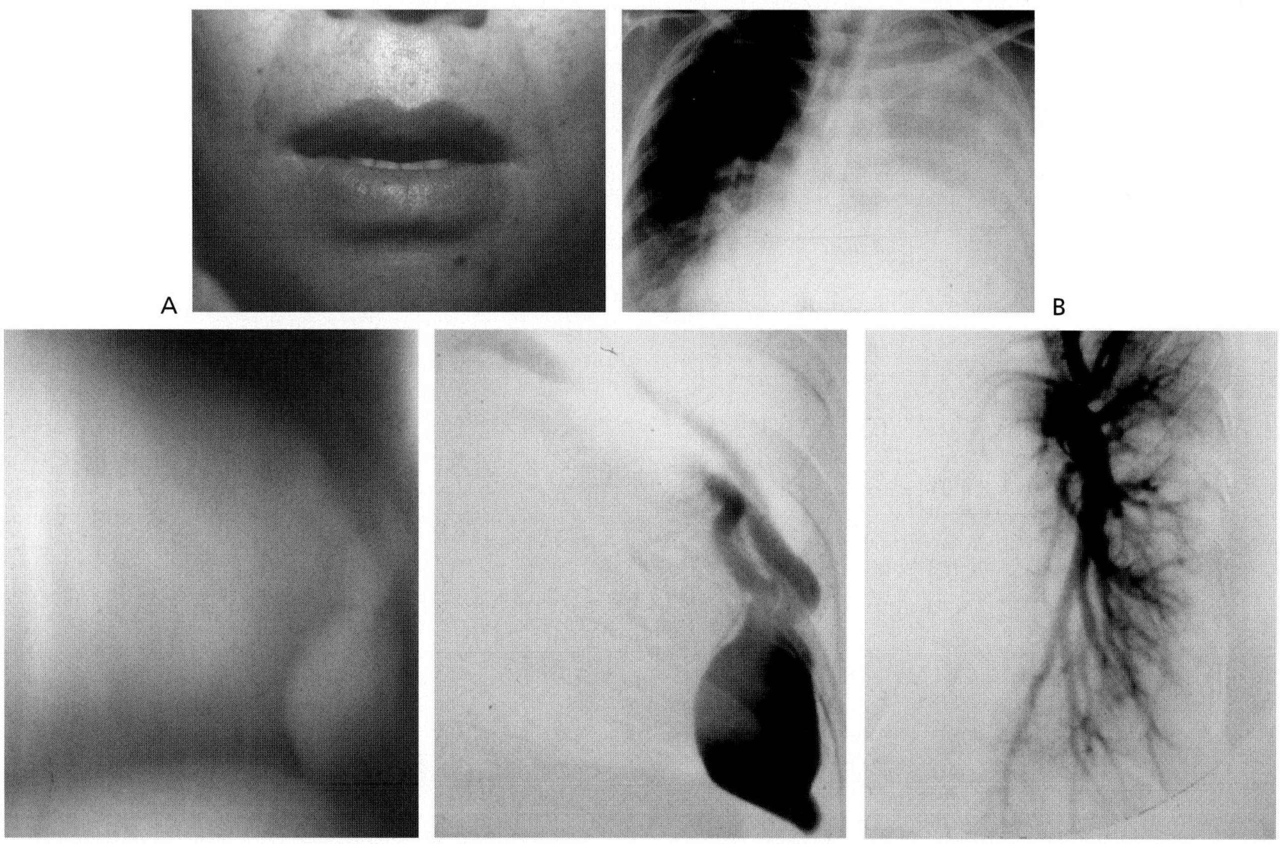

A B

C, D E

Figure 7.6

A: The patient's face presented multiple telangiectasia in the lips and face, which is consistent with the diagnosis of HHT. **B:** The chest x-ray film taken after delivery of her baby shows massive pleural fluid (hemothorax), which was drained with a large catheter at that time. **C:** Another chest x-ray film (not shown) and conventional planigram shows a peripheral nodule in the left lung. **D:** Pulmonary angiogram discloses an A-V fistula and aneurysm. **E:** Embolization was performed with a detachable balloon and security coil proximally. Pulmonary angiogram following embolization shows total occlusion of the fistula. **F,G:** Right hepatic artery arteriogram shows massive, enlarged, tortuous arteries and diffuse telangiectases (honeycomb parenchyma), and early filling of hepatic veins due to A-V shunts. Multiple collaterals from the superior mesenteric artery and adrenal arteries were connected with the main hepatic arteries. **H,I:** Left hepatic artery angiogram shows enlarged arteries and diffuse telangiectasis. Late phase shows A-V shunting with filling of hepatic veins **(I)**. **J,K:** Postembolization common hepatic angiogram shows remarkably reduced arterial flow through the liver, with reduction in A-V shunting. Segments V and VI were embolized with cyanoacrylate, and the rest of the liver was embolized with Ivalon 1,000 m in two stages. **L,M:** Histology of the liver shows massive telangiectasis, reduced capillaries and sinusoidal spaces, and direct connections between enlarged arteries and veins.

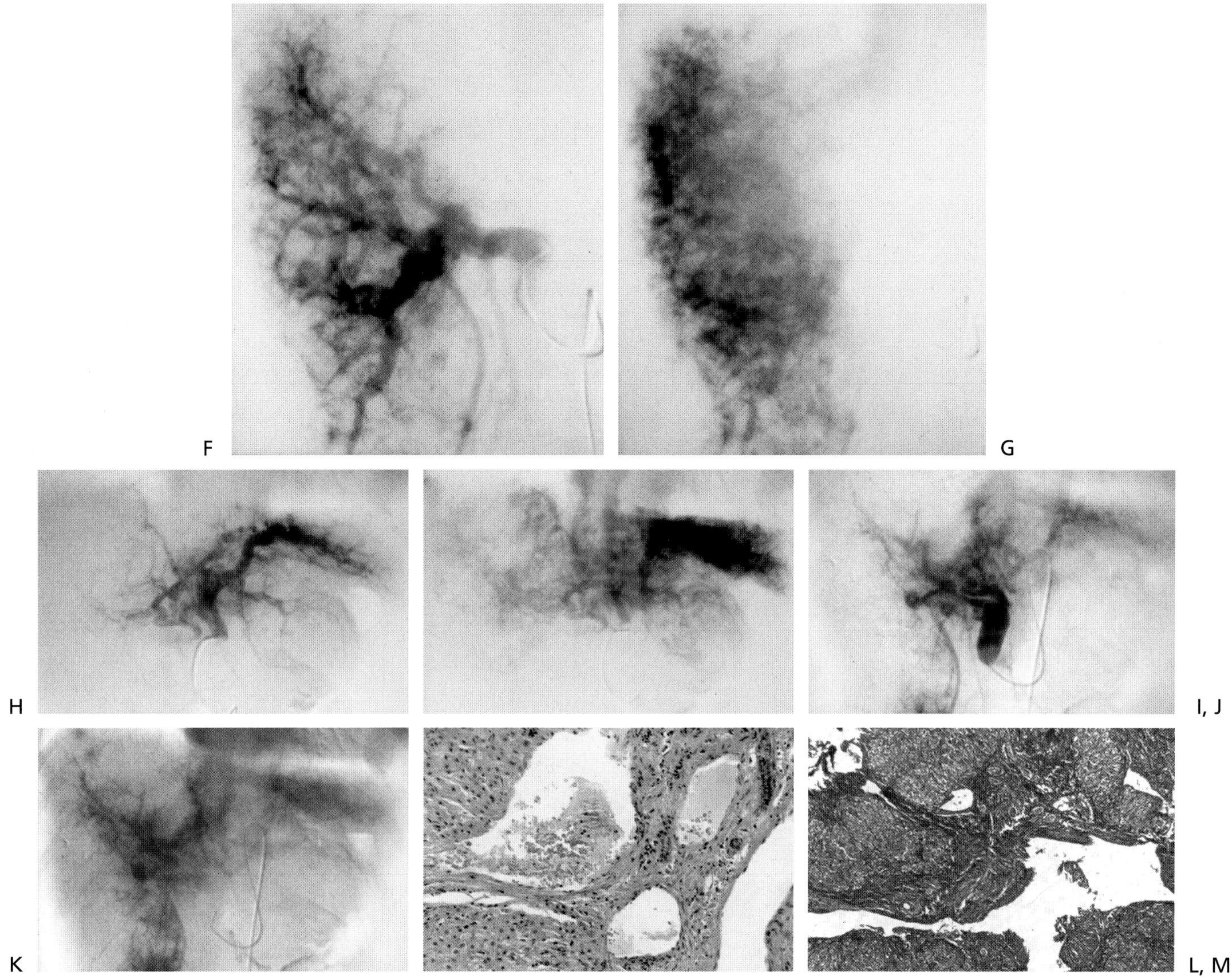

Figure 7.6 *(continued)*

Comment: HHT occurs more frequently than previously thought. It occurs in a variety of ethnic and racial groups, with a prevalence of 1 in 2,351 to 1 in 39,216 members of the population in one report and 1 in 100,000 in another report. The recognized manifestations of HHT are all due to abnormalities of the vascular structure, and telangiectasis are nearly universal. It is estimated that 60% of persons with pulmonary A-V malformations have HHT. Conversely, it is estimated that overall 5% to 15% of persons with HHT have pulmonary A-V malformations. Hepatic involvement occurs in 8% to 31% of cases. Pulmonary A-V malformations result in direct right-to-left shunts and may produce profound dyspnea, fatigue, cyanosis, or polycythemia. Liver A-V fistulas and telangiectases cause cardiac overload and heart failure with bruit. Current experience is much more extensive with pulmonary A-V malformation embolization. There is only half a dozen reported cases of embolized liver A-V fistulas. Embolization of the liver should be performed with larger than usual particles. For massive A-V fistulas, Gianturco coils can be used. For small-vessel, diffuse hepatic telangiectases with fistulas, 1.0-mm diameter Ivalon particles appear to work satisfactorily. Hepatic infarction has been reported following hepatic embolization treatment for HHT involvement. Another complication is ischemia of adjacent bowel structures, with development of ulcers and bleeding. Ivalon radiolabeled with technetium 99m (99mTc)–sulfur colloid can be used to evaluate the size of hepatic A-V fistulas, for proper selection of the size of the embolic material. Intrahepatic A-V fistulas appear to be subject to hormonal influence, and there is at least one report of two cases of functionally reversible hepatic A-V fistulas during pregnancy in patients with HHT. The patients recovered spontaneously after delivery, and congestive heart failure resolved within 6 months.

7.7 Embolization In The Chest And Lungs

Case 7.7:

A 35-year-old woman was treated surgically 7 years before the current admission for an ectopic pregnancy that caused severe hypotension and blood loss. At that time, a central venous catheter was inserted into the subclavian vein as a bedside procedure. The puncture reportedly was difficult, and advancement of the catheter was very hard. On the current admission, the patient complained of cervical edema, venous congestion, and exertional dyspnea due to heart failure. A cervical bruit was heard on physical examination. Angiography and possible treatment were requested.

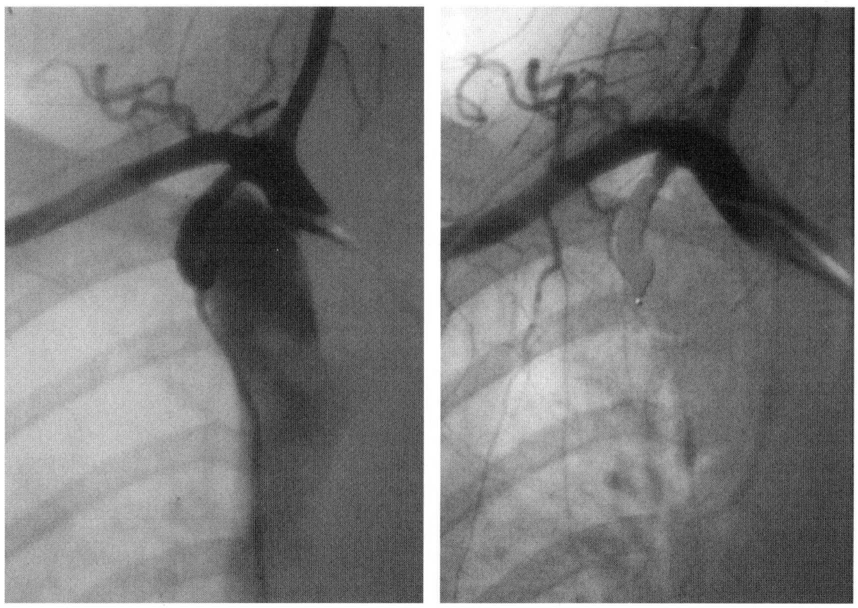

Figure 7.7

A: Right subclavian artery angiogram shows an A-V fistula between the IMA and brachiocephalic vein. Note the massive enlargement of the vein. **B:** Postembolization angiogram shows complete occlusion of the A-V fistula. A detachable latex balloon was used for embolization. Note bulging of the balloon at the fistulous rent and retrograde filling of the distal IMA, but total occlusion of the fistula.

Comment: Because of the close relationship between the IMA and subclavian and brachiocephalic veins, infraclavicular punctures with large-bore needles pose the risk of vein and artery laceration with subsequent bleeding or A-V fistula formation. To lacerate the IMA and the brachiocephalic vein at the same time, the stick has to be medial. Pneumothorax also is a risk for a puncture at that location. A-V fistulas involving the IMA may develop with neoplasms, trauma, and iatrogenic lesions. Mastectomy, indwelling pericardial catheters, sternotomy, and central venous cannulation are the main iatrogenic causes of this type of fistula. Many complications following central venous cannulation have been described, but A-V fistulas are relatively rare. In the few cases reported in the literature, surgery has been the main form of treatment. Embolization has been used in a few cases, and coils are the most frequent embolic agents used. Smaller embolic agents are not useful for this situation of high-flow, high-pressure A-V fistula, because these smaller agents would pass through the fistula and result in pulmonary embolization. Detachable balloons are flow oriented and permit fluoroscopic monitoring of the occlusion of the fistula through injection of dye through the guiding catheter, thus allowing adequate positioning of the balloon, preserving the main vasculature, and obviating surgical treatment. Although detachable coils are now available, we do not have sufficient experience in using them to treat A-V fistulas. Usually an 8F guiding catheter is used for balloon deployment, which requires that it be exchanged over a long guidewire. Superselective catheterization usually is not necessary due to the flow orientation, and only proximal positioning of the guiding catheter is required. Central venous access in the neck should be performed through the internal jugular vein and under ultrasound guidance.

7.8 Embolization In The Chest And Lungs

Case 7.8:

A 26-year-old immunocompromised woman presented with herpes zoster, diarrhea, dehydration, retinal detachment, and herpetic encephalitis. General therapeutic measures included placement of an intravenous central catheter through the right subclavian vein while she was in the intensive care unit. Difficult manipulation during the subclavian vein puncture led to mediastinal and intrathoracic bleeding. A chest x-ray film showed a large apical mass with intrathoracic extension and lateral displacement of the trachea. CT scan showed the mass to have mixed densities consistent with a large blood clot (hematoma). The patient was referred for angiography. She presented in a combative state and in poor condition, and she required general anesthesia for the procedure.

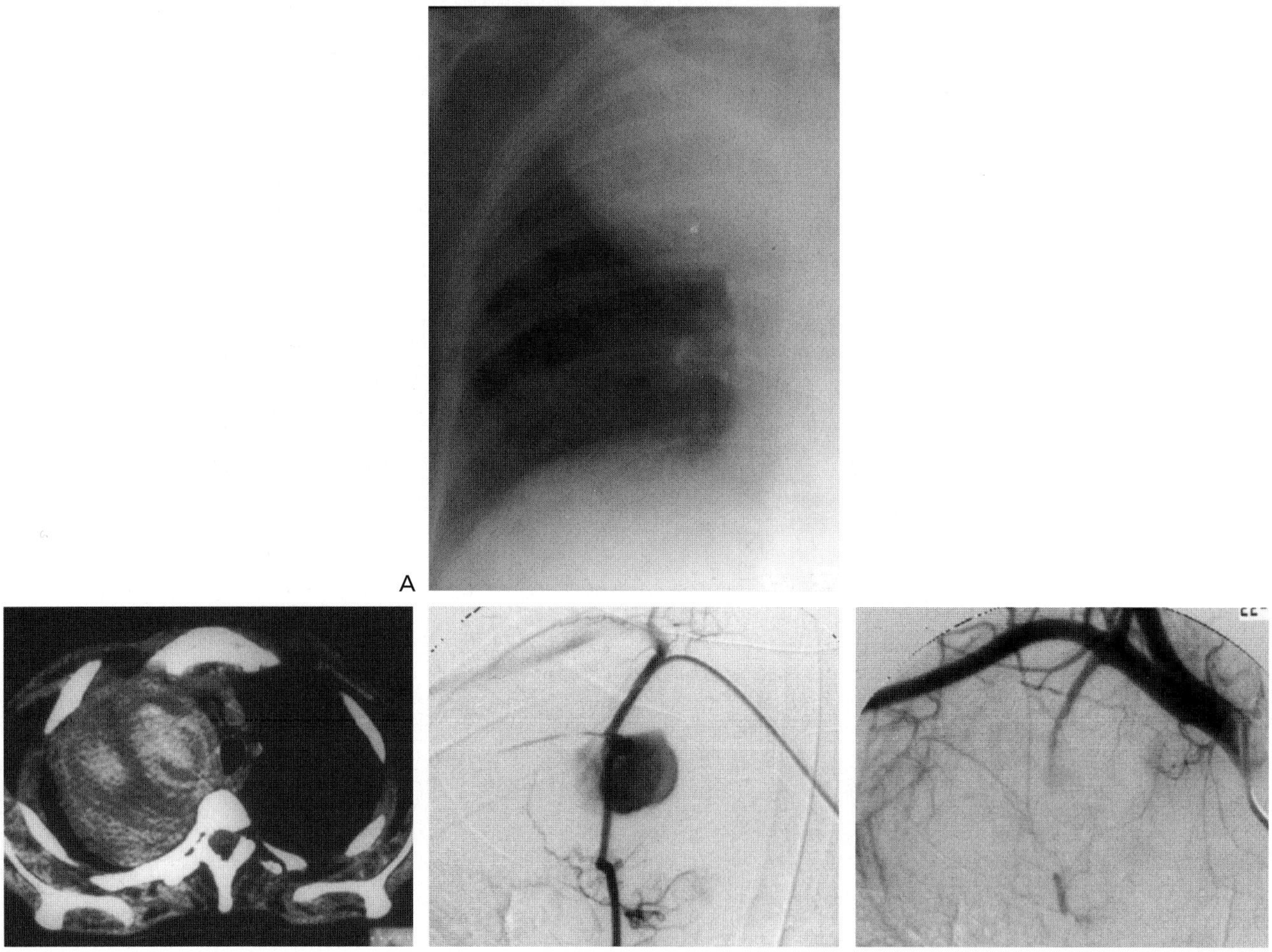

A

B, C

D

Figure 7.8

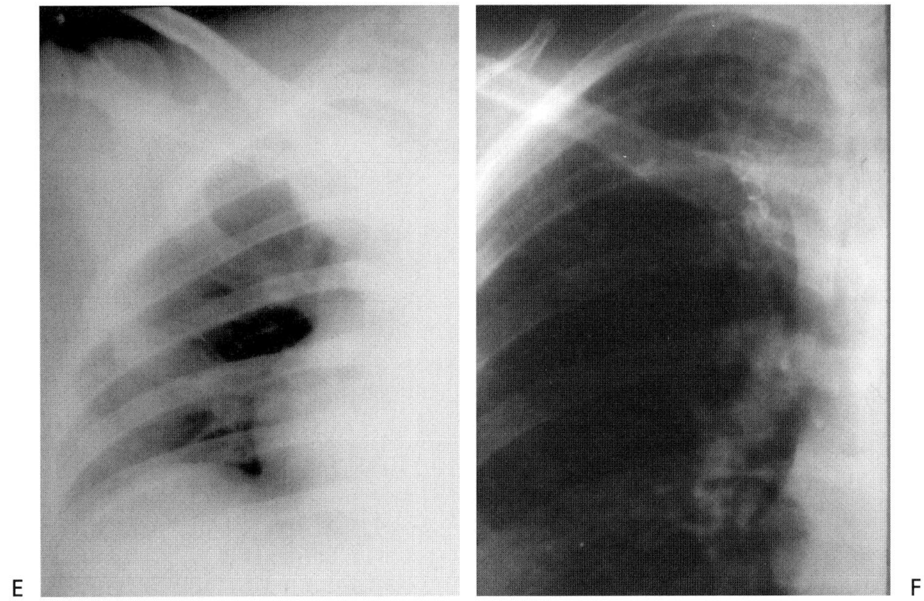

Figure 7.8 *(continued)*

A: Chest x-ray film shows a large apical mass displacing the trachea. **B:** CT scan shows the mass to have mixed densities inside, which is consistent with a hematoma and a central pseudoaneurysm. **C:** Emergency arteriogram shows a large pseudoaneurysm arising from the right IMA. **D:** Embolization with a Gianturco coil was performed, resulting in total occlusion of the IMA and the pseudoaneurysm. **E:** Chest x-ray film obtained about 1 month after embolization shows reduction mass size. The coil is barely seen inside the mass. Note extensive pleural effusion. **F:** Chest x-ray film obtained about 6 months after embolization shows complete resolution of the upper mediastinal mass. The patient was discharged about 2 months after embolization and was doing well.

Comment: This case posed a difficult problem of a very sick, noncooperative patient in an emergent situation. The hematoma was progressively enlarging, causing a drop in hematocrit and clinical deterioration that precluded surgical treatment. The diagnosis of the pseudoaneurysm was made by CT scan, and embolization was achieved easily by selective catheterization. The IMA was occluded by a spring coil. It is important to note that the coil was positioned along the IMA, occluding it below and above the pseudoaneurysm site, thus preventing retrograde filling of the pseudoaneurysm. Gelfoam and Ivalon are useful for smaller arteries, but for the size of artery in this case they are not indicated because of the potential for recanalization and the risk of inadequate occlusion. Little information on IMA trauma is available in the literature, and it should be noted that other percutaneous transthoracic interventions, such as biopsy and drainage procedures, may cause IMA lesions.

7.9 Embolization In The Chest And Lungs

Case 7.9:

A 49-year-old man presented with a thoracic wall mass, which biopsy revealed to be a myosarcoma. Embolization was requested as a preoperative measure.

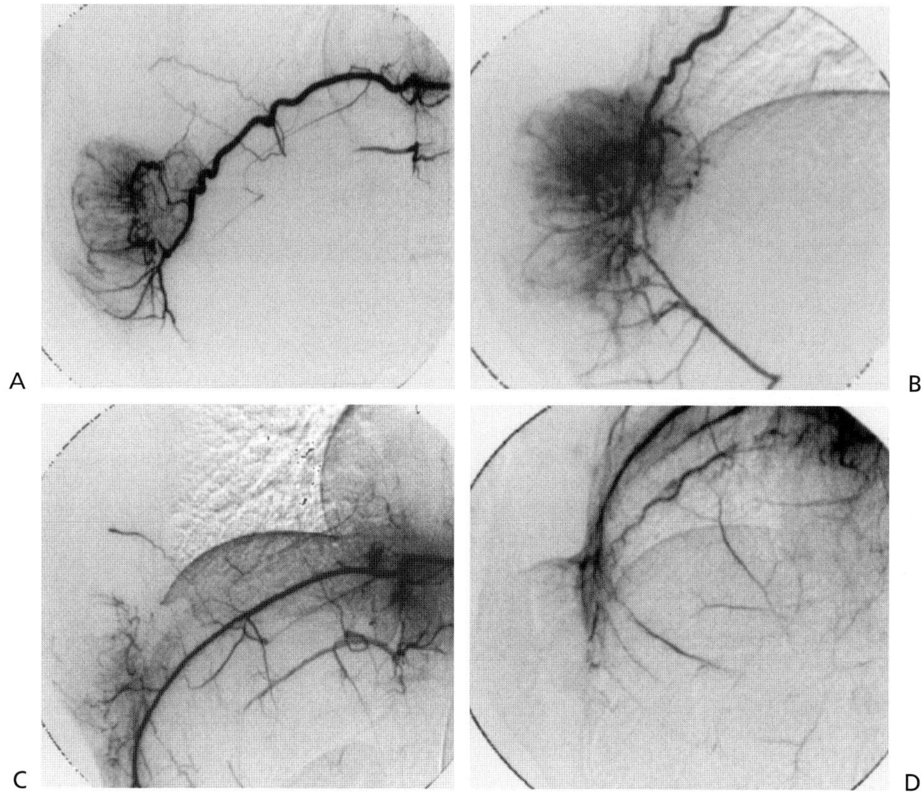

Figure 7.9

A,B: Selective angiograms performed at the eighth and ninth intercostal arteries show a large hypervascular mass in the thoracic wall, originating from the intercostal muscles. **C,D:** Postembolization angiogram above and below the level of the tumor shows marked reduction in the vasculature of the tumor. Ivalon 100 m was used for embolization.

Comment: The soft tissue mass presented by this patient required a large excision; therefore, embolization was performed as a preoperative measure. Remarkable control of bleeding was achieved with embolization. Pathologic examination after resection revealed nonviable cells. In a resectable tumoral lesion such as this, surgery is the only alternative; however, embolization may be an important aid in the management of the tumor, reducing blood loss and facilitating the surgical procedure. Embolization in similar lesions should be performed with nonabsorbable materials such as Ivalon. Gelfoam can be used more proximally to initiate or accelerate thrombosis. Devascularization may be so extensive that the tumor histology may not be recognizable following embolization.

Suggested Reading

Buscarini E, Buscarini L, Civardi G, et al. Hepatic vascular malformations in hereditary hemorrhagic telangiectasia: imaging findings. *AJR* 1994;163:1105–1110.

Derauf BJ, Hunter DW, Sirr SA, et al. Peripheral embolization of diffuse hepatic arteriovenous malformations in a patient with hereditary hemorrhagic telangiectasia. *Cardiovasc Intervent Radiol* 1987;10:80–83.

Dutton JA, Jackson JE, Hughes JM, et al. Pulmonary arteriovenous malformations: results of treatment with coil embolization in 53 patients. *AJR* 1995;165:1119–1125.

Gothlin JH, Nordgard K, Jonsson K, et al. Hepatic telangiectasia in Osler's disease treated with arterial embolization. Report of 2 cases. *Eur J Radiol* 1982;2:27–30.

Guttmacher AE, Marchuk DA, White RI. Hereditary hemorrhagic telangiectasia. *N Engl J Med* 1995;333:918–924.

Haitjenma T, ten Berg JM, Overtoom TT, et al. Unusual complications after embolization of a pulmonary arteriovenous malformation. *Chest* 1996;109:1401–1404.

Hardy C, Wong J, Young JN, et al. Balloon occlusion scintigraphy of aortopulmonary collaterals. *Pediatr Cardiol* 1994;15:241–245.

Hartnell GG, Jackson JE, Allison DJ. Coil embolization of pulmonary arteriovenous malformations. *Cardiovasc Intervent Radiol* 1990;13:347–350.

John PR, Procter AE. Bronchial artery embolization for life threatening haemoptysis from an iatrogenic chronic pulmonary abscess. *Clin Radiol* 1992;46:206–208.

Krowka MJ. Hepatopulmonary syndrome: what are we learning from interventional radiology, liver transplantation, and other disorders? *Gastroenterology* 1995;109:1009–1013.

Livneh A, Langevitz P, Morag B. et al. Functionally reversible hepatic arteriovenous fistulas during pregnancy in patients with hereditary hemorrhagic telangiectasia. *South Med J* 1988;81:1047–1049.

Lois JF, Gomes AS, Smith DC, et al. Systemic-to-pulmonary collateral vessels and shunts: treatment with embolization. *Radiology* 1988;169:671–676.

Moura R, Uflacker R, Yoshida WB, et al. Arteriovenous fistula between the right internal mammary artery and the subclavian vein: percutaneous closure with detachable balloon-catheter embolization. *Cardiovasc Surg* 1993;1:86–88.

Parker JA, Drum DE, Feldstein ML, et al. Lung scan evaluation of thrombolytic therapy for pulmonary embolism. *J Nucl Med* 1995;36:364–368.

Ramakantan R, Bandekar V, Gandhi M, et al. Massive hemoptysis due to pulmonary tuberculosis: control with bronchial artery embolization. *Radiology* 1996;200:691–694.

Remy-Jardin M, Wattinne L, Remy J. Transcatheter occlusion of pulmonary arterial circulation and collateral supply: failures, incidents, and complications. *Radiology* 1991;180:699–705.

René M, Sans J, Dominguez J, et al. Unilateral pulmonary artery agenesis presenting with hemoptysis: treatment by embolization of systemic collaterals. *Cardiovasc Intervent Radiol* 1995;18:251–254.

Roman CF, Cha SD, Incarvito J, et al. Transcatheter embolization of hepatic arteriovenous fistula in Osler-Weber-Rendu disease: a case report. *Angiology* 1987;38:483–488.

Uflacker R. Case of a patient with hemoptysis who suffered a bronchial embolization. *Cardiovasc Intervent Radiol* 1990;13:387.

Uflacker R, Kaemmerer A, Neves C, et al. Management of massive hemoptysis by bronchial artery embolization. *Radiology* 1983;146:627–634.

Uflacker R, Kaemmerer A, Picon PD, et al. Bronchial artery embolization in the management of hemoptysis: technical aspects and long-term results. *Radiology* 1985;157:637–644.

Uflacker R, Mourao GS, Piske RL. Treating complications of subclavian vein puncture by embolization of the internal mammary artery. *Cardiovasc Intervent Radiol* 1991;14:115–117.

Wedzicha JA, Pearson MC. Management of massive haemoptysis. *Respir Med* 1990;84:9–12.

White RI, Lynch-Nyhan A, Terry PB, et al. Pulmonary arteriovenous malformations: techniques and long-term outcome of embolotherapy. *Radiology* 1988;169:663–669.

White RI, Mitchell SE, Barth KH, et al. Angioarchitecture of pulmonary arteriovenous malformations: an important consideration before embolotherapy. *AJR* 1983;140:681–686.

Whiting JH, Morton KA, Datz FL, et al. Embolization of hepatic arteriovenous malformations using radiolabeled and non radiolabeled polyvinyl alcohol sponge in a patient with hereditary hemorrhagic telangiectasia: case report. *J Nucl Med* 1992;33:260–262.

Wong KP, Young N, Marksen G. Bronchial artery embolization to control haemoptysis. *Australas Radiol* 1994:38;256–259.

Yedlicka JW, Bjarnason H, Hunter DW, et al. Persistent pneumothorax following embolization of a pulmonary arteriovenous malformation. *J Vasc Interv Radiol* 1994;5:887–889.

CHAPTER 8

Embolization In Trauma

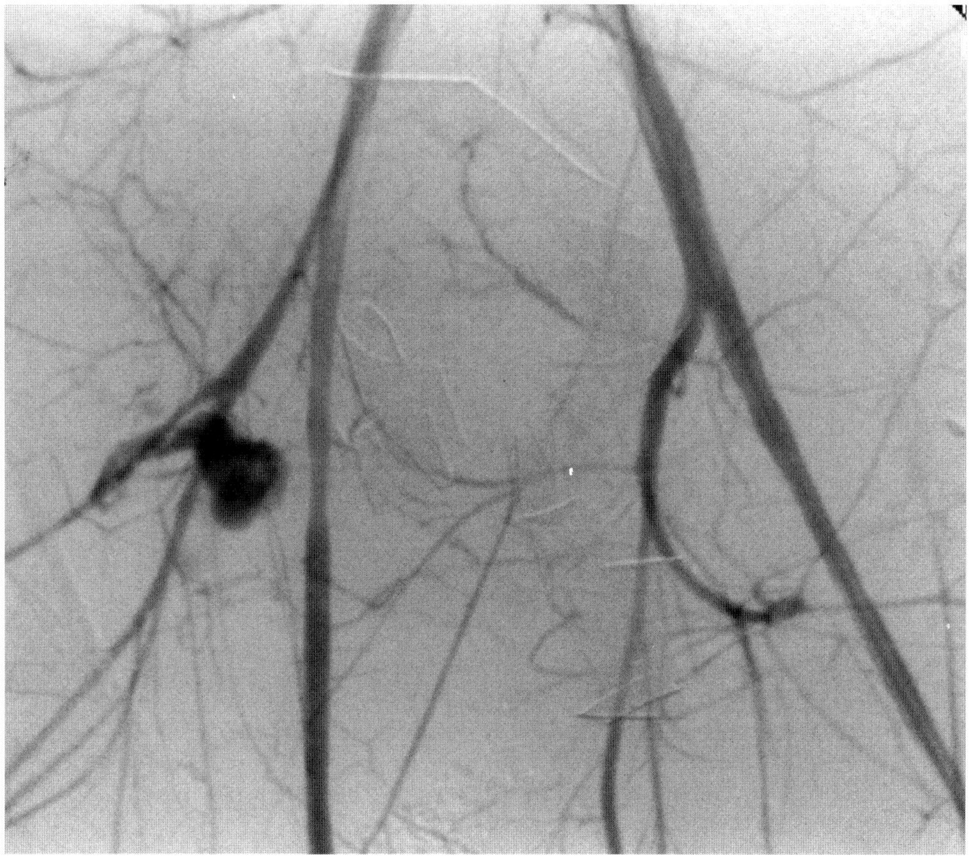

8.1 Embolization In Trauma

Case 8.1:

A 24-year-old man (weight approximately 200 lb) with gunshot injuries to the pelvis and right leg underwent exploratory surgery of the pelvis. No obvious arterial bleed was noted. The patient's hemodynamic condition worsened, which necessitated 8 units of packed red blood cells transfusion. Emergent angiogram and treatment were requested.

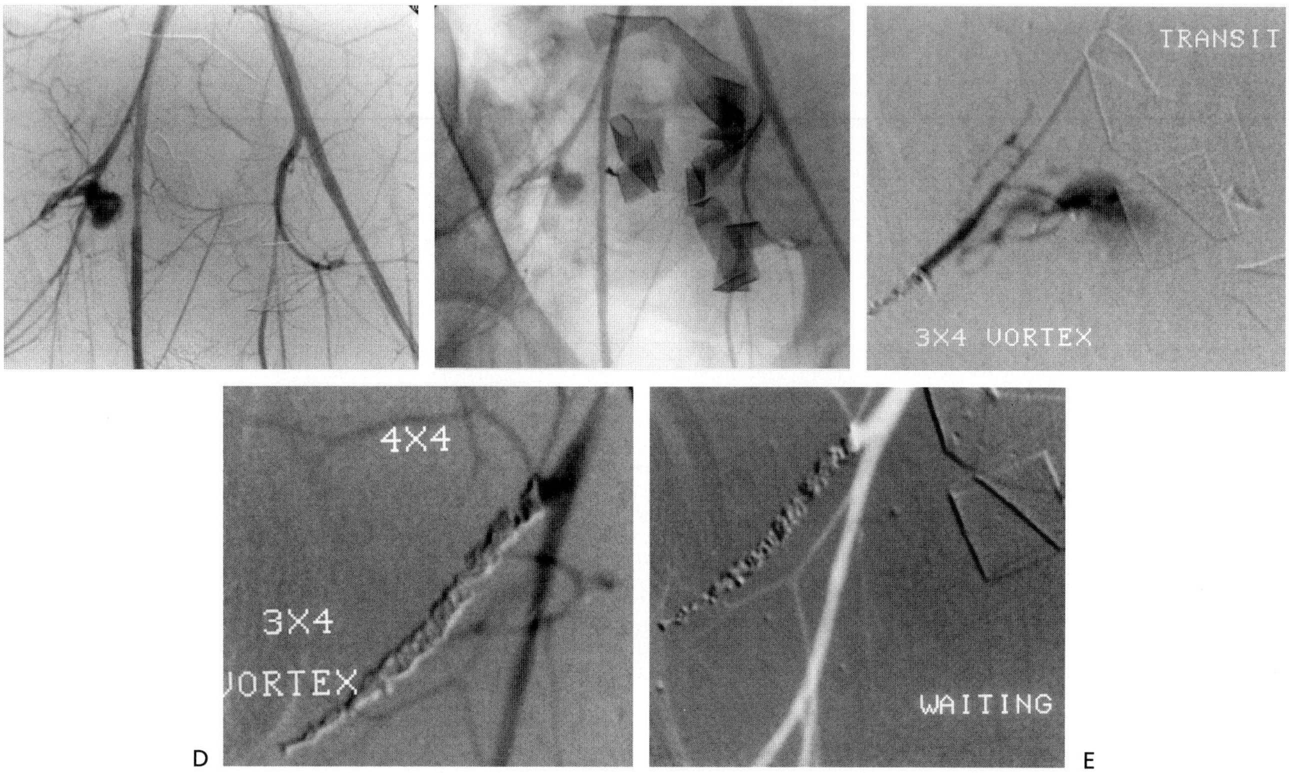

A, B C D E

Figure 8.1

A,B: Oblique view of the pelvis arteriogram with subtraction and bone windows shows active extravasation from the superior gluteal artery branch arising off the right internal iliac artery. Note the small caliber of the patient's arteries in comparison to his size, which reveals worsening shock and hypovolemic state. Through a 5F vascular sheath, a Omniflush catheter was used for pelvic angiography and subsequently helped in selecting the ipsilateral internal iliac artery by pulling the catheter down with the assistance of a soft-tip guidewire. **C:** An Omniflush catheter was exchanged over the wire for a 5F Cobra catheter, which was used to select the internal iliac artery. A smaller 3F Transit catheter was advanced into the gluteal artery. Angiogram shows the bleeding site. The catheter was advanced past the site of trauma into the superior gluteal artery. Multiple platinum vortex microcoils were placed distal to the lesion to cause obstruction and prevent collateral flow feeding of the lesion. **D:** Additional microcoils of larger dimension were placed proximally, covering the lesion site. Longer coils were not available at the time of the procedure. Injection shows a small amount of flow through the coils. **E:** Coagulation occurred after about 5 minutes, and the branch vessel was effectively occluded. Contralateral angiogram (not shown) was obtained to exclude collateral branches feeding the lesion site, as well as other bleeders.

Comment: Contrary to the traditional recommendation of using Gelfoam for embolization of vessels with traumatic tears or pseudoaneurysms, we advocate using coil embolization alone or with Gelfoam for massive bleedings, such as in this case. In two of our multiple cases of pelvic embolization for trauma, rebleeding occurred at or near the vessels that were embolized with Gelfoam alone and required a second embolization. These critically ill patients cannot tolerate continued bleeding often associated with other injuries; hence, it is important to embolize identifiable injuries in the initial setting. Thus, we advocate a more aggressive use of coil embolization. After the injured artery is identified, the microcatheter should be advanced carefully, past the extravasation site or pseudoaneurysm, and then the vessel should be packed with coils up to and proximal to the lesion. If the coils are not packed closely, there is a possibility of recanalization and rebleeding. Another useful technique is to use the "coil–Gelfoam sandwich," which is combination of Gelfoam packed between coils placed distal to and proximal to the lesion site. This technique, which is a modification of the "coil blockade" technique described by Panetta and Sclafani, allows selective isolation and occlusion of the injured vessel while sparing the distal collateral circulation.

8.2 Embolization In Trauma

Case 8.2:

A 45-year-old male patient underwent coronary angioplasty and stent placement, which was followed by a groin hematoma extending into the retroperitoneal area. A lesion in the femoral artery was suspected. Emergency arteriography was requested for possible embolization or stent graft placement.

A

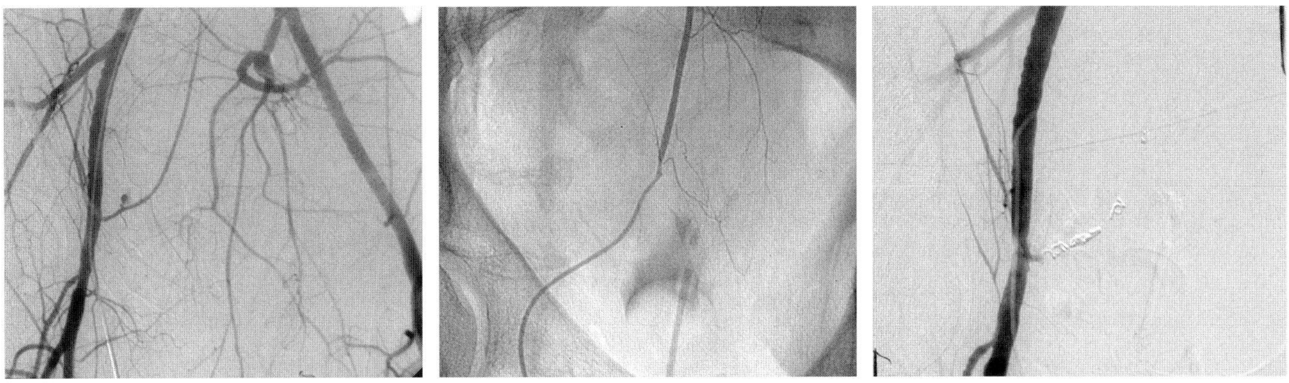

B, C

Figure 8.2

A: Pelvic arteriogram performed in the anteroposterior and oblique views shows the femoral and external iliac arteries are intact. A pseudoaneurysm was identified at the proximal segment of the right inferior epigastric artery, resulting from a very high femoral puncture. **B:** A KUMP catheter was used to selectively catheterize the inferior epigastric artery in an antegrade fashion. Embolization was performed with minicoils above and below the level of the pseudoaneurysm. **C:** Follow-up arteriogram of the right iliac artery shows occlusion of the inferior epigastric artery. Control of the bleeding was achieved. Pressure was held at the groin after the catheter was removed, and the patient did well.

Comment: Lesions in the common femoral artery, such as pseudoaneurysms and extravasations, are not common in conventional diagnostic angiography using the femoral approach. Development of more sophisticated interventional procedures requiring larger introducer catheters and full anticoagulation led to a more frequent rate of complications. Procedure-related complications are groin hematomas and, less frequently, pseudoaneurysms. Higher punctures at the level of the inguinal ligament or above may cause retroperitoneal hematomas. It is unusual for a high puncture to tear the inferior epigastric artery. Hematomas originating from that artery will spread in the retroperitoneal space and anterior abdominal wall, and they may be severe in course. Embolization of this type of complication is performed easily and controls the bleeding in most situations. The safety of femoral puncture is based on entrance into the common femoral artery below the inguinal ligament where the pulse is palpated best and the artery can be easily compressed for hemostasis. Occasionally, the inferior epigastric artery loop overlies the common femoral artery, and inadvertent puncture or laceration can be responsible for severe, unrecognized bleeding. The middle to lower common femoral artery should be chosen for safe puncture. Pseudoaneurysms of the common femoral artery are larger and not amenable to embolization, but they may be treated with compression using an ultrasound probe, thrombin injection or stent-graft placement. The use of closure devices reduced complications in fully heparinized patients.

8.3 Embolization In Trauma

Case 8.3:

A 55-year-old male patient was in a motorcycle accident and suffered head and pelvic trauma. Surgery for fixation of the pelvic fractures was performed. The patient developed symptoms of active pelvic bleeding while in the intensive care unit, and an emergency arteriogram for possible embolization was requested.

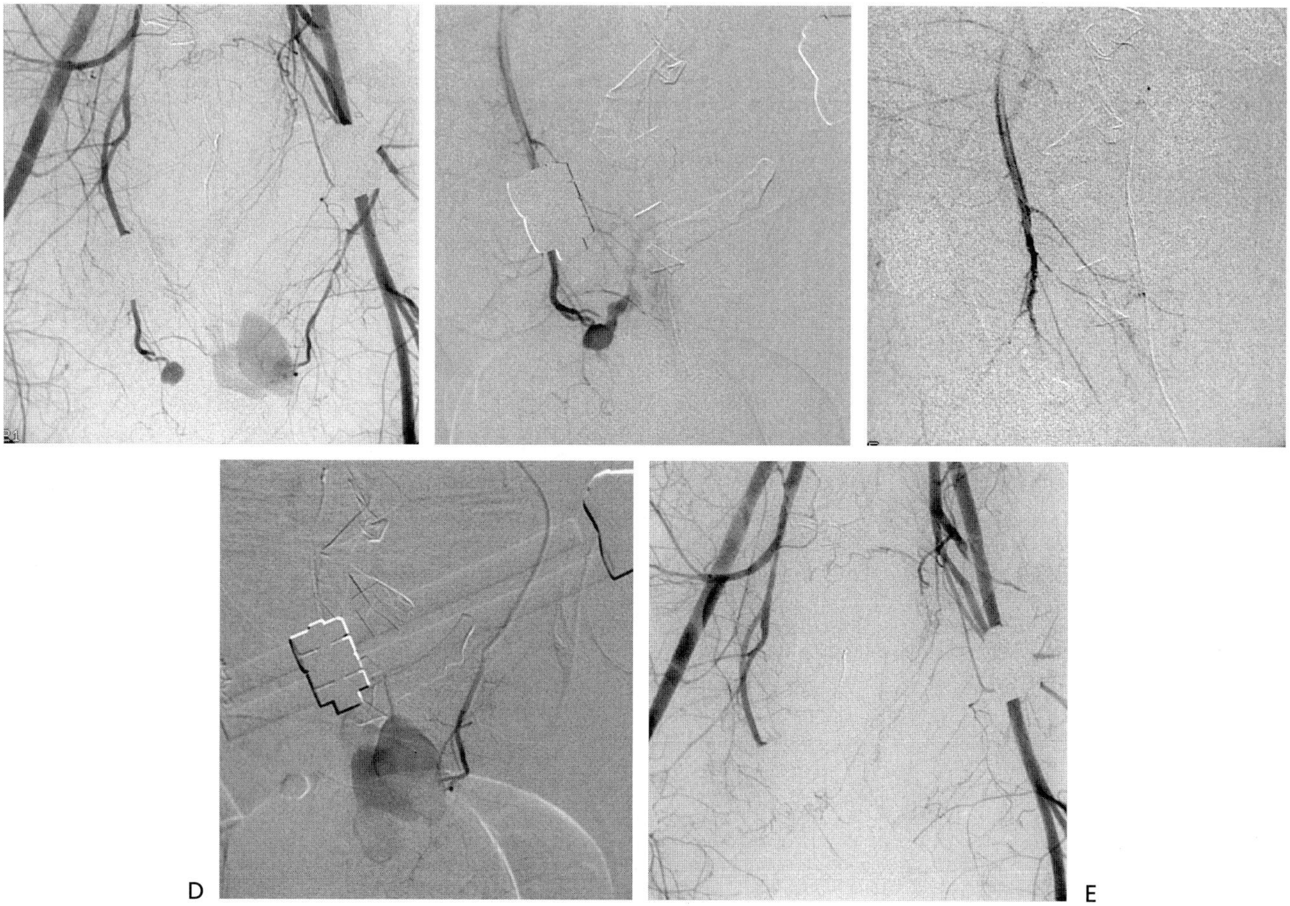

A, B C D E

Figure 8.3

A: Pelvic arteriogram shows bilateral active bleeding from the obturator arteries. Note the metal densities over the vessels due to the fixation devices. **B:** Selective injection in the anterior branches of the right internal iliac shows bleeding from the right obturator artery. **C:** Embolization with coils and Gelfoam resulted in total occlusion of the obturator artery. **D:** Contralateral injection of the left obturator artery shows massive active bleeding. Embolization with microcoils and Gelfoam was performed. **E:** Follow-up angiogram after embolization shows total occlusion with complete control of the bleeding, which allowed the patient to recover from the brain injury in a hemodynamically stable condition.

Comment: Pelvic fractures are common injuries of modern times; the majority are associated with motor vehicle accidents. The mortality rate is high, ranging from 5% to 25%. Complications, such as retroperitoneal hemorrhage, resulting from fractures of the pelvis may increase morbidity and mortality. The result of surgical ligation of the pelvic arteries for bleeding control have been very disappointing because of the extensive collateral arterial supply. The retroperitoneal space has an extraordinary capacity for accommodating large extravascular collections, and hypovolemia develops rapidly without other obvious symptoms. Embolization was attempted and proved useful for controlling pelvic bleeding in the early 1970s.

Diagnostic angiography should be used early in the course of complicated pelvic fractures or surgery, and embolization should be the natural extension of the procedure. Access through the usual femoral route may be difficult due to groin hematomas, making femoral pulse palpation difficult. A pelvic arteriogram should begin the survey, with the catheter located above the aortic bifurcation. However, a negative pelvic arteriogram is not sufficient to exclude bleeding. Small sites of bleeding can be visualized only with selective injections. The most frequent area of bleeding in the pelvis is the symphysis pubis; therefore, this area should be surveyed carefully. Selective hypogastric injections are mandatory, and extravasations should be embolized immediately with microcoils and/or Gelfoam. Coil embolization must be distal to reduce collateral filling of the distal vessels. More proximal occlusion should be performed with larger Gelfoam fragments. Arteriovenous (A-V) fistulas are encountered occasionally and should be addressed in a different manner, i.e., with a nonabsorbable occluding device and deployed very close to the vascular rent.

8.4 Embolization In Trauma

Case 8.4:

A 40-year-old female patient was in a motor vehicle accident and suffered a severe pelvic injury in the symphysis pubis. Surgery for fixation of the pelvic fracture was performed. Active pelvic bleeding developed 4 days after surgery, and an emergency arteriogram was requested for possible embolization.

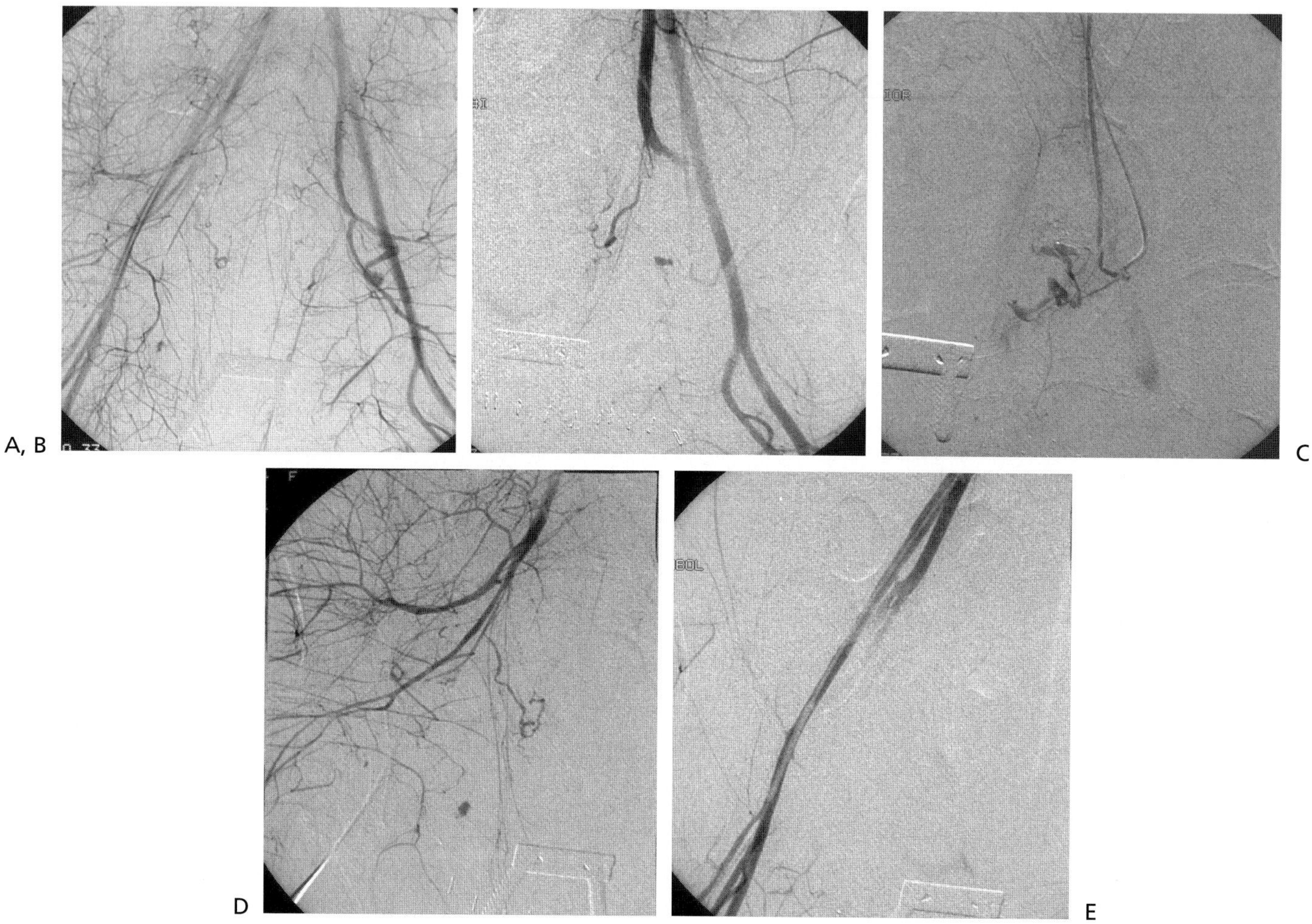

Figure 8.4

A: Pelvic arteriogram shows two areas of extravasation from the right and left internal iliac arteries. **B:** Postembolization angiogram of the left internal iliac artery shows a smaller but persistent area of bleeding originating from the left inferior epigastric artery, a branch of the distal external iliac artery. **C:** Selective injection into the left inferior epigastric artery shows bleeding from medial pubic branches. Embolization with Gelfoam was performed and controlled the bleeding. **D:** Selective right internal iliac angiogram shows a small but persistent point of bleeding that also was embolized with Gelfoam. **E:** A very selective catheterization was not possible, and the right internal iliac artery was embolized with Gelfoam, which controlled the bleeding.

Comment: Transcatheter embolization in pelvic trauma is indicated whenever angiography shows contrast extravasation occurring after accidental or surgical trauma. Angiography is indicated when there is clinical evidence of massive hemorrhage in the retroperitoneal space in patients with known pelvic fracture who fail to respond to initial volume replacement or when there is clinical evidence of bleeding in the soft tissues surrounding the area of trauma. When there is an unusual amount of bleeding from the wound in patients who recently underwent orthopedic surgery, a serious pelvic bleeding should be suspected.

Although the mortality of patients with pelvic bleeding continues to be high after embolization, it is mostly related to other injuries or complications and failure of other body systems. After embolization, there is a definite improvement in the rate of bleeding, and blood requirements usually are reduced to a minimum.

The arteries chosen for occlusion are preferably those showing active extravasation during examination. If anatomic considerations prevent superselective catheterization and embolization, the entire hypogastric artery may be closed off on the bleeding side. This may be done when several hypogastric branches are bleeding simultaneously and the patient cannot withstand a prolonged procedure. Ischemia of some pelvic organs may be disastrous, and potential nervous damage with sciatic paralysis with drop foot is a important complication that must be weighed against the morbidity and mortality of the bleeding.

8.5 Embolization In Trauma

Case 8.5:

A 52-year-old male patient was in a motor vehicle accident and suffered a severe pelvic injury involving both hips. There was severe disruption of the right hip with displacement of the head of the femur. A previous surgical attempt to fix the right hip was not successful, and the patient was transferred to our institution. Surgery for fixation of the pelvic fracture was to be performed, but we were requested to place an occlusion balloon catheter to reduce the risks of massive bleeding.

A, B

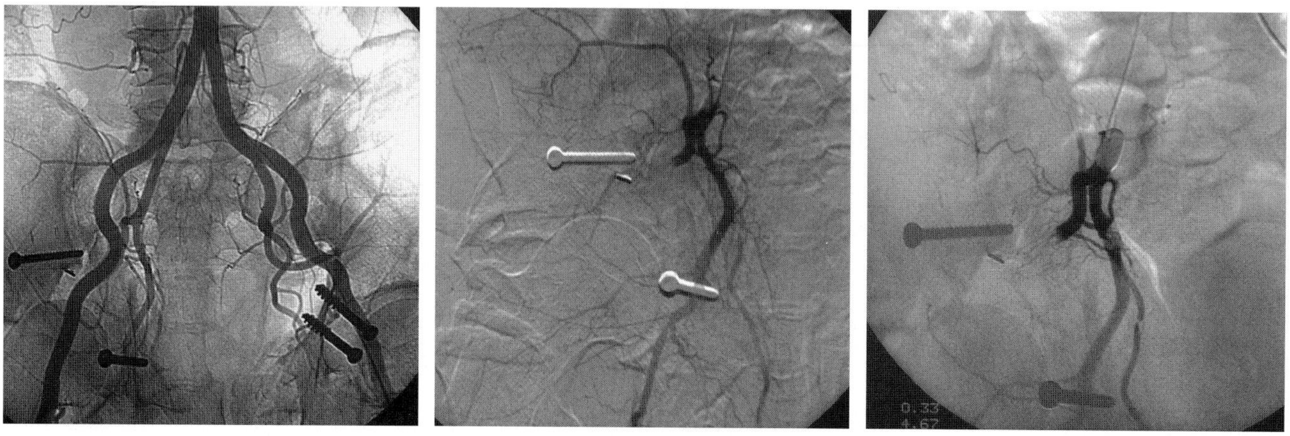

C

Figure 8.5

A: Pelvic arteriogram shows severe disruption of the bones and occlusion of the right gluteal artery. **B:** Selective right internal iliac artery angiogram shows no extravasation and thrombosis of the gluteal artery. **C:** An 8.5-mm balloon catheter was used to occlude the internal iliac artery. Surgery was performed successfully without significant bleeding.

Comment: Control of pelvic hemorrhage can be achieved by embolization alone using absorbable particles and balloon occlusion for temporary bleeding control or metal coils or detachable balloons for permanent occlusion. Several types of occlusion balloons can be used to temporarily occlude the target vessel. Initially, the Fogarty balloon catheter was used, but because it cannot be used over the wire, other occlusion balloons that can be used over the wire became preferable. More recently, Fogarty balloons that can be used over the wire have become available. Results with balloon occlusion are favorable, and the occlusion may be reversible.

8.6 Embolization In Trauma

Case 8.6:

A 49-year-old male patient was in a motor vehicle accident and suffered soft tissue and bone pelvic injury, particularly in the right gluteal muscle. Pain became intense, and an arteriogram was requested.

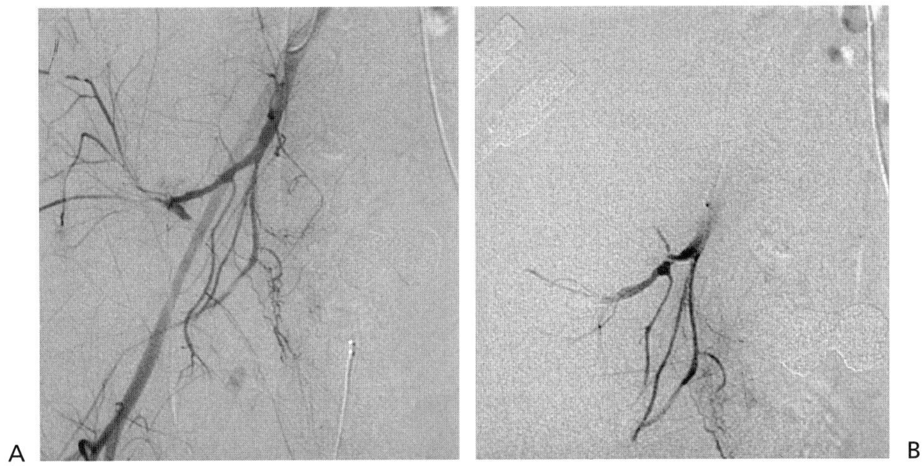

Figure 8.6

A: Right internal iliac artery angiogram shows active extravasation from the right superior gluteal artery. Late-phase arteriogram demonstrates residual extravasation at the injury site (not shown). **B:** Embolization of the superior gluteal artery with Gelfoam resulted in permanent cessation of bleeding.

Comment: Pelvic trauma with active bleeding usually is severe and associated with high morbidity and mortality. Embolization with particles is the easiest way to control the bleeding, with minimal invasion. Potential complications of embolization in such cases are ischemia of nontarget vessels; neurologic damage, with ischemic lesion of the sciatic nerve; and reflux of some of the particles from the hypogastric into the femoral artery, with distal ischemia. In patients who will remain in bed for long periods of time because of severe injuries, embolization of the superior gluteal artery is prone to cause sacral and buttock scars that may be difficult to treat.

Vasoconstrictor infusion is not an effective treatment for bleeding pelvic injuries, and embolization ultimately is necessary. Preservation of the internal pudendal arteries is important in younger men, and reabsorbable particles should be used to allow for recanalization of the embolized arteries.

8.7 Embolization In Trauma

Case 8.7:

A 48-year-old male patient fell and sustained a fracture of the humerus. Pain became intense with increased edema of soft tissues. An arteriogram was requested.

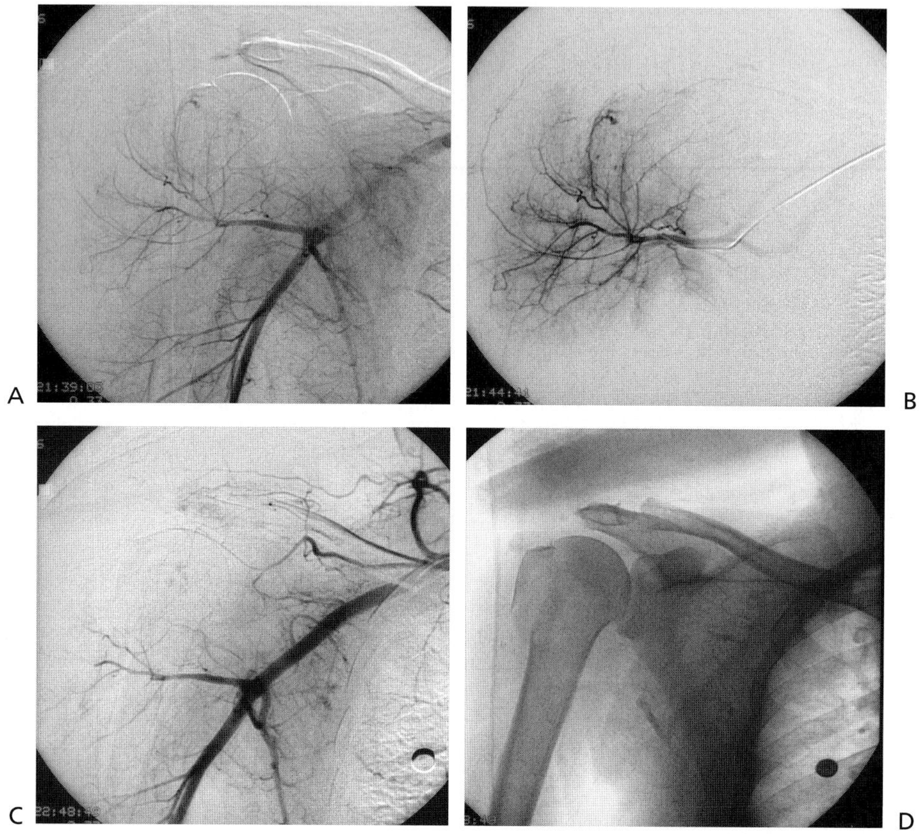

Figure 8.7

A: Arteriogram of the axillary artery shows a small area of bleeding just at the periphery of the humerus head originating from the humeral circumflex artery. **B:** Selective angiogram of the humeral circumflex artery shows several small points of extravasation. **C:** Embolization of the circumflex artery with polyvinyl alcohol particles and Gelfoam effectively controlled the bleeding. **D:** Unsubtracted x-ray film of the head of the humerus shows the fracture.

Comment: Traumatic lesions of the extremities, with active bleeding, usually are caused by penetrating wound. In rarer instances, such lesions are due to contusion or bone fracture, as in the case reported. Acute lesions are vascular lacerations with hemorrhage, thrombosis, or formation of acute pseudoaneurysms or A-V fistulas. These lesions are more common in the lower extremities. Chronic lesions usually are pseudoaneurysms and A-V fistulas that were missed at the first evaluation or developed over time. Traumatic A-V fistulas tend to have increased flow over time, causing distal ischemia due to flow stealing.

Acute bleedings can be problematic because of blood loss over a short period of time and can cause intense pain in expanding pseudoaneurysms and hematoma.

8.8 Embolization In Trauma

Case 8.8:

A 42-year-old male patient was involved in a motor vehicle accident. The pedestrian was hit by a car and developed a large hematoma in the thigh. Upon admission, his pain was very intense and an arteriogram was requested.

A, B

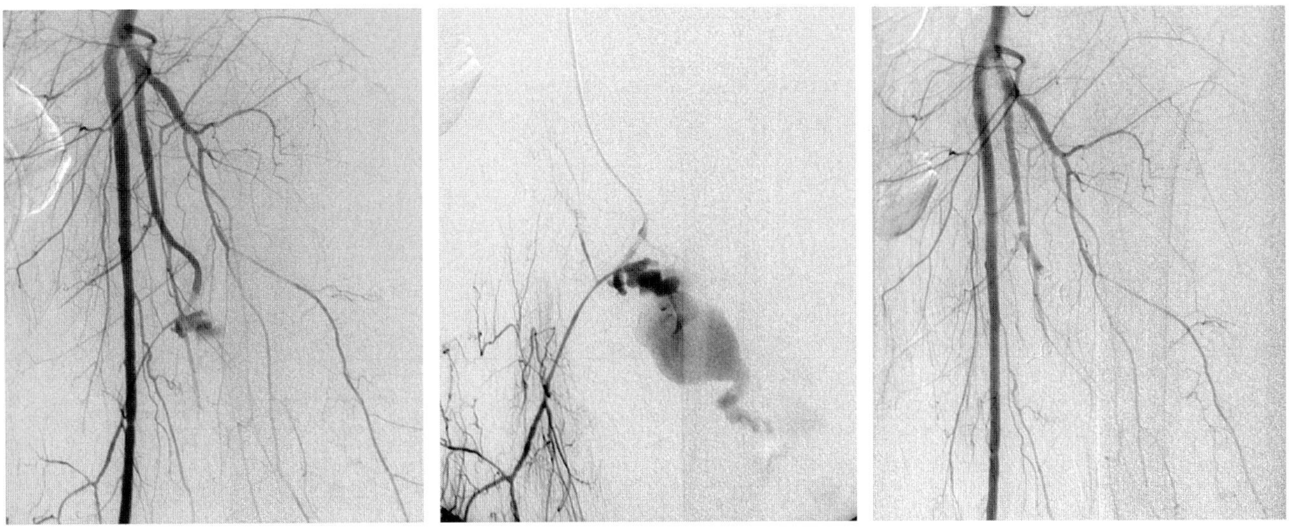

C

Figure 8.8

A: Selective angiogram of the left femoral and profunda femoris shows laceration of the profunda femoris associated with severe spasm. **B:** More selective injection shows massive extravasation with filling of a large pseudoaneurysm. **C:** Embolization was performed with four 3-cm × 5-mm minicoils. Total occlusion of the bleeding branch was achieved with control of the bleeding.

Comment: Penetrating lesions in the lower extremities are relatively common in the modern world, due to either motor vehicle accidents or trauma related to violent acts, such as stab wounds or gunshots. When the laceration is in a terminal or secondary muscular branch, embolization is easy and effective. In the case reported here, the arterial laceration was related to a contusion without penetration but produced a large pseudoaneurysm that was very painful and required immediate treatment. Surgical treatment without angiographic mapping requires extensive surgical investigation. Surgical exploration is never easy under the best of circumstances, and it is particularly difficult to identify a vascular lesion inside a large, uncontrolled hematoma that has evolved with extensive tissue infiltration. Compartment syndrome is another complication of closed bleeding that produces distal ischemia and requires surgical fasciotomy. More chronic limb lesions are A-V fistulas and/or pseudoaneurysms that were missed on the initial examination but which have developed progressively.

8.9 Embolization In Trauma

Case 8.9:

A 7-year-old female patient underwent minimally invasive surgical correction of pectus excavatum deformity using a temporary Walter Lorenz metal strut that traverses the chest behind the sternum and in front of the rib cage. In this surgery, the sternum was not inverted or removed. A few days after surgery, the patient developed left chest pain and an enlarging hematoma in the chest wall. Emergency angiogram was requested for possible embolization.

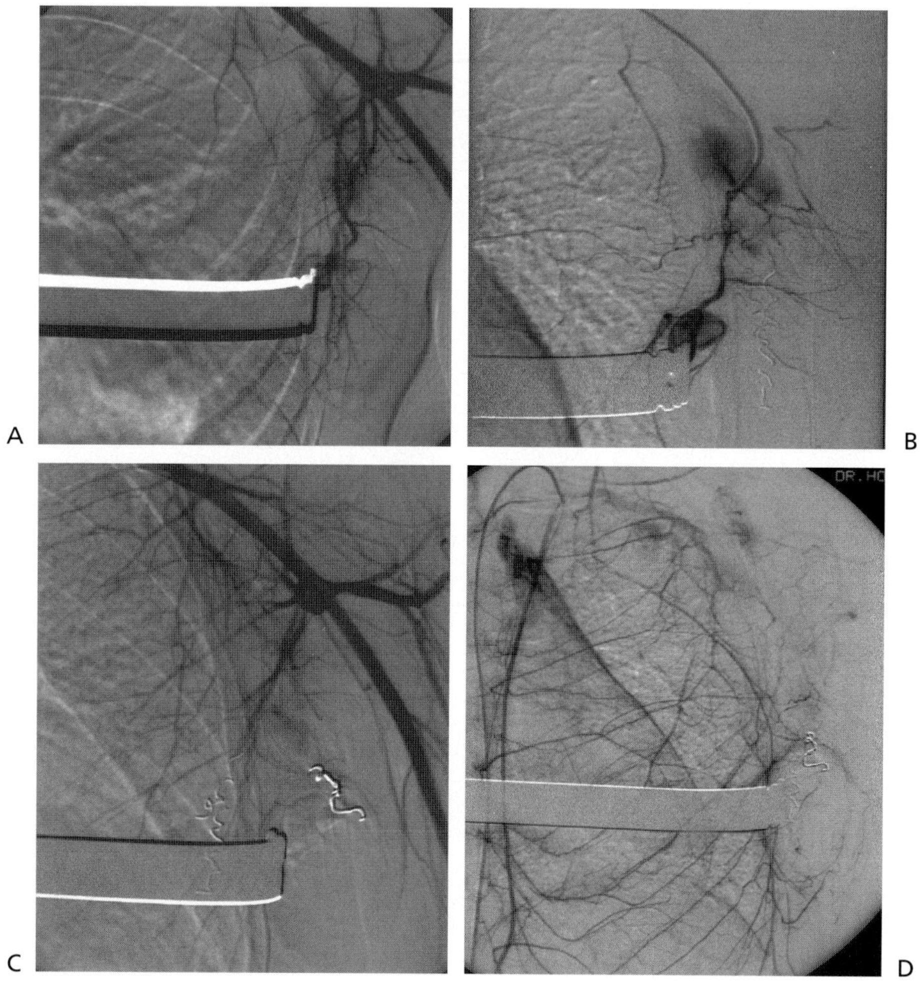

Figure 8.9

A: Left subclavian artery angiogram was performed and shows a pseudoaneurysm originated from a lateral thoracic artery. **B:** Superselective angiogram of the branch with the pseudoaneurysm shows the large lesion next to the metal edge. Note the coils in the branches of the dorsal thoracic artery, which was embolized to reduce the possibility of pseudoaneurysm filling through collaterals. **C:** Postembolization angiogram shows occlusion of the pseudoaneurysm and control of the bleeding. **D:** Postembolization angiogram of the left internal mammary artery shows filling of the anterior intercostal arteries and the hematoma surrounded by normal branches. There is no filling of the pseudoaneurysm through other collaterals. Note the coils.

Comment: Traumatic laceration of the internal thoracic artery caused by this new device is a problem with serious consequences. This is the first such lesion described. The Walter Lorenz metal strut is introduced behind the sternum and anteriorly to the rib cage in a subcutaneous position. Use of this device supposedly is safer than regular surgery. The bar is retrieved after 1 to 2 years. Identification of the lesion was key in the treatment decision. Embolization was safe and quickly controlled the bleeding, with minimal invasiveness.

The procedure required general anesthesia because of the young age of the patient, but it was performed in only a few minutes. The pain was controlled immediately following the procedure, and there were no sequelae.

8.10 Embolization In Trauma

Case 8.10:

A 16-year-old male patient was treated for pectus excavatum using conventional surgical procedure with sternum inversion and support by a metal bar behind the sternum. Four days after surgery, the patient developed a hematoma in the thoracic wall and severe pain. Angiography was requested for possible embolization.

A 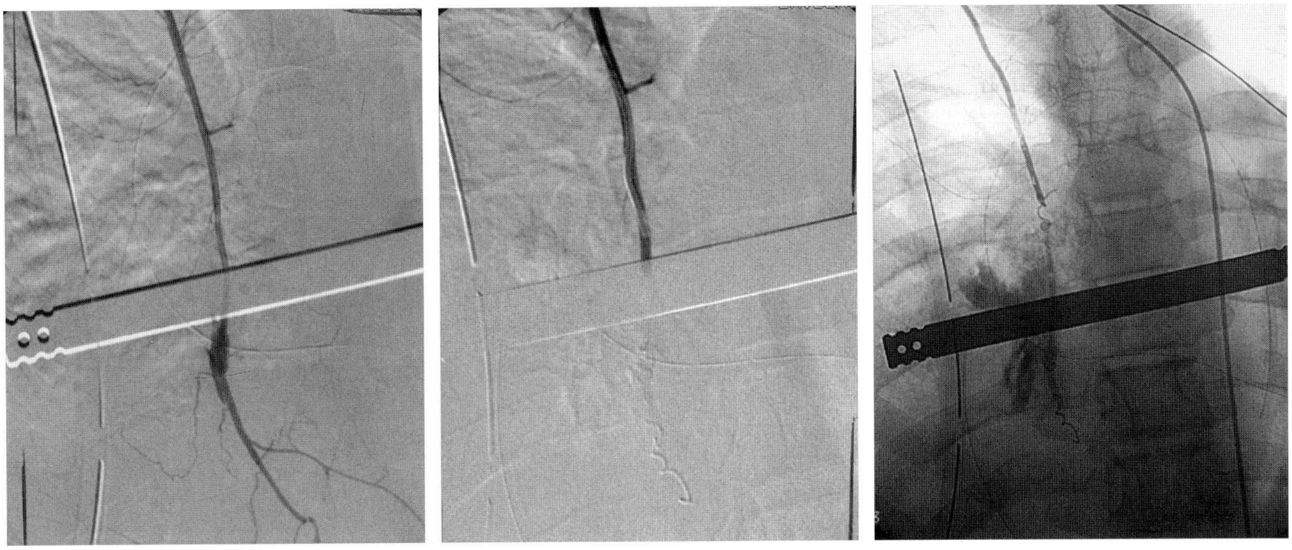 B, C

Figure 8.10

A: Initial aortogram with panoramic view of the chest wall did not show any abnormality (not shown). After selective injection into the right internal mammary artery, a fusiform pseudoaneurysm of the mammary artery was identified, just below the metal bar. **B:** Embolization of the internal mammary artery performed beyond and before the level of the pseudoaneurysm achieved occlusion of the pseudoaneurysm. **C:** Injection in the contralateral internal mammary artery did not show any midline anastomosis or filling of the pseudoaneurysm. Note the residual perivascular extravasation in the unsubtracted picture following embolization.

Comment: Lesions of the internal mammary artery are rare. Surgery of the sternum and percutaneous transthoracic needle biopsies are the most traumatic events in the area and can cause unintentional vascular laceration with bleeding into the thoracic cavity or chest wall. Surgical management requires open chest surgery with its associated morbidity. Selective embolization is the easiest and less invasive way to treat such trauma. Computed tomographic (CT) scan of the chest in this case shows a parasternal hematoma (not shown), but did not provide specific information about the arterial laceration. Another cause of internal mammary lesion is percutaneous transthoracic needle biopsy using an anterior parasternal approach. It is important to note on the CT scan the location of the internal mammary vessels and avoid them during the procedure. The internal mammary arteries are very superficial in the internal aspect of the thoracic cage and covered only by thin soft connective tissue and the parietal pleura. Bleeding into the thoracic cavity may be massive if the source is not identified in time.

Case 8.11:

A 22-year-old male patient who was unrestrained when he involved in a head-on motor vehicle collision suffered a direct blow to the chest by the steering wheel. Fracture of the sternum was identified by CT scan (not shown), and there were signs of mediastinal hemorrhage and enlargement. An emergency trauma arch arteriogram was requested to locate a thoracic aorta laceration.

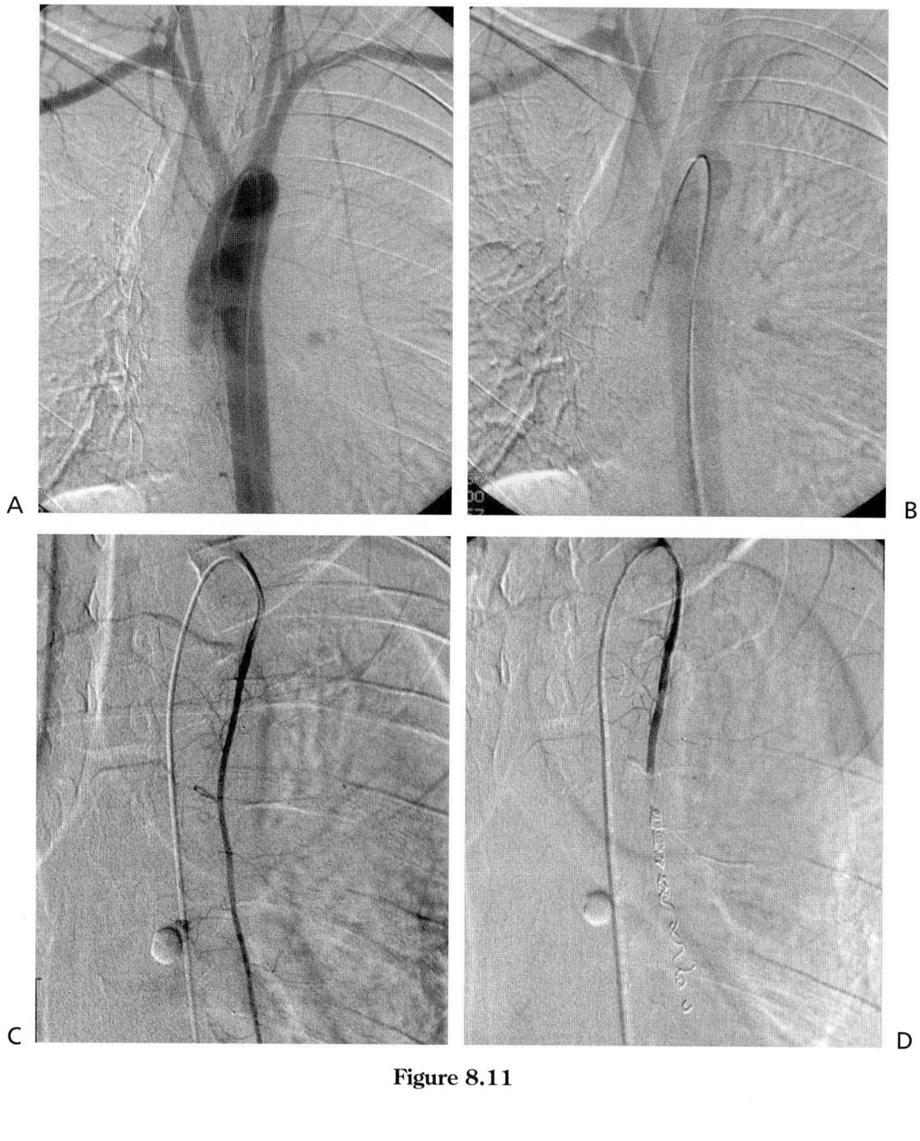

Figure 8.11

A: Right anterior oblique view of the thoracic aortogram did not show any traumatic lesion to the aorta; however, a small area of contrast extravasation is observed between the sternum and the left internal mammary artery. **B:** Late-phase angiogram demonstrates contrast accumulation in the soft tissues. **C:** Selective injection in the left internal mammary artery shows the extravasation is related to the sternal bone and supplied by a small medial branch from the left internal mammary artery. Note the anterior intercostal arteries are severely spastic. **D:** Embolization with coils was performed. Postembolization angiogram shows occlusion of the left internal mammary artery, and control of the bleeding was achieved. Embolization using a 2.8F microcatheter to deploy several microcoils was performed to occlude the middle segment of the left internal mammary artery at the level of the bleeder branch.

Comment: Direct trauma to the sternum is another cause of bleeding in the mediastinum. Blood supply to the sternum originates from the internal mammary artery, epigastric arteries, adjacent pleural arterioles, and mediastinal branches from the pericardium and bronchial arteries. Major suppliers are related to the internal mammary arteries. Vascular laceration may cause bleeding in the surrounding structures of the mediastinum, with severe symptoms and potential morbidity in multiply traumatized patients, as the patient reported here, concomitant to a head trauma. Angiography rapidly identified the site of bleeding and allowed the hemorrhage to be treated by embolization alone.

8.12 Embolization In Trauma

Case 8.12:

A 39-year-old male patient who was involved in a car accident suffered a direct contusion of the left chest wall. A large hematoma developed in the subcutaneous tissues, but no rib fracture was identified. Emergency angiogram was requested for diagnosis and possible embolization.

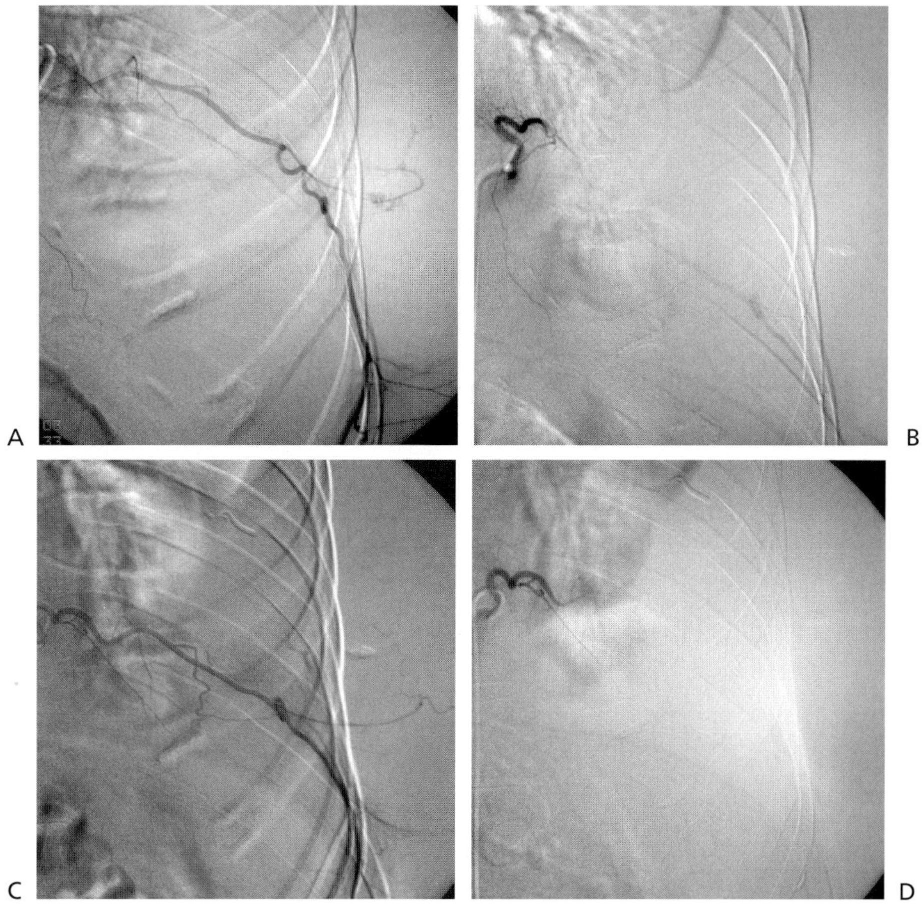

Figure 8.12

A: Aortogram did not show any active bleeding (not shown). Selective injections into the seventh, eighth, and ninth intercostal arteries were performed. Injection into the eighth intercostal artery shows peripheral subcutaneous branches bowed by the chest wall hematoma and a pseudoaneurysm in the middle. **B:** Embolization with Gelfoam was performed with the catheter located proximally in the origin of the artery. Follow-up angiogram shows occlusion of the eighth intercostal artery. **C:** Injection of the ninth intercostal artery shows no bleeding, but embolization was performed. **D:** Embolization was performed above (seventh) and below (ninth) the level of bleeding.

Comment: Contusion to the chest wall usually cause fractures of the ribs, and bleeding usually is related to the fracture. A pseudoaneurysm is less likely to occur, as in this case. Embolization with Gelfoam particles was performed in the traumatized artery (eighth intercostal). The arteries above and below also were embolized to reduce the risks of reconstitution of flow into the distal eighth intercostal artery. The intercostal arteries are in communication with extensive collateral circulation at all levels, and a pseudoaneurysm or distal branch can easily pick up blood flow from a parallel artery above or below the level of trauma.

8.13 Embolization In Trauma

Case 8.13:

A 42-year-old male patient suffered a stab wound on the left posterior aspect of the chest about the level of the sixth intercostal space. Pneumothorax developed, followed by hypotension. Upon arrival in the emergency room, a chest tube drain was placed to treat the pneumothorax, but there was significant hemorrhage through the tube. It was believed that the aorta had been cut by the knife. Emergency angiography was requested for diagnostic.

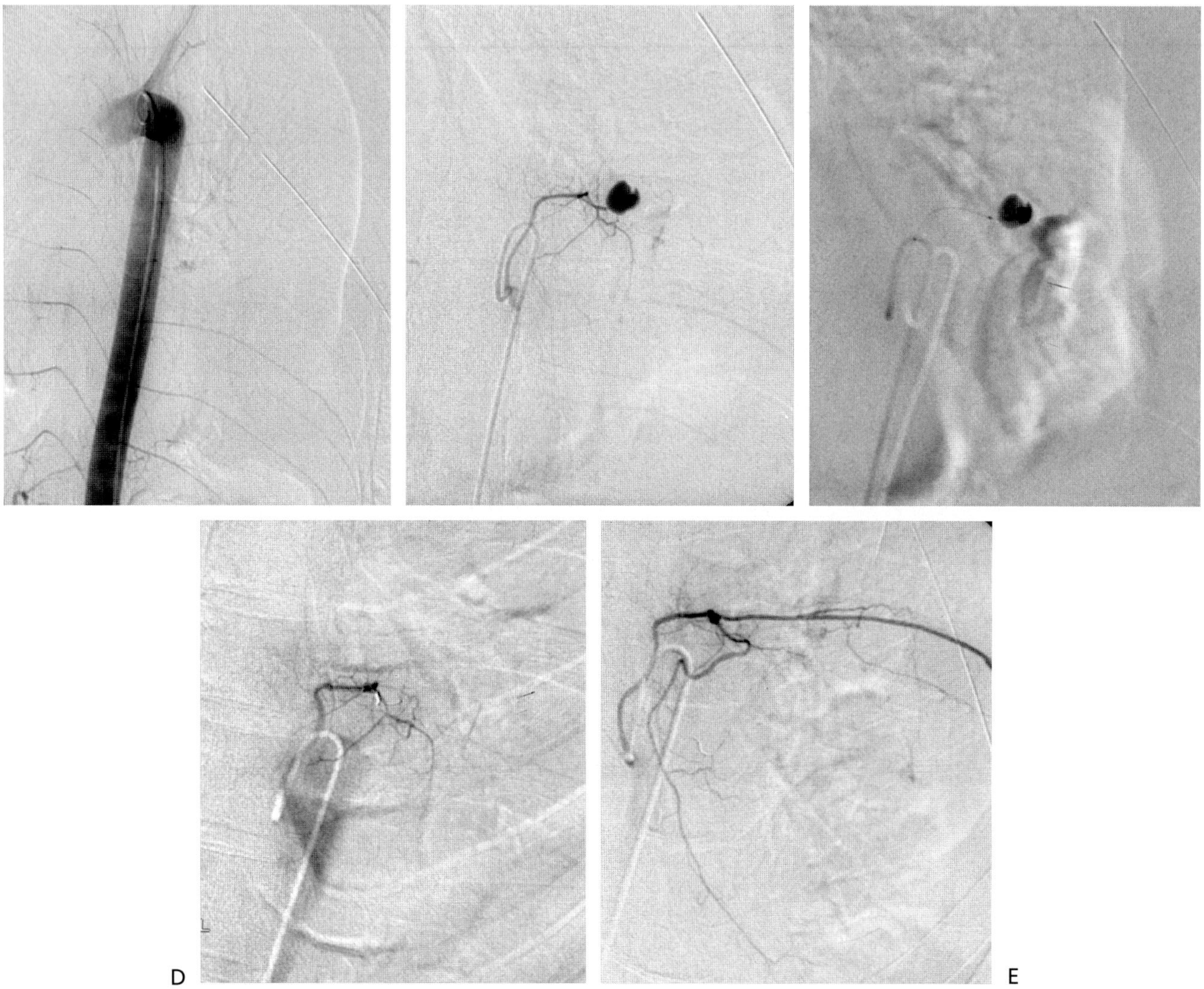

A, B

C

D

E

Figure 8.13

A: Thoracic aortogram shows bleeding from the left sixth intercostal artery. **B:** Selective arteriogram of the sixth intercostal artery shows a pseudoaneurysm in the proximal segment of the intercostal artery. **C:** Late-phase arteriogram shows extravasation of contrast into the thoracic cavity. Note the microcatheter located right at the edge of the lesion. **D:** Embolization was performed with two curved short microcoils. Postembolization angiogram shows occlusion of the torn artery. **E:** Angiograms were performed below and above the lesion level to locate any anastomosis that could feed the pseudoaneurysm. The angiogram shown is from the fifth intercostal level. Bleeding was controlled, and the patient improved following embolization.

Comment: Fortunately in this patient, the aorta was not subject to trauma and only an intercostal artery was torn. Massive bleeding ensued following the stab wound. The chest tube decompressed the chest cavity and the patient became unstable, necessitating an emergency arteriogram. Embolization could be performed relatively quick and effectively. Embolization of this kind of lesion, with active bleeding, must be managed with a low-pressure delivery system, such as coils, to minimize the bursting of bleeding during embolization. Coils usually are good devices for embolization in such situations. They can be delivered precisely with a low-pressure system and are thrombogenic enough to control the bleeding. Gelfoam particles are more thrombogenic, but they allow much less control of the delivery and are prone to fragmentation. However, when recanalization of the artery is desired, it is preferred to use reabsorbable particles, such as Gelfoam.

Suggested Reading

Ben-Menachem, Coldwell DM, Young JWR, et al. Hemorrhage associated with pelvic fractures: causes, diagnosis and emergent management. *AJR* 1991;157:1005–1014.

Berger JJ, Britt LD. Pelvic fracture hemorrhage. Current strategies in diagnosis and management. *Surg Ann* 1995;27:107–112.

Feliciano DV, Bitondo CG, Mattox KL, et al. Civilian trauma in the 1980's: a 1 year experience with 456 vascular and cardiac injuries. *Ann Surg* 1984;199:717–721.

Moura R, Uflacker R, Yoshida WB. et al. Arteriovenous fistula between the right internal mammary artery and the subclavian vein: percutaneous closure with detachable balloon-catheter embolization. *Cardiovasc Surg* 1993;1:86–88.

Panetta T, Sclafani SJA, Goldstein AS, et al. Percutaneous transcatheter embolization for massive bleeding from pelvic fractures. *J Trauma* 1985;25:1021–1029.

Saueracker AJ, McCroskey BL, Moore EE, et al. Intraoperative hypogastric artery embolization for life-threatening pelvic hemorrhage: a preliminary report. *J Trauma* 1987;27:1127–1129.

Sclafani SJA, Shaftan GW, Scalea TM, et al. Nonoperative salvage of computed tomography-diagnosed splenic injuries: utilization of angiography for triage and embolization for hemostasis. *J Trauma* 1989;39:818–825.

Selby JB. Interventional radiology of trauma. *Radiol Clin North Am* 1992;30:427–439.

Seppänen SK, Leppänen MJ, Pimenoff G, et al. Microcatheter embolization of hemorrhages. *Cardiovasc Intervent Radiol* 1997;20:174–179.

Uflacker R, Mourao GS, Piske RL. Treating complications of subclavian vein puncture by embolization of the internal mammary artery. *Cardiovasc Intervent Radiol* 1991;14:115–117.

Uflacker R. Transcatheter embolisation of arterial aneurysms. *Br J Radiol* 1986;59:317–324.

CHAPTER 9

Embolization In The Organs Of The Pelvis And Lower Genitourinary Tract

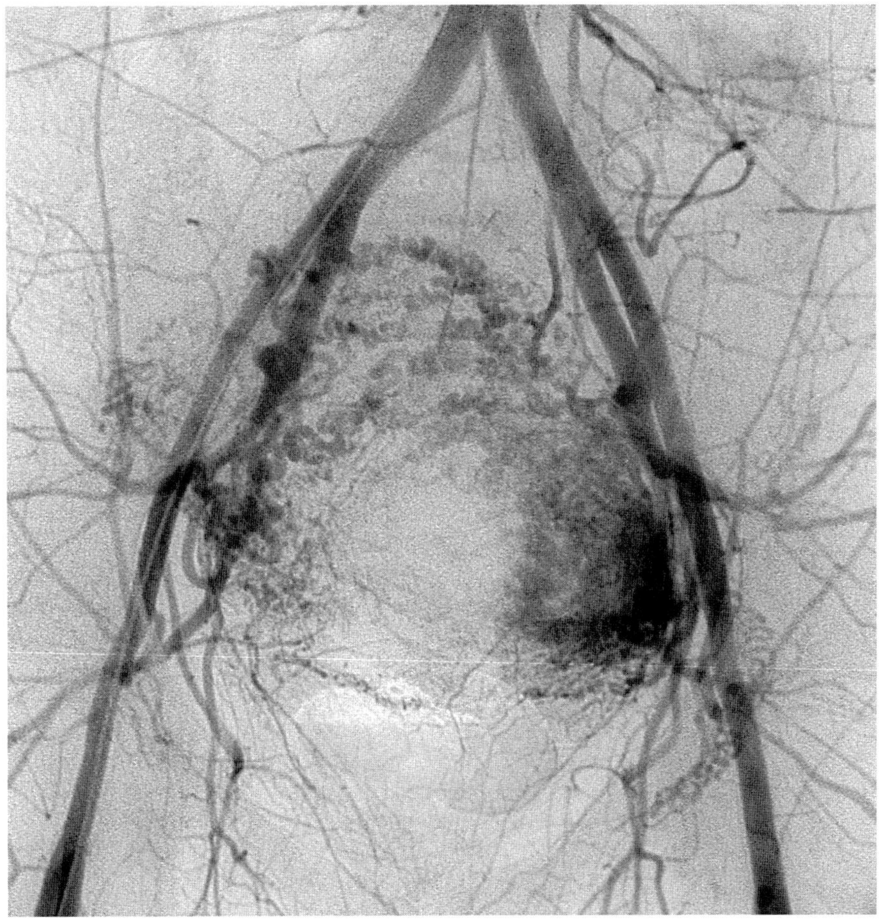

9.1 Embolization In The Pelvis And Genitourinary Tract

Case 9.1:

Selective arterial embolization of idiopathic high-flow priapism was performed in a 39-year-old man.

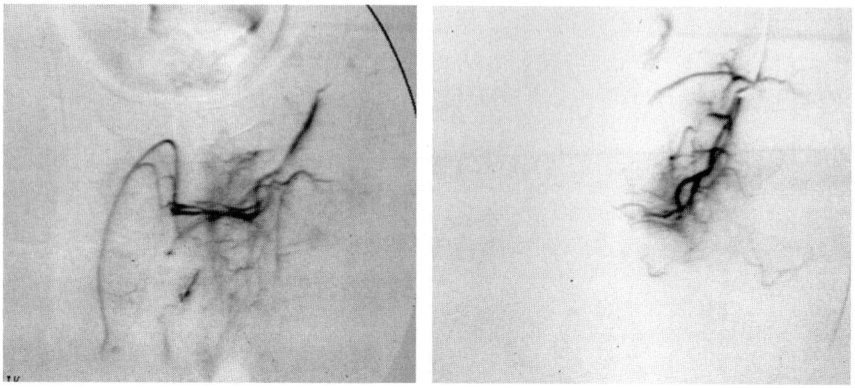

A B

Figure 9.1

Selective digital substraction angiography of the cavernous arteries. **A:** Preembolization study of the cavernous arteries. **B:** Embolization with Gelfoam demonstrates occlusion of the cavernous arteries.

Comment: Priapism is a long-term sustained erection (more than 6 hours) unaccompanied by sexual desire. There are two main forms of priapism: (i) venoocclusive and (ii) high flow or arterial. Venoocclusive priapism is more common than arterial-dependent priapism. In arterial (high-flow) priapism, there usually is a direct communication between the arterial system and the corpus cavernosum after trauma. The etiology in low-flow (venous) priapism is different and includes some type of occlusive problem. Most frequent causes include hypercoagulability states, intravenous drug abuse, sickle cell anemia, leukemia, vasculitis, and steroid, antipsychotic, or antihypertensive therapy. Some of these causes also may play a role in high-flow priapism. The diagnosis of idiopathic priapism is made by history and exclusion of other possibilities. Priapism leads to tissue ischemia and acidosis, causing ulceration and gangrene, and may lead to amputation of the penis. Treatment of priapism in the early period is aspiration and irrigation of the corpus cavernosus. If these attempts fail, epidural anesthesia or intracavernosal ketamine may be used. Surgical shunt therapies are reserved for unresponsive cases and have mixed results. Embolization treatment is relatively new and was first performed in 1977 by Wear et al. Autologous clot or Gelfoam may be used as embolizing agents. Both agents are absorbable, and some patients obtain erectile function a few months after treatment. The presented case had no history of trauma, drug, or any other cause. Embolization therapy was performed after failure of aspiration, irrigation, as well as local and general anesthesia. There was immediate improvement after embolization. Penile erection returned within 2 months, which allowed restoration of normal sexual activity.

9.2 Embolization In The Pelvis And Genitourinary Tract

Case 9.2:

A 31-year-old man with a history of direct perineal trauma 3 months earlier developed high-flow priapism. Doppler ultrasound revealed focal areas of high-flow turbulence inside the corpora cavernosa.

A 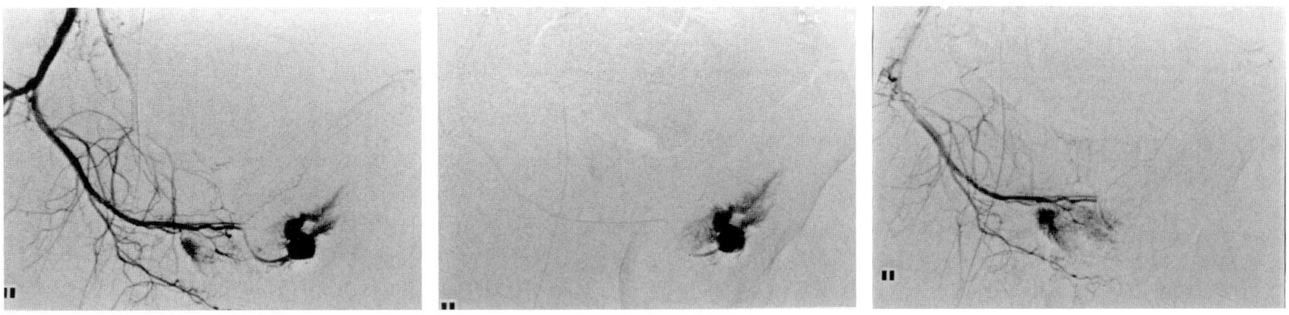 B, C

Figure 9.2

A: Selective right internal pudendal arteriogram shows contrast material extravasation rising from the cavernous artery and into the corpora cavernosa. **B:** A 2.5F Tracker catheter was advanced coaxially into the cavernous artery prior to embolization. Superselective injection shows contrast material extravasation. **C:** After selective embolization with a 2-mm Gelfoam pledget, active extravasation was no longer present. The dorsal artery of the penis and the bulbar artery remained relatively intact. Sexual function was restored several months later.

Comment: Priapism is defined as prolonged and often painful erection, may be incomplete but constantly rigid, and is unrelated to sexual stimulation. Hemodynamically, most cases of priapism occur as a result of engorgement of the corpora cavernosa from intrinsic or extrinsic venous outflow obstruction, termed "veno-occlusive" priapism. However, in a small number of patients, the cause is related to uncontrolled arterial inflow, usually due to direct perineal or penial trauma and laceration of one of the cavernosal arteries with extravasation into the surrounding erectile tissue lacunae (creating an arterial-lacunar fistula). This form of priapism has been called "high-flow" or arterial priapism. Arterial priapism occurs in the absence of neurogenic-mediated relaxation and is sustained by high oxygen tension and shear stress associated with cavernosal artery laceration. In patients with posttraumatic priapism, a high-flow arterial cause should be considered and appropriately investigated by color flow Doppler ultrasound and confirmed by a selective pudendal arteriogram. Prompt diagnosis may prevent unnecessary shunt surgery and permits treatment with selective embolization therapy. The effective treatment for high-flow priapism ideally should abolish the abnormal, uncontrolled arterial inflow while preserving normal erectile function. Selective embolization therapy with temporary particulate embolic material (autologous clot or Gelfoam) offers effective management of the pathophysiology with rapid restoration of blood flow, minimizing complications and potentially allowing recovery of normal sexual function.

9.3 Embolization In The Pelvis And Genitourinary Tract

Case 9.3:

A 25-year-old woman developed postpartum intrapelvic and abdominal wall bleeding following a cesarean section. Arteriogram of the pelvis was requested for possible embolization.

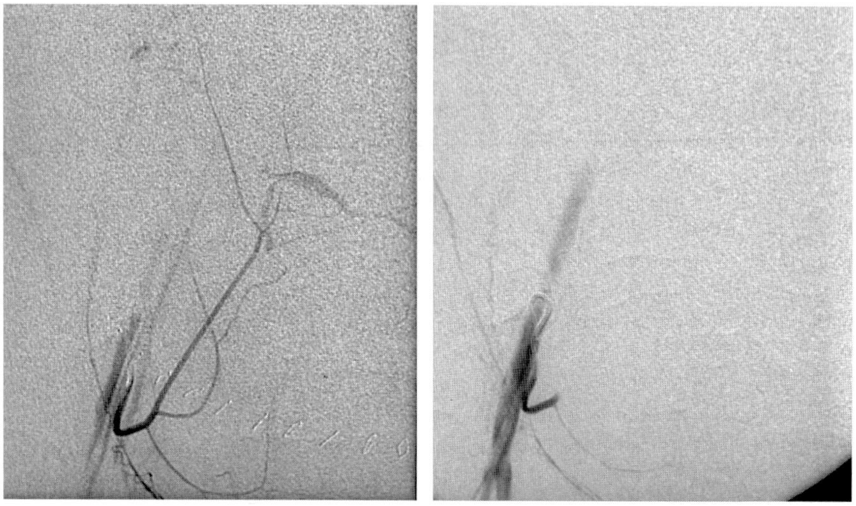

A B

Figure 9.3

Iliac arteriography did not show any bleeding related to the hypogastric arteries (not shown). **A:** Right external iliac artery angiogram shows bleeding from the right inferior epigastric artery within the abdominal wall along the cesarean section wound and not in the uterus. **B:** Superselective catheterization of the inferior epigastric artery with an Sos Omni catheter was used for embolization with particles of Gelfoam. Control of bleeding was obtained. Recurrence of vaginal bleeding occurred about 12 hours after embolization of the inferior epigastric artery, and embolization of the right internal iliac artery was necessary (not shown).

Comment: Postpartum hemorrhage is relatively uncommon following delivery. Bleeding may be devastating and lead to coagulopathy and death. Angiography can detect the site of bleeding and the catheter at the same procedure used for embolization. Transcatheter embolization of the pelvic vessels has proved particularly useful in cases of clinically uncontrolled vaginal hemorrhage, and in cases where surgery is not feasible, viable, or desirable. In this particular case, the initial picture was abdominal wall bleeding related to a lesion in the inferior epigastric artery, which was treated by embolization.

The superiority of embolization over surgical ligature of hypogastric arteries for control of pelvic and uterine hemorrhage has long been recognized. Selective catheterization allows occlusion of pathologic small-diameter vessels, thus eliminating the plexus of collaterals.

9.4 Embolization In The Pelvis And Genitourinary Tract

Case 9.4:

A 38-year-old woman with a history of cesarean section 1 day earlier developed vaginal bleeding due to a noncontracted uterus. Ultrasound shows a distended uterine cavity that was full of clots. Angiography was requested for possible embolization.

A

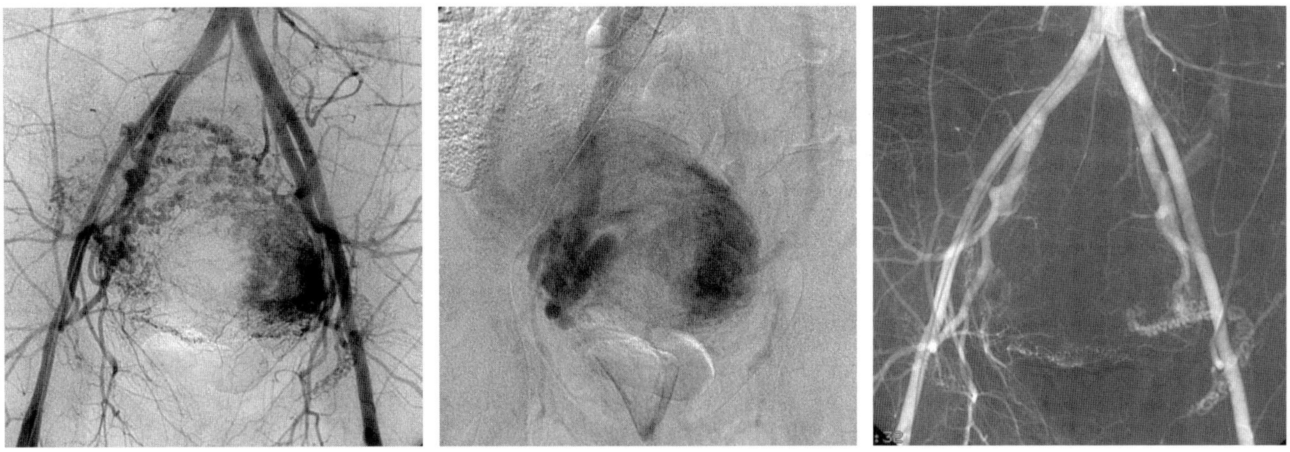

B, C

Figure 9.4

A: Pelvic arteriography shows an enlarged uterus with massive hypervascularity due to the thickened uterine mucosa, which originated from both uterine arteries. **B:** Late-phase arteriogram shows uterine mucosal enhancement and large draining veins. **C:** Embolization of both internal iliac arteries was performed with Gelfoam, and significant reduction in vascularity was obtained, followed by control of the bleeding.

Comment: Burchel has shown that, after bilateral surgical ligation, pulse pressure drops by 85%, but blood flow is only reduced by 48%, due to abundant collateral circulation present in the pelvis. Uterine embolization should be performed early to reduce the possibility of the patient developing a coagulopathy, which would cause the situation to become more severe and difficult to control. The anatomy of the pelvic vessels facilitates transcatheter embolization; however, more nontarget peripheral branches may be occluded by the same procedure. Excessive occlusion of peripheral pelvic arteries may cause ischemia of organs and lead to conditions such as necrosis of bladder wall and ischemic injury to the sciatic nerve. The more proximal the embolization, the greater the possibility of reflux into the systemic circulation.

9.5 Embolization In The Pelvis And Genitourinary Tract

Case 9.5:

A 26-year-old woman with a history of cesarean section for delivery of twins developed postpartum massive vaginal bleeding. Pelvic arteriogram and embolization were requested.

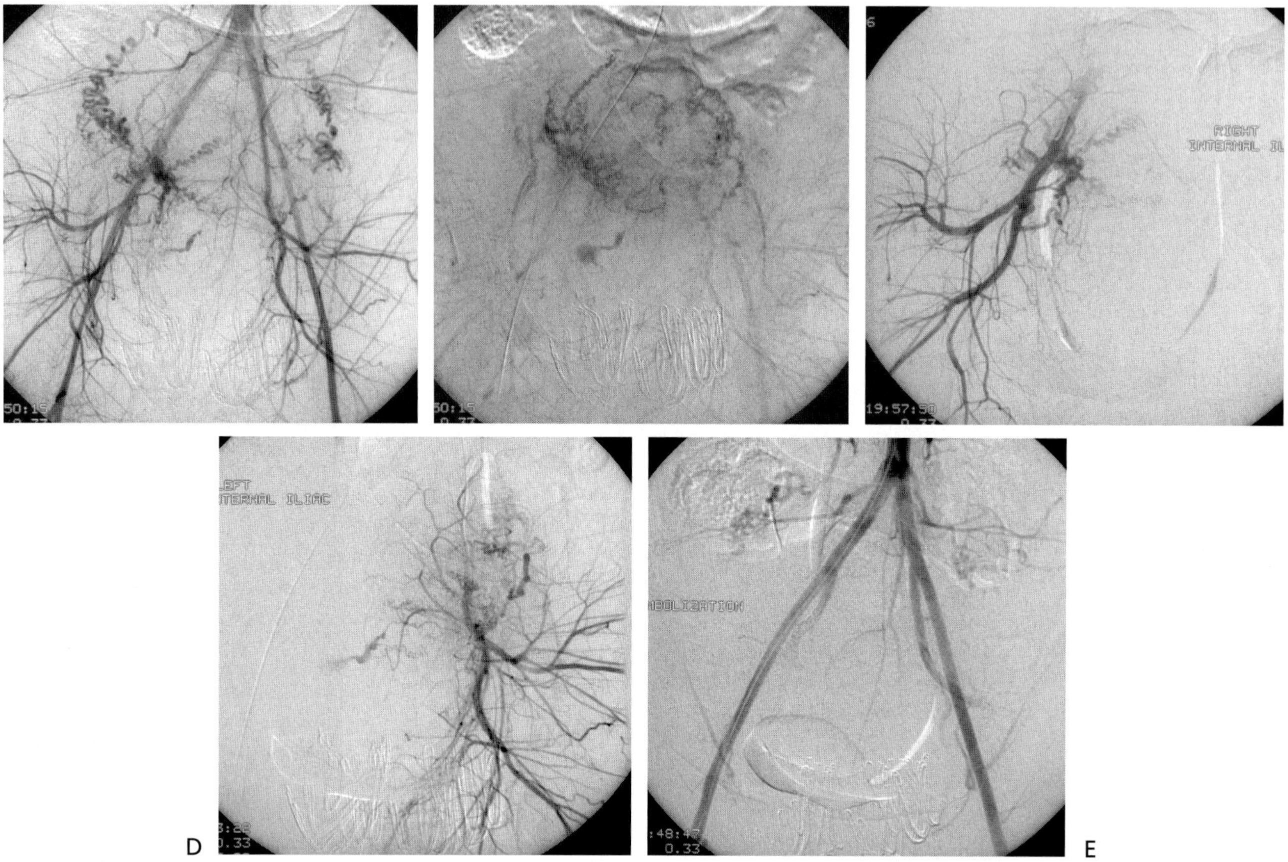

A, B C D E

Figure 9.5

A: Pelvic arteriogram shows an enlarged uterus with large vessels and active bleeding near the colon of the uterus, with feeders from both sides. **B:** Late-phase pelvic angiography shows the spread of bleeding into the uterine cavity and some enhancement of the thickened uterine mucosa. **C:** Selective injection into the right internal iliac artery did not show active bleeding. **D:** Selective injection into the left internal iliac artery shows active bleeding from the left uterine artery. **E:** Embolization with Gelfoam and coils was performed mostly in the anterior segment of both internal iliac arteries. Successful control of the bleeding spared the patient a hysterectomy. Pelvic arteriogram shows occlusion of both internal iliac arteries.

Comment: Catheterization technique should be accurate and spare the posterior segment of the internal iliac artery whenever possible. Embolization preferably should be unilateral. Control of the bleeding almost always is possible. Complications from embolization are dependent on the embolic material and are anatomically related. Possible complications are lower limb ischemia, necrosis of gluteal muscles, bone necrosis, and neurologic damage to the sciatic and femoral nerves. Future pregnancies are possible because of the significant enlargement of collaterals.

9.6 Embolization In The Pelvis And Genitourinary Tract

Case 9.6:

An 8-year-old female patient with a history of acute appendicitis treated by surgical appendectomy presented with a pelvic abscess causing fever and pain. Computed tomographic (CT)-guided transgluteal drainage was performed and the catheter maintained for 1 week. Massive hemorrhage occurred after catheter removal. Emergency arteriography was performed for hemorrhage control.

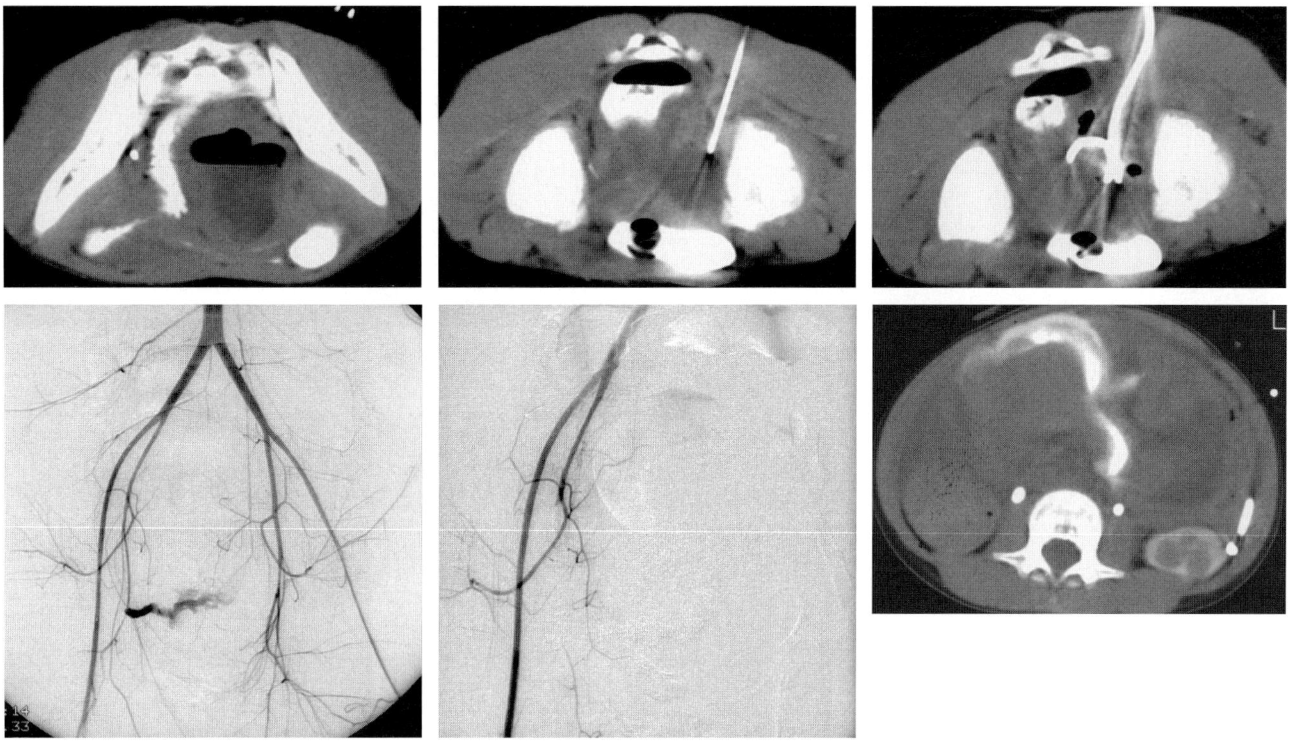

Figure 9.6

A: CT scan of the pelvis with the patient in the prone position shows a large fluid collection with an air–fluid level within. Note the radiopaque marker on the right buttock at the level of the iliac bone. **B:** Transgluteal puncture with an 19-gauge needle allowed access for drainage. Note that the needle was introduced more laterally than it should have been. The correct path would be closer to the sacral bone coursing just lateral to the rectum wall, to avoid the pelvic nerves and vessels. The incorrect positioning of the needle was not recognized at the time of drainage. **C:** Postdrainage CT scan shows the 8F catheter within the abscess effectively draining the collection. After 1 week of drainage, there was improvement of the infection and the catheter was removed. Significant bleeding ensued after catheter withdrawal through the puncture hole. Significant intraperitoneal bleeding and hypotension developed, which required blood replacement and fluids. **D:** Emergency pelvic arteriography was performed and massive bleeding from the inferior gluteal artery was identified. Immediate catheterization of the inferior gluteal artery using a microcatheter and embolization using microcoils were performed. **E:** Total occlusion of the bleeding artery was obtained, with complete control of the bleeding and stabilization of blood pressure. **F:** CT scan following embolization shows the peritoneal cavity full of blood clots and extravasated contrast material. Laparotomy eventually was performed for blood evacuation due to development of fever 2 days after the embolization. The patient was discharged 7 days following embolization.

Comment: Faulty technique used for transgluteal pelvic abscess drainage caused this major unnecessary complication. Although there is a possibility that infection or catheter contact may have caused the arterial lesion, it is less likely in this case. Development of a pseudoaneurysm would be the more likely scenario if the infection was the cause of the vascular lesion. Acute bleeding such as that seen in this patient more likely is related to direct puncture by the needle and catheter placement. Extreme care should be exercised when puncturing a pelvic fluid collection from the transgluteal approach. Risks are twofold: damage to the pelvic arteries, as demonstrated in this case; and neurologic injury to the sciatic nerve or branches. Careful, progressive puncture through the greater sciatic foramen, just above the piriformis muscle, and close to the sacral bone is the correct technique, preferably guided by fluoroscopic CT. The drainage catheter probably tamponaded the arterial lesion, and massive bleeding ensued at withdrawal. Superselective embolization of the inferior gluteal artery controlled the bleeding, which otherwise would have been very difficult to treat surgically. Use of microcoils was a good option, as it is fast and permanent. Unfortunately, surgical evacuation of the abdominal cavity was necessary due to development of fever.

9.7 Embolization In The Pelvis And Genitourinary Tract

Case 9.7:

A 38-year-old man was involved in a motorcycle accident and suffered abdominal trauma with splenic and hepatic injuries and pelvic fracture, which evolved with osteomyelitis of the iliosacral joint. Intrapelvic fluid collection was identified on an outside CT scan, and CT-guided transgluteal drainage was requested.

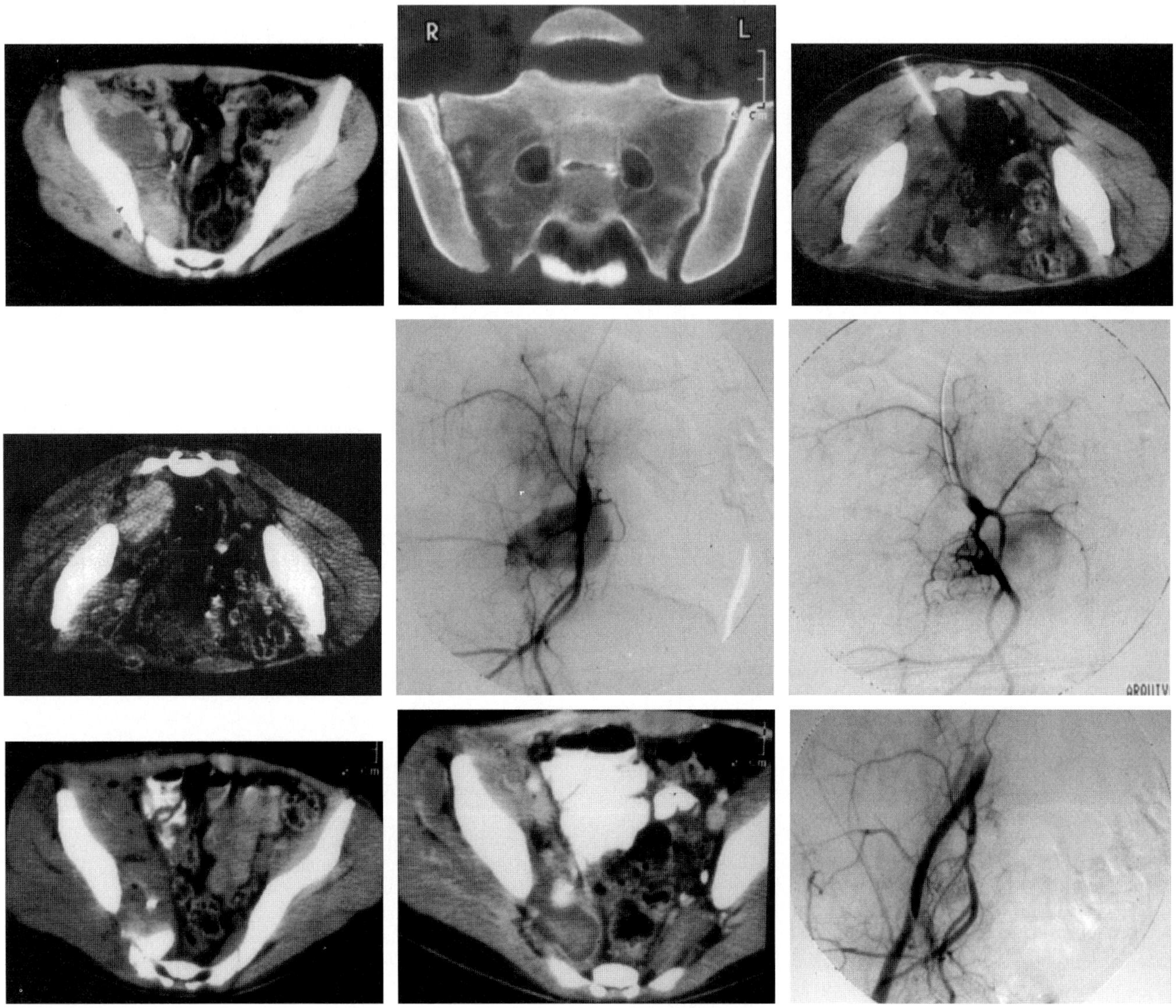

A, B C

D, E F

G, H I

Figure 9.7

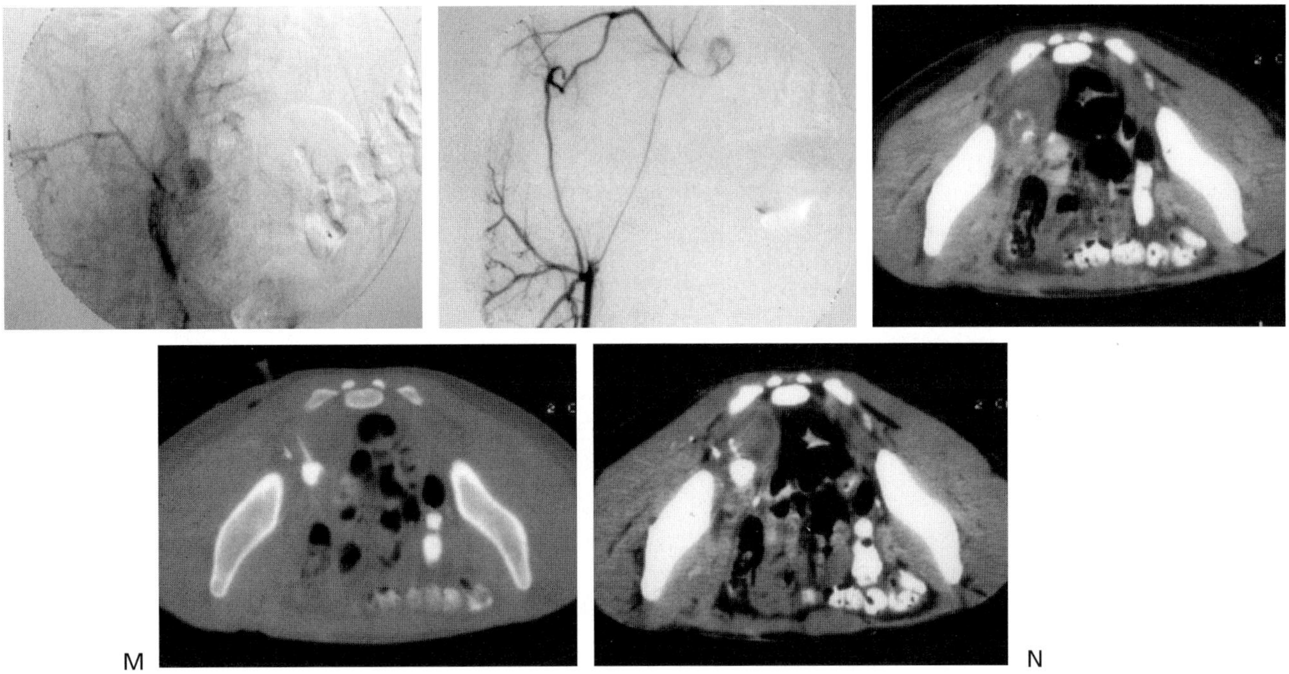

J K, L

M N

Figure 9.7 *(continued)*

A,B: CT scan of the pelvis and sacrum shows pelvic fluid collection and bone erosions, consistent with osteomyelitis of the iliosacral joint. Ten days later, septic arteritis of the right knee was diagnosed and drained percutaneously (not shown). Due to increasing pelvic pain extending to the right leg, drainage of the pelvic collection was requested about 10 days after knee drainage. **C:** Direct transgluteal puncture of the fluid collection produced pulsatile bright red blood consistent with arterial blood. **D:** Repeat contrast-enhanced CT scan shows dense enhancement of the lesion, which suggested it to be a pseudoaneurysm. **E:** Immediately following the diagnosis, an angiogram was obtained, which shows a large pseudoaneurysm of the superior gluteal artery. Embolization with coils was performed. **F:** Follow-up angiogram demonstrates no filling of the pseudoaneurysm, and the patient's pain gradually improved. **G:** Follow-up CT scan obtained the next morning shows no flow within the pseudoaneurysm and residual contrast within the cavity. The patient improved and was discharged 3 days following embolization. Pain developed over the next several days and gradually became worse. **H:** About 20 days after the embolization, the pain worsened to a degree that the patient could not stand up, walk, or lay on his back. The patient was readmitted, and new CT scan with intravenous contrast was obtained. The scan shows a partially resolved hematoma with an adjacent pseudoaneurysm of smaller dimensions. **I,J:** New angiogram was obtained immediately, which demonstrates no filling of the pseudoaneurysm through the gluteal artery, but filling through smaller collaterals. **K:** Injection into the iliac circumflex artery shows filling of the pseudoaneurysm via retrograde flow from the distal branches of the superior gluteal artery. Embolization through the collaterals was attempted but failed to occlude the pseudoaneurysm. CT-guided direct puncture of the pseudoaneurysm was performed, and embolization was attempted. **L:** Direct puncture of the pseudoaneurysm was performed with an 18-gauge needle. Note the tip of the needle within the pseudoaneurysm. **M:** Embolization with Histoacryl mixed with lipiodol was performed. Note the tip of the needle within the lesion and the pseudoaneurysm full of radiopaque glue. **N:** Follow-up CT scan 2 days after embolization shows the pseudoaneurysm full of glue and the tract of the needle with the radiopaque material. Following embolization, the patient improved remarkably and resumed his professional activities within 30 days. Follow-up is now 8 years and the patient still is doing well.

Comment: This case demonstrates the usefulness of less invasive procedures in patients with severe traumatic lesions of difficult surgical resolution. Osteomyelitis caused the vascular lesion, with development of the pseudoaneurysm in the gluteal artery, in an area of difficult access for surgical treatment. The diagnosis was not made initially, and an inadvertent puncture of the pseudoaneurysm was performed. Transarterial embolization occluded the pseudoaneurysm; however, there was recanalization of the lesion cavity through the distal branches of the superior gluteal artery, with recurrence of symptoms and increased risk of bleeding and neurologic damage. The second embolization attempt failed due to the difficulty in access through the collaterals. A direct approach with transgluteal puncture was chosen for direct embolization. Histoacryl was used for embolization and permanently occluded the pseudoaneurysm cavity. Histoacryl is now approved for use in United States, and is an excellent permanent occluder for embolization and proved to be the best option in this case. No tissue necrosis or other complication occurred. An alternative would be the use of multiple coils deployed inside the pseudoaneurysm. Percutaneous drainage of the pyogenic arthritis also was a unique procedure that has not been reported previously and proved very efficient.

9.8 Embolization In The Pelvis And Genitourinary Tract

Case 9.8:

A 77-year-old man presented with pelvic pain and claudication in the left leg. Angioplasty of the left superificial femoral artery was performed to treat the claudication. An aortobiiliac bypass had been placed several years earlier for treatment of an abdominal aortic aneurysm.

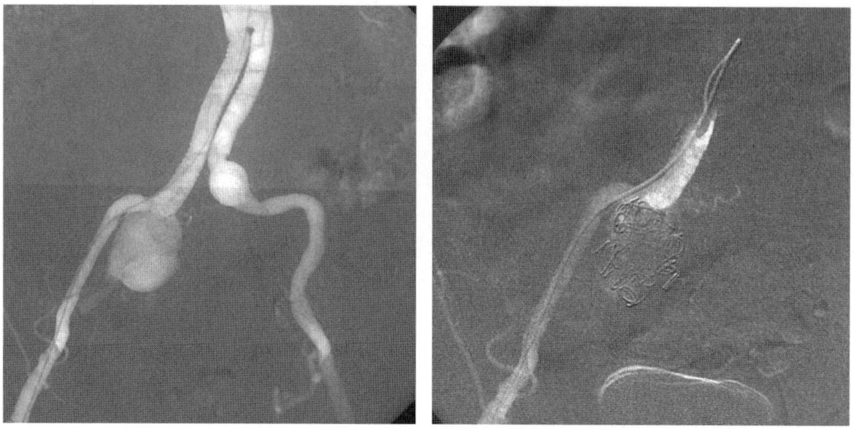

A B

Figure 9.8

A: Iliac arteriography shows a large pseudoaneurysm in the right internal iliac artery, in continuity with the distal branches. The total external diameter of the lesion seen on a diagnostic CT scan was much larger than the lumen demonstrated by angiography, which explains the symptoms of pelvic pain. **B:** Selective catheterization of the aneurysm was followed by deployment of 20 Gianturco coils of several sizes, with total occlusion of the aneurysm. Postembolization iliac arteriogram shows total occlusion of the aneurysm, with resolution of the pain over the next several days.

Comment: Large internal iliac aneurysms may be symptomatic due to enlarging size and pulsatile compression of surrounding structures. Nerve compression may be disabling and cause severe pain. The other great risk of this type of lesion is rupture. Progressive enlargement of the iliac aneurysm may result in rupture or sudden enlargement with or without distal embolism causing blue toe syndrome and ischemia of the gluteal muscles and skin.

Embolization is usually effective in treating this type of lesion and may effectively isolate the aneurysm from the main parent vessel. A large number of coils is necessary for occlusion of the aneurysm, and the distal arterial outlet should be specially occluded. Even if a stent graft or covered stent is used to isolate the aneurysm from the parent artery, it is necessary to occlude and pack the aneurysm with coils or detachable balloons.

9.9 Embolization In The Pelvis And Genitourinary Tract

Case 9.9:

A 24-year-old woman with chronic renal failure received a kidney transplant in the right side of the pelvis, which eventually required nephrectomy due to rejection. A new kidney was transplanted to the left pelvis. The patient presented with pelvic pain several weeks following surgery. In one of the posttransplant follow-up ultrasound examinations, a pseudoaneurysm was identified in relation to the right external iliac artery. An angiogram and possible treatment were requested.

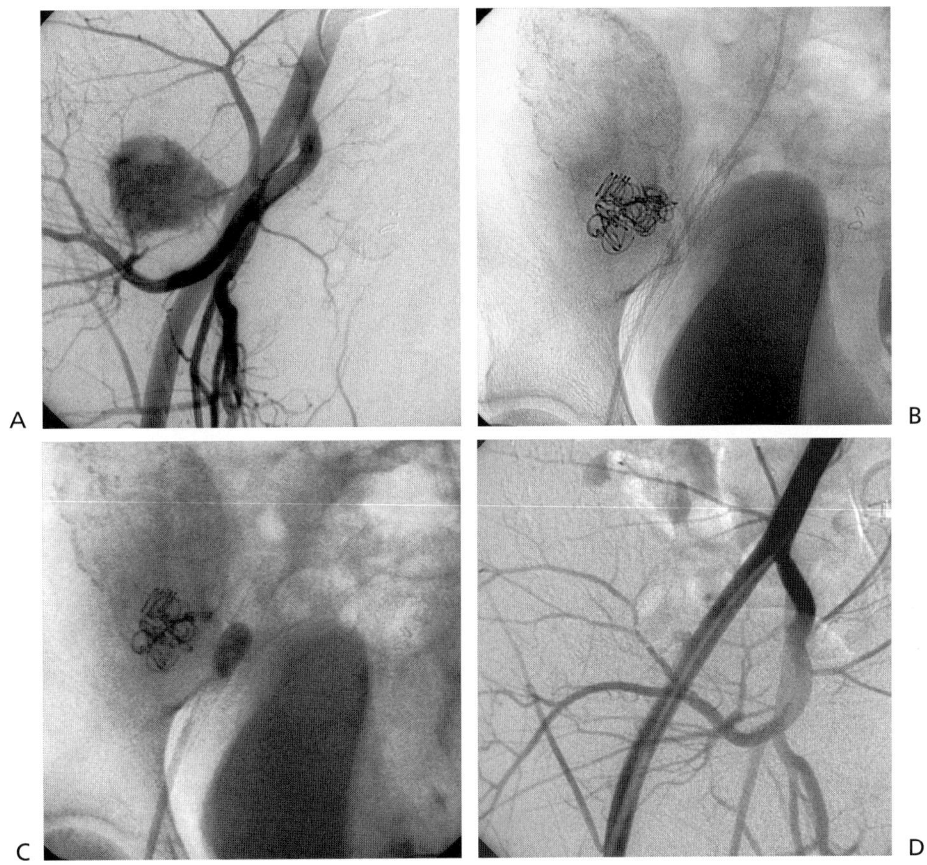

Figure 9.9

A: Contralateral femoral catheterization with selective injections in the right common iliac artery allowed identification of a large pseudoaneurysm in the right external iliac artery, related to the anastomotic site of the first transplanted kidney. **B:** The catheter was introduced into the pseudoaneurysm through the mesh wall of a 12-mm × 40-mm Wallstent using an ipsilateral approach, and multiple coils were deployed within the cavity. **C:** The occlusion balloon was used to block flow at the level of the mouth of the pseudoaneurysm for 20 minutes and allow thrombosis of the pseudoaneurysm. **D:** Postembolization angiogram of the right iliac artery shows occlusion of the pseudoaneurysm, which was followed by control of pain.

Comment: This is a typical example of a case where a covered stent, if available, would be the best device for treating the pseudoaneurysm and maintaining patency of the parent vessel. The option of embolizing the lumen of the pseudoaneurysm and protecting the neck of the pseudoaneurysm and the lumen of the parent vessel with a bare stent is feasible; however, there is no guarantee that the pseudoaneurysm will thrombose because there is still communication with the arterial blood flow/pressure. A large number of coils is necessary to fill the lumen of this type of lesion, but there is always the risk of not treating adequately the neck of the pseudoaneurysm. Stasis promoted by balloon occlusion of the parent artery flow also helps in developing thrombosis.

9.10 Embolization In The Pelvis And Genitourinary Tract

Case 9.10:

A 24-year-old woman with cancer of the uterus was treated with radical surgery followed by radiation therapy. Dehiscence of the suture resulted, followed by transvaginal hemorrhage and bleeding through the surgical wound. Surgical inspection demonstrated a pseudoaneurysm from the right external iliac artery that was treated by ligation of the external iliac artery above and below the lesion. Further deterioration of the patient's condition included transvaginal bleeding and fecal leakage through the suture wound. The patient became hemodynamically unstable, and an arteriogram was requested for possible embolization because of the difficulty of surgical intervention.

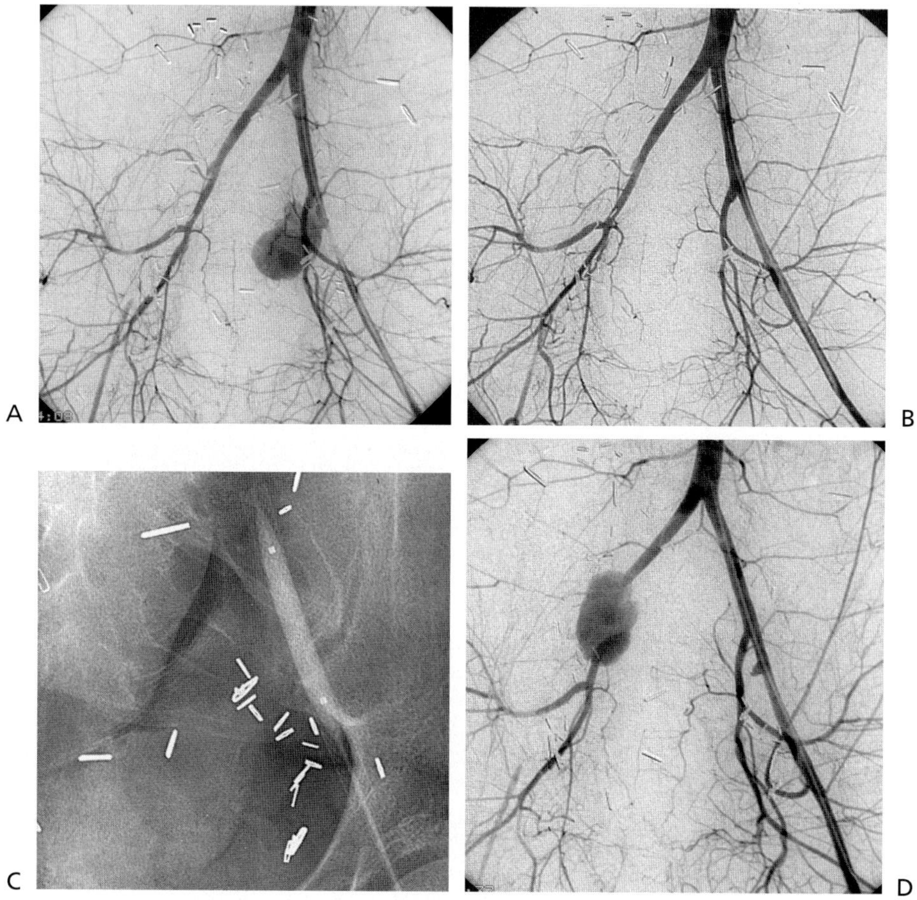

Figure 9.10

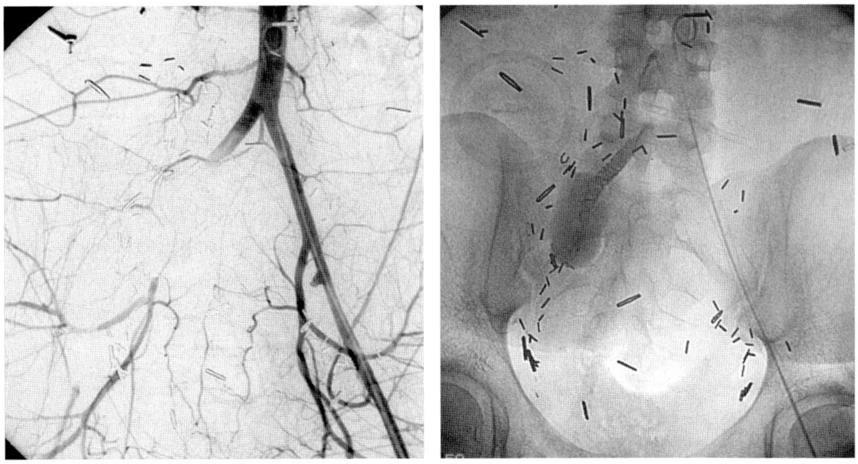

E F

Figure 9.10 *(continued)*

A: Pelvic arteriogram shows occlusion of the right external iliac artery that was previously ligated. A large pseudoaneurysm identified in the left external iliac artery was associated with severe spasm of the parent artery in the most proximal segment. **B:** A Wallstent (8 mm × 40 mm) was placed within the artery at the level of the pseudoaneurysm. Note total occlusion of the pseudoaneurysm. **C:** Angioplasty balloon was used to occlude the flow within the artery and pseudoaneurysm for 20 minutes. **D:** Recurrence of hemorrhage occurred about 1 week after stent placement. New pelvic arteriogram shows occlusion of the left pseudoaneurysm, with filling of a small segment of the neck. There was a new large pseudoaneurysm from the stub of the ligated right external iliac artery, with patency of the internal iliac artery and reconstitution of the right common femoral artery. **E:** From the contralateral approach, the pseudoaneurysm, the short stub of the right external iliac artery, and the proximal right internal iliac artery were embolized with multiple coils. Follow-up angiogram shows total occlusion of the pseudoaneurysm and maintenance of flow into the internal iliac and common femoral arteries. **F:** Unsubtracted picture of the pelvis shows residual contrast material within the pseudoaneurysm and the coils in the occluded vessels. Despite control of bleeding, the patient developed renal failure and untreatable sepsis, and she died 25 days after the embolization.

Comment: Arterial pseudoaneurysms supposedly are better treated by covered stent grafts; however, covered stents are not yet universally available. Also, it is not known if covered stents are effective and safe in the presence of infection, as was obvious in the case of this patient. Bare stents with a tight mesh can be used across the orifice of an aneurysm or pseudoaneurysm and act as a wall, allowing thrombosis to develop within the lesion. It is of benefit to occlude flow in the parent vessel and within the aneurysm. In this case, the bare stent proved to be effective in controlling the bleeding; unfortunately, the patient developed a second pseudoaneurysm in a different location that required embolization therapy. Embolization can be performed through the mesh of the stent, as demonstrated in Figure 9.9D, which is much safer. Filling the cavity of the pseudoaneurysm with glue, coils or balloons are alternatives that may be used in different clinical settings. Embolization of the parent vessel also is very effective when the distal blood flow provided by the artery is negligible or unimportant to the surrounding tissues. In this patient, the surgical alternative was not an option due to the significant changes in the pelvis related to radiation therapy, infection, and bleeding. Embolization played a significant role in prolonging somewhat the life of this patient.

Suggested Reading

Bastuba MD, Saenz de Tejada I, Dinlenc CZ, et al. Arterial priapism: diagnosis, treatment, and follow-up. *J Urol* 1994;151:1231–1237.

Belgrano E, Puppo P, Quattrini S, et al. Percutaneous temporary embolization of the internal pudendal arteries in idiopathic priapism: 2 additional cases. *J Urol* 1984;131:756–758.

Carmignani G, Belgrano E, Puppo P. Idiopathic priapism successfully treated by unilateral embolization of internal pudendal artery. *J Urol* 1984;131:553–554.

Cohen G, Braunstein L, Ball D, et al. Selective arterial embolization of idiopathic priapism. *Cardiovasc Intervent Radiol* 1996;19:47–49.

Hollis H, Luethke J, Yakes W, et al. Percutaneous embolization of an internal iliac artery aneurysm: technical considerations and literature review. *J Vasc Interv Radiol* 1994;5:449–451.

Ito M, Matsui K, Mabe K, et al. Transcatheter embolization of pelvic arteries as the safest method for postpartum hemorrhage. *Int J Gynaecol Obstet* 1986;24:373–378.

Lazinger M, Beckman C, Cossi A, et al. Selective embolization of bilateral arterial cavernous fistulas for posttraumatic penile arterial priapism. *Cardiovasc Intervent Radiol* 1996;19:281–284.

Puppo P, Belgrano E, Germinale F, et al. Angiographic treatment of high-flow priapism. *Eur Urol* 1985;11:397–400.

Walker WJ. Case report: successful internal iliac artery embolisation with glue in a case of massive obstetric haemorrhage. *Clin Radiol* 1996;51:442–444.

Walker TG, Grant PW, Goldstein I, et al. High-flow priapism: treatment with superselective transcatheter embolization. *Radiology* 1990;1053–1054.

Wear JB, Crummy AB, Munson BO. Post traumatic priapism: successful treatment with autologous clot embolization. *AJR* 1979;133:329–334.

Winter CC, McDowell G. Experience with 105 patients with priapism: update review of all aspects. *J Urol* 1988;140:980–983.

Yamashita Y, Harada M, Yamamoto H, et al. Transcatheter arterial embolization, of obstetric and gynaecological bleeding: efficacy and clinical outcome. *Br J Radiol* 1994;67:530–534.

CHAPTER 10

Embolization, Blood Flow Reduction, And Infusion In The Treatment Of Lesions Of The Musculoskeletal System

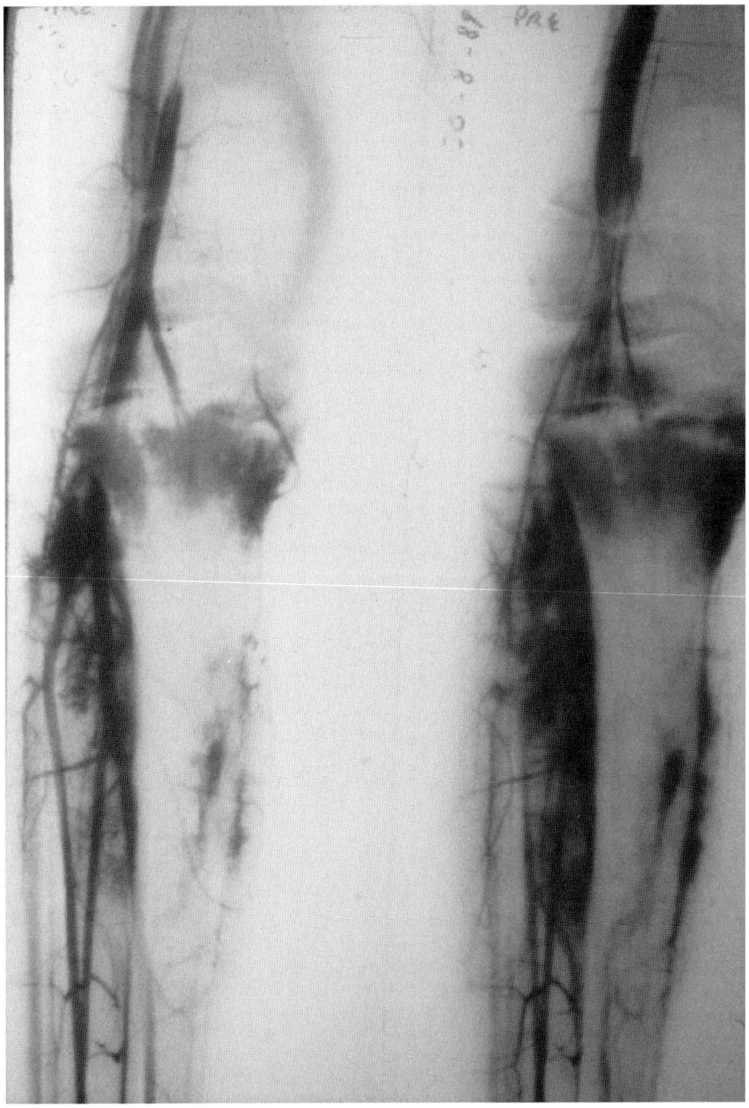

10.1 Embolization In The Musculoskeletal System

Case 10.1:

A 13-year-old male patient presented with osteosarcoma of the right tibia with severe pain and difficult deambulation.

A, B

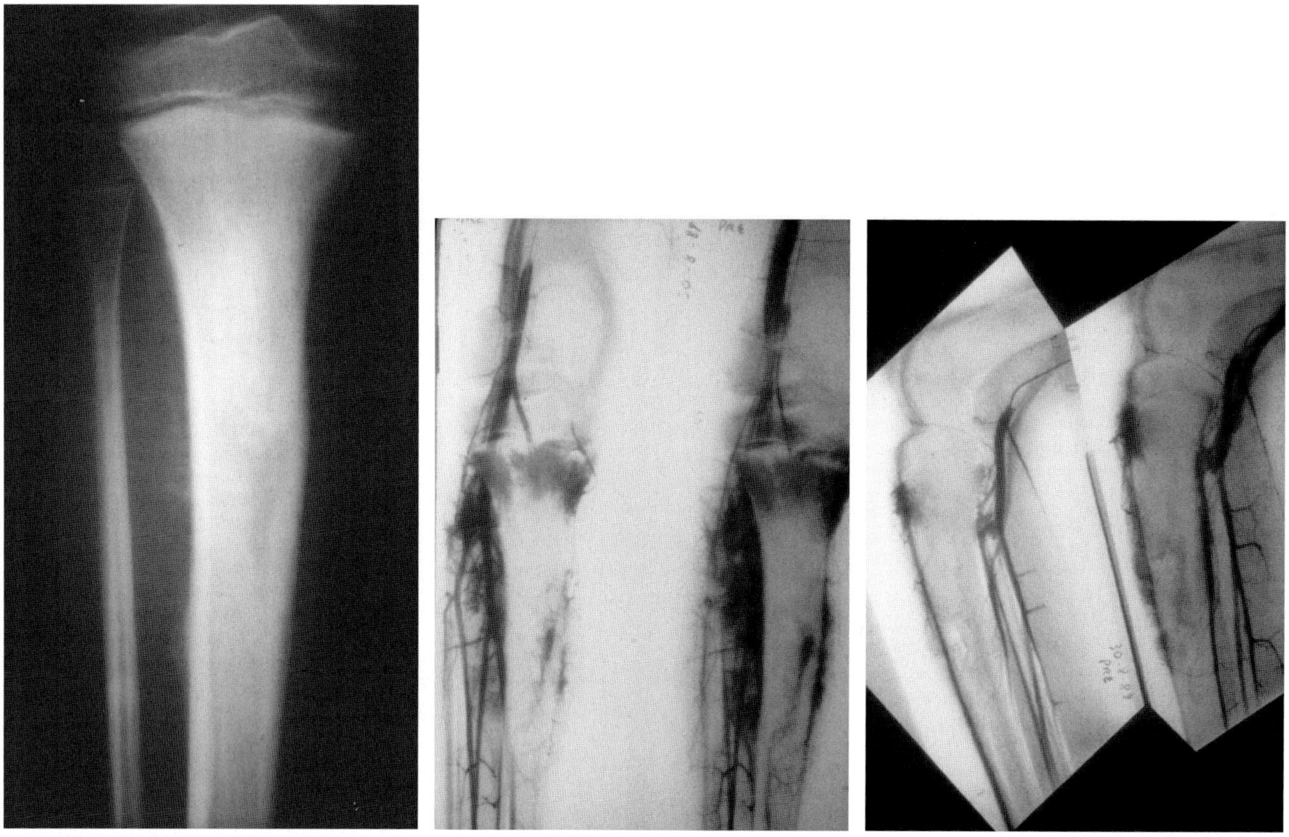

C

Figure 10.1

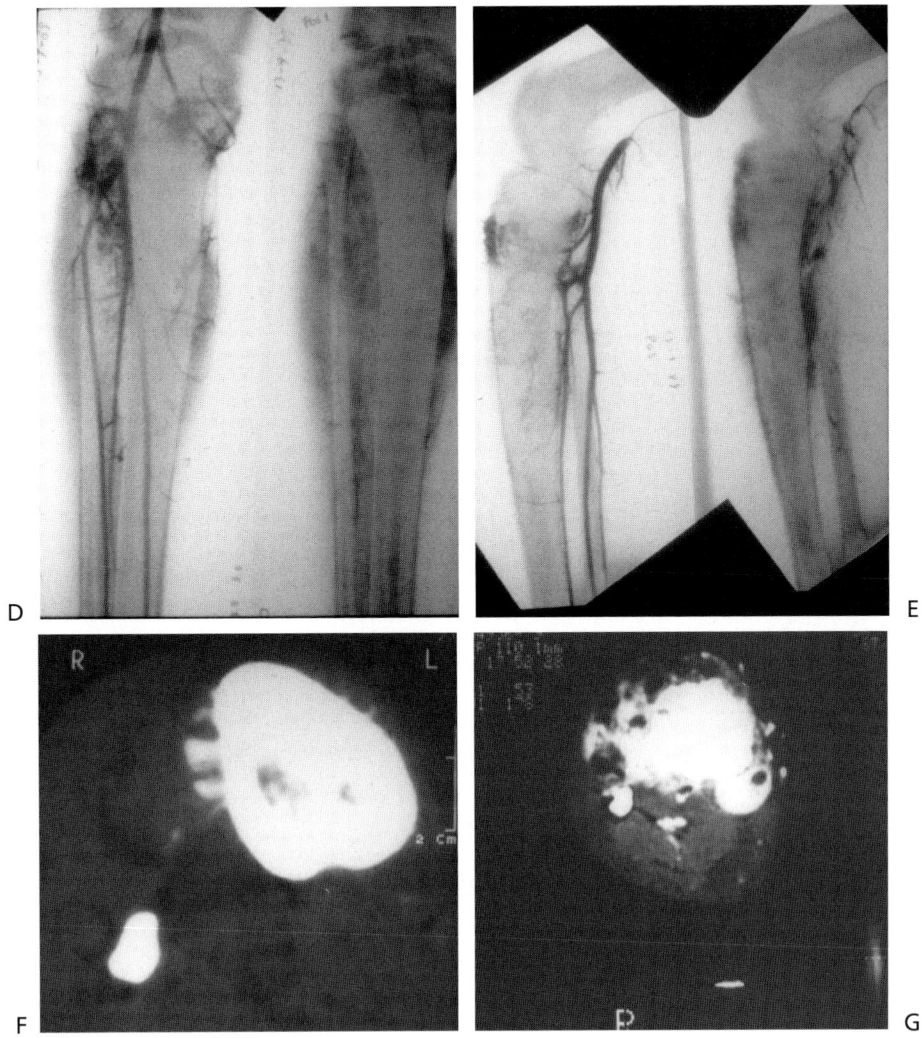

Figure 10.1 *(continued)*

A: Plain x-ray film of the leg shows the bone mass with calcification. **B,C:** Preinfusion arteriogram in the anteroposterior and lateral views show the large hypervascular neoplasm of the proximal tibia. **D,E:** Following the second infusion of cisplatin, the arteriogram demonstrates a significant decrease in neovascularity. **F,G:** Computed tomographic (CT) scans before and after cisplatin infusion show reduction neoplasm size and increase in lesion calcification. The preexisting pain improved markedly following treatment.

Comment: The 3-year disease-free survival rate of patients with medullary osteosarcoma treated by surgery alone or in combination with radiation therapy usually is 20% and may not be more than 40%. Chemotherapy delivered systemically, utilizing high-dose methotrexate with a combination of other factors or doxorubicin (Adriamycin) as a single agent or in a multiagent regimen, has resulted in the eradication of established metastases, destruction of primary tumor, and increase in disease-free survival to 55% in 3 years. Selective intraarterial infusion of certain chemotherapeutic agents that are effective systemically have the potential to increase effectiveness, allowing limb salvage with removal of the tumor-bearing bone and insertion of an internal prosthesis. Patients with medullary osteosarcoma of the extremities are considered candidates for limb salvage procedure after intraarterial infusion of chemotherapy. Fifty-seven percent of the patients have angiographic improvement, defined as decrease or disappearance of tumor vascularity, indicating partial or complete remission, and compares favorably to the systemically administered cis-diaminedichloroplatinum. In another series of patients treated by chemotherapy (cisplatin) and conservative surgery, there was improvement of pain in the majority of patients and limb salvation in 24 of 40 patients; 72% of patients were disease-free in 2 years of follow-up. Cisplatin doses are 120 to 200 mg/m^2 in 300 mL of saline solution, infused in 2 to 24 hours every 2 weeks, and up to 5 to 7 times. Hydration is necessary, and forced diuresis is done with mannitol during drug infusion.

10.2 Embolization In The Musculoskeletal System

Case 10.2:

A 24-year-old female patient presented with osteosarcoma of the proximal tibia. Severe pain precluded deambulation.

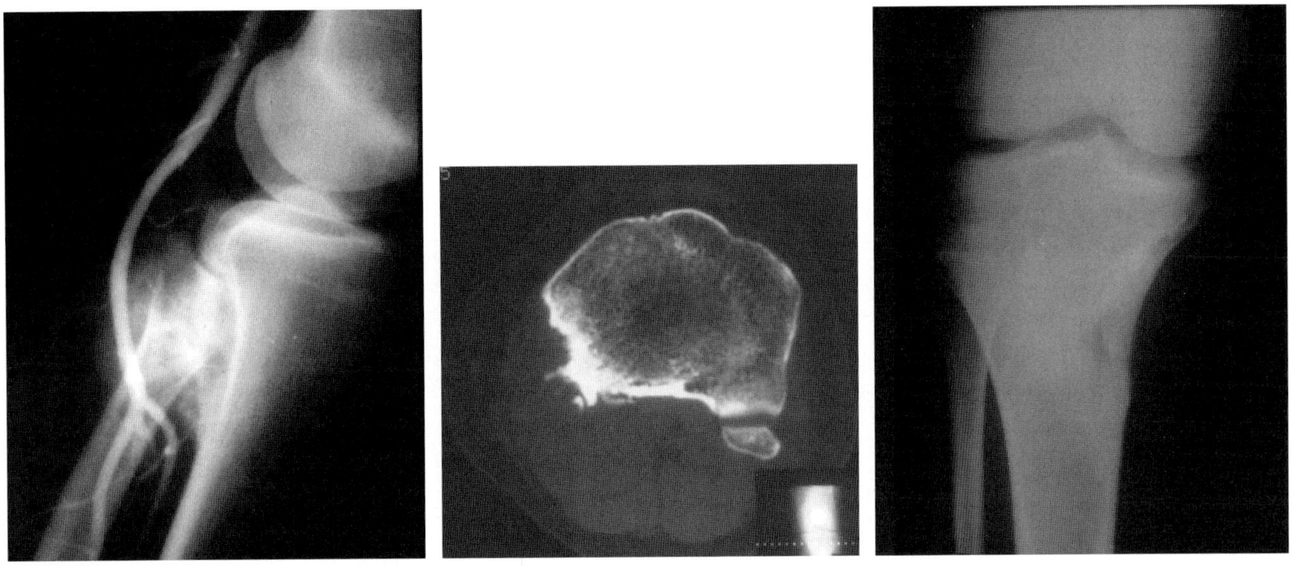

A

B, C

Figure 10.2

A: Lateral view of an arteriogram shows the neoplasm below the knee. Note the hypervascularity. Infusion of cisplatin was performed. **B:** Follow-up CT scan shows reduction of the mass and increased calcification. **C:** Plain film of the proximal tibia shows increased density of the lesion and reduction in size.

Comment: It is difficult to define response to treatment in bone tumors. The response to intraarterial infusion as determined by clinical examination is seen as heat, tenderness, decreased pain, and decreased mass size; by conventional radiography and CT scan as change in soft tissue mass and increased calcification; by angiography as change in tumor vascularity and tumor stain density; and by histopathologic examination as percentage of tumor destruction and fibrovascular regeneration.

Complete remission is defined as disappearance of all signs and symptoms of tumor plus 60% to 100% tumor destruction with evidence of fibrovascular activity. Partial remission is defined as 50% or greater decrease in soft tissue mass, together with unequivocal improvement seen on angiography or CT scan.

Intraarterial infusion for osteosarcoma treatment is accomplished by subselective catheterization of the feeding vessels. Systemic heparinization is used to minimize thromboembolism. Toxic effects of cisplatin infusion include renal impairment, hematologic depression, high-frequency hearing loss, nausea, and vomiting.

10.3 Embolization In The Musculoskeletal System

Case 10.3:

A 20-year-old male patient presented with fibrosarcoma of the right leg. A large mass was present, with associated pain and soreness. Embolization was requested as a preoperative measure to reduce bleeding and facilitate resection.

A, B

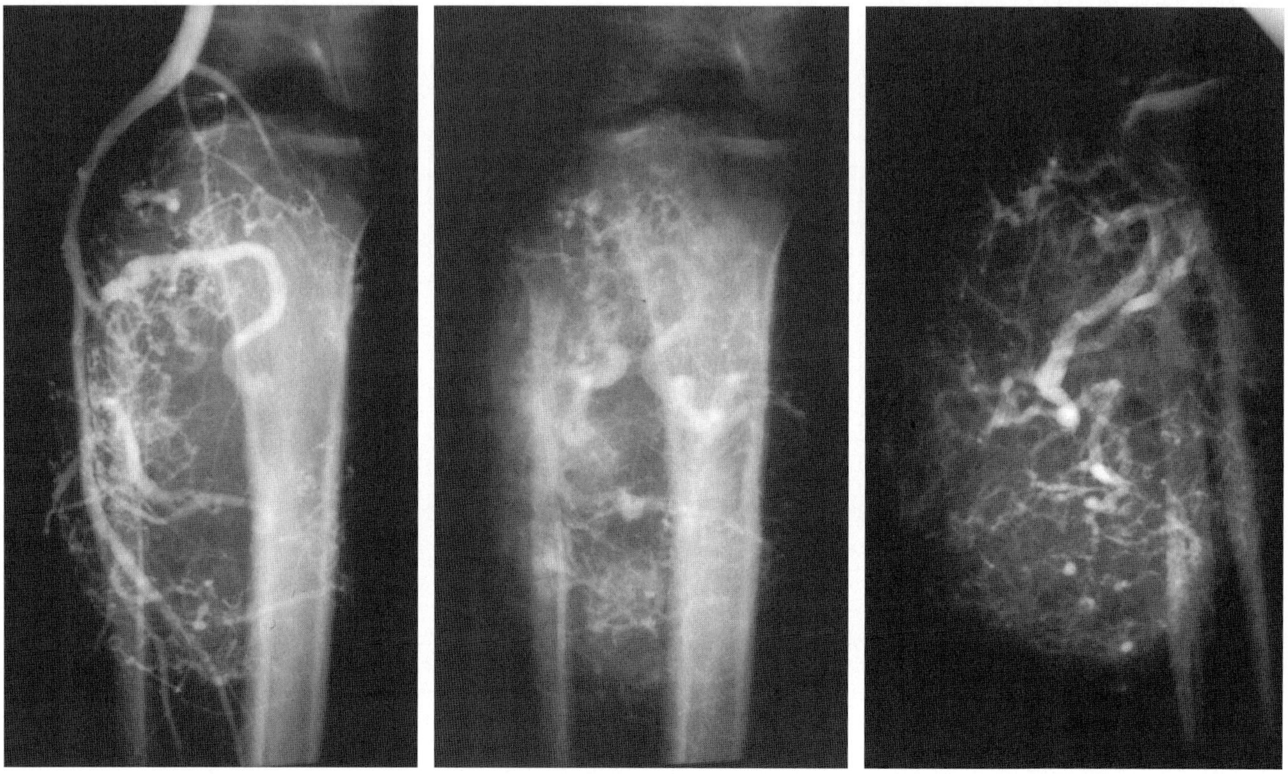

C

Figure 10.3

D 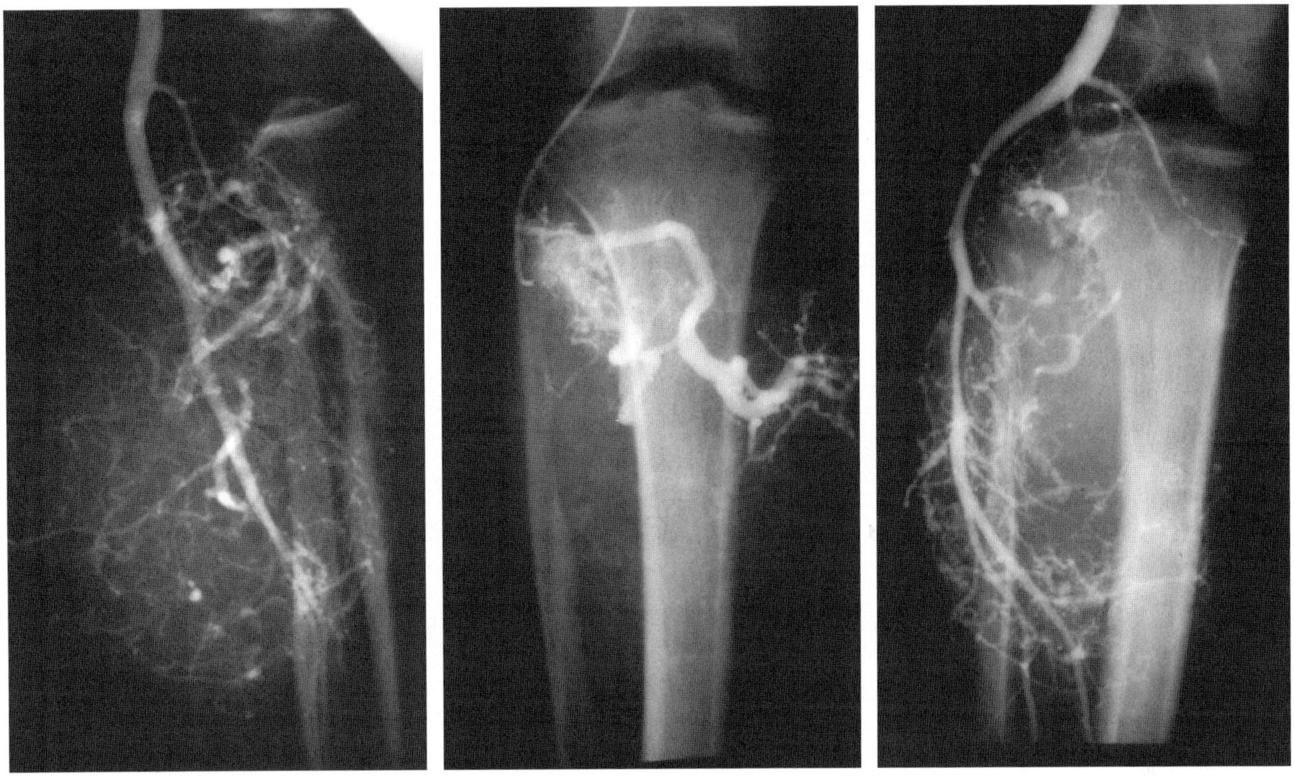 E, F

Figure 10.3 *(continued)*

A: Arteriogram of a large soft tissue mass in the thigh shows hypervascularity and tumoral vessels. **B:** Late-phase arteriogram shows vascular lakes and venous return. **C–E:** Selective injections were performed and followed by embolization with Ivalon and Gelfoam particles. **F:** Postembolization angiogram shows marked reduction in vascularity within the tumor. Extensive surgical resection was performed, with reduced loss of blood.

Comment: The mechanism of action of arterial occlusion in the management of neoplasms of bone is not obvious. It is believed, especially with regard to hypervascular neoplasms, that the occlusion decreases the size of the tumor and slows its progression. This action, in turn, decreases the pressure of expansion or stretching of the adjacent strictures, such as the periosteum containing the nerve fibers, that are partly responsible for the pain. The main role of embolization in soft tissue tumors is to improve resectability; however, major or total necrosis of the lesion can be achieved in some cases.

10.4 Embolization In The Musculoskeletal System

Case 10.4:

A 45-year-old male patient presented with plasmocytoma of the sacrum. Severe pain and instability precluded normal activities. Percutaneous biopsy and embolization were requested.

A, B C D, E F

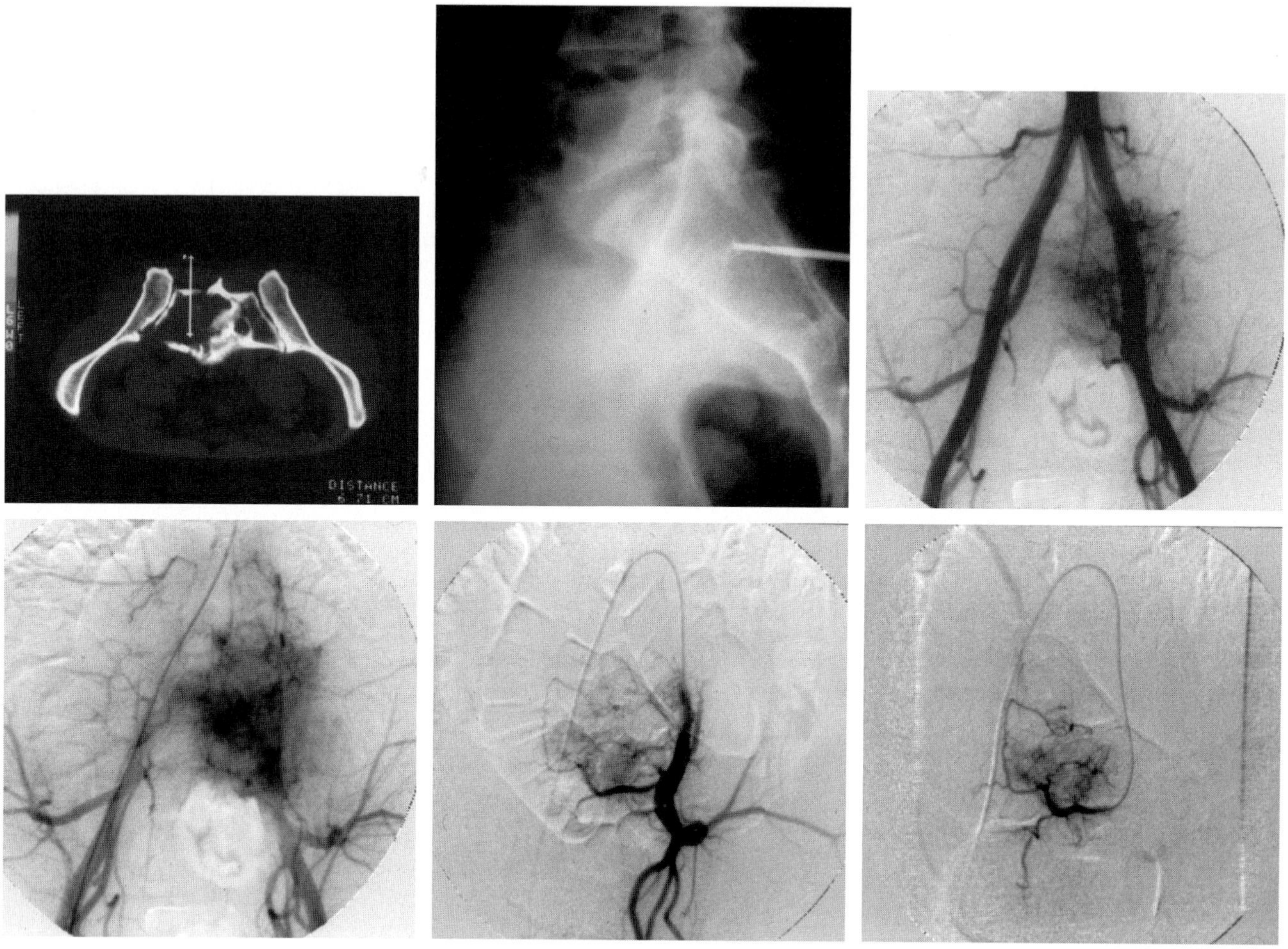

Figure 10.4

G 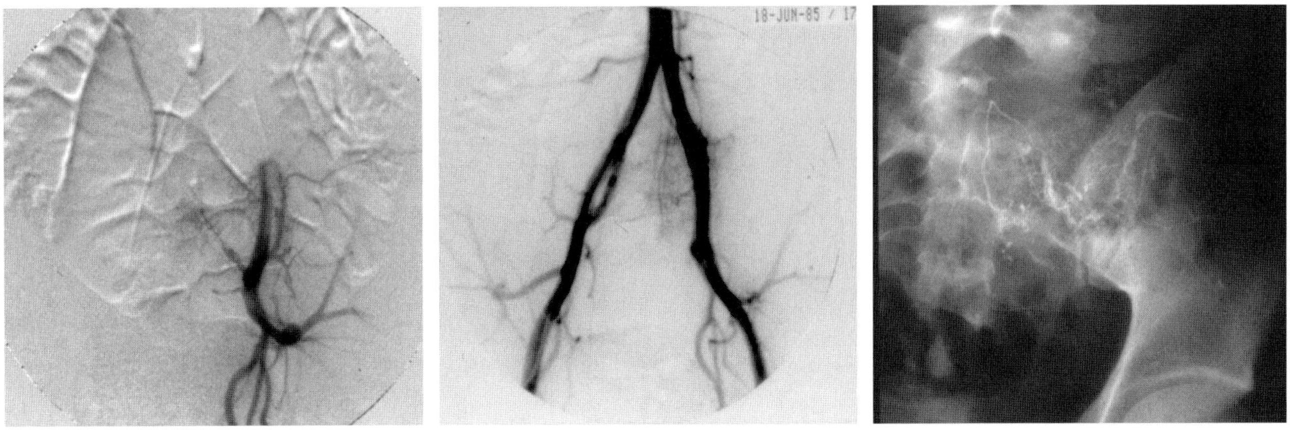 H, I

Figure 10.4 *(continued)*

A: CT scan of the sacrum was obtained for bone biopsy. Note the large osteolytic lesion in the left sacral wing. **B:** Lateral view of the sacrum with the bone biopsy needle in place. **C,D:** Pelvic arteriogram shows the large hypervascular bone mass in the left sacrum. **E,F:** Selective angiogram of the left internal iliac artery and branches was followed by embolization with cyanoacrylate. **G:** Postembolization left internal iliac artery injection shows marked reduction in the vascularity of the tumor mass. **H:** Pelvic arteriogram demonstrates total devascularization of the sacral tumor. **I:** Plain film of the pelvic bones shows the radiopaque cyanoacrylate in the tumoral vessels. Surgical resection followed embolization, and metal braces were used to stabilize the spine and pelvis.

Comment: Angiography makes it possible to locate vascularized vertebral and spine tumors and to determine their size and especially their extraosseous extension. The angiographic differential diagnosis, however, is limited. Metastases, sarcomas, and myelomas are hypervascular and supplied by irregular arteries with blood pools and arteriovenous shunts. Other tumors, such as hemangiopericytomas, aneurysmal bone cysts, and giant cell tumors, may present a similar angiographic pattern. Vertebral hemangiomas are angiographically typical, seen as blood pools that fill from the ipsilateral and contralateral hemivertebra.

Selective angiographic evaluation is followed by embolization with small particles, such as Ivalon, dura mater, or cyanoacrylate. Embolization of vascularized spine tumors usually is performed to facilitate surgery or improve symptoms as a palliative measure to reduce compression of adjacent structures or the spinal cord. Regression of spinal malignancies may be achieved, sometimes with recalcification of the affected bone structure.

10.5 Embolization In The Musculoskeletal System

Case 10.5:

A 35-year-old male patient presented with a chondrosarcoma of L2. Pain was severe with evidence of medullary compression. Preoperative embolization was requested.

A, B

C

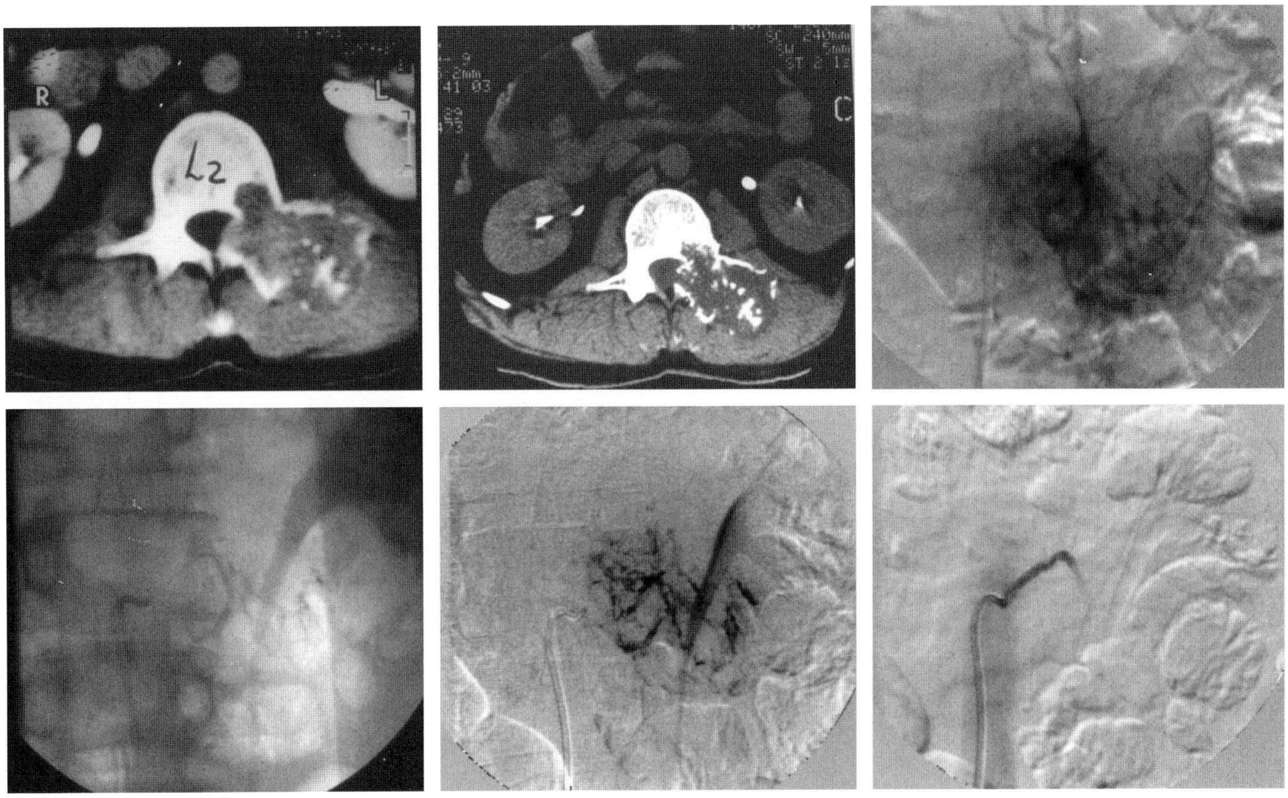

D, E

F

Figure 10.5

A: Preembolization CT scan shows the L2 mass with calcifications within. **B:** Postembolization CT scan shows the radiopaque cyanoacrylate within the lesion. **C:** Selective injection in the second left lumbar artery shows a hypervascular mass extending beyond the bone edges. **D:** A microcatheter was advanced into the lumbar artery for embolization with cyanoacrylate. **E:** Embolization was performed, and occlusion of the tumor vessels was achieved. **F:** Postembolization angiogram shows total occlusion of the tumor vessels. Surgery with tumor resection was performed a few days after embolization.

Comment: Embolization is an important adjuvant for treatment of bone tumors. Embolization most commonly is performed to facilitate surgical resection. Palliative treatment also is important, because a number of these tumors will respond to embolization. Alleviation of symptoms may be achieved by embolization alone, and actual necrosis of the tumor may develop. Calcification of the necrotic tumor is helpful to maintain stability and reduce pressure of the tumor over adjacent structures.

10.6 Embolization In The Musculoskeletal System

Case 10.6:

A 35-year-old female patient presented with giant cell tumor of the pubic bone extending into the right hip joint, with severe pain and difficult deambulation.

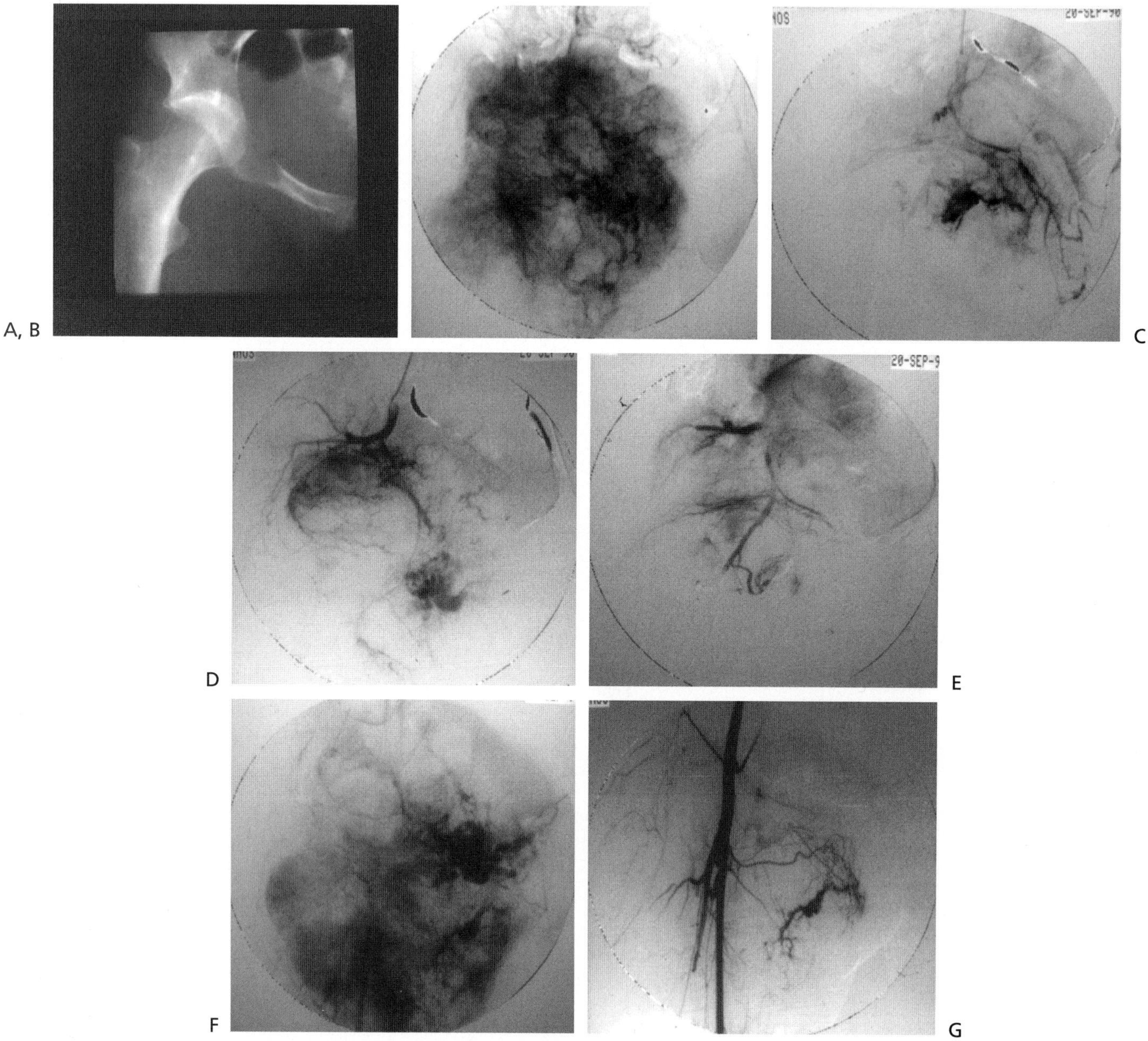

Figure 10.6

A: Plain x-ray film of the right hip shows a sharply defined osteolytic lesion associated with a large soft tissue mass. **B:** Right internal iliac artery angiogram reveals a massively hypervascular mass. **C:** Embolization was performed with Ivalon and Gelfoam. **D:** Superior gluteal artery angiogram demonstrates the upper part of the hypervascular mass. **E:** Embolization with Ivalon and Gelfoam was performed. **F:** Injection at the common femoral artery shows the lower component of the mass is still open and has significant hypervascularity. **G:** Embolization of several branches was performed with Ivalon and Gelfoam.

Comment: Embolization is effective in controlling symptoms of giant cell tumors of the bone. Relief of pain is obtained in a large number of patients who do not respond to previous treatment, such as surgery, radiation therapy, or chemotherapy. Pain alleviation usually is obtained within 1 week after embolization, with tumoral response in size and increased calcification. Surgical resection may be feasible following embolization due to reduction in size. In a series of 21 patients with giant cell tumor of the bone, 67% of patients responded to treatment. There was symptom control in 42% of patients for 1 to 7 years (mean 25 months), although recurrence was observed in 4 patients at an average of 45 months. There was only improvement of symptoms in 19% of the cases.

Suggested Reading

Ekelund L, Laurin S, Lunderquist A. Comparison of a vasoconstrictor and vasodilator in pharmacoangiography of bone and soft-tissue tumors. *Radiology* 1977;122:95.

Feldman F, Casarella WJ, Dick HM, et al. Selective intra-arterial embolization of bone tumors: a useful adjunct in the management of selected lesions. *AJR* 1975;123:130.

Loring L, Hallisey M. Arteriography and interventional therapy for diseases of the hand. *Radiographics* 1995;15:1299–1310.

Wallace S, Granmayeh M, de Santos LA, et al. Arterial occlusion of pelvic bone tumors. *Cancer* 1979;43:322.

CHAPTER 11

Embolization In Hemangiomas, Arteriovenous Malformations, And Arteriovenous Fistulas

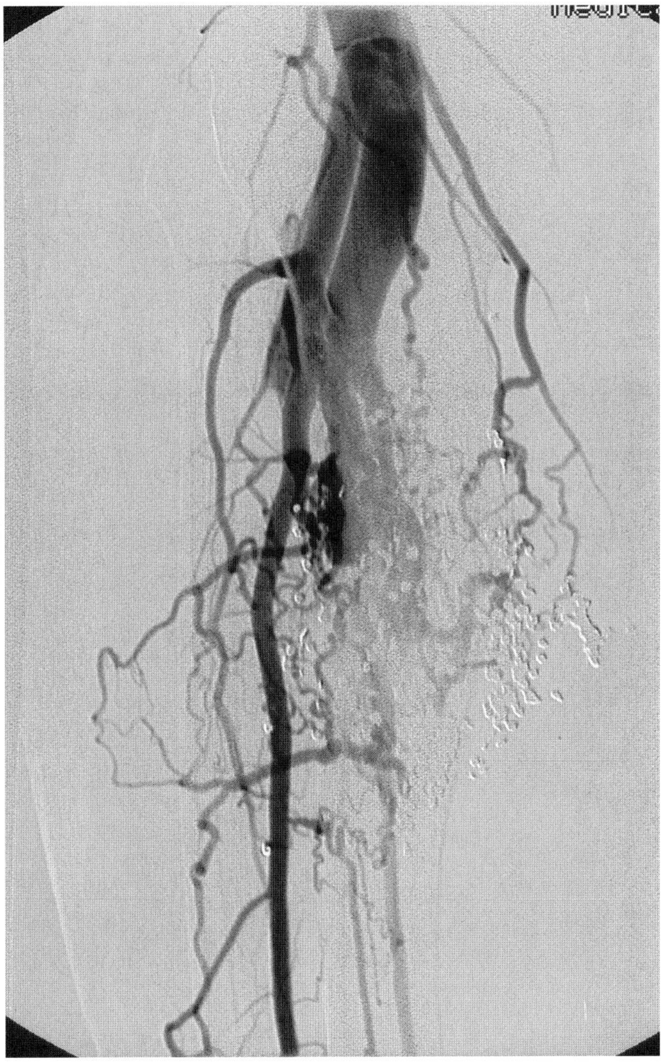

11.1 Embolization In Arteriovenous Malformations And Fistulas

Case 11.1:

A 42-year-old woman underwent surgery for discal hernia at L5–S1. Months after surgery, a murmur was heard on the pelvis, associated with left leg venous stasis. An arteriogram was requested for diagnosis, to be followed by surgical treatment.

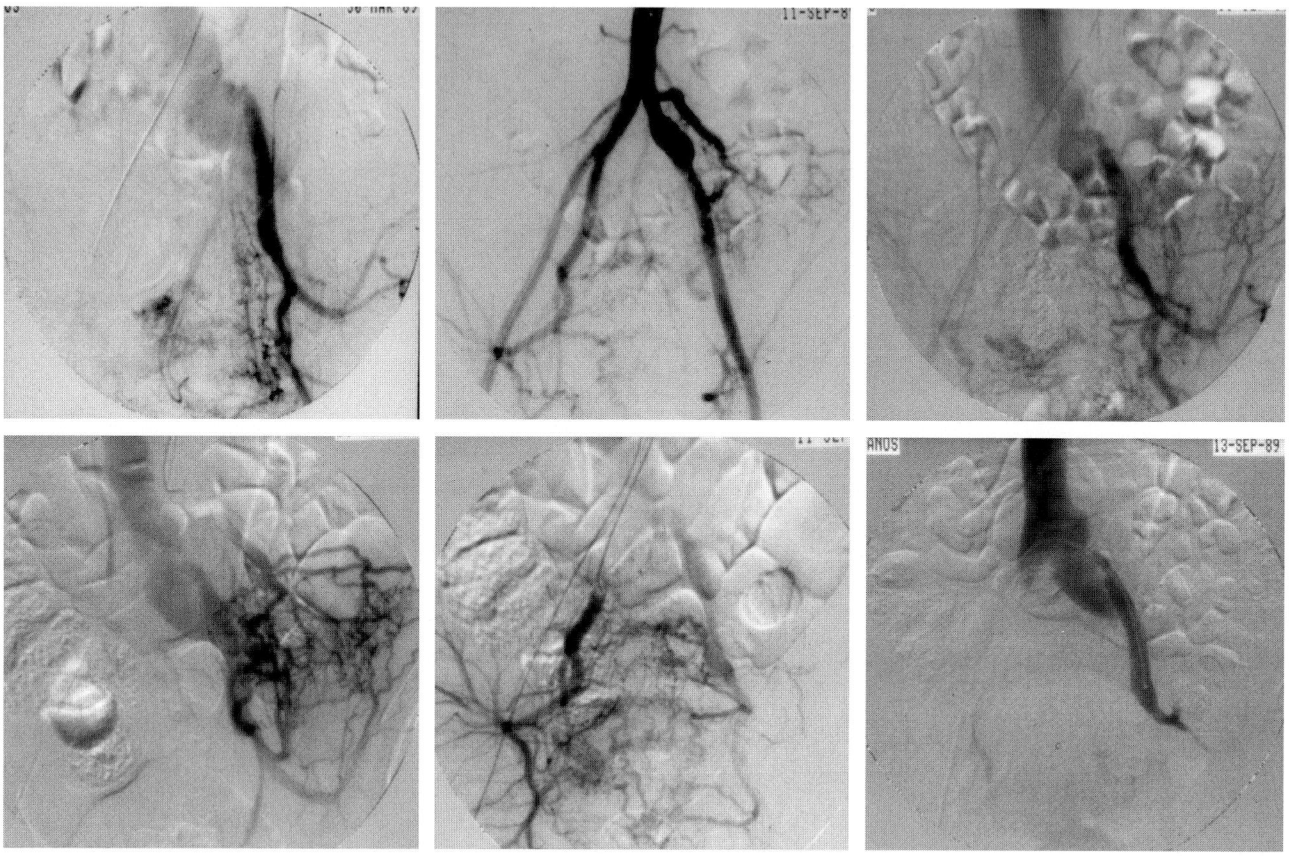

A, B

C

D, E

F

Figure 11.1

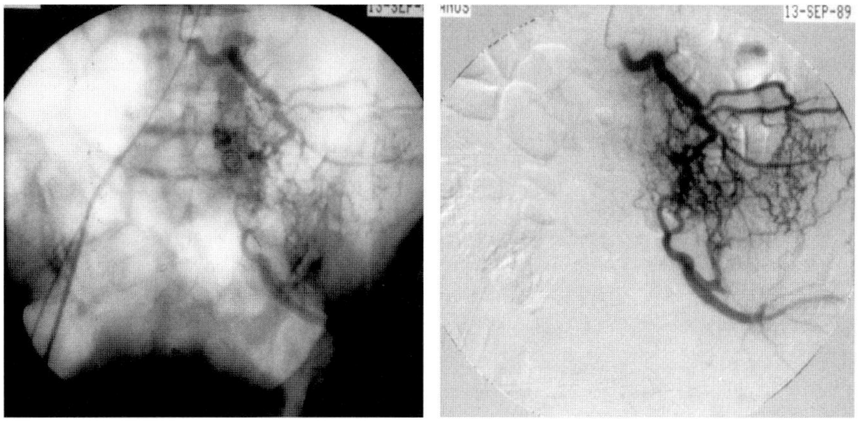

G H

Figure 11.1 *(continued)*

A: Pelvic arteriogram shows a direct arteriovenous (A-V) fistula between the left internal iliac artery and left common iliac vein. Late-phase angiogram demonstrates retrograde filling of the distal left internal iliac artery and the connection with the common iliac vein by the A-V fistula. At this time, with the diagnosis of A-V fistula, a decision was made to take the patient to surgery and to suture a polytetrafluoroethylene (PTFE) patch at the origin of the left internal iliac vein to close the A-V fistula. **B:** Six months after surgery, the patient presented with recurrent symptoms of A-V fistula in the pelvis. Pelvic arteriogram shows occlusion of the origin of the left internal iliac artery with aneurysmatic dilation of the common left iliac artery. **C:** Postsurgical late-phase arteriogram shows retrograde filling of the distal left internal iliac artery, now isolated from the orifice in the iliac artery, with flow originating from an enlarged left lumbar artery and draining into the A-V fistula. **D:** Selective injection of the fourth left lumbar artery shows filling of the superior gluteal artery and left internal iliac artery, as well as the A-V fistula. **E:** Injection into the right internal iliac artery shows contralateral filling of branches of the left internal iliac artery and the A-V fistula. **F:** Without access for embolization through the arterial side of the circulation, a venous approach was used. Through the right iliac vein, a catheter was advanced over the confluence of the iliac veins; through the fistulous orifice the catheter was advanced into the isolated left internal iliac artery. Note the stenosis at the level of the fistulous tract. **G:** Embolization with coils was performed in the arterial segment of the A-V fistula beyond the fistulous tract. The unsubtracted arteriogram shows the coils within the artery. **H:** Postembolization selective injection of the fourth left lumbar artery shows filling of the superior gluteal artery and left internal iliac artery and occlusion of the A-V fistula. The coils are barely visible.

Comment: A-V fistulas are abnormal communications between the arteries and veins. Congenital A-V fistulas are due to an arrest in embryonic development at a later fetal stage than the formation of hemangiomas. Acquired A-V fistulas usually are caused by trauma due to a penetrating wound. Congenital lesions usually do not cause significant heart failure due to high output, although other local effects may occur and are related to A-V fistula location. Traumatic A-V fistulas more frequently cause heart failure due to overload, and treatment may become an urgent need. Treatment of A-V fistulas may be surgical or interventional. Surgical ligation of the A-V fistula may require extensive dissection, and the fistulous rent must be sutured or closed with a patch, as was done initially in the case presented. If the vessels are not separated and careful analysis of the anatomy is not considered, the procedure may fail and the A-V fistula may remain open. The reported case was a side-to-side A-V fistula from the left internal iliac artery with the internal iliac vein. Surgery addressed only the orifice of the internal iliac artery and not the actual rent of the fistula. In occluding the hypogastric artery orifice, surgery in this case precluded what could have been a direct approach for embolization. The interventional treatment of a lesion, such as this one, may be performed using two different technologies. One method is direct embolization of the fistulous tract (not the case for this patient) or embolization of the parent vessel. The other method is placement of a covered stent that will occlude the rent of the fistula, mainly applicable to side-to-side fistulas. When the A-V fistula involves a terminal vessel or there is a tract that may have connections with collaterals, embolization of the tract up to the fistulous rent is more advisable. In this case, there was no direct access from the arterial side after surgery; therefore, a venous approach was used to occlude the artery, retrogradely through the A-V communication. Embolization of the artery with Gianturco coils achieved A-V fistula occlusion.

11.2 Embolization In Arteriovenous Malformations And Fistulas

Case 11.2:

A 43 year-old-man suffered a gunshot wound in the right leg and developed an A-V fistula, venous congestion, edema, and ulceration at the ankle. A bruit was heard over the lesion, associated with severe swell. An arteriogram was requested for diagnosis and possible embolization.

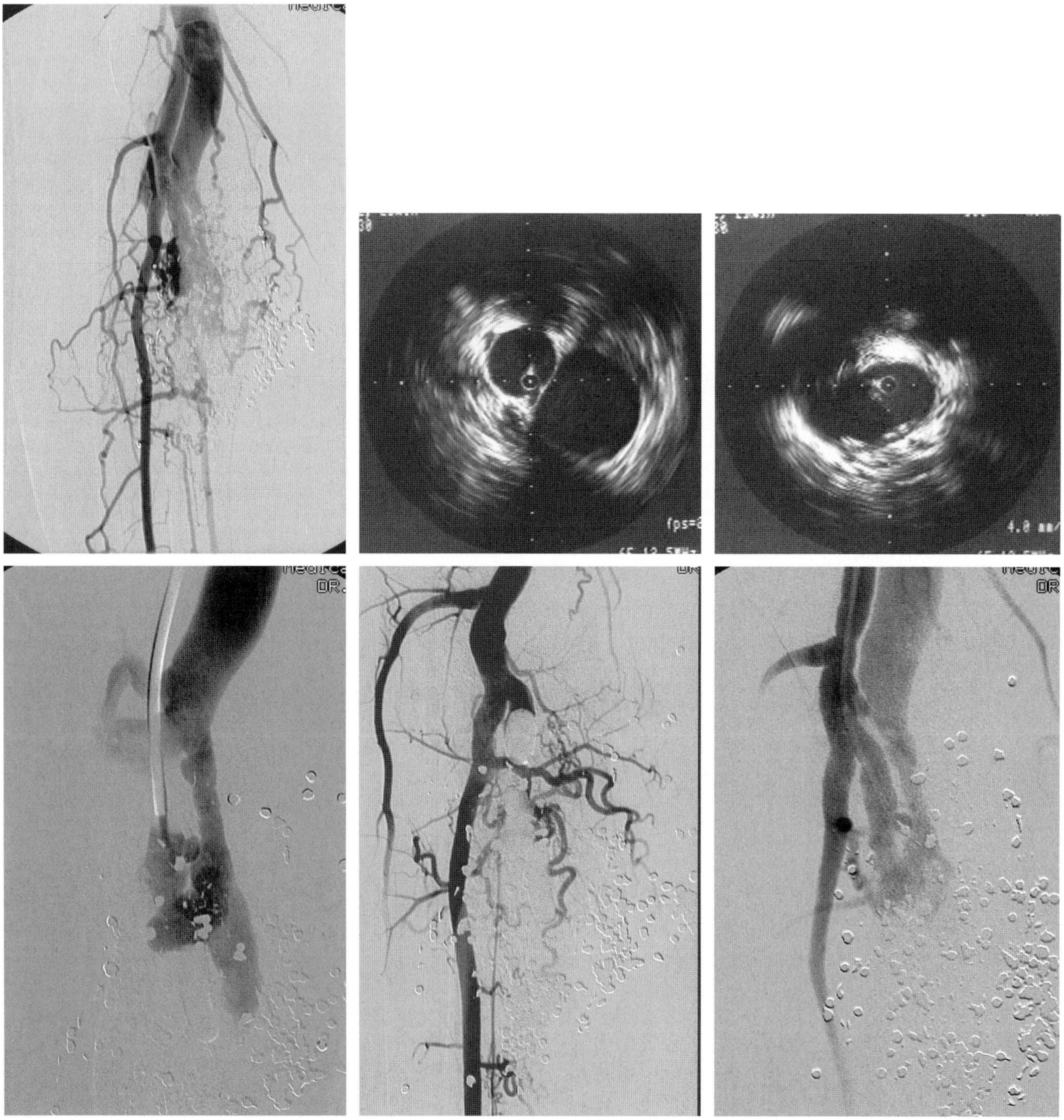

A, B C

D, E F

Figure 11.2

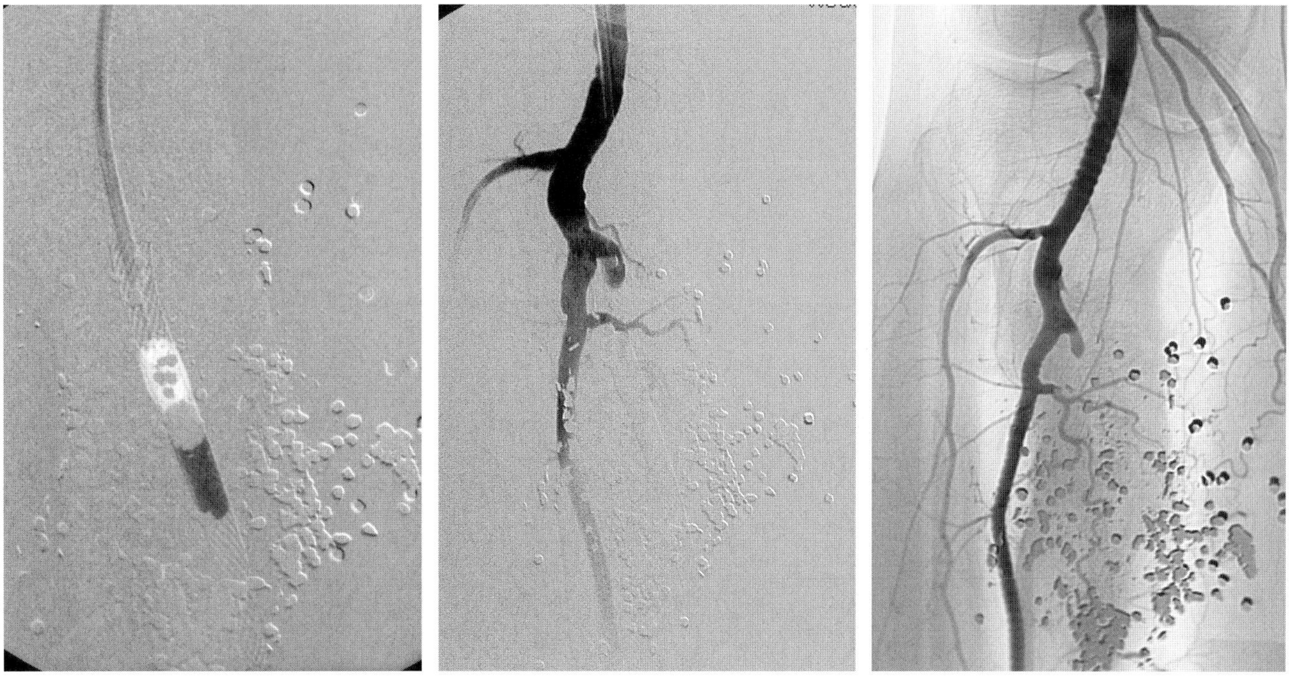

G H, I

Figure 11.2 *(continued)*

A: Antegrade approach to the right femoral artery to perform the angiogram demonstrates a massive side-to-side A-V fistula between the posterior tibial artery and one posterior tibial vein. Note the multiple lead pellets around the vascular lesion. The decision to use detachable balloons was made because of the large size of the communication between the artery and vein. **B:** Intravascular ultrasound shows the enlarged artery and vein. **C:** Note the direct communication between the artery and vein measuring more than 8 mm. **D:** The distal segment of the posterior tibial artery was patent. One detachable balloon was deployed at the distal level, beyond the fistulous rent. Injection through the 7F guiding catheter shows the large size of the fistula. **E:** Three balloons were used to occlude the fistula. Note total occlusion with one balloon distal to the fistula, one at the level of the fistula and one above the fistulous communication. The only remaining distal artery is the anterior tibial artery. **F:** There was recurrence of symptoms. One-month follow-up angiogram shows the open A-V fistula and no balloons. One balloon migrated to the left lower pulmonary artery. This balloon was deflated by percutaneous puncture with a 23-gauge, 15-cm Chiba needle. A new embolization was performed. **G:** A Wallstent 8 mm × 6 cm was used to bridge the gap of the arterial wall, and the detachable balloons were deployed within the stent. **H:** Postembolization angiogram shows total occlusion of the A-V fistula without filling of the vein. Note the shadow of the stent in the posterior tibial artery. **I:** Three-month follow-up angiogram shows the fistula is permanently occluded. There was marked improvement in the edema of the right lower extremity with partial healing of the ankle ulceration at the time of follow-up.

Comment: Direct, side-to-side A-V fistulas pose a difficult problem to the interventionalist. When there is a tract between the two vessels, it usually is possible to treat the fistula with coils or balloon embolization, without sacrificing the parent vessel. In that case, when a tract is present, the embolic material is deployed into the tract, occluding the communication but sparing the artery and vein. When a tract is not present, as in the presented case, occlusion of the fistula by embolization is only possible by occluding the parent artery. More recently, the covered stents became available and are ideal devices to occlude side-to-side A-V fistulas, thus preserving the parent artery. When covered stents or stent grafts are not available, a bare stent can be used to constrain the detachable balloons within the desired area, without passing through the rent of the fistula. The parent artery will be occluded, but it is still a safe method to treat permanently the A-V fistula and avoid the risk of passage of the embolic material through the rent of the fistula, as occurred in the first attempt.

11.3 Embolization In Arteriovenous Malformations And Fistulas

Case 11.3:

A 16-year-old girl presented with a lump in her back, which initially was described as related to heavy exercise during a workout. The exercise may or may not have been related to trauma, but the lesion became painful and required treatment. A bruit was heard over the lesion, and the diagnosis of A-V fistula or arteriovenous malformation (AVM) was established. An arteriogram was requested for diagnosis, to be followed by embolization.

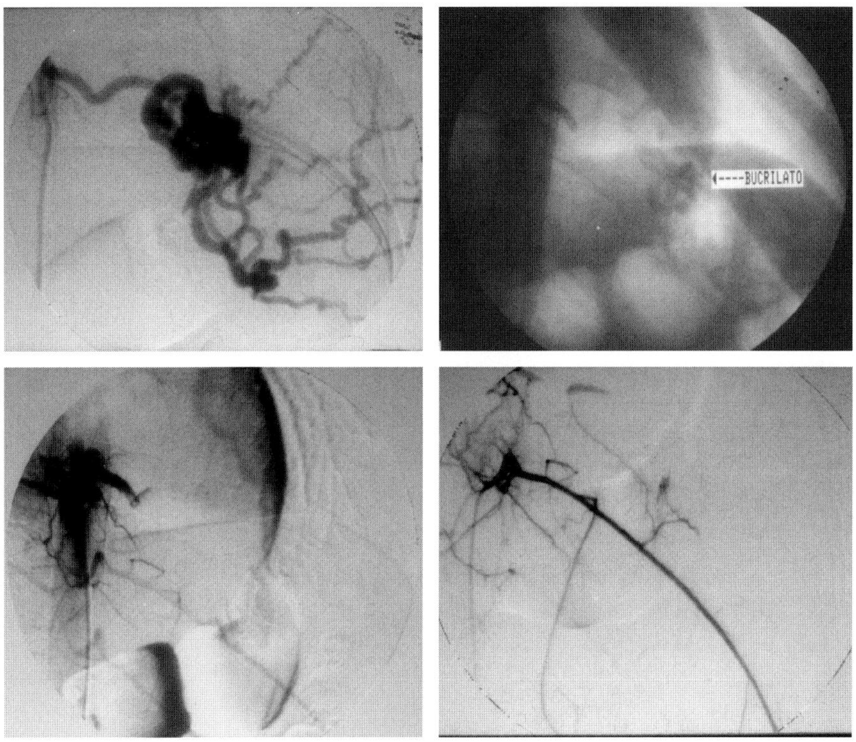

Figure 11.3

A: Selective injection in the ninth left intercostal artery shows a massive A-V fistula with a single artery feeder that drains into a complex, enlarged intercostal vein and communicates with multiple, more superficial draining veins. **B:** Bucrylate was used to occlude the fistula using an 1.8F microcatheter. Note the radiopacity of the polymer, which was used with lipiodol. **C:** Postembolization angiogram shows total occlusion of the A-V fistula. **D:** Postembolization angiogram in the eighth and tenth intercostal arteries did not show any communication with the A-V fistula.

Comment: This is an example of a congenital A-V fistula that may have became symptomatic after heavy exercise. It is unlikely, however, that trauma was the cause of the fistula. In addition, the patient was young, and hormonal changes may have been responsible for enlargement of the fistula. This type of lesion is best treated by embolization, although surgery also is an option. The young patient refused to have the lesion treated surgically due to esthetic concerns. Gianturco coils could have been used as well. Cyanoacrylate was the embolic material selected in this case and was very effective, resulting in instantaneous occlusion of the fistula.

11.4 Embolization In Arteriovenous Malformations And Fistulas

Case 11.4:

A 9-year-old boy presented with an A-V fistula in the neck at the base of the skull. The fistula was located between the left vertebral artery and left vertebral vein. Pain was present, and a constant bruit was heard in the left ear.

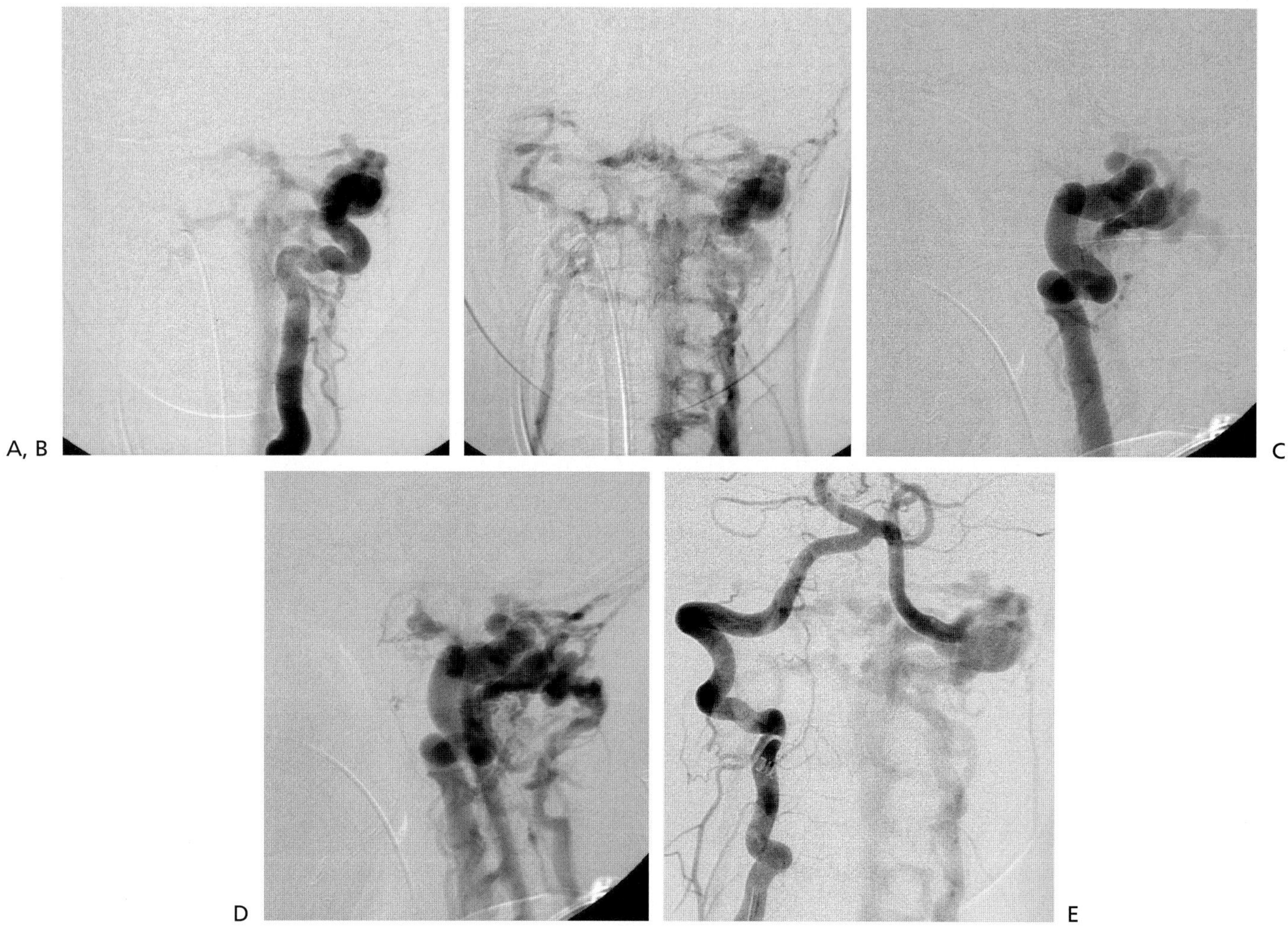

Figure 11.4

F 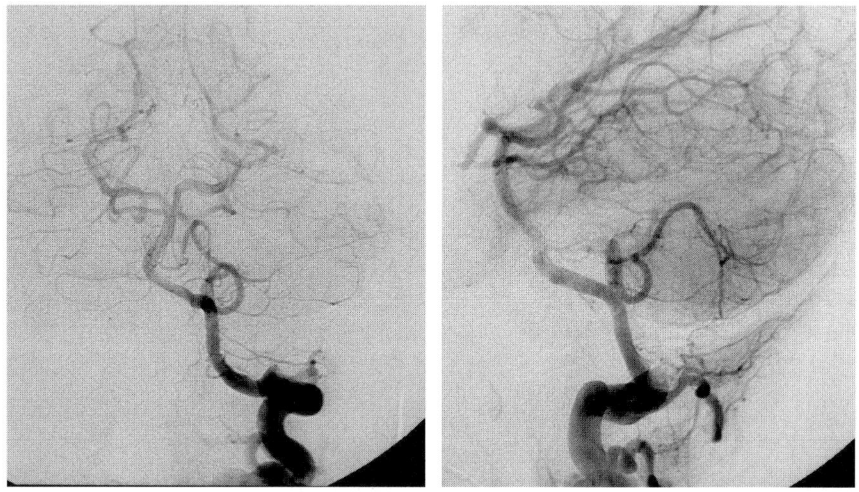 G

Figure 11.4 *(continued)*

A: Selective left vertebral artery angiogram shows the massive A-V fistula draining into the left vertebral vein. **B:** Later-phase angiogram shows filling of the paravertebral cervical venous system. **C,D:** Lateral view of the left vertebral angiogram shows the A-V fistula and massive venous drainage. **E:** Contralateral vertebral angiogram shows retrograde filling of the left distal vertebral artery and the A-V fistula. Note the large venous aneurysm. **F:** A detachable balloon was used to occlude the A-V fistula. Note reconstitution of antegrade flow into the brain and occlusion of the fistulous rent in the anteroposterior view of the left vertebral artery. **G:** Lateral view of the left vertebral artery angiogram shows total occlusion of the fistula and no filling of the venous system.

Comment: This case demonstrates the ideal situation for embolic treatment of an A-V fistula. There is a high-flow communication between the artery and vein but an interposed short tract, which allowed deployment of the detachable balloon. In this type of fistula, it is possible to preserve the parent artery and flow into the brain. Due to the tortuosity of the vertebral artery, use of a covered stent to treat this vessel would have been more difficult. Occlusion of the parent vessel also is an alternative; however, one must be sure that the contralateral artery will be sufficient to supply the brain with blood flow. When the parent artery is occluded, it is important to ensure that there are no collateral branches or communications beyond the occlusion and the fistulous rent that would maintain the fistula open. Therefore, it is important to perform a test occlusion to check the embolization before definitive deployment of the balloon. Detachable balloons are the only devices that allow adequate test occlusion. Coils are useful, but even the more modern detachable coils do not allow good test occlusion, because occlusion of the A-V fistula is not immediate when coils are used.

11.5 Embolization In Arteriovenous Malformations And Fistulas

Case 11.5:

A 51-year-old woman presented with a large AVM of the third finger of the right hand. The finger was very dysfunctional and sore, and there were signs of ischemia of the tip, with marked atrophy and discoloration. Embolization was requested in an attempt to avoid amputation.

A, B

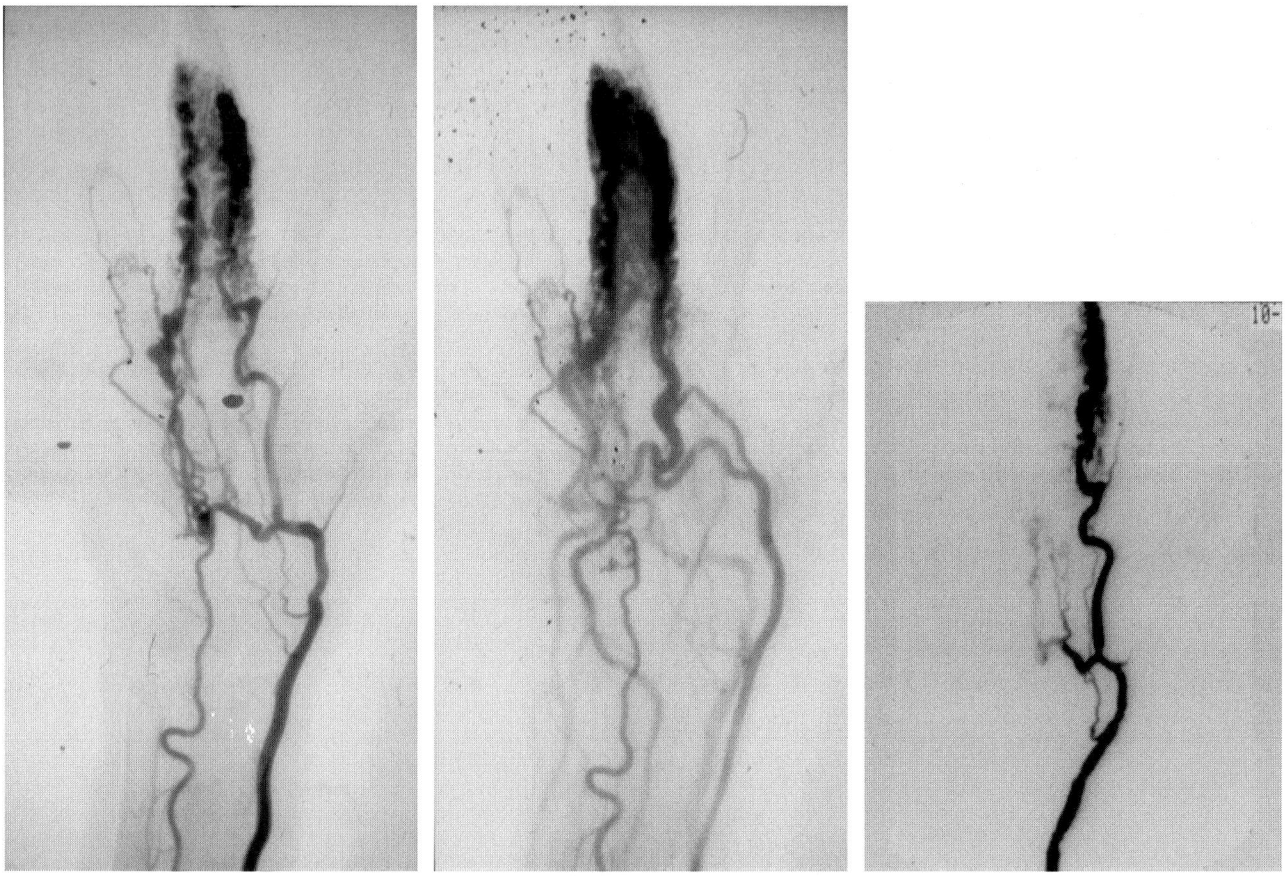

C

Figure 11.5

D E, F G H, I

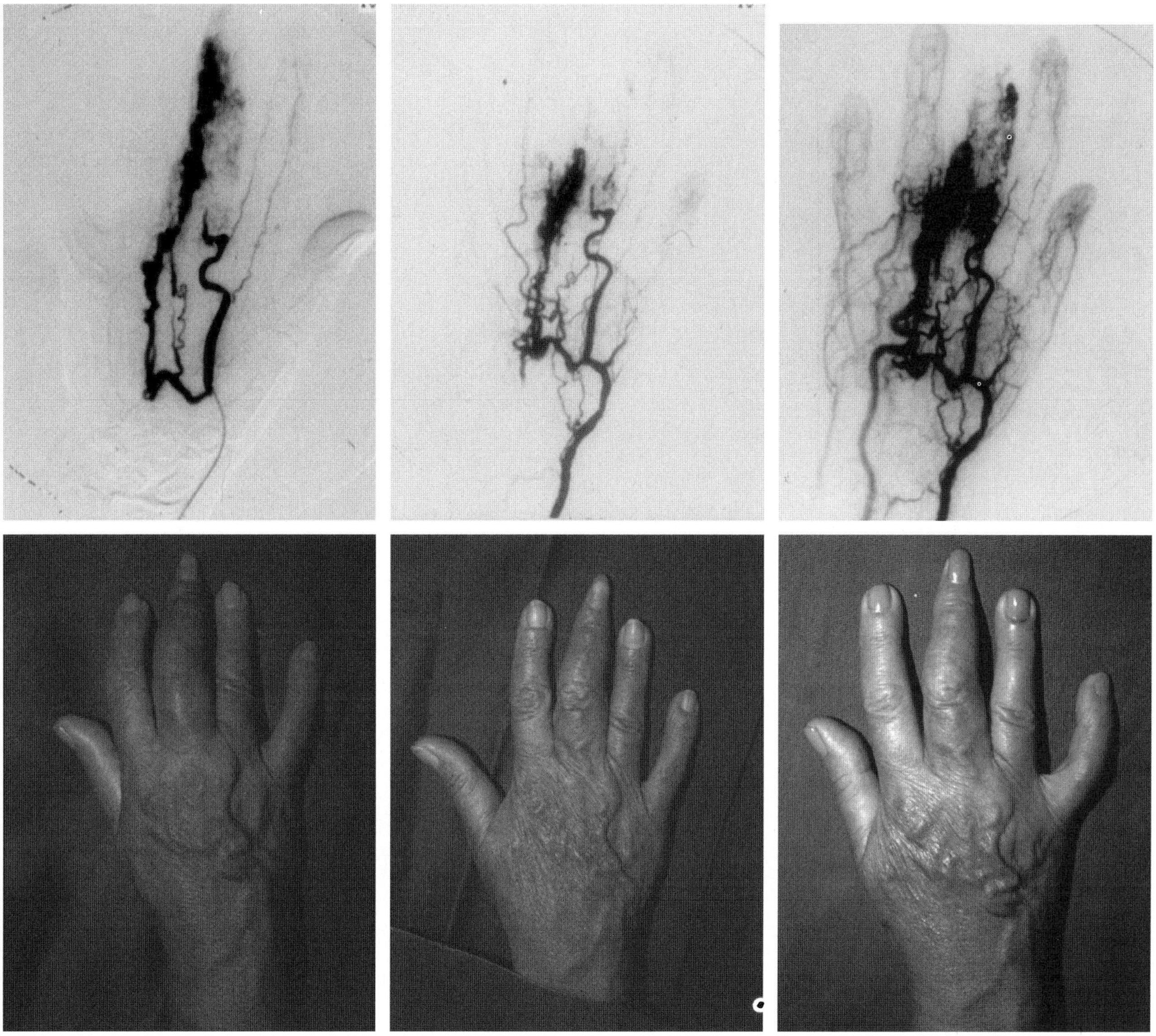

Figure 11.5 *(continued)*

A: Initial angiography of the right hand shows the massive hypervascular AVM in the third finger, with flow still from the tip of the finger. **B:** Venous phase of the hand arteriogram shows dense stain and numerous draining vein. **C:** Superselective injection in the digital artery was followed by embolization with Ivalon particles. **D:** Lateral digital artery injection following embolization shows marked reduction in flow. **E:** Postembolization angiogram of the major feeders shows reduction of flow. **F:** Final postembolization angiogram shows proximal filling of the AVM but improvement in the filling of normal distal vessels in the tip of the third finger. **G:** Preembolization photograph of the right hand. Note the enlarged finger with a very thin tip. **H:** One-month postembolization angiogram shows improvement in size and mobility of the finger. **I:** Six months after two embolizations, the finger is functional and of acceptable size.

Comment: AVMs constitute some of the most difficult diagnostic and therapeutic dilemmas in the practice of medicine. It is important to make a differential diagnosis between hemangiomas and AVMs. Hemangiomas usually are not present at birth and have a bright scarlet color that gradually disappears. Hemangiomas are benign vascular tumors of infancy and histologically characterized by masses of proliferating endothelial cells. Vascular malformations are defects of vascular morphogenesis, or vascular anomalies. AVMs have a persistent color depending on the dominant arterial, capillary, venous, or lymphatic component. Magnetic resonance can accurately distinguish between high-flow and low-flow malformations. In addition, the relationship to adjacent anatomic structures, such as muscles, nerves, and organs, is easily determined. High-flow malformations typically demonstrate signal void on most sequences. To assess if therapy is warranted, a number of factors should be evaluated. Control of symptoms and restoration of physiologic functions should be the most important criteria for therapeutic decisions, rather than esthetic indications. Treatment of grossly deforming AVMs can and should be attempted in well-selected patients. The case presented illustrates a good indication for treatment in a patient with gross deformity of the finger, with pain and distal ischemia from a high-flow AVM. Embolization in this case was performed with Ivalon particles. Occlusion of most of the malformed vessels improved the pain and swelling, and was followed by significant functional improvement.

11.6 Embolization In Arteriovenous Malformations And Fistulas

Case 11.6:

A 40-year-old man presented with a massive AVM of the right hand. The hand was very dysfunctional and sore, and there was a bleeding large ulceration of the dorsal aspect of the hand due to ischemia. Two fingers were previously amputated. Embolization was requested in an attempt to improve the ulceration, control the bleeding, and avoid further amputations.

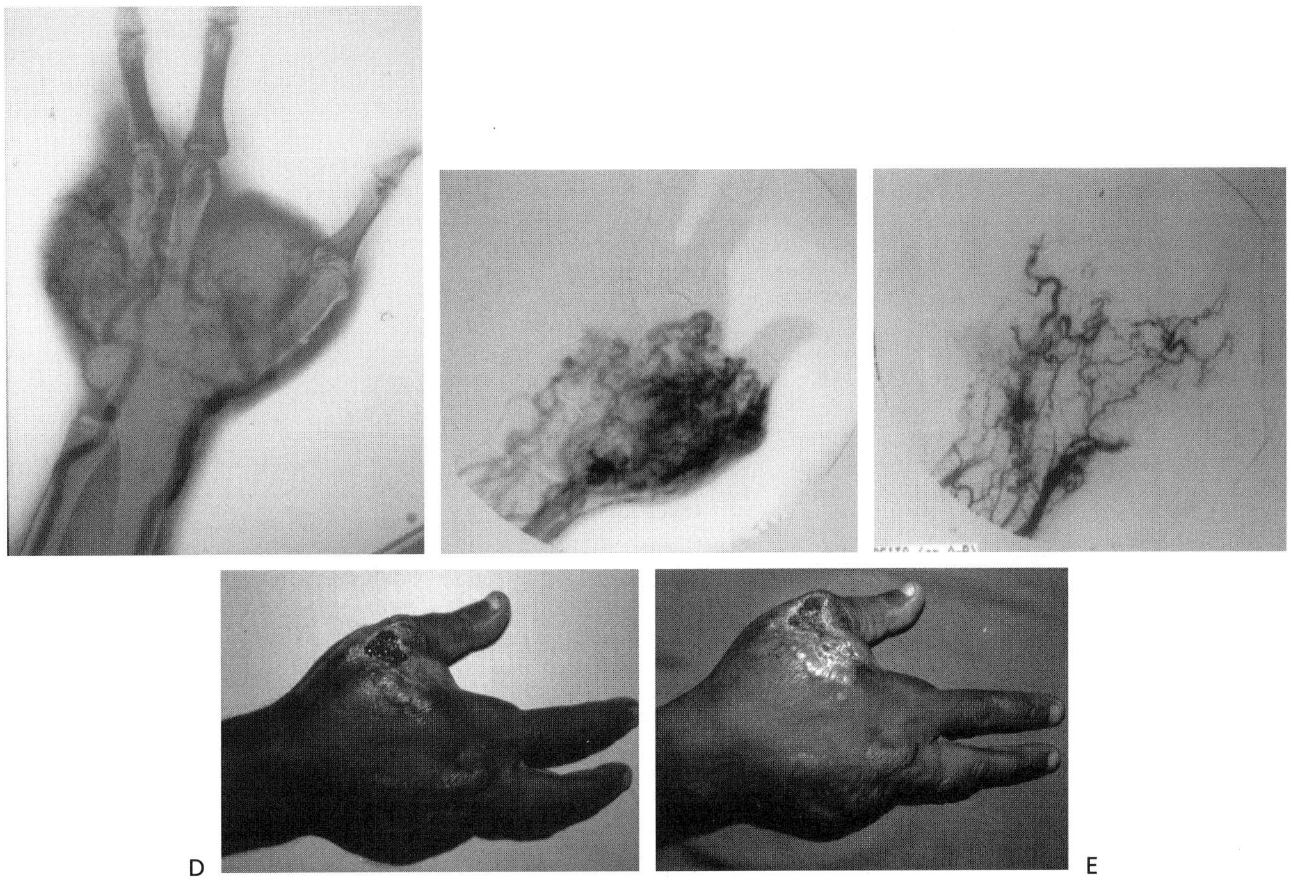

A B, C D E

Figure 11.6

A: Late phase of an older angiogram of the right hand shows the massive hypervascular lesion located predominantly in the lateral aspect. Note the two missing digits. **B:** Selective catheterization of the radial artery shows the large and complex nidus of the AVM. **C:** Embolization with cyanoacrylate was performed, with occlusion of most of the nidus originating from the radial artery. **D:** Preembolization photography of the right hand shows the large ulceration in the dorsal aspect. **E:** Postembolization photography shows improvement in ulceration, with progressive healing and control of bleeding. Another embolization was performed and resulted in further improvement.

Comment: Embolization in this case was indicated to control bleeding and to improve the ulceration. Occlusion of a significant part of the nidus usually is sufficient to reduce blood steal from the skin and improve the ischemic ulceration. Small microcatheters are used to reach distal branches, to allow injection of tissue adhesive. Care should be exercised to reduce the risk of occlusion of normal vessels in the fingers. Although cyanoacrylate glue was used in this case, a number of options are available. Direct puncture and alcohol injection into the nidus is an effective alternative. When injecting absolute alcohol into large AVMs, Swan-Ganz and arterial line monitoring should be performed. Pulmonary artery pressures are monitored consistently during the injection. Decadron (dexamethasone sodium phosphate) 10 mg is given intravenously to all adult patients prior to the procedure. Cardiopulmonary collapse is a rare but dreadful sequela, and pulmonary artery pressure monitoring is essential. Pulmonary hypertension, which is caused by precapillary spasm, is a transient but potentially lethal phenomenon. Nitroglycerin injection is helpful in reducing elevated pulmonary pressure.

11.7 Embolization In Arteriovenous Malformations And Fistulas

Case 11.7:

A 38-year-old-man presented with a large and very painful AVM of the left hand extending into the first and second fingers. The second finger was very dysfunctional, rigid, and sore, and was causing work-related difficulties for this patient. The distal phalanx of the second finger had been amputated, and the wound would not heal. There was extensive ulceration in the skin covering the metacarpal segment of the left hand extending over the first and second fingers. Embolization was requested in an attempt to avoid surgical amputation.

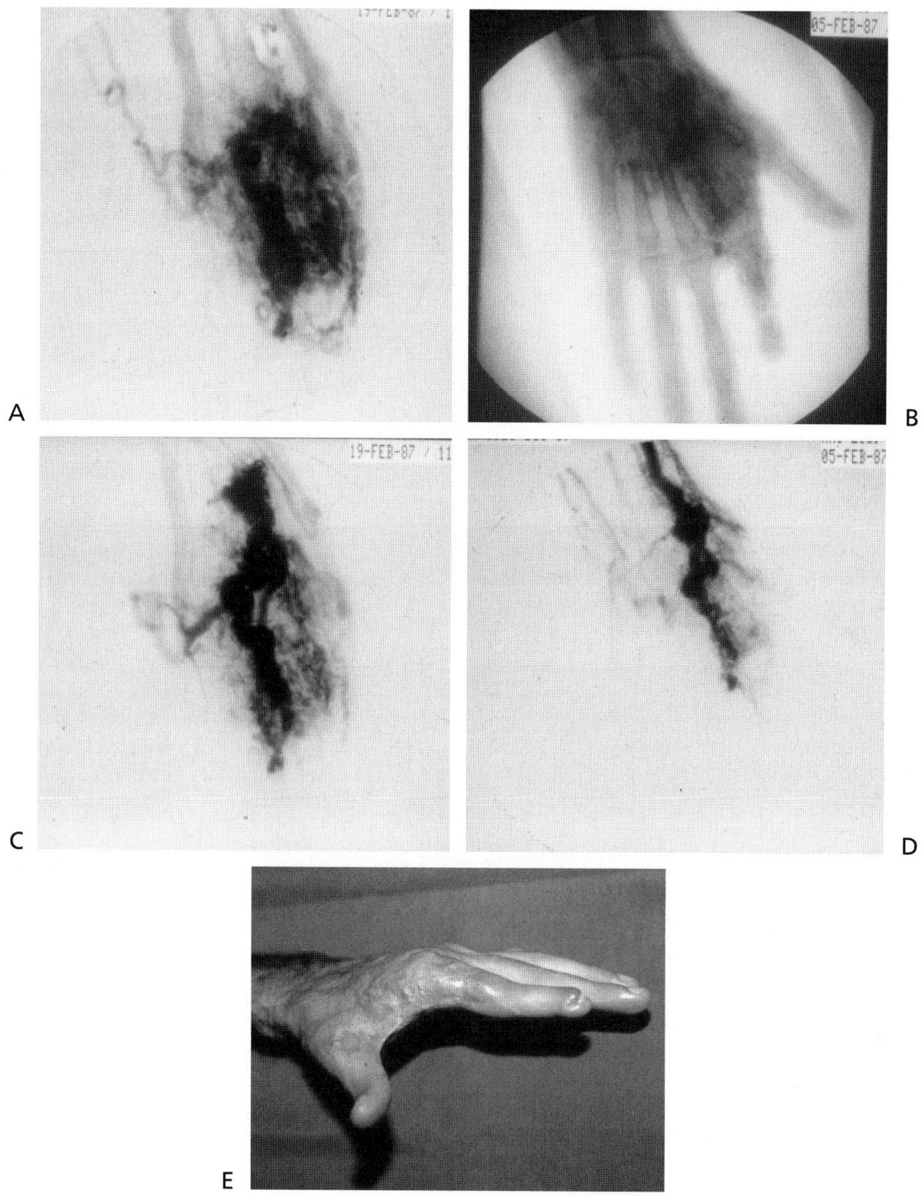

Figure 11.7

A: Late arterial phase of the left hand angiogram shows the hypervascular nidus of the lesion extending from the carpal to metacarpal segments and second finger of the left hand. There was no filling of the digital arteries of the first, second, and third fingers, due to steal from the hyperflow in the AVM. **B:** Unsubtracted view of the left hand shows the location of the AVM in relation to the fingers. **C:** Superselective catheterization of the arterial feeders shows dysplastic arteries within the AVM. **D:** Embolization with Ivalon was performed, which resulted in significant reduction in the vascularity of the nidus, as seen in the follow-up angiogram. There was improvement in the flow into the digital arteries, not demonstrated in this view. **E:** Two months after embolization, the tip of the second finger and the skin in the metacarpal area of the left hand are healed.

Comment: Angiography is always advisable to define the angioarchitecture of the AVM before a decision is made regarding treatment. The locations of the lesion, the feeding arteries, and the draining veins are important considerations for treatment strategy. Puncture of the branchial artery was selected to gain access to the hand vascular system. A microcatheter was used to catheterize the hand branches from the radial and ulnar arteries. Multiple superselective injections were performed to define the feeder vessels. Ivalon was used for embolization in this patient in an attempt to reduce the hypervascularity of the AVM. Significant reduction in flow was achieved, which allowed the distal digital arteries to be visible on the angiogram. Ivalon is a nonabsorbable particle that plugs the vessels with a distribution in a flow-oriented fashion. There was marked improvement in perfusion of the fingers and the areas of skin ulcerations, which promoted healing of the lesions, the tip of the second finger, and the metacarpal area. The 2-month follow-up clinical inspection showed healing of all lesions and improvement of the pain and of movements of the hand. With physical therapy, the patient regained control of the hand and could use the opposition of first and second fingers for grabbing objects and working. A surprising finding in the evolution of this lesion was the exteriorization of some of the Ivalon particles through the hand skin. It is not possible to see in the black-and-white photograph above, but the small white granules were observed in small vesicles. It is possible that the lesion was recanalizing itself.

11.8 Embolization In Arteriovenous Malformations And Fistulas

Case 11.8:

A 42-year-old woman presented with a painful AVM of the medial and plantar aspect of the left foot. The foot was functional, but walking was difficult. Embolization was requested in an attempt to improve symptoms.

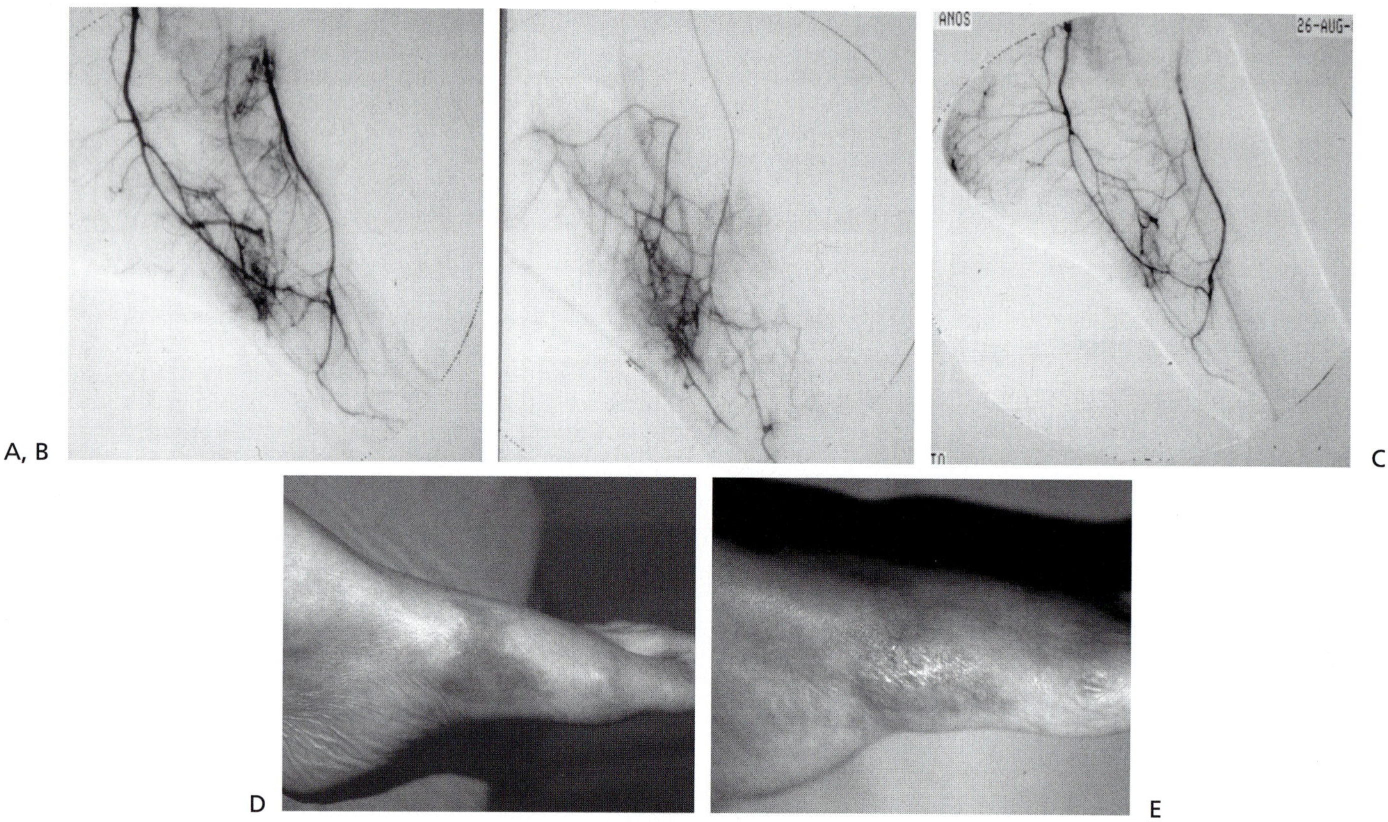

Figure 11.8

A: Selective angiography of the anterior tibial artery and dorsalis pedis shows a moderately hypervascular AVM in the medial aspect of the foot, supplied predominantly by the medial tarsal artery. **B:** Superselective angiography of the medial tarsal artery was followed by embolization with Ivalon 100m particles. **C:** Postembolization angiography injected through the dorsalis pedis artery shows patency of the plantar arch and lateral plantar artery, but the lesion was mostly ablated. **D:** Pre-embolization aspect of the AVM in the right foot. **E:** Postembolization aspect of the AVM in the right foot seen 2 weeks after the procedure.

Comment: The case reported illustrates a relatively difficult situation to treat. Superselective catheterization of several smaller arteries and embolization with small particles was required. Occlusion of adjacent normal vessels is dangerous in this situation because of the proximity of the digital arteries, which could cause toe ischemia. Flow-directed embolization with small particles was the best option for treatment of this lesion. Glue could be used, but would require extra care to avoid reflux in adjacent arteries. Microcoils are not a good choice in this case because it was paramount to preserve the parent arteries and occlude the nidus. Other fluids, such as ethanol, would be too dangerous due to the risk of causing muscle and skin necrosis. Note the hyperchromia of the skin in Figure 11.8D. Two-month follow-up photograph showed improvement, with shrinking of the cutaneous lesion and change of color. There was marked improvement of symptoms.

Suggested Reading

Gomes AS, Busutil RW, Baker JD, et al. Congenital AVMs: the role of transcatheter arterial embolization. *Arch Surg* 1983:118:817–825.

Jackson JE. Successful management of pelvic arteriovenous malformation by repeated particulate intra-arterial embolization. *Br J Urol* 1996;77:169–172.

Kaufaman SL, Kumar AAJ, Roland JMA, et al. Transcatheter embolotherapy in the management of congenital arteriovenous malformations. *Radiology* 1980;137:21–29.

Uflacker R, Saadi J. Transcatheter embolization of superior mesenteric arteriovenous fistula. *AJR* 1982;139:1212–1214.

Widlus DM, Murray RR, White RI, et al. Congenital arteriovenous malformations: tailored embolotherapy. *Radiology* 1988;169;511–516.

Yakes W, Rossi P, Odink H. Arteriovenous malformation management. *Cardiovasc Intervent Radiol* 1996;19:65–71.

Yakes WF, Haas DK, Parker SH, et al. Symptomatic vascular malformations: ethanol embolotherapy. *Radiology* 1989;170:1059–1066.

Yakes WF, Parker SH, Gibson MD, et al. Alcohol embolotherapy of vascular malformations. *Semin Interv Radiol* 1989;6:146–161.

Yakes WF, Pevsner PH, Reed MD, et al. Serial embolization of an extremity arteriovenous malformation with alcohol via direct percutaneous puncture. *AJR* 1986;146:1038–1040.

CHAPTER 12

Embolization In Lesions Of The Head And Neck

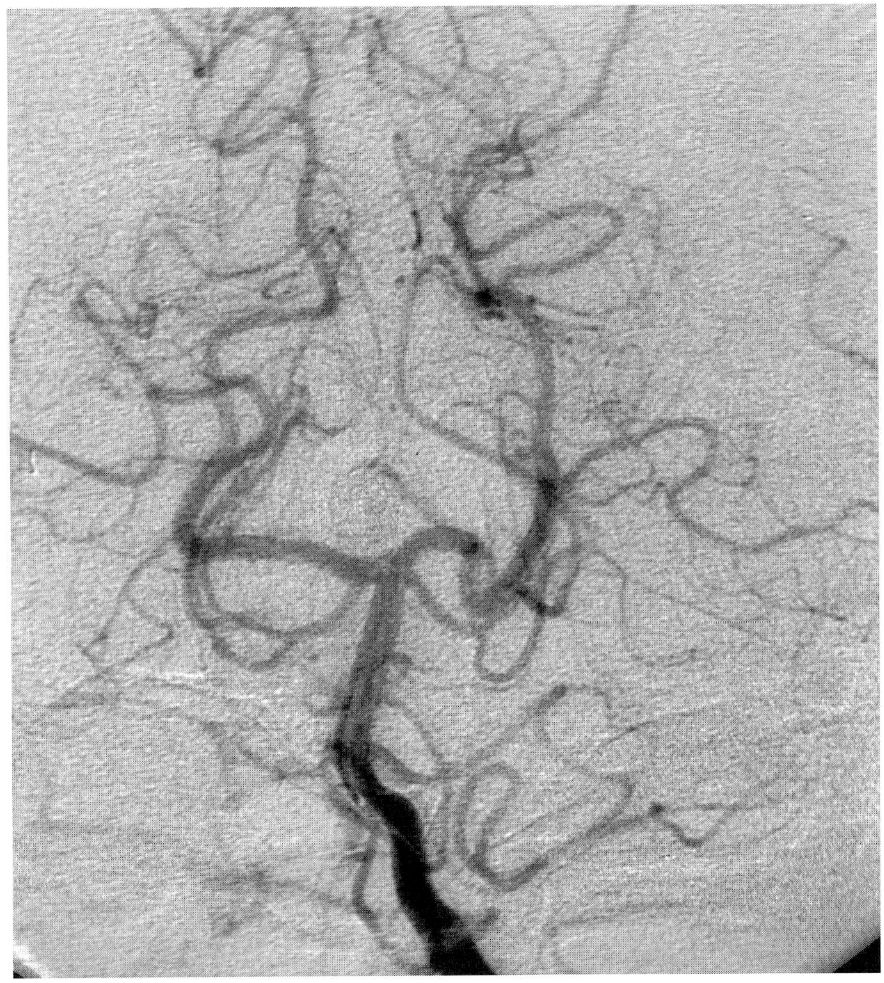

12.1 Embolization In Lesions Of The Head And Neck

Case 12.1:

A 61-year-old man with subarachnoid hemorrhage and a large saccular aneurysm in the anterior communicating artery was sent for angiography and embolization. Guglielmo detachable coils (GDC) were used to embolize the aneurysm.

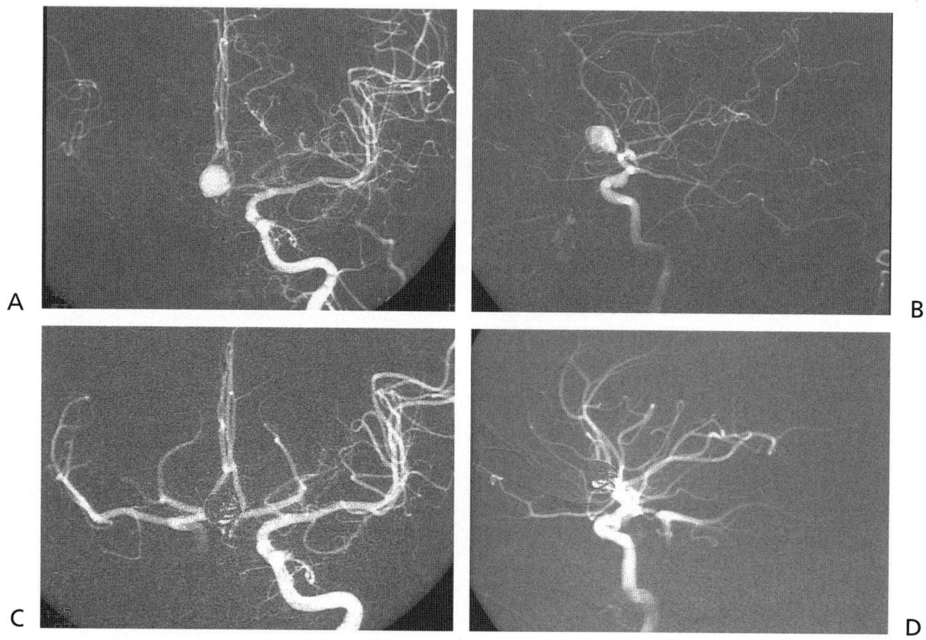

Figure 12.1

A: Selective left internal carotid arteriogram in the anteroposterior (AP) view shows a large aneurysm in the anterior communicating artery. **B:** Selective left internal carotid arteriogram in the oblique view shows the large aneurysm directed anteriorly and the small neck of the aneurysm. **C:** Left carotid angiogram with right carotid compression shows postembolization occlusion of the aneurysm with the GDC. Note patency of the anterior communication artery and good perfusion of the intracerebral circulation. **D:** Lateral view of the left carotid angiogram demonstrates the occluded aneurysm.

Comment: Aneurysmal subarachnoid hemorrhage has a high fatality rate of up to 50%. Much of the poor outcome is caused by cases of rebleeding, many of which occur within 24 hours and require early diagnosis and treatment. Surgery is the time-honored treatment for cerebral aneurysms. More recently, coil embolization has been a less invasive alternative to surgery, with a relatively high success rate, for larger aneurysms with narrow necks. It is important to occlude the whole lumen of the aneurysm, as any space within the aneurysm may perpetuate the risk of bleeding.

12.2 Embolization In Lesions Of The Head And Neck

Case 12.2:

A 35-year-old man who presented with acute subarachnoid hemorrhage and coma required tracheal intubation. Surgery failed to exclude the aneurysm.

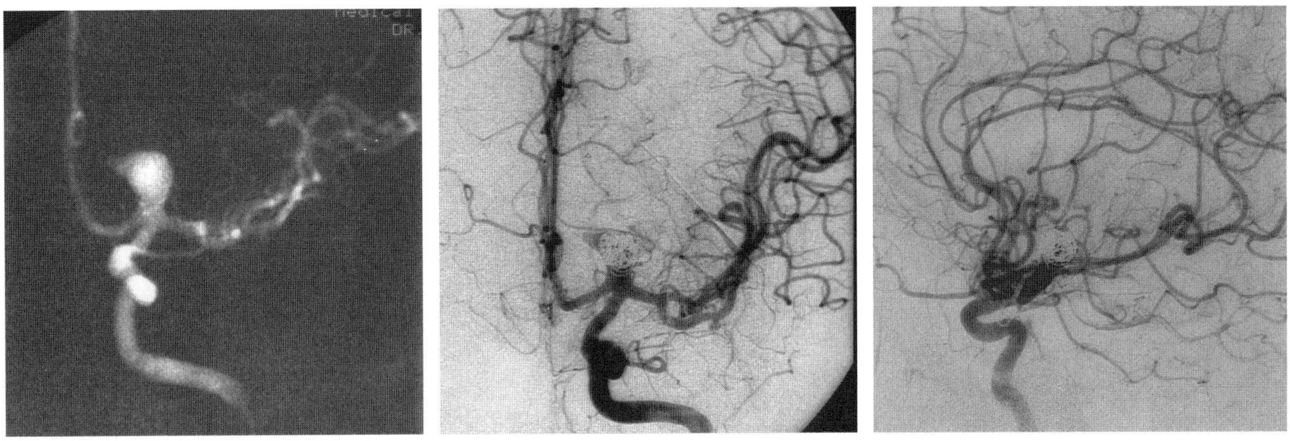

A B, C

Figure 12.2

A: Selective catheterization of the left internal carotid artery was performed through a cutdown in the neck at the level of the common carotid artery. Arteriography shows a large saccular aneurysm at the bifurcation of the left internal carotid artery, with infundibular dilation. Note irregularity of the medial aspect of the aneurysm. Embolization was performed. **B:** AP view of left carotid arteriogram after GDC embolization. The aneurysm is only partially filled by the coils. There is an excessive space in the medial aspect of the aneurysm. **C:** Lateral view of the aneurysm in the postembolization angiogram. Note the metal clip near the artery.

Comment: Aneurysms with irregular contours are more prone to rebleeding than cerebral aneurysms with regular contours. The large neck of this aneurysm represents a serious limitation to intravascular treatment because the chances of aneurysm thrombosis are reduced. The patient never recovered from the coma and died 2 days after embolization.

12.3 Embolization In Lesions Of The Head And Neck

Case 12.3:

A 44-year-old man with a basilar tip aneurysm presented with headaches but no bleeding.

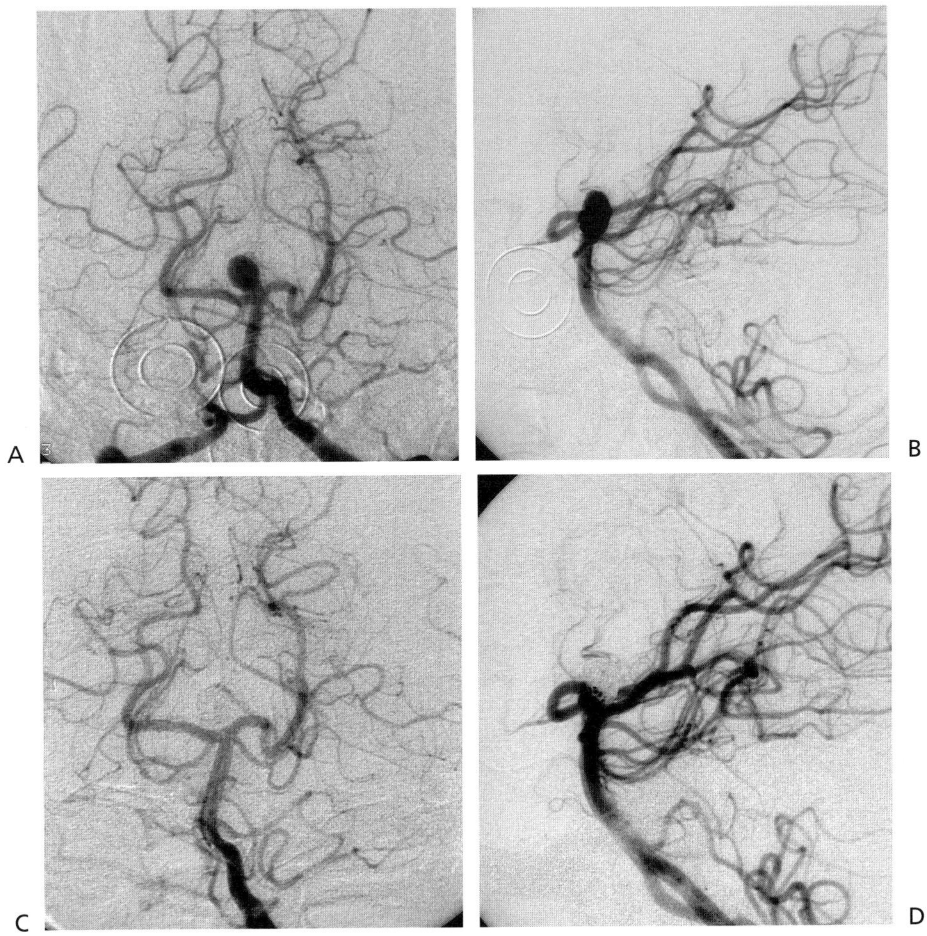

Figure 12.3

A: Digital selective left vertebral artery angiogram in the AP view shows a large basilar tip aneurysm without intraluminal thrombus and a relatively large neck. **B:** Lateral view of the basilar artery shows the basilar tip aneurysm directed upward. **C:** Postembolization angiogram of the basilar artery and posterior cerebral arteries shows total occlusion of the aneurysm by the GDC. A 30-cm long × 10-mm diameter GDC was used for embolization. **D:** Lateral view of the basilar artery arteriogram shows exclusion of the basilar tip aneurysm.

Comment: Surgical treatment of basilar tip aneurysm is very risky and carries high morbidity and mortality rates. Coil embolization currently is the preferred treatment for this type of aneurysm. The success rate of embolization is high, and it is a straightforward procedure when the anatomy is adequate. Spasm of the access artery is the most important cause of failure of GDC embolization, as it makes placement of the coil impossible.

Case 12.4:

A 36-year-old woman with a carotid cavernous fistula (CCF) 2 months following facial trauma due to a gunshot wound was referred for embolization.

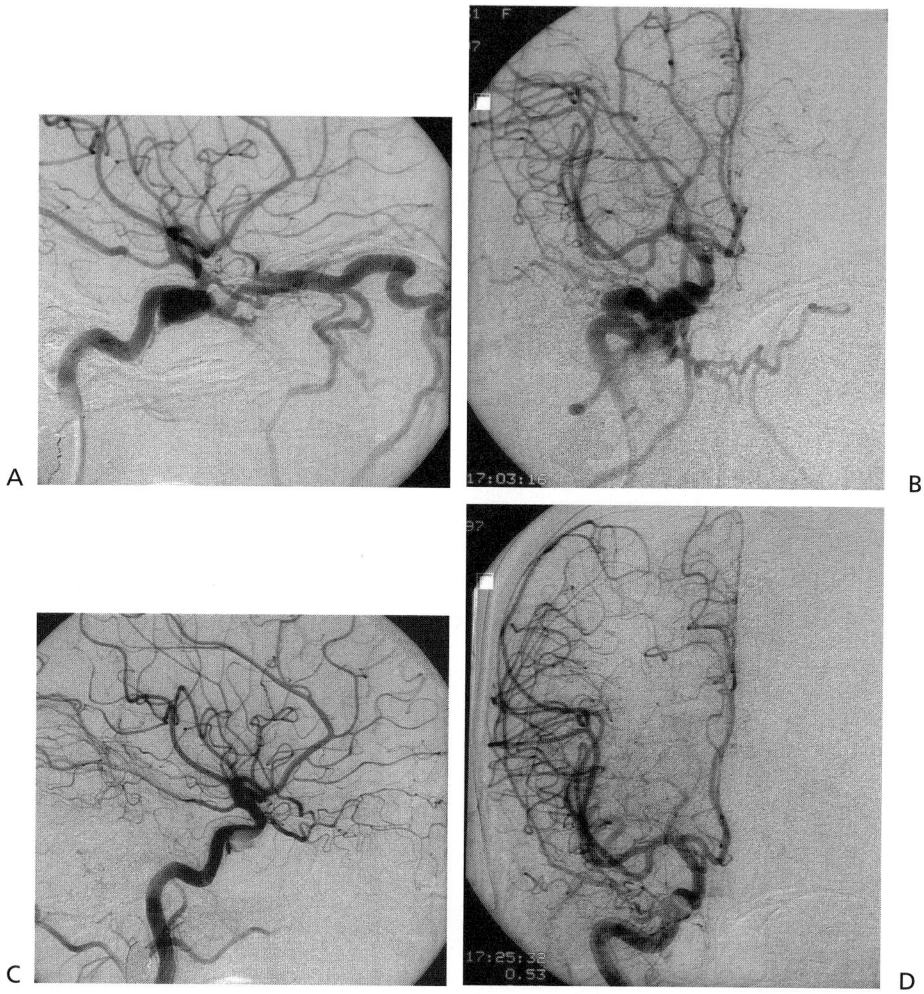

Figure 12.4

A: Lateral view of a right internal carotid angiogram shows a pseudoaneurysm at the level of the intracavernous segment of the internal carotid artery and direct communication with the cavernous sinus and centrifugal flow in the ophthalmic vein and facial vein. Note the faint image of the bullet behind the internal carotid artery at the bottom of the photograph. **B:** AP view of the right internal carotid angiogram shows the CCF and the veins of the face, with filling of the contralateral facial veins. **C:** Postembolization angiogram in the lateral view shows total occlusion of the CCF after occlusion of the rent of the fistula with an ITC silicone detachable balloon. Note a small leak around the balloon filling the pseudoaneurysm but not the fistula. **D:** AP view of the carotid angiogram after embolization of the CCF. Note total occlusion of the fistula without filling of the facial veins.

Comment: CCFs are abnormal direct communications between the intracavernous segment of the internal carotid artery and the cavernous sinus, with or without fracture of the base of the skull. Carotid rupture inside the cavernous sinus results in injection of high-flow/high-pressure blood into a low-pressure venous compartment. Reversal of venous flow in the ophthalmic veins causes venous hypertension in the face and orbit, creating pulsatile exophthalmos, visual deficit, and chemosis. Due to the proximity of cranial nerves III, IV, and VI, paralysis of the eye ensues. Angiographic protocol should include injections in both the internal and external carotid arteries and the vertebral artery. It is necessary to evaluate the patency of the anterior communicating artery. If it becomes necessary to sacrifice the internal carotid artery during treatment, information on whether the brain will be adequately fed by a single carotid will be available. The efficacy of embolization is high, and total cure may be obtained by embolization alone. The most important precaution is to keep the parent vessel open while the CCF is occluded. A retrograde approach through the ophthalmic vein by puncture or disection is also very effective for embolization.

12.5 Embolization In Lesions Of The Head And Neck

Case 12.5:

A 29-year-old woman with CCF 2 months following facial trauma due to a motor vehicle accident was referred for diagnostic angiography and embolization.

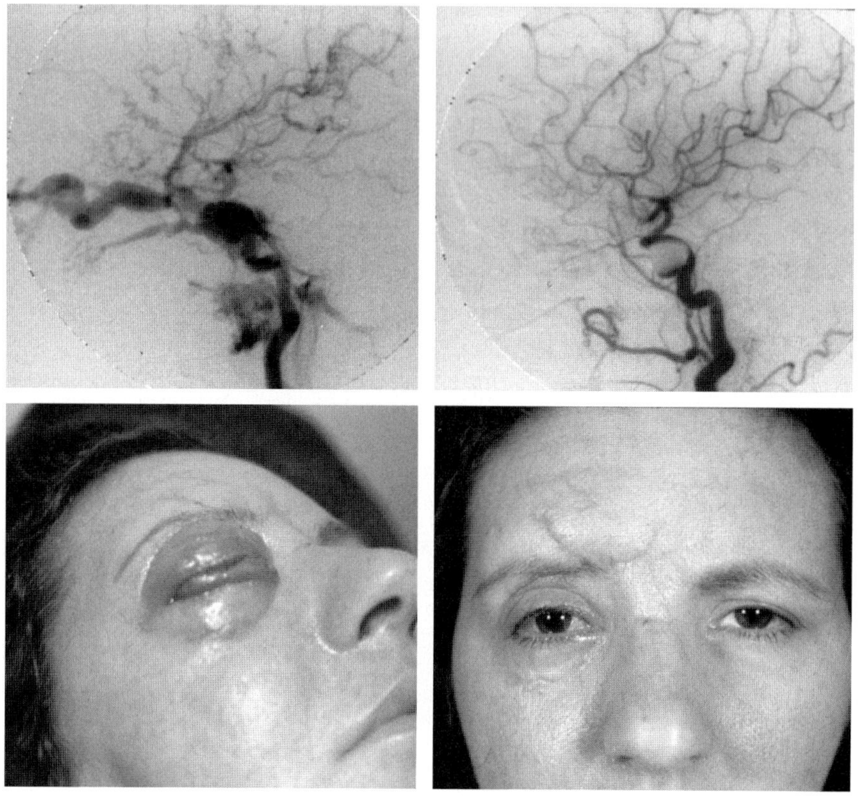

A B C D

Figure 12.5

A: Right carotid angiogram shows the CCF with massive filling of the ophthalmic veins through the cavernous sinus and retrograde filling of the petrosal sinus. **B:** Detachable balloon embolization occluded the rent of the CCF and maintained patency of the internal carotid. However, a filling defect resulting from the size and high density of the balloon is observed. Note improvement of intracerebral circulation. **C:** The patient's face shows orbital edema and chemosis. **D:** After treatment, the patient's face shows regression of the edema and chemosis. Subtle paralysis of the eye was still present. Note the scars from the trauma on the forehead.

Comment: The therapeutic objective in CCF is to occlude the fistulous tract while maintaining intact carotid flow. Surgical treatment of CCF is difficult. Surgical ligation of the intracavernous and supracavernous internal carotid (trapping procedure) may be useful in some cases; however, the procedure is very invasive and not as reliable as detachable balloon embolization. Embolization using a 6F or 7F guiding catheter and detachable balloons is the treatment of first choice. More than one balloon often is necessary to occlude the CCF. It is not always possible to preserve carotid flow. When occlusion of the carotid is necessary, proper identification of patent communicating arteries is mandatory. Spectacular clinical results are obtained if the therapy is adequate. There is regression of the edema and chemosis within a few hours, and the patient may be cured within a few days. In case of previous arterial ligation, the CCF can be approached by the retrograde venous route through surgical exposure of the superior ophthalmic vein on the upper medial orbital border. Blindness usually regresses within several days or weeks as the eyeball is decompressed. Nerve paralysis and double vision may persist for long periods of time or may be permanent.

12.6 Embolization In Lesions Of The Head And Neck

Case 12.6:

A 26-year-old woman presented with posttraumatic frontal arteriovenous (A-V) fistula.

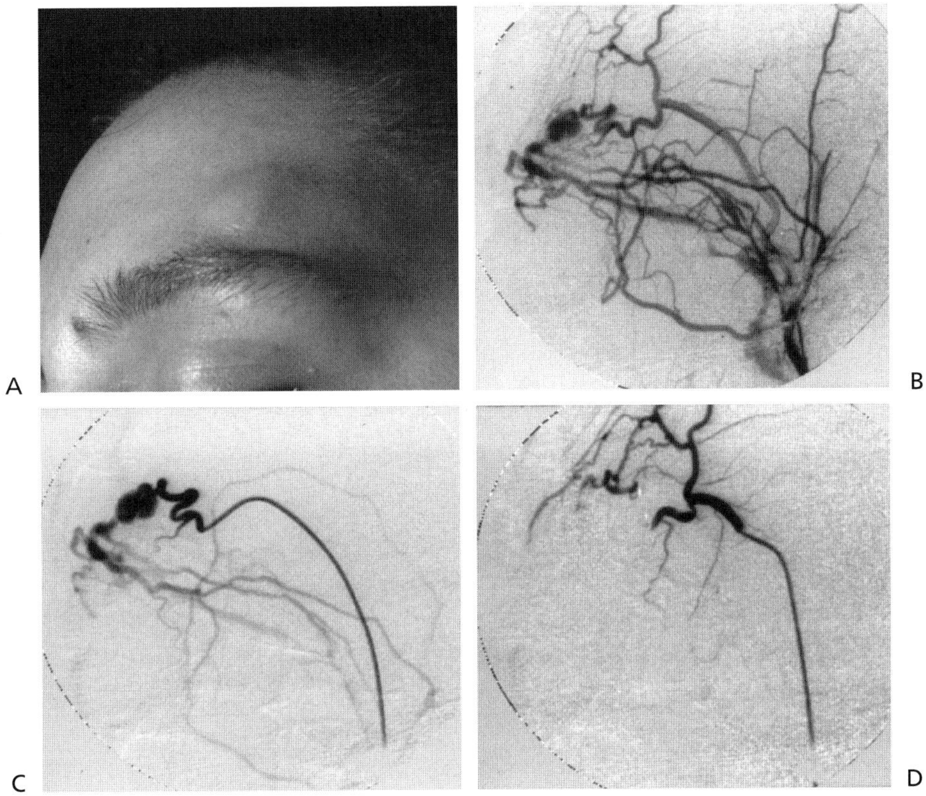

Figure 12.6

A: Lesion on the forehead of the patient. **B:** External carotid artery angiogram shows the A-V fistula supplied by the temporal superficial artery. **C:** Selective temporal superficial arteriogram. **D:** Superselective catheterization and angiogram of the afferent pedicle. A small area of skin ulceration developed a few days after the embolization, but healed without significant scar formation.

Comment: Traumatic A-V fistulas of the face are relatively rare. High-flow lesions will cause enlargement of draining veins and deformity of the skin contour. The thrill in the A-V fistula may cause intracranial noise, as was the case with this young patient. Direct embolization of the A-V fistula requires superselective catheterization and embolization of the fistulous tract. Microcatheters were not available at the time of the procedure; therefore, a 4F catheter was used. Microcoils were a possible alternative in this case; however, the volume of the coils would have been perceptible underneath the skin. Cyanoacrylate probably is the best alternative for treatment in such a situation. The thin 4F catheter was used to get as close as possible to the lesion, and the glue was injected using the flow to direct the embolization. Cyanoacrylate requires injection using a nonionic solution to push the glue through the catheter.

12.7 Embolization In Lesions Of The Head And Neck

Case 12.7:

A 2-year-old child presented with dural vascular malformation with A-V fistula.

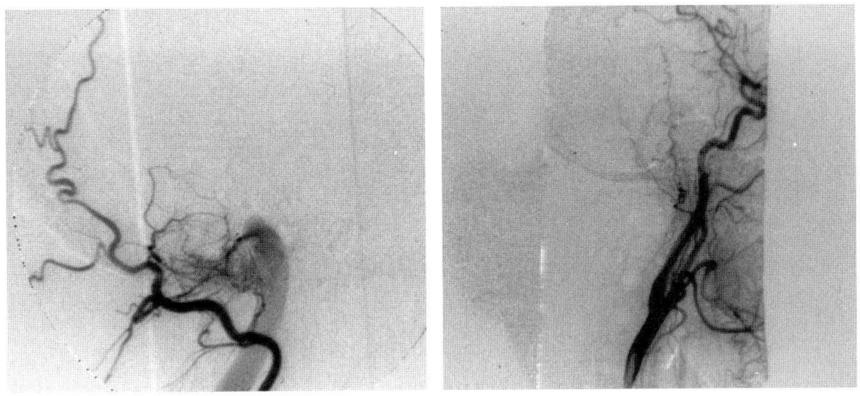

A B

Figure 12.7

A: Superselective arteriogram in the right occipital artery shows the direct A-V fistula from the occipital artery to the sigmoid sinus, through meningeal branches. **B:** Postembolization angiography of the right common carotid artery shows occlusion of the A-V dural fistula. Embolization was performed with a collagen compound.

Comment: Dural A-V fistulas are relatively common and have a variety of presentations. Embolization is the best treatment, and cyanoacrylate glue probably is the best option. Collagen compound in an investigational protocol was used in this case.

12.8 Embolization In Lesions Of The Head And Neck

Case 12.8:

A 23-year-old man presented with a massive bleeding pseudoaneurysm of the internal carotid artery following transsphenoidal surgery for pituitary adenoma.

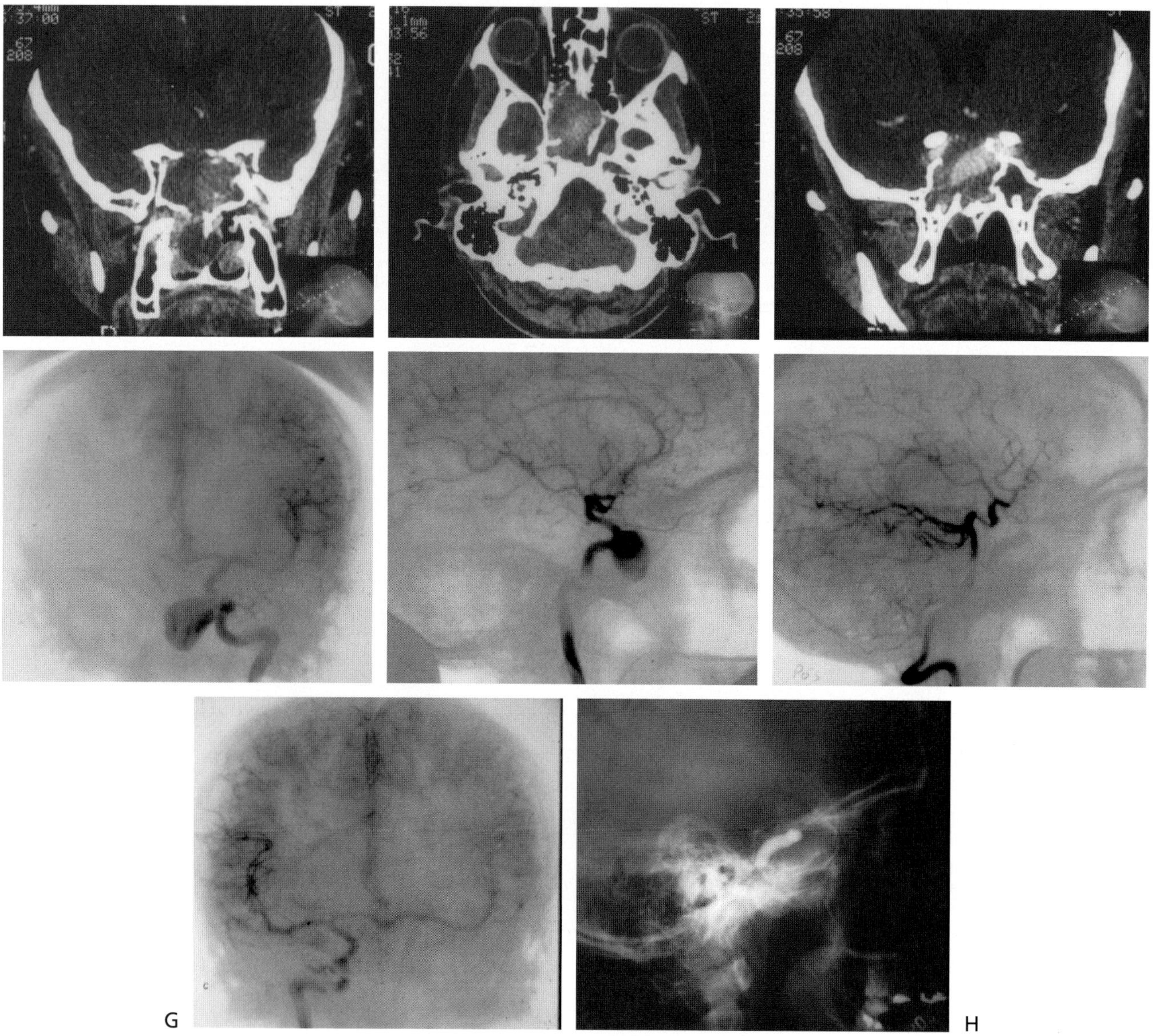

A, B C D, E F G H

Figure 12.8

A–C: CT scans in the axial and coronal views shows the pseudoaneurysm and bleeding inside the sella turcica. **D:** Left carotid arteriogram in the AP view shows the large pseudoaneurysm arising from the internal carotid artery at the level of the sella turcica. **E:** Lateral view of the left carotid angiogram shows the pseudoaneurysm pointing forward. **F:** Embolization with a detachable balloon to occlude the internal carotid artery was performed. Injection of the vertebral artery shows patency of the posterior communicating artery and filling of the left middle cerebral artery. **G:** Right carotid arteriogram shows patency of the anterior communication artery and filling of the left middle cerebral artery. Note no reflux into the occluded left internal carotid artery. **H:** Embolization was performed with a detachable latex balloon, which occluded the internal carotid artery at the level of the pseudoaneurysm, and a safety occlusive detachable balloon lower down in the internal carotid artery. The bleeding was controlled, and the patient recovered fully without any neurologic sequelae.

Comment: A large bleeding pseudoaneurysm of the internal carotid artery that develops a few days after transsphenoidal surgery of the hypophysis is a life-threatening situation. Bleeding is usually in the nasopharynx and readily perceptible. Embolization with preservation of patency of the internal carotid artery is impossible with current techniques. A low-profile stent graft, if available, would be a possible alternative in such case; however, the tortuosity of the internal carotid and the length of the artery from the groin may be severe limitations to success of this technique.

12.9 Embolization In Lesions Of The Head And Neck

Case 12.9:

A 62-year-old woman with a large hypophyseal tumor developed nasopharyngeal bleeding after transsphenoidal surgery.

A, B

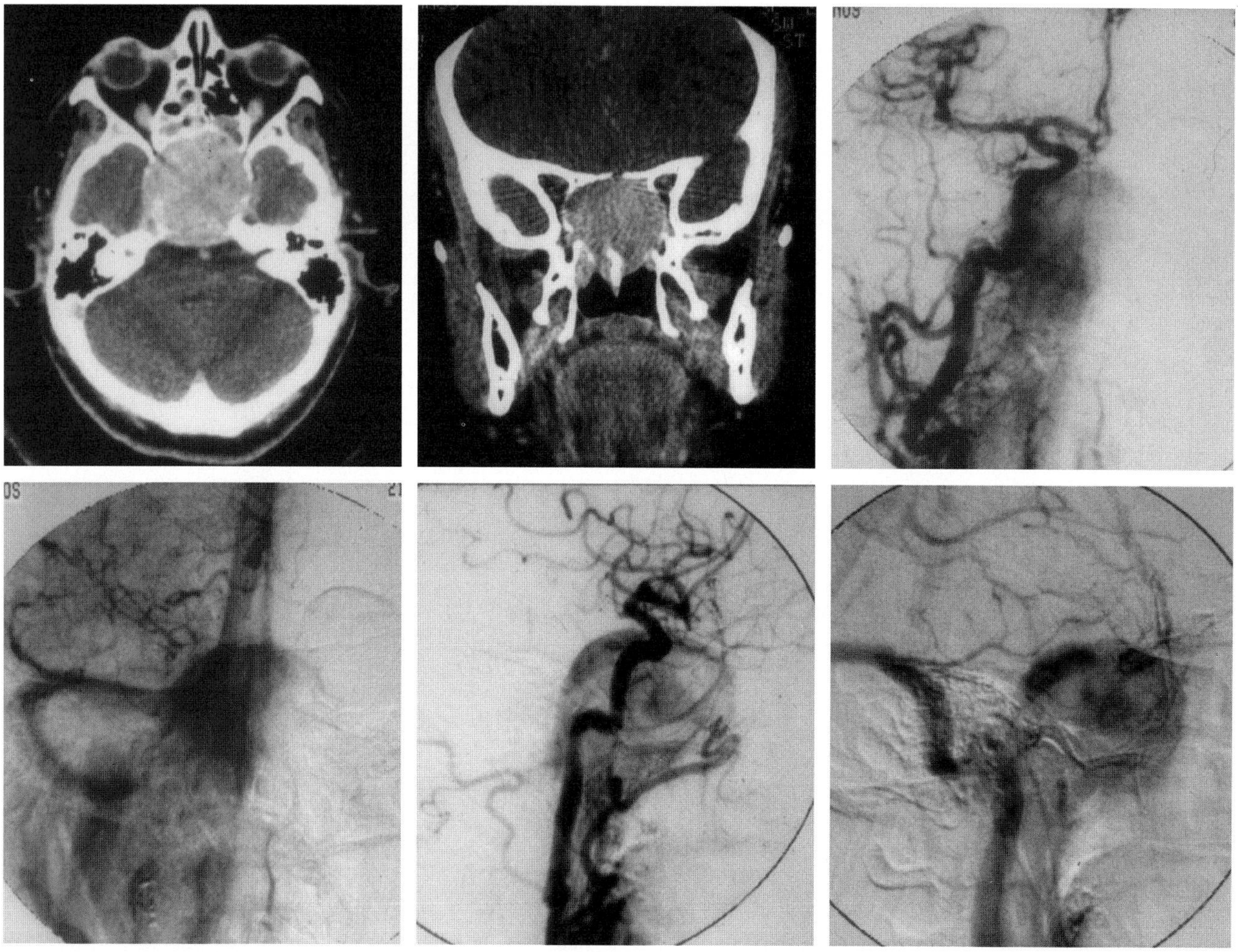

C

D, E

F

Figure 12.9

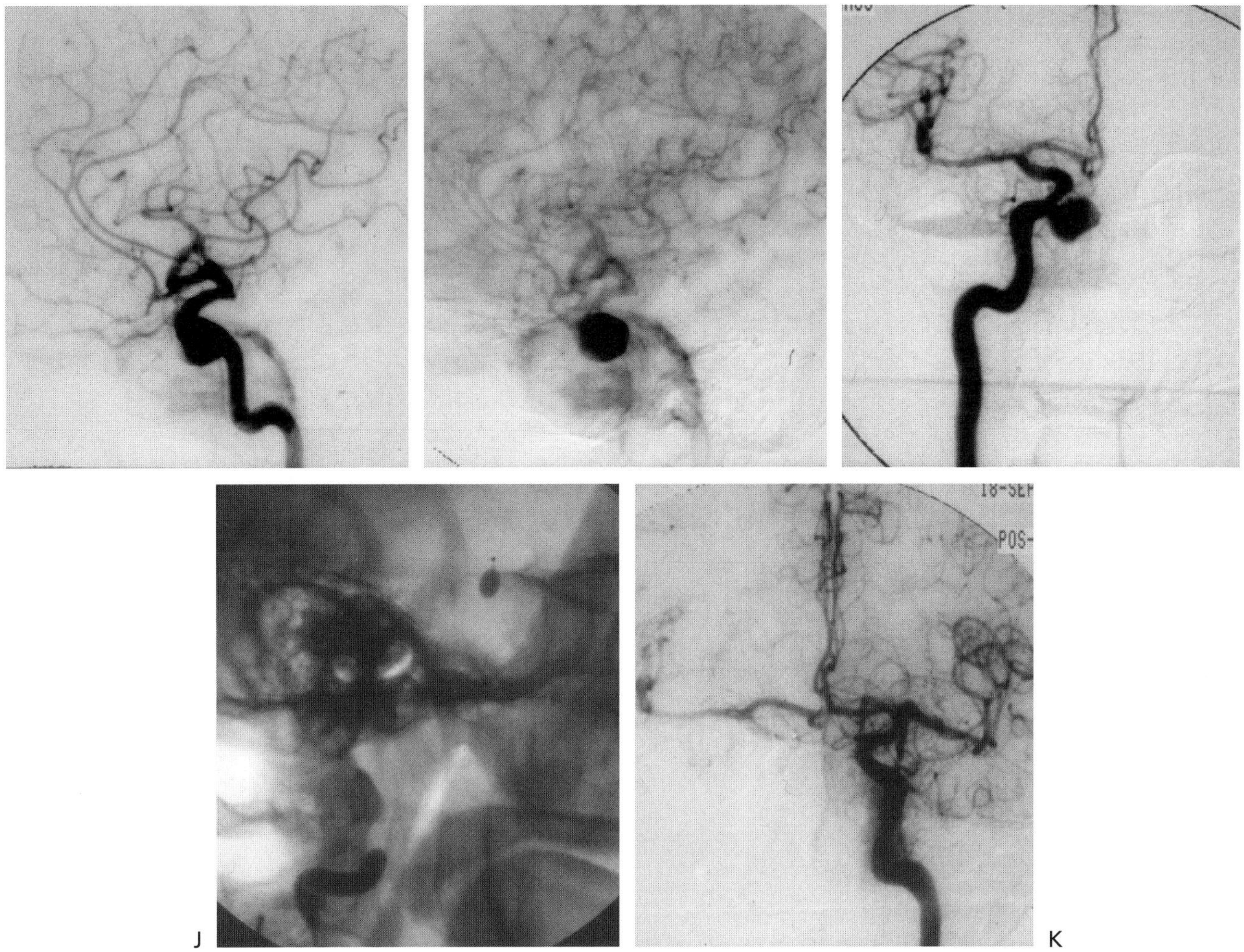

Figure 12.9 *(continued)*

A,B: CT scans in the axial and coronal views show a large hypophyseal tumor. **C–F:** Angiograms of the right carotid artery in the AP and lateral views show the hypervascularity of the sellar tumor. Transsphenoidal surgery was performed and resulted in ablation of the tumor, but a pharyngeal bleeding complication developed. **G,H:** Right carotid angiogram in the lateral view shows the pseudoaneurysm arising from the internal carotid artery at the level of the sella turcica. **I:** Anterior view of the right carotid arteriogram shows the pseudoaneurysm protruding medially. **J:** X-ray film of the skull in the lateral view shows the smaller balloon occluding the distal internal carotid artery close to the bifurcation and a larger safety balloon located proximal in the internal carotid artery. **K:** Postembolization left carotid arteriogram in the AP view shows occlusion of the right carotid and filling of the right middle cerebral artery through the anterior communicating artery.

Comment: Detachable balloon occlusion of the internal carotid artery was adequate to treat this pseudoaneurysm, despite sacrificing the patency of the carotid. It is important to document the patency of the posterior and anterior communicating arteries to provide enough blood flow to the brain. The larger the sellar lesion, the higher the chances of major vascular trauma. Although rare, this type of vascular lesion must be anticipated when a patient develops nasopharyngeal bleeding after transsphenoidal surgery.

12.10 Embolization In Lesions Of The Head And Neck

Case 12.10:

A 60-year-old man with massive bleeding in the naso-oropharynx after surgical resection of the right tonsil was referred for diagnostic angiography.

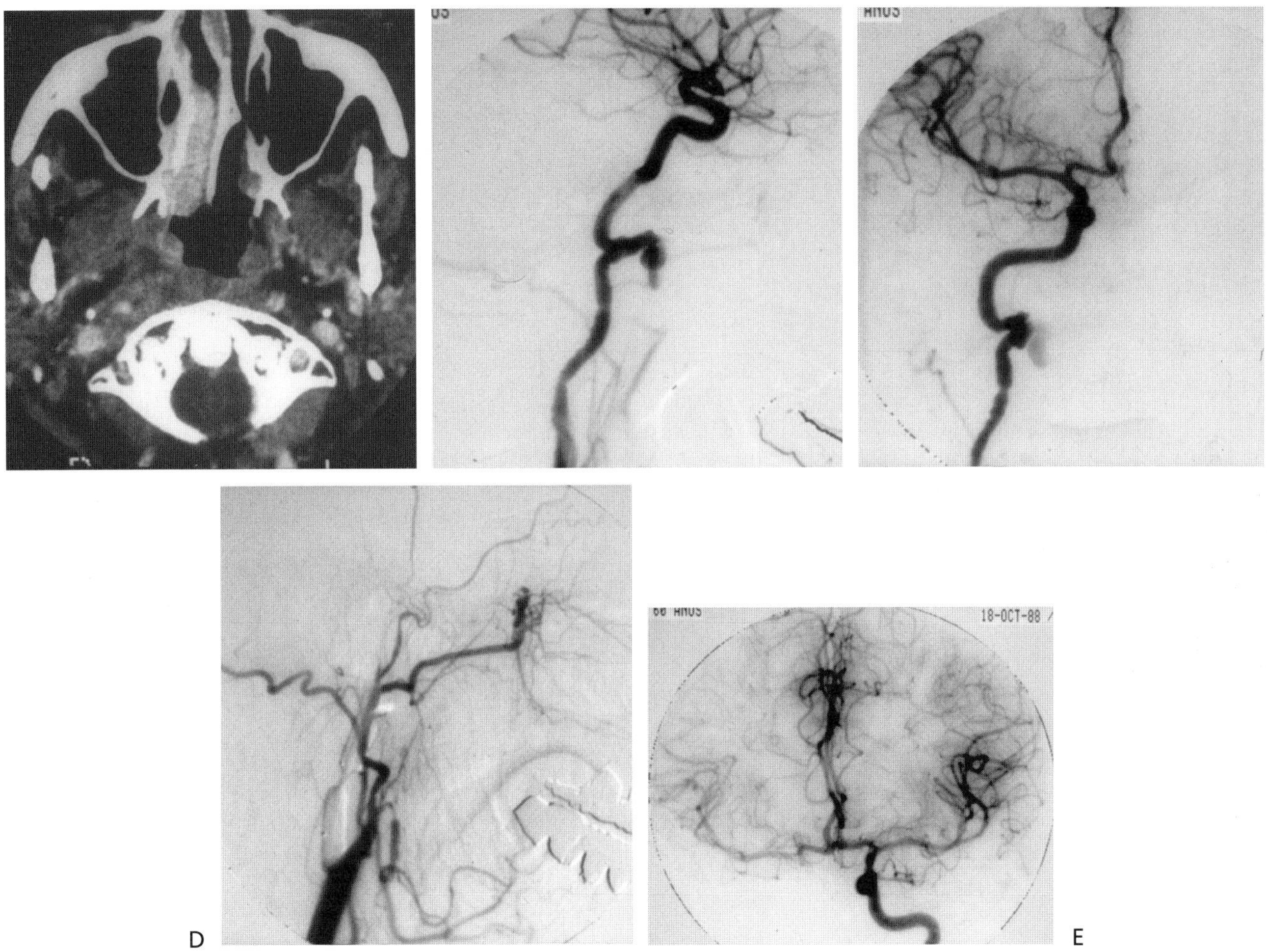

A B, C

D E

Figure 12.10

A: CT scan of the base of the skull in the axial view shows tissue swelling in the retropharynx. **B:** Lateral view of the right carotid angiogram shows a prominent anteriorly directed pseudoaneurysm of the internal carotid artery. **C:** AP view of the carotid angiogram shows the pseudoaneurysm protruding medially. **D:** Embolization of the internal carotid artery with detachable balloons controlled the bleeding. Note filling of the external carotid artery and the two balloons at two levels. **E:** Intracerebral circulation shows normal filling through an angiogram performed in the left carotid, demonstrating patency of the anterior communicating artery.

Comment: Direct trauma of the internal carotid caused by surgical resection resulted in a severe vascular lesion in this case. Note that the artery is tortuous and the pseudoaneurysm is at the tip of the vascular loop, which was very superficial behind the right tonsil. The possibility of a small-profile stent graft or covered stent, if available, would be attractive to treat such a lesion, especially without infection. Detachable balloon embolization was the best alternative at the time.

12.11 Embolization In Lesions Of The Head And Neck

Case 12.11:

A 44-year-old female presented with a severe infection in the retropharynx and development of a pseudoaneurysm of the left internal carotid artery.

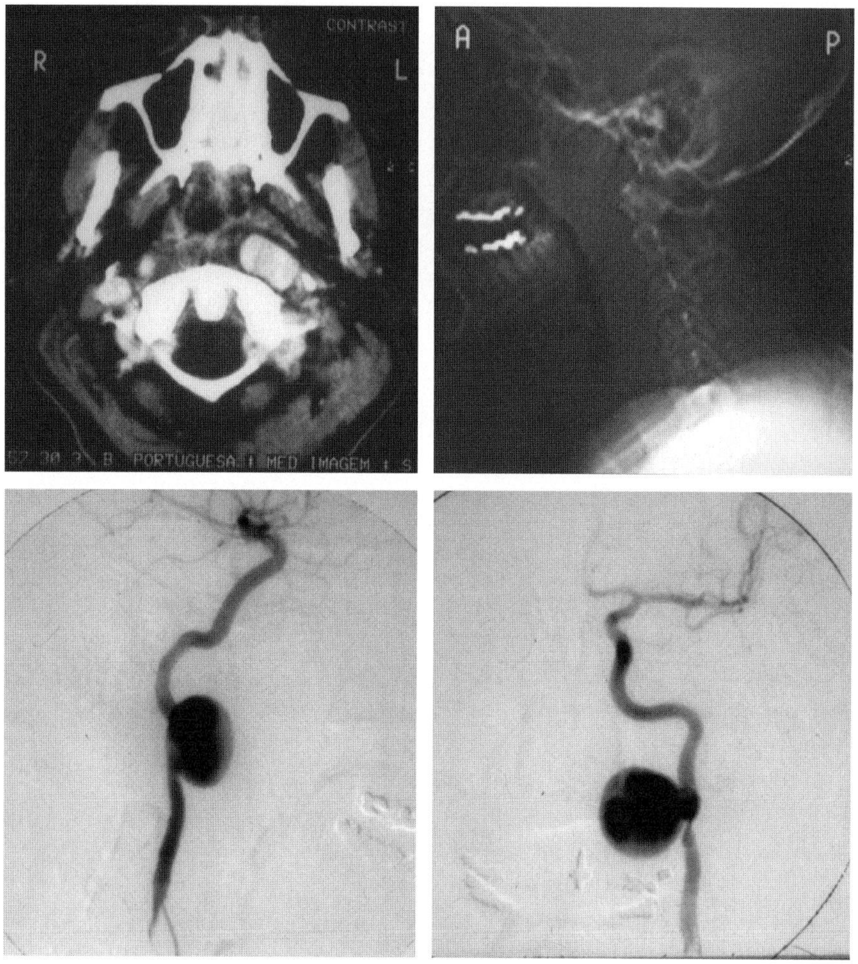

A B C D

Figure 12.11

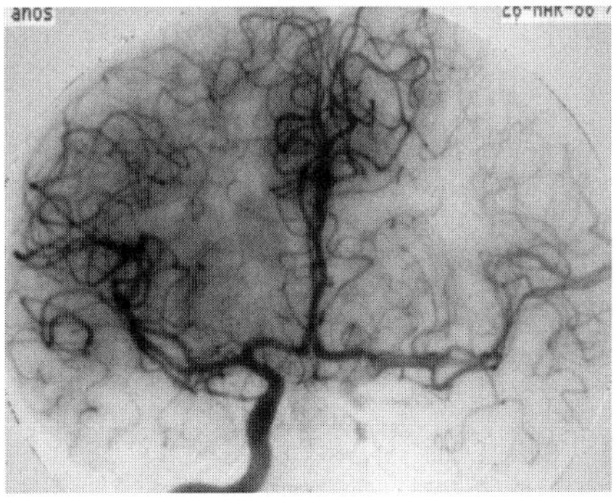

E

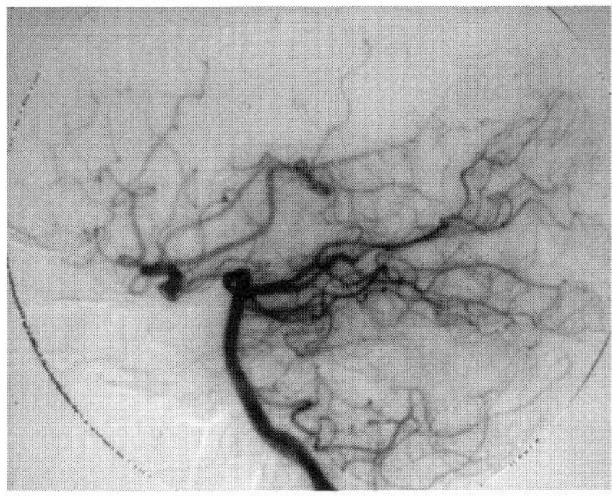

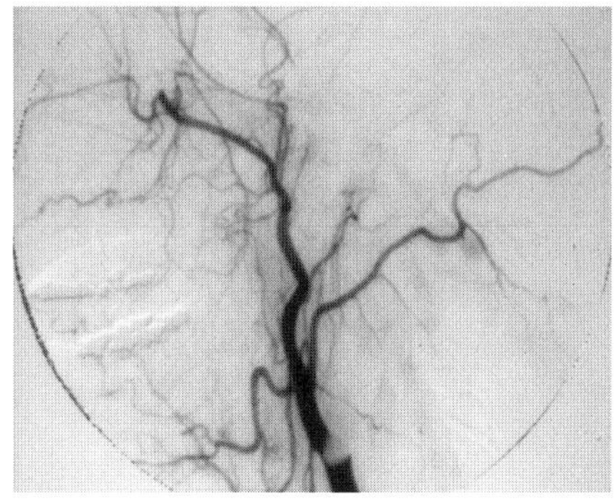

F, G

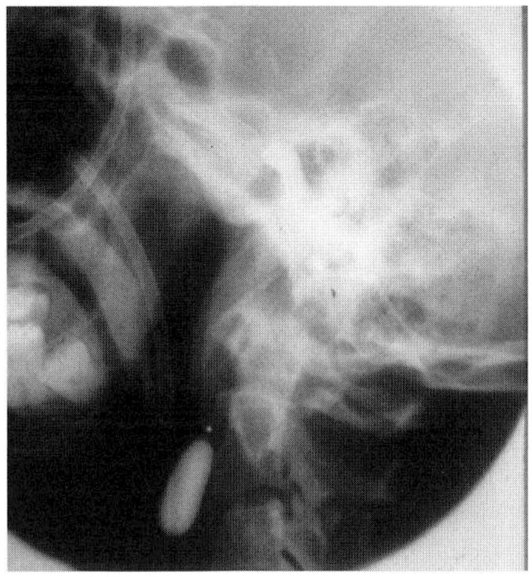

H

Figure 12.11 *(continued)*

A: CT scan in the axial view shows thickening of the retropharyngeal tissues and a contrast-enhanced structure simultaneously with the vessels, suggesting a pseudoaneurysm. **B:** Lateral view of a digital x-ray film of the cervicocranial region shows marked thickening of the soft tissues. **C:** Lateral view of a carotid arteriogram shows a large pseudoaneurysm of the internal carotid artery at the level of the skull base. **D:** Anterior view of an internal carotid angiogram shows the pseudoaneurysm protruding medially. **E:** After embolization of the internal carotid aneurysm with a detachable balloon, angiogram of the right carotid artery shows patency of the anterior communicating artery and filling of the left middle cerebral artery. **F:** Lateral view of the vertebral artery shows patency of the posterior communicating artery and filling of some of the branches of the left middle cerebral artery. **G:** Postembolization angiogram of the left carotid shows patency of the external carotid artery and a small filling defect in the bifurcation of the common carotid artery. **H:** Postembolization x-ray film shows the two detachable balloons above and below the level of the aneurysm. Note marked reduction of the thickness of the soft tissues in the retropharynx.

Comment: Infection can be a cause of arterial lesion and pseudoaneurysm formation, as in this young female patient. Although a stent graft would have been an excellent alternative for treatment in this case, it was not available at the time. Embolization with detachable balloons was the best option available. A balloon above and another balloon below the lesion was believed to be necessary for adequate treatment and thrombosis of the pseudoaneurysm.

12.12 Embolization In Lesions Of The Head And Neck

Case 12.12:

An 11-year-old boy with a gunshot wound in the neck presented with massive bleeding and shock.

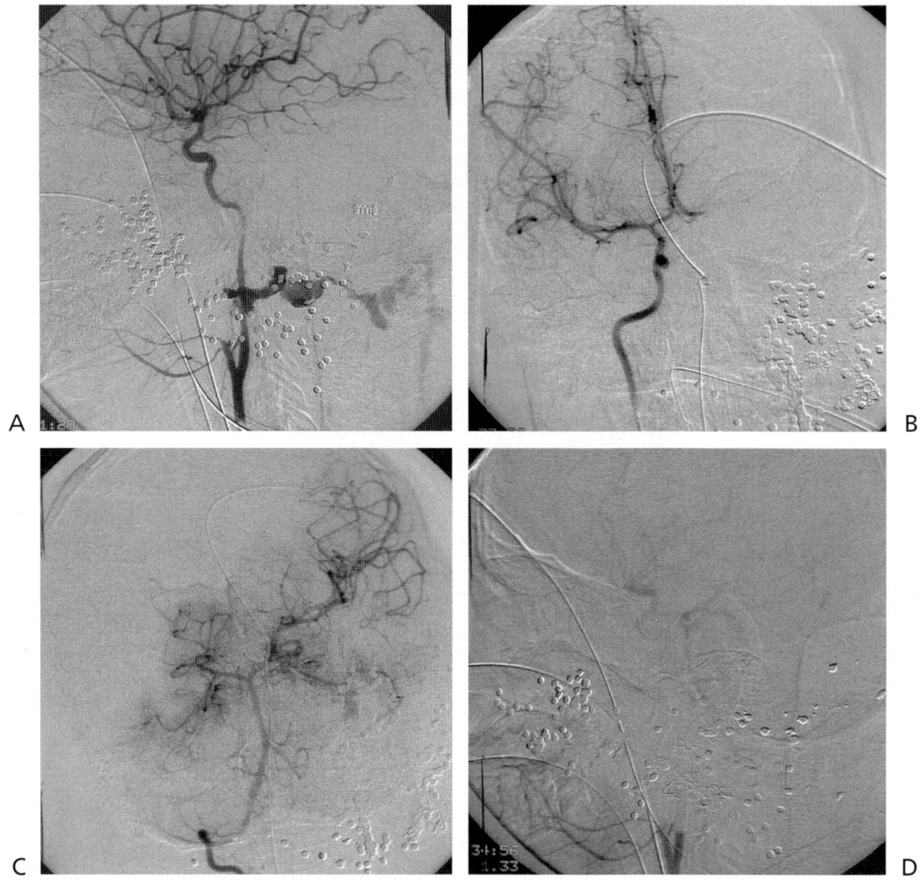

Figure 12.12

A: Lateral view of the left common carotid arteriogram shows occlusion of the external carotid artery, severe spasm of the internal carotid artery, and proximal rupture of the internal carotid artery with contrast material extravasation, running in the direction of the back of the neck and accumulating on the angio table surface. **B:** Right carotid arteriogram shows patency of the anterior communicating artery. **C:** Vertebral arteriogram shows patency of the posterior communicating artery with filling of the peripheral branches of the middle cerebral artery. **D:** Embolization of the left internal carotid artery with multiple coils was performed and resulted in total occlusion of the carotid. Lateral view of the left common carotid angiogram shows occlusion. Note coils in the vessel, around the vessel, and into the soft tissues. There is faint filling of the intracerebral vessels by reflux of contrast material into the left vertebral artery.

Comment: This was a life-threatening situation with massive hemorrhage through an open wound. Although less desirable, embolization of the carotid artery was the quickest way to achieve hemostasis and control of the situation. No neurologic sequelae ensued after the embolization; however, the patient required several units of blood and developed some degree of renal failure.

A stent graft or a covered stent, if available at that time, probably would have been a good option to seal off the vascular rupture.

Suggested Reading

Cognard C, Pierot L, Boulin A, et al. Intracranial aneurysms: endovascular treatment with mechanical detachable spirals in 60 aneurysms. *Radiology* 1997;202:783–792.

Tournade A, Courtheoux P, Sengel C, et al. Saccular intracranial aneurysms: endovascular treatment with mechanical detachable spiral coils. *Radiology* 1997;202:481–486.

Uflacker R, Lima S, Ribas GC, et al. Carotid-cavernous fistulas: embolization through the superior ophthalmic vein approach. *Radiology* 1986;159:175–179.

Vinuela F, Duckwiler G, Mawad N. Guglielmi detachable coil embolization of acute intracranial aneurysms: perioperative anatomical and clinical outcome in 403 patients. *J Neurosurg* 1997; 86:475–482.

PART II

Nonvascular Percutaneous Therapy

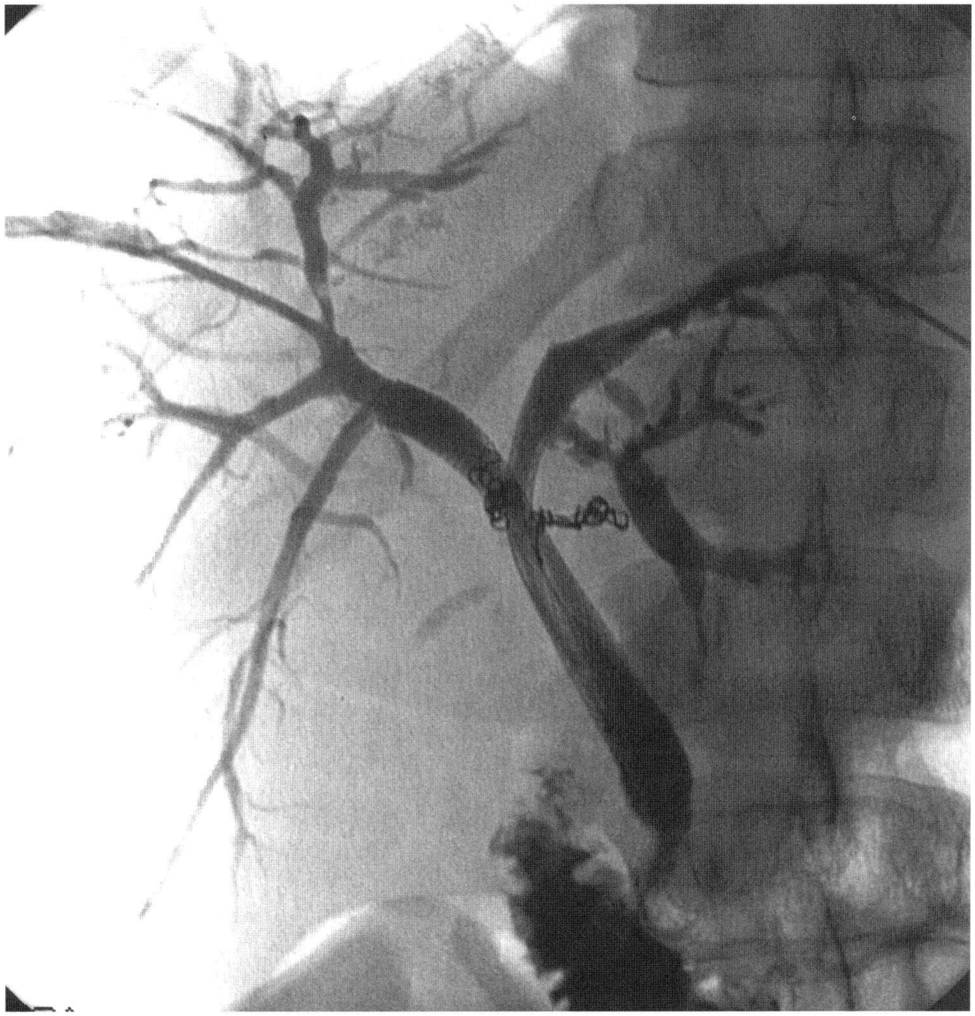

CHAPTER 13

Interventional Uroradiology

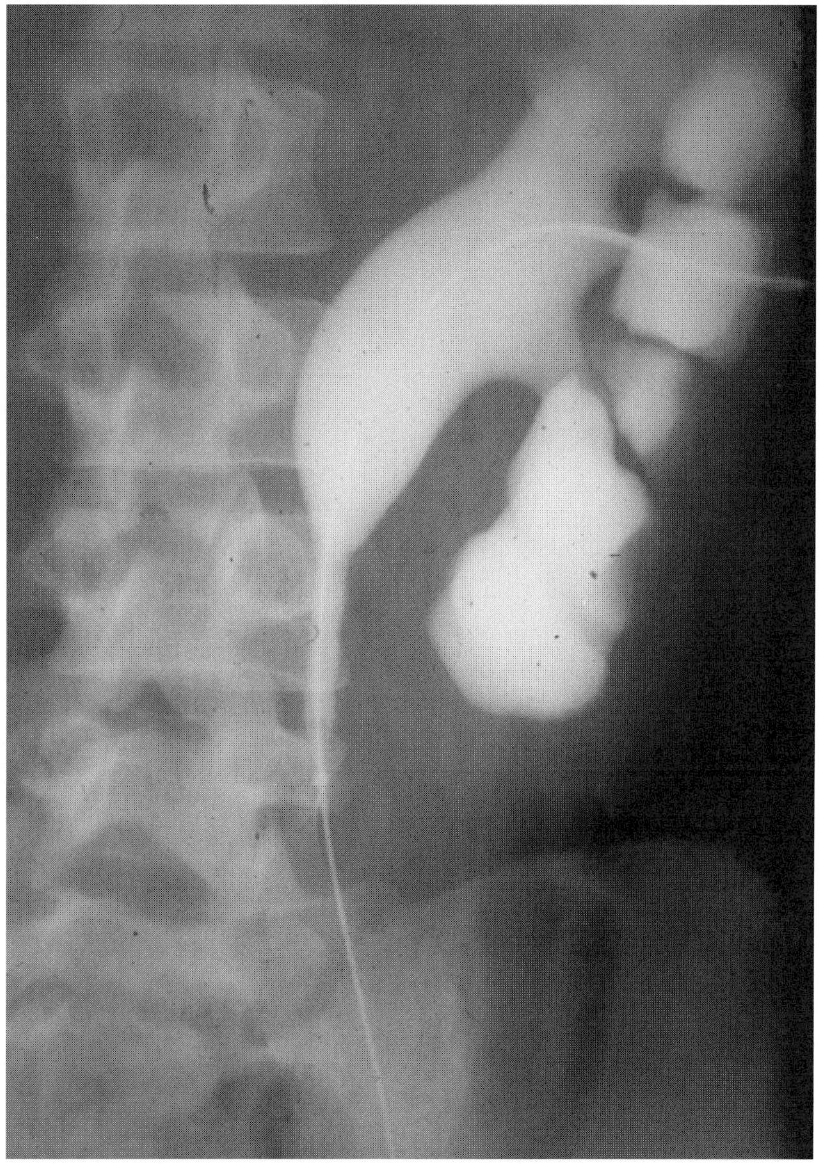

13.1.1 Percutaneous Nephrostomy

Case 13.1.1:

A 34-year-old female patient with a large kidney stone in the right lower calix required percutaneous access for lithotripsy.

A, B

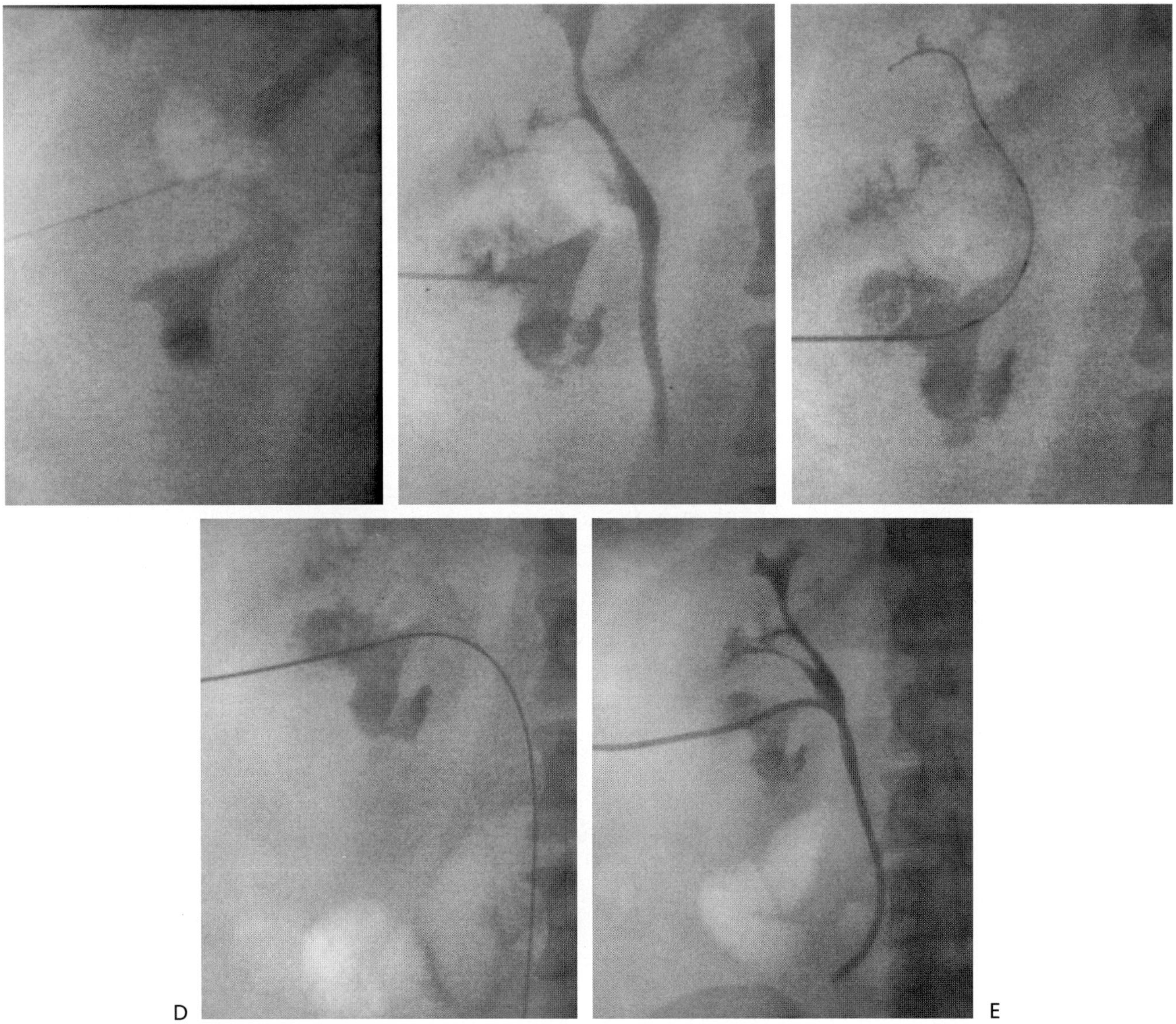

C

D

E

Figure 13.1.1

A: Percutaneous nephrostogram performed with a 23-gauge Chiba needle shows a dilated right lower calix with an infundibular stenosis. **B:** An 18-gauge trocar needle was used to directly stick the lower calix and allow introduction of the guidewire. **C:** A steerable Lunderquist guidewire was used to reach the small-sized pelvis. **D:** Catheterization of the ureter was performed. **E:** An 8F catheter was advanced into the ureter and left in place for surgical access the next morning. The catheter was exchanged over the wire and the tract was dilated to 24F.

Comment: With the aid of cross-sectional imaging and fluoroscopy, access to the collecting system of the kidney can be obtained for introduction of a catheter or drain. As in this case, the percutaneous nephrostomy procedure is merely the first step in a more sophisticated interventional uroradiologic technique for treatment of renal stones. However, simple urinary drainage remains a common indication for nephrostomies. Nephrostomy for kidney access for endourologic procedures has been used for many years. The development of new instruments and the refinement of older techniques allowed for the virtual replacement of open stone operation, even for large stones. The percutaneous access must follow certain guidelines:

1. Stay below the twelfth rib, if possible.
2. Puncture through the posterolateral edge of the paravertebral muscle but avoid going too far laterally, especially if above the twelfth rib, in order to avoid the colon, liver, and spleen.
3. For renal pelvic and ureteral calculi, puncture through a posterior calix, preferably at a middle group level.
4. For caliceal calculi, puncture the affected calix at the medial edge of the calculus.
5. Specific guidelines depend on renal anatomy, calculus location and size, and whether there are multiple or staghorn calculi.

As demonstrated in this case, a large calculus occupies the whole lower caliceal group. The pelvis is very small and the ureteropelvic junction (UPJ) is widely open. However, the infundibulum of the lower group of calices is narrow and probably one of the reasons for stone buildup. Direct puncture of the lower calix is the natural access for this specific type of stone. Note that the ureter was catheterized to provide safer access for percutaneous surgery in the operating room. The catheter provided access and allowed adequate nephrolithotomy.

13.1.2 Percutaneous Nephrostomy

Case 13.1.2:

A 9-year-old male patient with UPJ stenosis developed hydronephrosis and infection, with perirenal abscess.

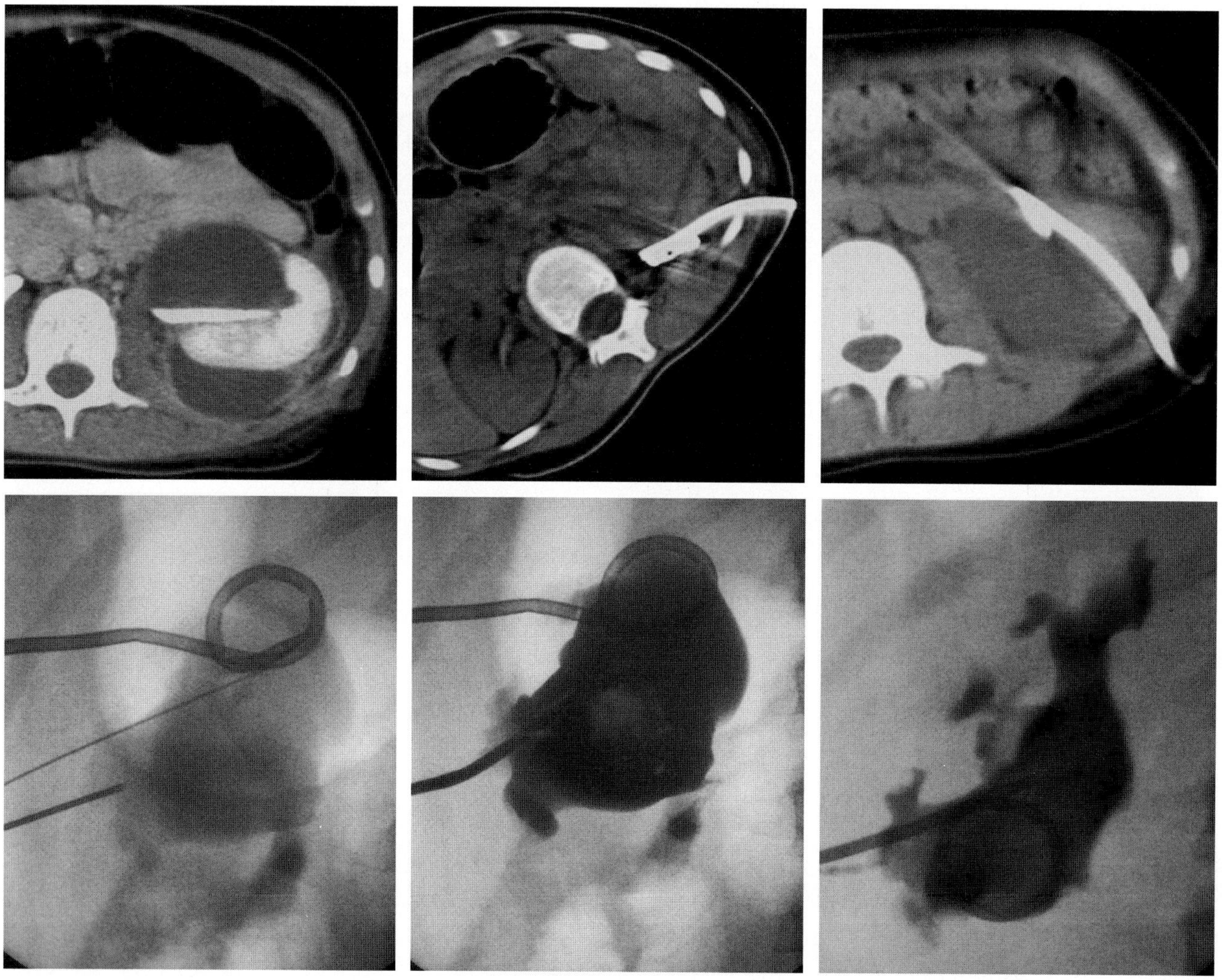

A, B C

D, E F

Figure 13.1.2

A: Computed tomography (CT) of the abdomen demonstrates adequate nephrostogram effect with delayed excretion of the left kidney, into a markedly enlarged pelvis, and a 5 × 6-cm perirenal fluid collection. **B:** CT-guided drainage of the perirenal abscess was performed. Purulent material was aspirated. **C,D:** Following abscess drainage, percutaneous nephrostomy was performed under fluoroscopic guidance. A fine needle was used for the antegrade pyelogram, followed by access through a lower calix puncture. **E:** Note the extremely dilated pelvis. A 10F nephrostomy catheter was placed. **F:** Catheter nephrostogram performed 4 weeks after nephrostomy shows a moderately dilated pelvis with normal calices. Despite resolution of the infection, no ureteral visualization was observed at this point, but the catheter was removed on the request of the attending physician, against our advice. Follow-up CT scan 6 months after catheter removal (not shown) shows delayed nephrogram effect on the right kidney, and dilated calices and pelvis.

Comment: Indication for percutaneous nephrostomy is basically related to the presence of urinary obstruction of benign or malignant origin. It also is part of diagnostic and therapeutic maneuvers. It has virtually replaced surgical nephrostomy for relief of supravesical obstruction because it is easier and has far lower morbidity and mortality rates, and it provides rapid access for intrarenal therapy.

Common indications for percutaneous nephrostomy are as follows:

1. Obstruction with dilation or azotemia
2. Ureteral stricture or fistula as a prelude to ureteral stent insertion
3. Urodynamic studies
4. Prior to stone removal
5. Nephroscopy for biopsy or tumor resection
6. Foreign body removal
7. Allograft evaluation and management
8. Infusion of solvents and drugs
9. Access for intrarenal surgery

Benign or malignant obstruction of the urinary tract is the most common indication for placement of a nephrostomy catheter. Urinary diversion with percutaneous nephrostomy is indicated by symptoms, such as persistent colic, high temperature, uremia, and hydronephrosis caused by stones. Percutaneous nephrostomy is successful in almost 100% of cases, regardless of the degree of collecting system dilation. Retrograde ureteral stents can be placed successfully in about 80% of the patients. Comfort and successful decompression are better in patients with fever and hydronephrosis, when treated by percutaneous nephrostomy. Nephrostomies performed for reasons unrelated to infection, renal failure, or solitary kidney usually can be performed on an outpatient basis. When there is infection, such as in the case reported here, admission to the hospital and aggressive antibiotic therapy should be pursued. Extravasation of infected urine, particularly in patients with failed pyeloplasty for UPJ obstruction, is devastating and associated with severe morbidity and symptomatology. Drainage of the infected urinoma is essential for management of the problem. Revision of the pyeloplasty may be necessary in the majority of the patients, after the infection and hydronephrosis are controlled.

13.1.3 Percutaneous Nephrostomy

Case 13.1.3:

A 75-year-old female patient with a severely prolapsed uterus and a large transitional cell carcinoma of the bladder developed bilateral hydronephrosis and azotemia. Bilateral nephrostomy was attempted. Nephrostomy of the left kidney was performed without problems; the right nephrostomy was more complex.

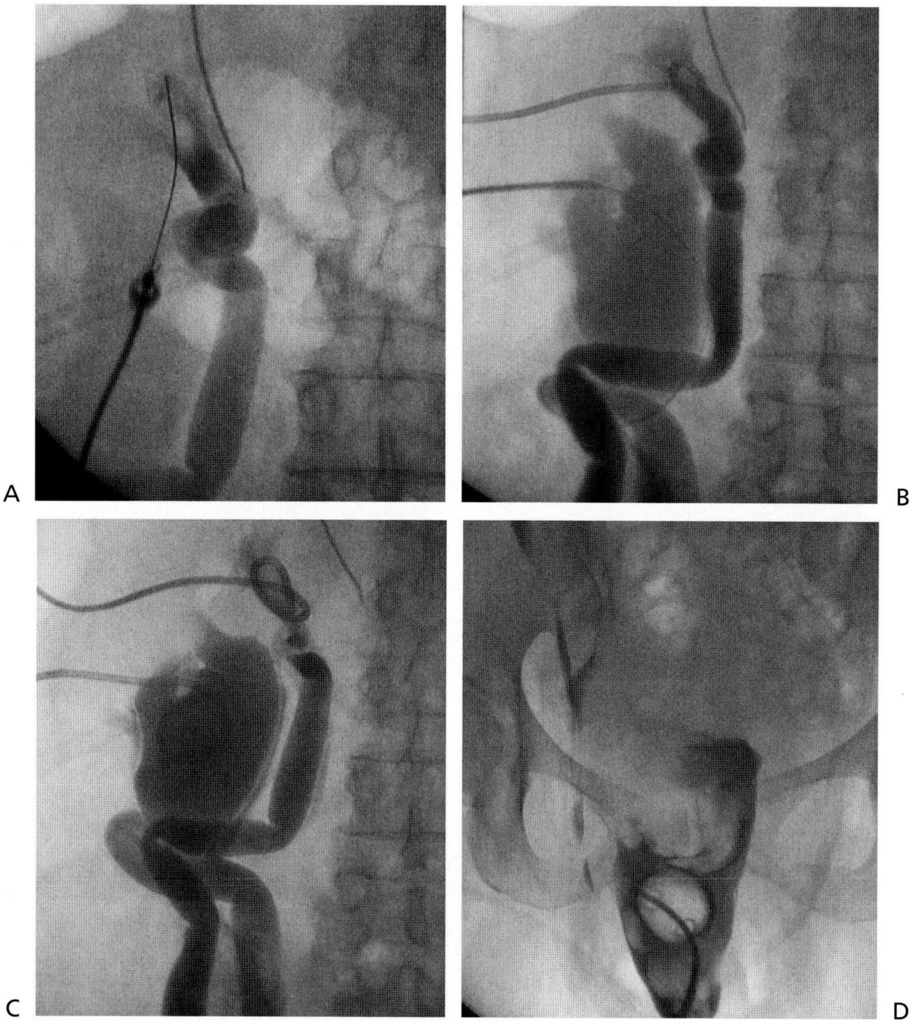

Figure 13.1.3

A: Fine-needle puncture of the right kidney for a nephrostogram shows a small collecting system drained by a significantly dilated ureter. **B:** An 8F nephrostomy catheter was placed for drainage. It was know from a previous ultrasound (US) study that there was a much more dilated collecting system, suggesting a duplication. Nephrostogram of the larger collecting system shows a large pelvis with dilated calices. **C:** A second nephrostomy catheter was placed in the main collecting system. Both catheters were open to external drainage. **D:** A cystogram associated with injection through both catheters shows complete duplication of the right pelvic/ureteric system and obstruction at the level of the bladder wall. Despite initial improvement, the patient developed pneumonia requiring tracheal intubation, gram-negative sepsis, and coagulopathy, probably secondary to urinary tract infection. The patient died about 2 weeks after drainage.

Comment: Most of the indications for percutaneous nephrostomy vary from institution to institution. Oligoanuria and pyonephrosis are common indications. Almost half of ureteral obstructions are caused by malignancies. Lithiasis is the main etiology in subjects with benign disease, causative of oligoanuria and pyonephrosis. Percutaneous nephrostomies are achieved successfully in almost every case, even in nondilated collecting systems. There is improvement of renal function and infection in most cases. Aggressive treatment of the infection is advised, and adequate drainage is necessary. However, the overall immunocompromise in cancer patients may cause worsening of the clinical picture and perpetuate renal infection. Multiple catheters often are necessary, especially when there is stone or stenotic obstruction of the caliceal infundibula, duplication of the collecting system, or caliceal diverticulum.

13.1.4 Percutaneous Nephrostomy

Case 13.1.4:

A 52-year-old female patient presented with kidney stones and horseshoe kidneys. She complained of pain in the left flank and groin. Previous intravenous pyelogram (IVP) showed at least two stones in the dilated pelvis of the left kidney and a highly inserted ureter. Percutaneous nephrolithotomy was indicated.

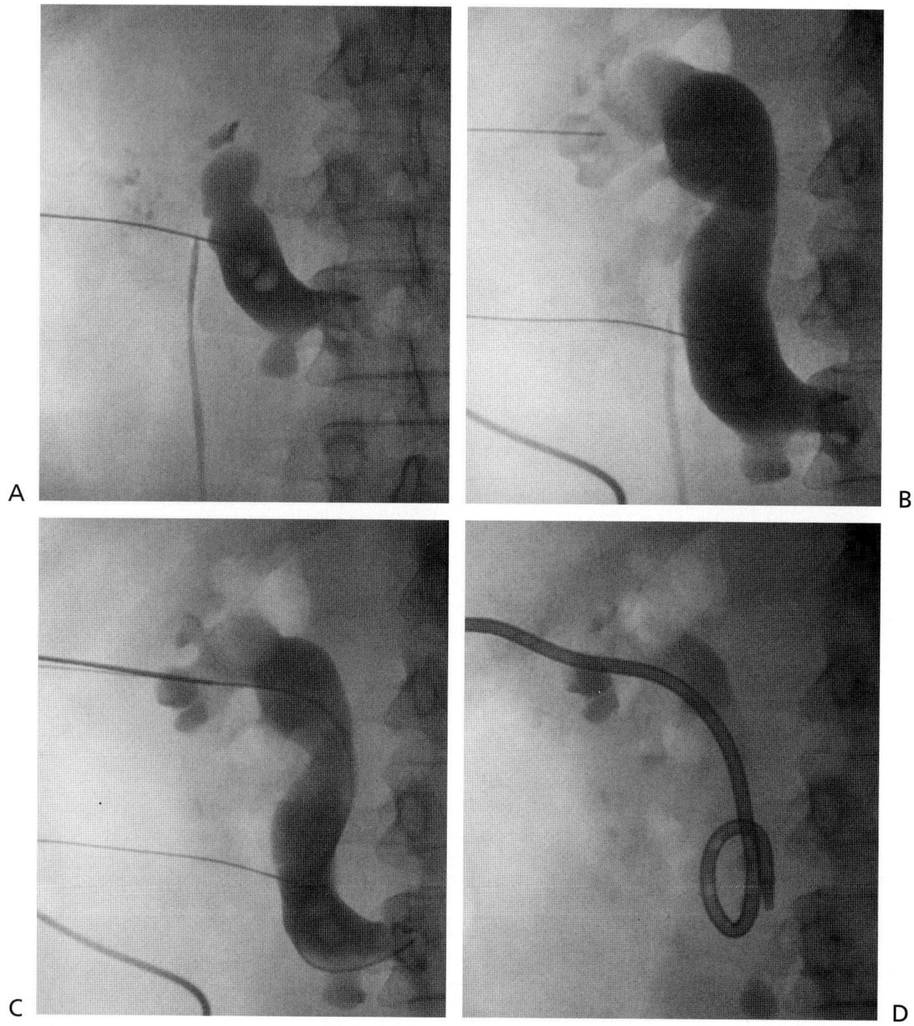

Figure 13.1.4

A: Left percutaneous fine-needle nephrostogram with the patient in the prone position shows a dilated collecting system in a horseshoe kidney. Note the significant dilation of the collecting system with two round stones and high insertion of the ureter. **B:** The fine needle was introduced in the dilated pelvis. Once a dilated upper calix was identified, another 23-gauge fine needle was used to puncture the upper calix. Carbon dioxide (CO_2) was injected for better delineation of the upper calices. An 18-gauge needle was used for direct puncture of the edge of the papilla. **C:** A guidewire was introduced into the collecting system. **D:** A 10F nephrostomy catheter was introduced for external drainage and percutaneous lithotripsy access.

Comment: Because of the extremely anterior position of the lower pole in horseshoe kidneys, a puncture of the upper calices provides the shortest tract possible from which almost any location can be reached. The upper pole of the horseshoe kidney is in direct contact with the posterior wall of the abdomen. When the patient is in the prone position, injection of gas within the collecting system will preferentially opacify the upper pole calices. Due to variation in anatomy, the horseshoe kidney is more prone to vascular complications and bleeding during percutaneous procedures. Because of the anomalous implantation of the ureter, there is either an aberrant angle or stenosis, causing dilation and stone formation.

13.1.5 Percutaneous Nephrostomy

Case 13.1.5:

A 45-year-old female patient with severe iodine allergy presented with a large pelvic stone. Percutaneous lithotripsy was indicated, but a CO_2 technique was used for percutaneous access because of her allergy.

A, B

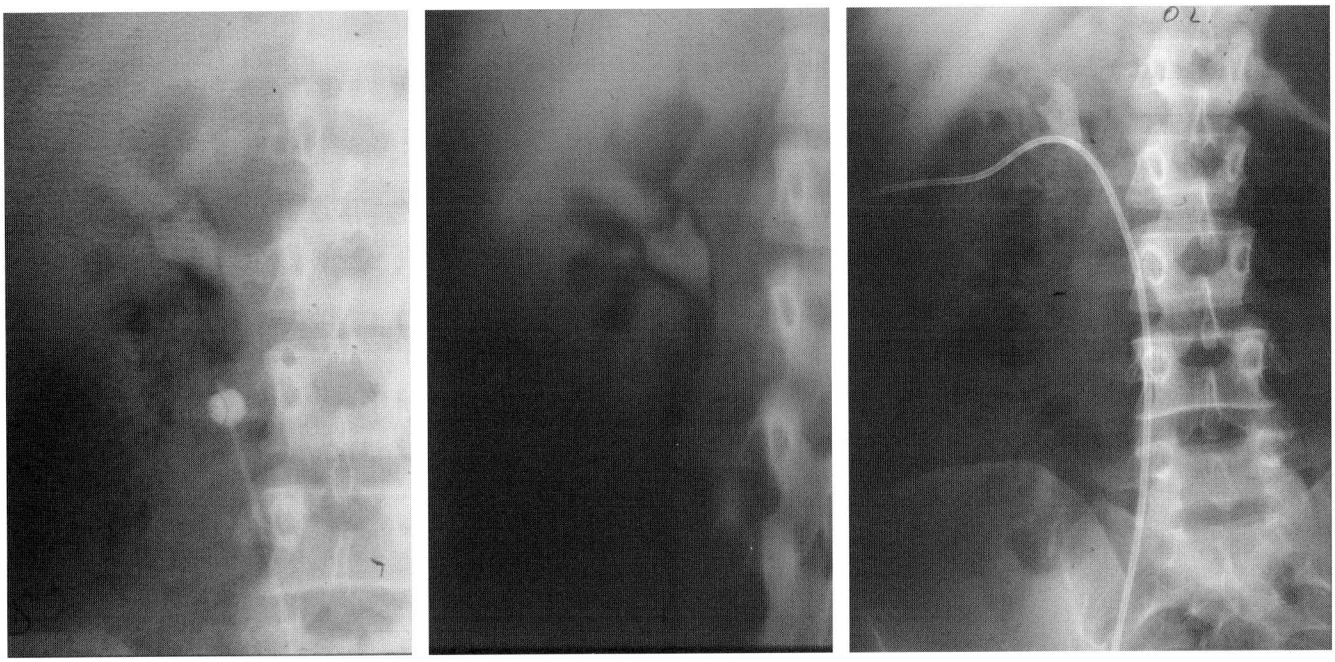

C

Figure 13.1.5

A: A balloon catheter was placed in the right ureter via cystoscopy. **B:** The patient was placed in the prone position, and CO_2 was injected to opacify the collecting system. **C:** A middle group calix was punctured, and a percutaneous nephrostomy was performed with placement of a straight catheter into the ureter.

Comment: Opacification of the collecting system and localization of stones within the renal pelvis or calices is crucial for successful lithotripsy, because appropriate selection of the entry site is necessary. An antegrade pyelogram usually can be performed by direct fine-needle puncture of the collecting system for contrast material injection. Retrograde injection of iodinated contrast medium through the ureteral catheter also can be used for collecting system opacification to provide percutaneous access. Iodine-allergic persons are at low risk when injection of the contrast material is limited to the collecting system; however, contrast extravasation, pyelovenous backflow, and overdistention of the renal pelvis with contrast may precipitate anaphylactic reactions. Although reactions to contrast tend to be mild in these patients, an option of collecting system opacification with CO_2 through a ureteral catheter is available. To guide the percutaneous procedure, a balloon occlusion catheter is introduced via a cystoscope, up into the ureter. With the balloon inflated, CO_2 is injected to opacify the caliceal system. Because the patient is in the prone position, the dorsal calices are well delineated by this technique and the puncture is easily selected.

13.1.6 Percutaneous Nephrostomy

Case 13.1.6:

A 15-day-old premature male baby with a stricture of the penile and bulbous urethral junction, bilateral renal dysplasia, and functional right single kidney presented with anuria, hydronephrosis, and sepsis. Emergency percutaneous nephrostomy was requested.

A B

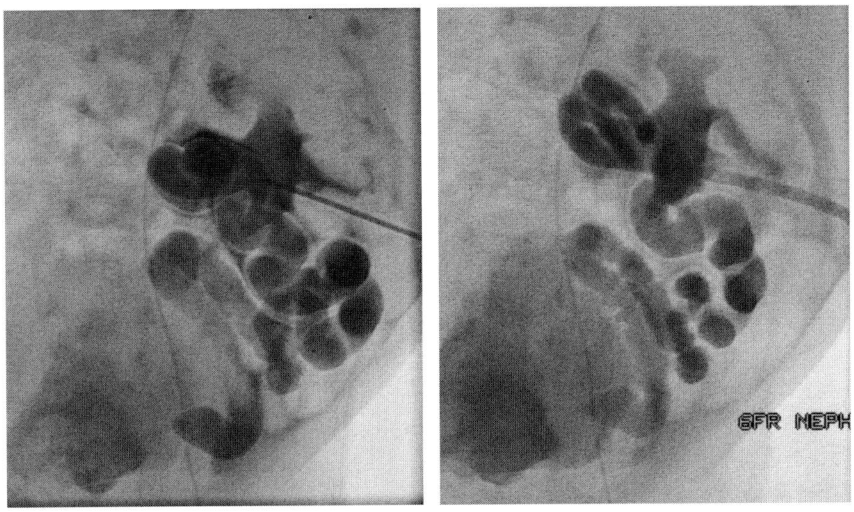

Figure 13.1.6

A: With the patient under general anesthesia and in the prone position, a 23-gauge fine needle was used to puncture the right kidney collecting system. Injection of contrast material shows significant dilation of the pelvis and ureter. The ureter is extremely dilated and redundant. **B:** A 6F nephrostomy catheter was placed within the collecting system for external drainage. Significant improvement in renal function and infection followed the nephrostomy. Surgery of the ureter eventually was performed, with resection of a stenosis. The patient presented several problems related to prematurity in the following 6 months, but renal function was within normal limits.

Comment: Percutaneous nephrostomy is performed in infants for diagnostic and temporizing purposes. Diagnostic antegrade urography provides clear definition of the anatomy and, in association with dynamic studies, permits better evaluation of the physiologic problem. Kidneys in infants and young children lie lower than in adults. The soft tissues in the renal fossa are less developed than in adults, and the kidneys are closer to the skin. Less renal parenchyma is available, and the tract is not properly formed. General anesthesia usually is necessary. Use of small tubes, 6F or 5F, is necessary to minimize renal damage and vascular injury. The pediatric kidney usually is much more mobile than in adults, and it may be difficult to dilate the tract once the collecting system is cannulated. Common indications are posterior urethral valves, congenital hydronephrosis, and megaureter with and without stenosis. Other indications are postoperative strictures, pyonephrosis, obstructed allografts, fistulas, renal calculi, and neoplastic obstruction. Drainage of an infected obstructed megaureter in a sick baby is best treated by percutaneous nephrostomy.

13.2.1 Percutaneous Ureteral Manipulations And Stenting

Case 13.2.1:

A 22-year-old male patient presented with oliguria, worsening renal function, and a large palpable kidney. US and CT scans showed a huge single kidney with UPJ obstruction. Nephrostomy was requested.

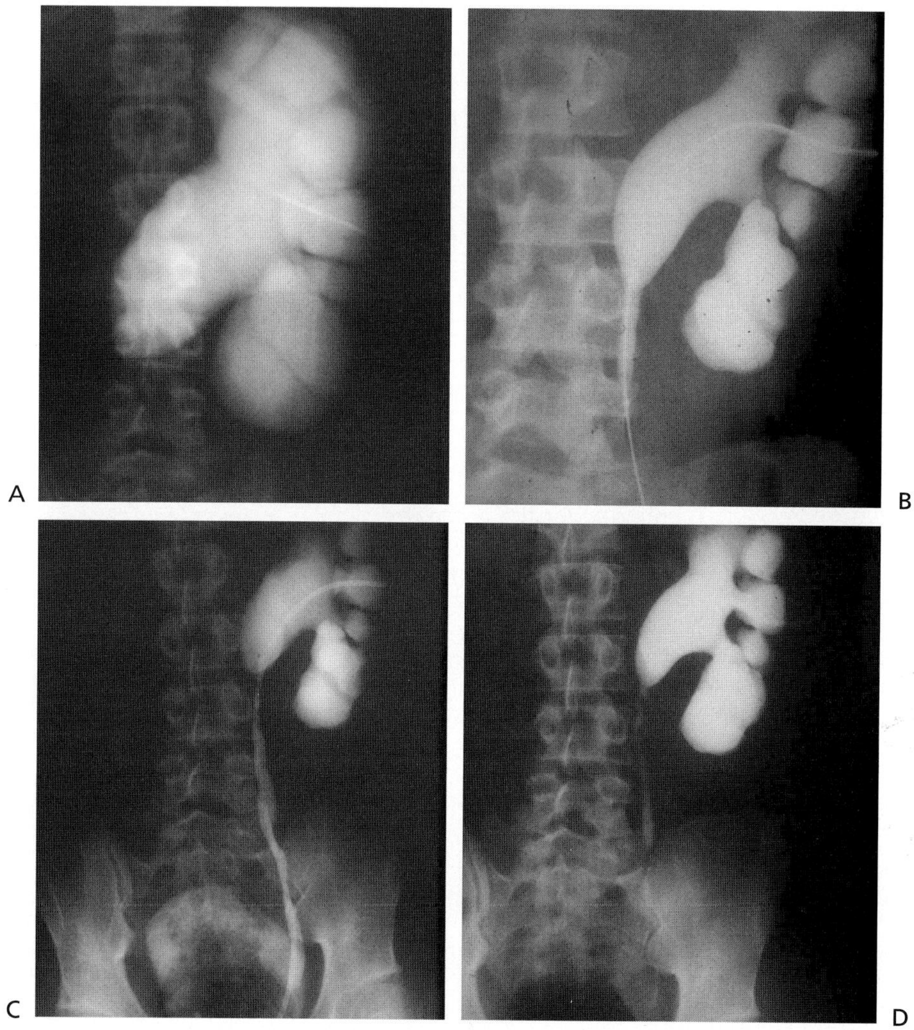

Figure 13.2.1

A: Fine-needle antegrade pyelogram shows a huge left single kidney with total UPJ obstruction. Note the remarkable ballooning of the calices. No ureter was visualized. **B:** A middle calix was selected, and an 18-gauge needle was used for access. Catheterization of the ureter through the stenosis was performed, and a 6- and 8-mm balloon was used for plasty of the UPJ. **C:** A ureteronephrostomy catheter was placed and maintained through the stenosis for 3 months, with two additional balloon plasties of the stenosis performed in the mean time. **D:** Follow-up nephrostogram, prior to nephrostomy removal, shows adequate patency of the UPJ, with significant reduction in the size of the left kidney. There was flow within the ureter. The catheter was removed, and the patient did well in follow-up of more than 5 years.

Comment: The best access to the UPJ obstruction is percutaneous, and the balloon pyeloplasty is the easiest treatment to perform, as long as the ureter is catheterized. The middle or upper calices are selected for puncture, using US and fluoroscopic guidance. From the middle calices, the UPJ is easily accessible, and it is easier to cross the obstruction. When it is not possible to cross the obstruction from above, it is necessary to try a retrograde transureteral approach using a ureteroscope. A hydrophilic wire usually easily passes the stenosis and into the pelvis, where the wire can be snared and exteriorized through the percutaneous tract. In that case, a pull-through system should be available to introduce rigid dilators or balloons. It may be not necessary to rupture the ureter to treat the stenosis, but overdilation is expected to have a better result than underdilation. The case reported here is a clear example of the success of the technique, with resolution of the UPJ stenosis in a quite critical patient with single kidney. Immediate decompression of the kidney reverses the loss of renal function in most cases. When infection is associated, the loss of renal function may be more difficult to reverse. Long-term follow-up is necessary, as recurrences require either redilation or more aggressive endopyelotomy. Stents should be maintained within the ureter, across the stenosis, for 6 to 8 weeks in some cases. In children, when renal function is less than 10% and there is no renal function improvement after percutaneous nephrostomy, nephrectomy may be an option if it is not a solitary kidney. In most patients, split renal function improves about 30%, which suggests that pyeloplasty should be attempted, with higher chances of success. There usually is further improvement over a period of 2 to 3 years after pyeloplasty. A trial of split renal function should always be tried before the decision for nephrectomy is made.

13.2.2 Percutaneous Ureteral Manipulations And Stenting

Case 13.2.2:

A 45-year-old male patient presented with pyonephrosis due to UPJ obstruction. Initial drainage was performed percutaneously, and control of the infection was achieved in a few days. Stenosis of the UPJ was treated by balloon plasty.

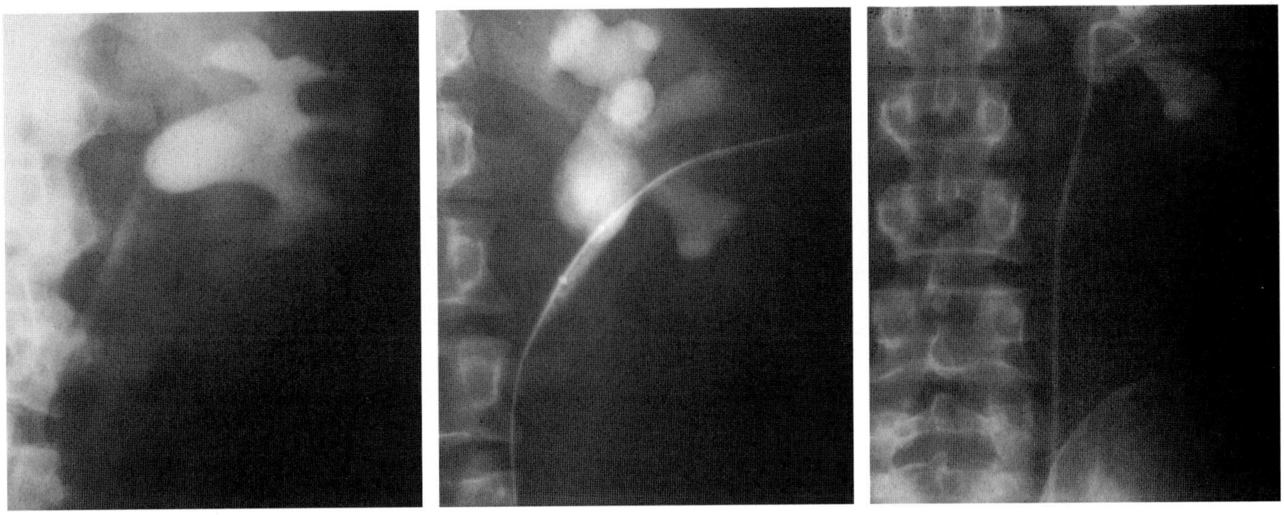

A B, C

Figure 13.2.2

A: Nephrostogram shows a moderately dilated collecting system. Drainage was done previously to treat pyonephrosis. **B:** Catheterization of the UPJ was performed, and dilation was achieved with a 6-mm balloon. **C:** The ureteral stent was placed for 3 weeks and then removed by cystoscopy. Renal function returned to normal levels.

Comment: Pyonephrosis can be defined as the presence of purulent material in a dilated urinary tract. Clinical presentation symptoms are fever and flank pain, combined with radiographic evidence of urinary obstruction. The diagnosis can be confirmed by aspiration, pyelogram, and nephrostomy. Although nephrectomy is curative for the problem, the morbidity associated with the procedure is very high, and the patient loses a kidney. Preoperative nephrostomy and vigorous antibiotic therapy may be a life-saving procedure in many patients and may obviate nephrectomy. Following control of the infection, the clinical status of the patient and the determination of residual renal function must be assessed. Effective drainage should improve the patient's clinical status in 24 to 48 hours and allow for additional treatment. To reduce the risks of septicemia, a pyelogram should be performed using the minimum of contrast medium to determine if the calix was punctured. The drain should be placed with as little manipulation as possible, and no attempts to pass the obstruction should be made. Increases in intrapelvic pressure can introduce germs into the bloodstream and produce septicemia. A full diagnostic nephrostogram can be performed 48 hours after drainage, when the risks of infection are lessened, without significant risk. Percutaneous nephrostomy compares favorably with internal retrograde ureteral stenting and surgery to treat pyonephrosis, although some patients will require other surgery for urinary tract obstruction. Major complications, such as sepsis and bleeding, may occur in up to 9% of patients. Treatment of the obstructive problem can be performed with endoluminal procedures, such as balloon dilation of the UPJ stenosis or surgical endopyelotomy.

Case 13.2.3:

A 40-year-old male patient presented with UPJ obstruction and recurrent infection. Percutaneous approach for pyeloplasty was attempted.

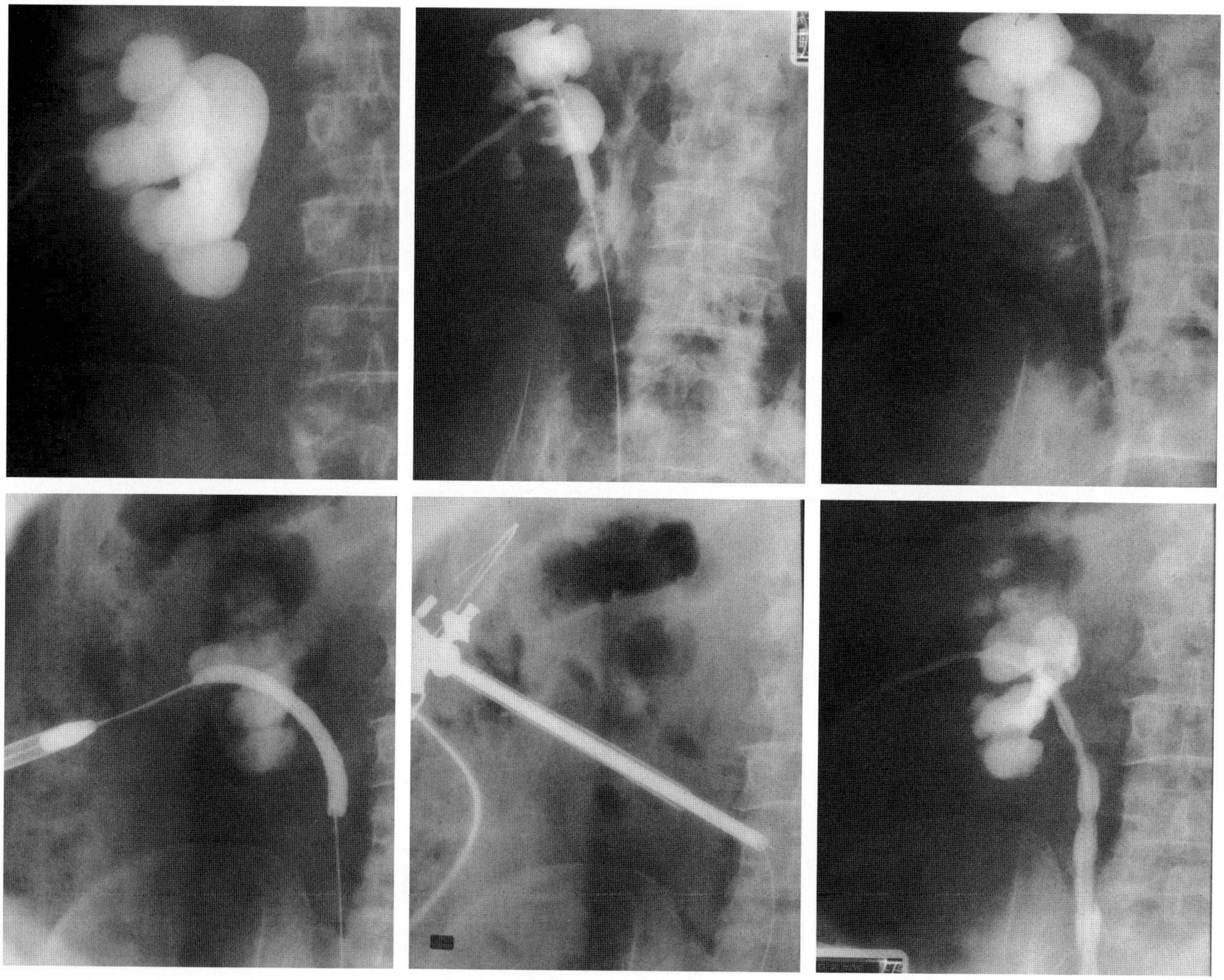

A, B — C — D, E — F

Figure 13.2.3

A: Percutaneous antegrade pyelogram shows a significantly dilated collecting system with no visualization of the ureter. **B:** Following decompression, it was possible to catheterize the ureter and perform balloon angioplasty with a 6- and 7-mm balloon. Note extravasation of contrast due to rupture of the ureteric wall. **C:** Follow-up nephrostogram after 3 weeks shows a persistent stenosis with a filling defect in the pelvic wall. **D:** A more aggressive approach was decided, using percutaneous access for an endopyelotomy. After dilating the tract, a 10-mm balloon was used to dilate the stenosis. **E:** Endopyelotomy was performed over the wire using a Sacks knife. **F:** An 8F ureteral double J stent was left in place. Final nephrostogram shows adequate patency of the UPJ.

Comment: Surgical open pyeloplasty has been the procedure of choice for treatment of UPJ stenosis; however, it is subject to a number of complications, such as fistulization, suture dehiscence, and reobstruction, due to damage to the periureteral blood supply. The percutaneous technique was introduced in 1983 and has a success rate of 87%. Endopyelotomy has been the procedure of choice for primary or secondary UPJ obstruction. Technically it requires percutaneous access, as for nephrostomy, through a mid-zone calix. Catheterization of the stenosis or occluded UPJ is necessary for success of the procedure. Cannulization of the UPJ can be achieved from above using a steerable guidewire. If the guidewire cannot be passed down the ureter, it can be coiled in the pelvis and used for access only. Alternatively, a guidewire can be passed retrogradely through the ureter into the renal pelvis and, using a Dormia basket or snare, retrieved through the percutaneous tract. Once the guidewire is positioned firmly within the ureter across the UPJ, the percutaneous access can be used for the procedure. A balloon catheter and/or urethrotome may be used for dilation and incision of the UPJ stenotic wall. Balloon dilation may suffice to correct the UPJ stenosis. When using the urethrotome, the relationship of the UPJ to the retroperitoneal vascular structures must be considered. In 53% of cases, there is a close relationship between the anteroinferior segmental artery and the anterior aspect of the UPJ. In 40.6% of cases, there is a close relationship between an important tributary of the renal vein, draining the inferior pole of the kidney. In several instances, the UPJ is embraced by an artery or a vein anteriorly and posteriorly simultaneously. Therefore, it is only acceptable to incise the UPJ stenosis in its lateral aspect, or the so-called "nonvascular area" of the UPJ.

13.2.4 Percutaneous Ureteral Manipulations And Stenting

Case 13.2.4:

A 45-year-old female patient presented with UPJ obstruction and stones. Surgical pyelolithotomy was undertaken. A large urinary fistula developed through a leak in the UPJ. Percutaneous nephrostomy was requested.

A 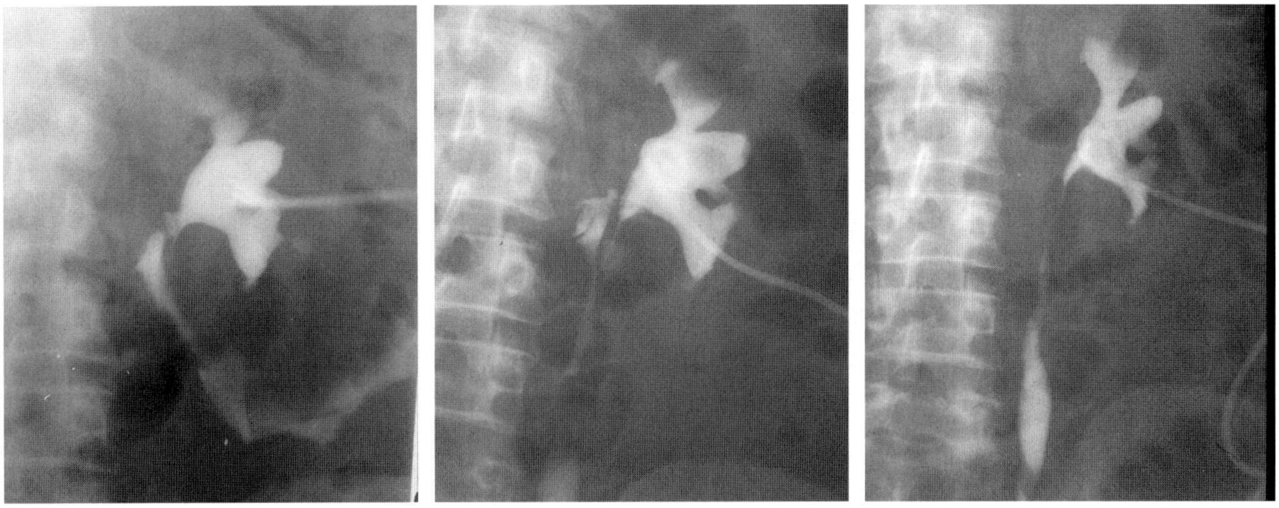 B, C

Figure 13.2.4

A: Percutaneous nephrostomy was performed. Injection of the collecting system shows a large leak from the UPJ incision. Note that the fistulous tract surrounds the kidney and drains through the cutaneous incision. Nephrostomy was performed with a 10F catheter and open to gravity drainage. **B:** One week of continuous drainage improved the leak, and the incision dried out. Injection of contrast shows a small persistent leak. **C:** Follow-up nephrostogram obtained 3 weeks after drainage shows total resolution of the leak, without significant stricture of the ureter.

Comment: Leaks from the urinary tract usually are related to a surgical procedure or trauma. Fistulas may occur in patients with advanced neoplastic disease following radical surgery or radiation therapy. Some forms of inflammatory bowel disease may cause pelvic or ureteral fistulas. Percutaneous nephrostomy by itself can drain the urinary tract by diverting urine flow away from the fistula, allowing it to heal if it is small. If the fistula is associated with a stricture, the nephrostomy tract will provide access for stenting and balloon dilation of the stricture. When the fistulas are larger, they are more likely to develop stenosis and large perirenal cavities (urinomas) that may require separate drainage.

13.2.5 Percutaneous Ureteral Manipulations And Stenting

Case 13.2.5:

A 65-year-old male patient with bladder cancer was treated with an ileal conduit. Six months after surgery, the patient developed bilateral hydronephrosis and increased creatinine levels. Bilateral nephrostomies were requested.

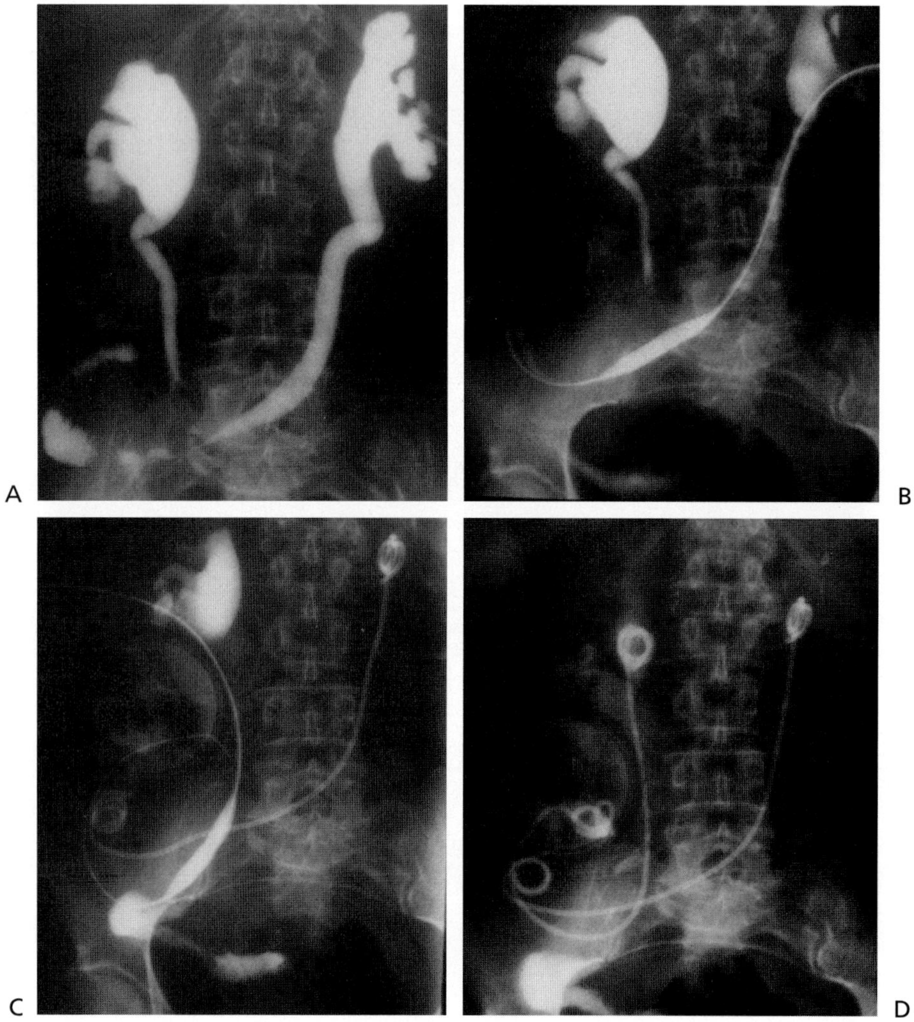

Figure 13.2.5

A: Bilateral nephrostograms show hydronephrosis in both kidneys, with almost total occlusion of the ureteral anastomoses with the ileal conduit. A decision was made to dilate the stenoses. **B:** The left ureter was catheterized, and the stenosis was crossed using a Lunderquist steerable wire. A 6-mm balloon catheter was used to dilate the stenosis. An 8F ureteral stent was introduced between the left renal pelvis and the ileal conduit, reestablishing drainage of the left kidney. **C:** The right ureter was catheterized, and a 6-mm balloon was used to dilate the stenosis. A ureteral stent was placed across the stenosis. **D:** Final photograph of the bilateral 8F stents in place shows some residual contrast within the ileostomy bag in the abdominal wall.

Comment: Anastomotic ureteral obstructions with ileal conduit are relatively common. Fortunately, they can be treated easily with endoluminal techniques. Surgical revision of the anastomosis can be reserved for more severe cases or patients who do not respond to balloon dilation. The main cause of stenosis in these cases is an inflammatory process and/or ureteral ischemia following surgery. Balloon dilation, followed by stent placement, is very effective in resolving the stricture, but may require repeated procedures. Irradiation of the retroperitoneum or pelvis can cause early or late ureteral obstruction. Percutaneous balloon dilation also has been useful in the management of this complication. The ileal conduit is an adequate receptacle for urine, but it requires continuous use of an ileostomy bag to collect urine output. The Charleston pouch has a larger capacity and the ostomy is much smaller, which allow the patient to intermittently self-catheterize for pouch evacuation.

13.2.6 Percutaneous Ureteral Manipulations And Stenting

Case 13.2.6:

A 44-year-old black male patient with neurogenic bladder secondary to T4 paraplegia was treated with an ileal conduit that failed. He then was treated with a gastrocolic urinary diversion (Charleston pouch). The patient developed stenosis of the anastomosis of the ureter, with hydronephrosis and infection. The right kidney was seen to be more dilated on US. Percutaneous nephrostomy and stenting were requested.

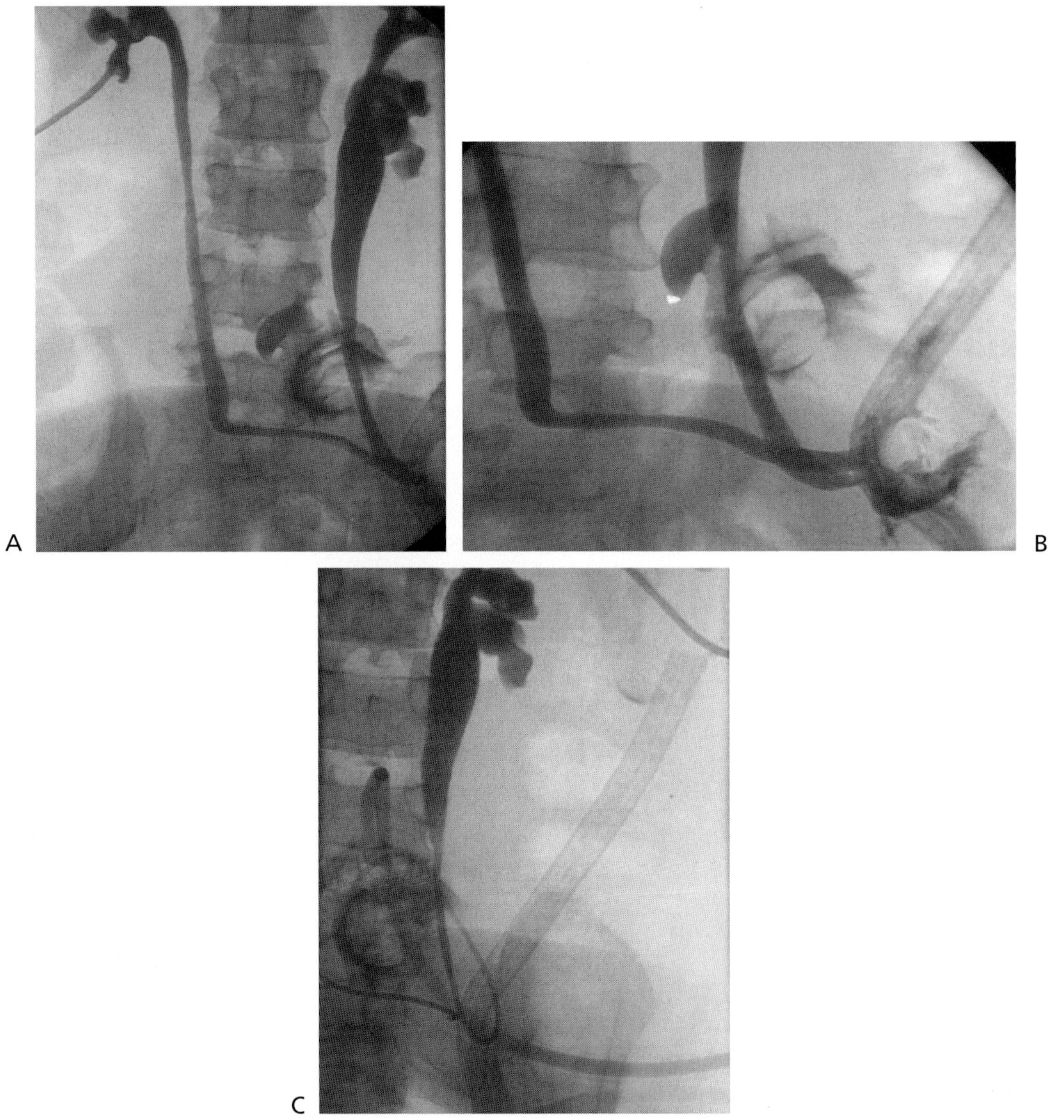

Figure 13.2.6

A: Bilateral nephrostomies were performed. There is significant dilation of the left ureter. **B:** Close-up view demonstrates stenosis of the left ureteric anastomosis. The right ureter was normal. **C:** Nephrostogram performed after balloon dilation of the left ureter anastomosis and placement of a ureteral stent. The right nephrostomy was pulled.

Comment: The procedure performed for treatment of ureteral strictures in urinary diversion begins with a nephrostogram and access through a nephrostomy. Bilateral nephrostomies usually are required when the stenosis is bilateral, which is the most frequent situation. Catheterization of the ureter and crossing of the obstruction are the next steps. When there is infection, careful treatment with drainage and antibiotic therapy should precede stricture treatment. Crossing the obstruction is not always straightforward, because fibrosis can be very extensive and the stenosis very hard. Usually, however, there is a small tract that can be catheterized with a steering guidewire or hydrophilic wire. Dilation with a Teflon catheter usually is advisable to facilitate passage of the plasty balloon. Despite being occluded, the anastomotic site can be very mobile and difficult to cross. In a number of cases, a small fistula will be opened during catheterization attempts and extravasation may jeopardize the procedure. In some cases, it is adequate to stop the procedure and wait a couple of days before making another attempt. Once the obstruction is passed, the balloon, usually slightly oversized, is introduced across the stenosis and inflated until the waist disappears. An 8F to 10F ureteral stent should be left in place for healing of the anastomosis, for at least 3 weeks. In some patients, a wire-mounted cold-knife can be pulled through the stricture area under fluoroscopic control. After stent removal, an 8F external stent is left in place for 6 to 8 weeks to maintain the ureteroenteric anastomotic area in 70% to 80% of cases. Failures are related to previous radiation therapy, among other causes. The gastrocolic urinary diversion (Charleston pouch) is a large receptacle with a small ostomy hole through which the patient can self-catheterize and drain the urine. The presence of the stent within the pouch is not important. It is not necessary for the patient to carry an ileostomy bag all the time.

13.2.7 Percutaneous Ureteral Manipulations And Stenting

Case 13.2.7:

A 64-year-old female patient with gynecologic cancer who previously was treated with surgery, radiation, and chemotherapy presented with azotemia and fever. IVP showed delayed excretion of the right kidney. Nephrostomy was requested.

A

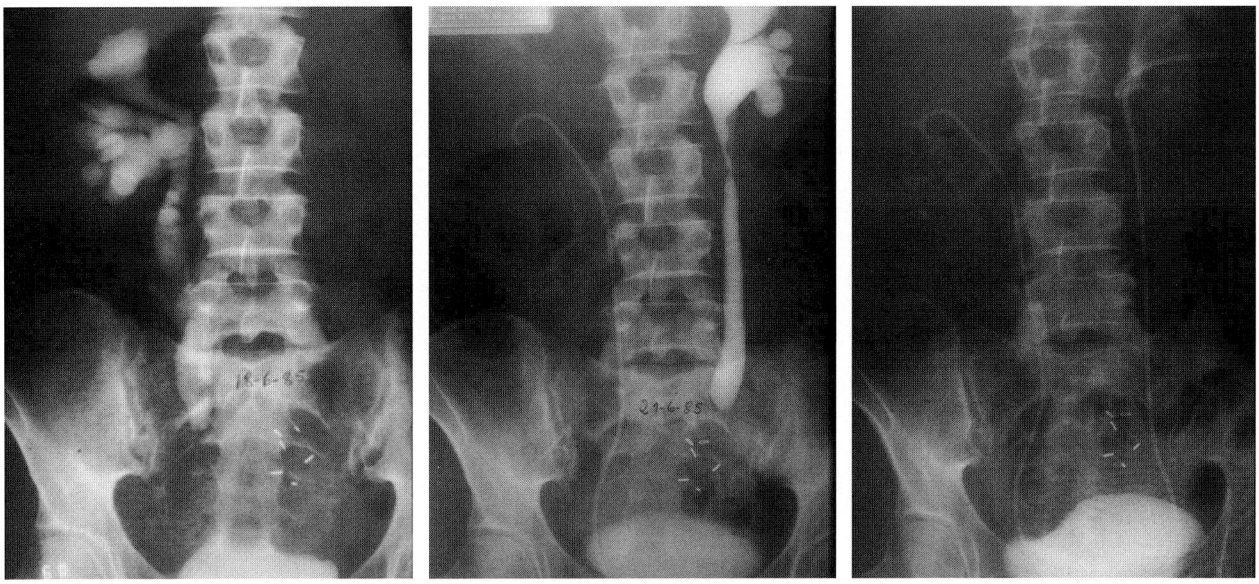

B, C

Figure 13.2.7

A: IVP 60-minute film shows a dilated right renal collecting system with obstructed ureter. **B:** Percutaneous access was obtained for a nephrostomy, and a double J ureteral stent was placed for decompression. The left kidney subsequently became obstructed, and nephrostomy and ureteral stent were placed. **C:** Final film of the abdomen shows bilateral ureteral stents, with adequate decompression of both kidneys.

Comment: Obstruction by genitourinary or any other malignancy causing uropathy and azotemia may be one of the leading indications for percutaneous nephrostomy and ureteral stenting, which now is the preferred method of treatment because it is faster, safer, and effectively drains the obstructed kidneys in critically ill cancer patients. This technique relieves the obstruction, allowing time for effective chemotherapeutic agents or radiation treatments. In the presence of an inoperable or otherwise untreatable malignancy, internal drainage can be established by inserting a double J ureteral stent. Reestablishment of drainage reverses the azotemia and may prolong the patient's life for months to 1 year.

13.2.8 Percutaneous Ureteral Manipulations And Stenting

Case 13.2.8:

A 65-year-old black male patient presented to the emergency room with abdominal pain of increasing severity. He had a history of stroke, myocardial infarction, and aorto-bifemoral bypass, left nephrectomy several years before and left above-the-knee amputation (AKA) 1 year before. Clinical and laboratory examinations and CT scan showed urinary infection, elevated creatinine, and a periaortic/perigraft mass, consistent with a pseudoaneurysm. Surgery was undertaken to treat the pseudoaneurysm, but it was not believed that the renal function problem needed to be addressed at that time. Several weeks later, renal function deteriorated and the patient was admitted for treatment of hydronephrosis and ureteral obstruction.

A, B

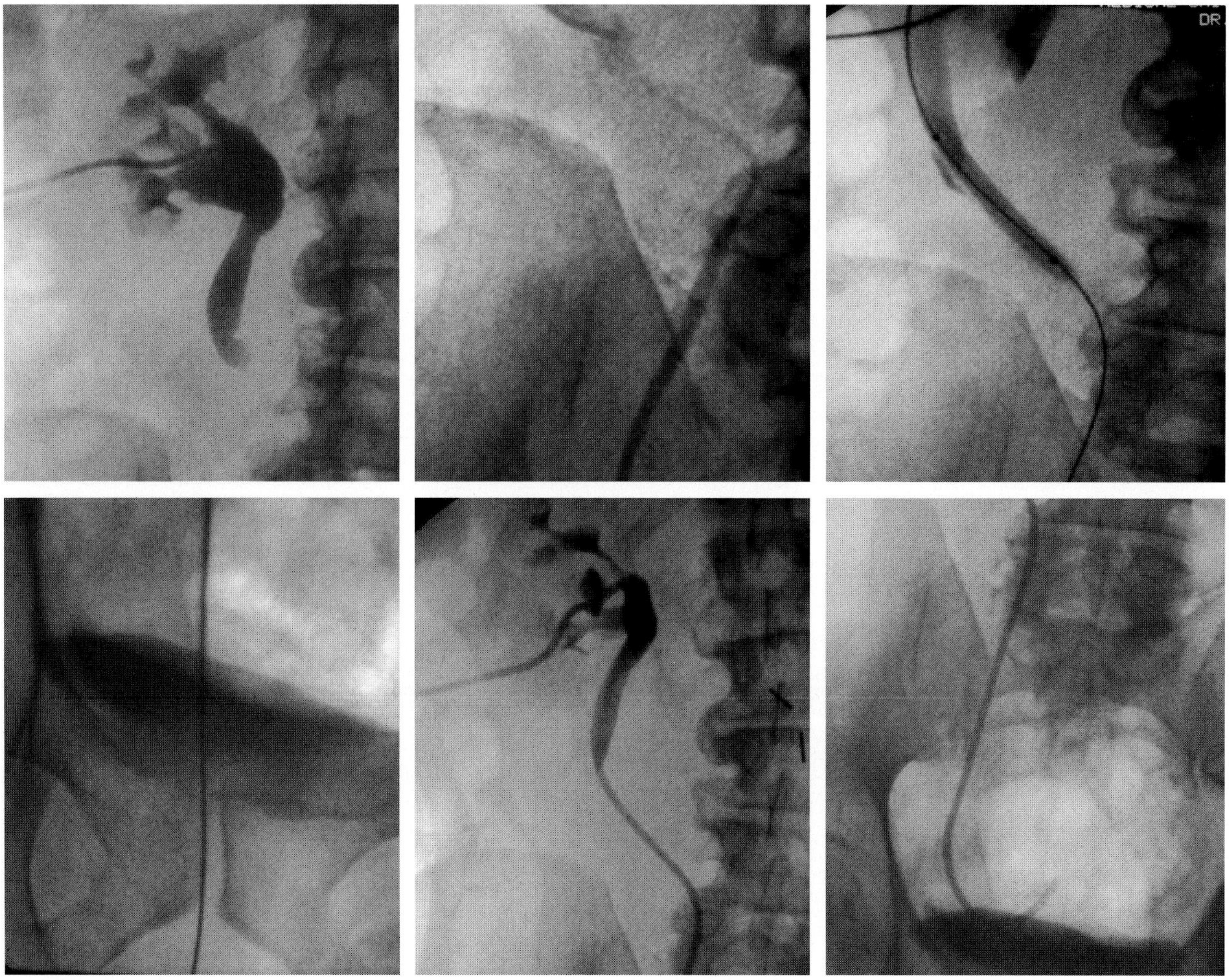

C

D

E, F

Figure 13.2.8

A: Percutaneous nephrostogram of the right kidney shows a moderately dilated collecting system with occluded mid-ureter. **B:** More selective catheterization of the ureter shows a distorted right ureter with a long segment of stenosis, possibly related to retroperitoneal fibrosis generated by the aortic pseudoaneurysm. **C:** Balloon dilation was performed with a 6-mm balloon catheter. It was difficult to advance the balloon through the tight stenosis, and a pull-through guidewire introduced into the penile urethra was used. Once the external segment of the wire was available outside the penis, the balloon was easily advanced for dilation and the stent introduced. **D:** Note the distal wire through the bladder and urethra. **E,F:** Radiography obtained after stent placement shows the ureteral stent in a good position. Renal function returned to normal, and the stent was removed through a cystoscope 3 months later.

Comment: Ureteral strictures secondary to periureteral fibrosis, anastomotic fibrotic strictures, and ischemia can be dilated. Diffuse strictures secondary to rejection (in renal allografts) or necrosis cannot be dilated. Access to the kidney in such cases should be from the upper pole or a mid-kidney calix to facilitate the antegrade approach to the ureter. A high-pressure, 6- to 8-mm diameter, angioplasty balloon over a super-stiff guidewire should be used. Crossing the stenosis can be challenging; the antegrade as well the retrograde approach should be considered. A number of steerable and hydrophilic wires and devices currently are available, and very few stenoses will pose significant resistance to catheterization. Predilation with a 10F catheter/dilator facilitates passage of the balloon. Hydrophilic coated balloons help in crossing the generally tight stenosis of obstructed ureters. After balloon dilation, an external-internal stent can be left for acute drainage. It can be replaced with a larger-bore, double J stent as soon as the urine clears and bleeding stops. The stents can remain in place for 3 to 4 months. The stent can be exchanged by cystoscopy or less frequently by percutaneous access. When strictures are very difficult to negotiate or the wire is not stable enough to advance the catheter/balloon, the urethra can be catheterized and the guidewire exteriorized for performance of a pull-through maneuver. A coat hanger (stiff) wire should be used, and any size of catheter or system can be pushed safely across the stricture. Catheterization of the urethra in females is easier than in men because of the short length of the female urethra. In men, it may be easier to catheterize the urethra retrogradely and snare the wire inside the bladder, pulling the wire externally for the pull-through maneuver.

13.3.1 Percutaneous Lithotripsy

Case 13.3.1:

A 43-year-old male patient had a left renal pelvic stone. Percutaneous lithotripsy was planned.

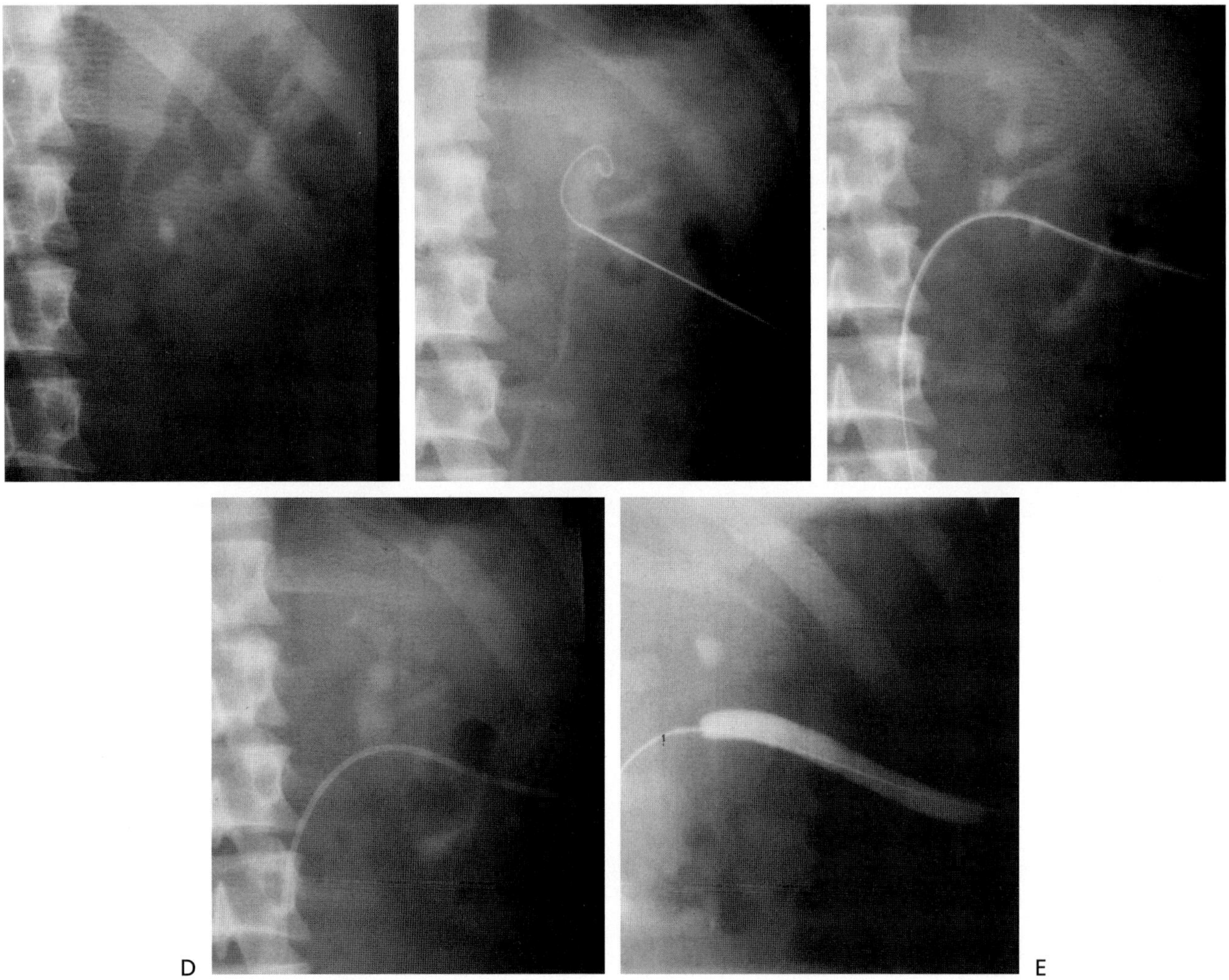

A, B C D E

Figure 13.3.1

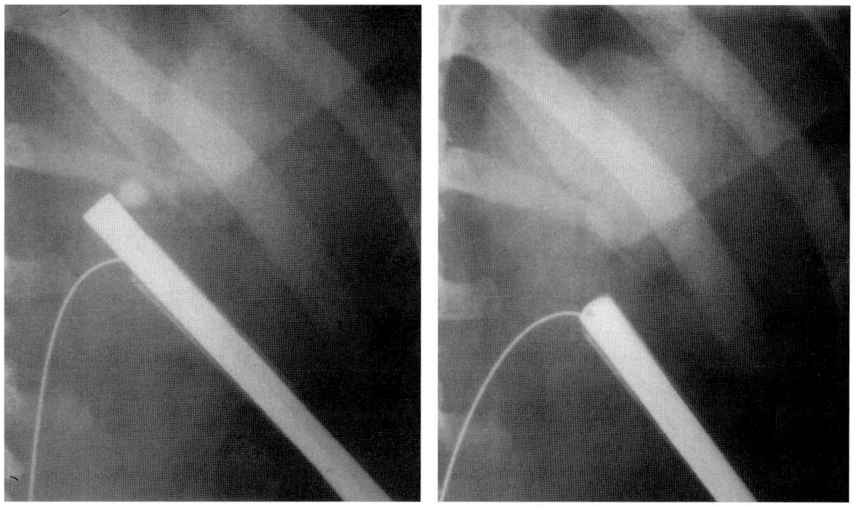

F G

Figure 13.3.1 *(continued)*

A: Film of the left kidney shows a 10 × 6-mm pelvic stone. **B:** Needle puncture of the lower pole calix. **C:** Using a KMP catheter, the ureter was selectively catheterized. **D:** A 6F catheter was left in place for access, with the tip within the ureter. The patient was sent to surgery the next morning. **E:** The tract was dilated with a 10-mm balloon and the sheath was introduced. **F:** The plastic 24F sheath was introduced, and the nephroscope was used for stone fragmentation and retrieval. Note the safety wire parallel to the sheath. **G:** Final photograph after lithotripsy shows the pelvis is free of stones.

Comment: Access to the urinary tract for lithotripsy uses percutaneous nephrostomy. A variety of techniques are used for stone treatment. Mechanical dislocation of small stones (3 to 4 mm) can be accomplished easily without significant tract dilation. Larger stones require disintegration, pulverization, crushing, basketing, snaring, or use of forceps and aspiration for stone extraction. Dilation of the tract up to 24F to 26F is required for adequate access to the stones by lithotripsy instruments. Percutaneous nephrostomy for stone management may have to be performed in nondilated renal pelvis. About 80% of renal calculi can be treated successfully by extracorporeal shock-wave lithotripsy (ESWL); nevertheless, about 20% of patients will require percutaneous procedures alone or complementary to ESWL. The percutaneous approach combines multiple methods of access and stone fragmentation, using a nephroscope and instrumentation within the collecting system. Almost all renal stones and caliceal, pelvic, or staghorn calculi can be treated percutaneously. When ESWL fails to break hard stones or there is difficulty in releasing the stones due to impaction, the percutaneous approach is useful. When large amounts of stone fragments are impacted in the pelvis, nephrostomy and percutaneous access may be able to remove the fragments in a single procedure. Contraindications are uncorrectable hemorrhagic diathesis, active infection, extreme obesity, and renal tuberculosis.

13.3.2 Percutaneous Lithotripsy

Case 13.3.2:

A 36-year-old male patient with a right kidney stone was a candidate for percutaneous lithotripsy. A retrograde ureteral stent was placed by cystoscope.

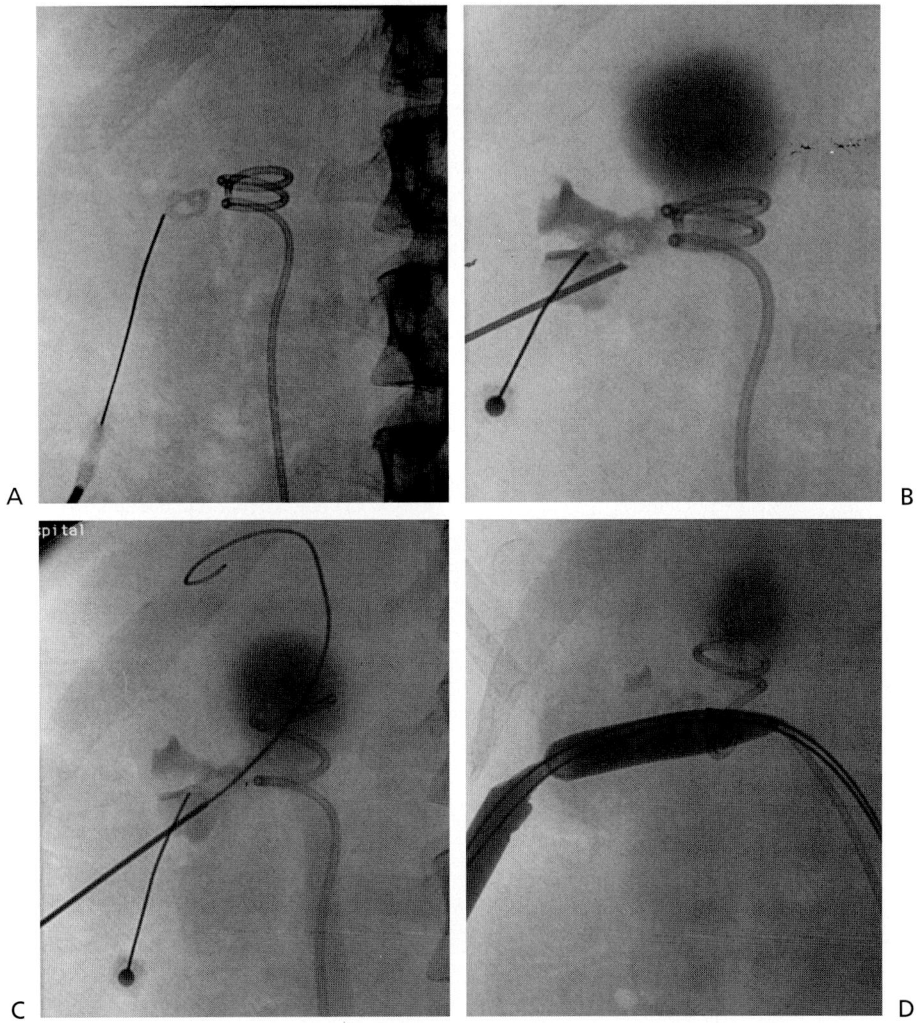

Figure 13.3.2

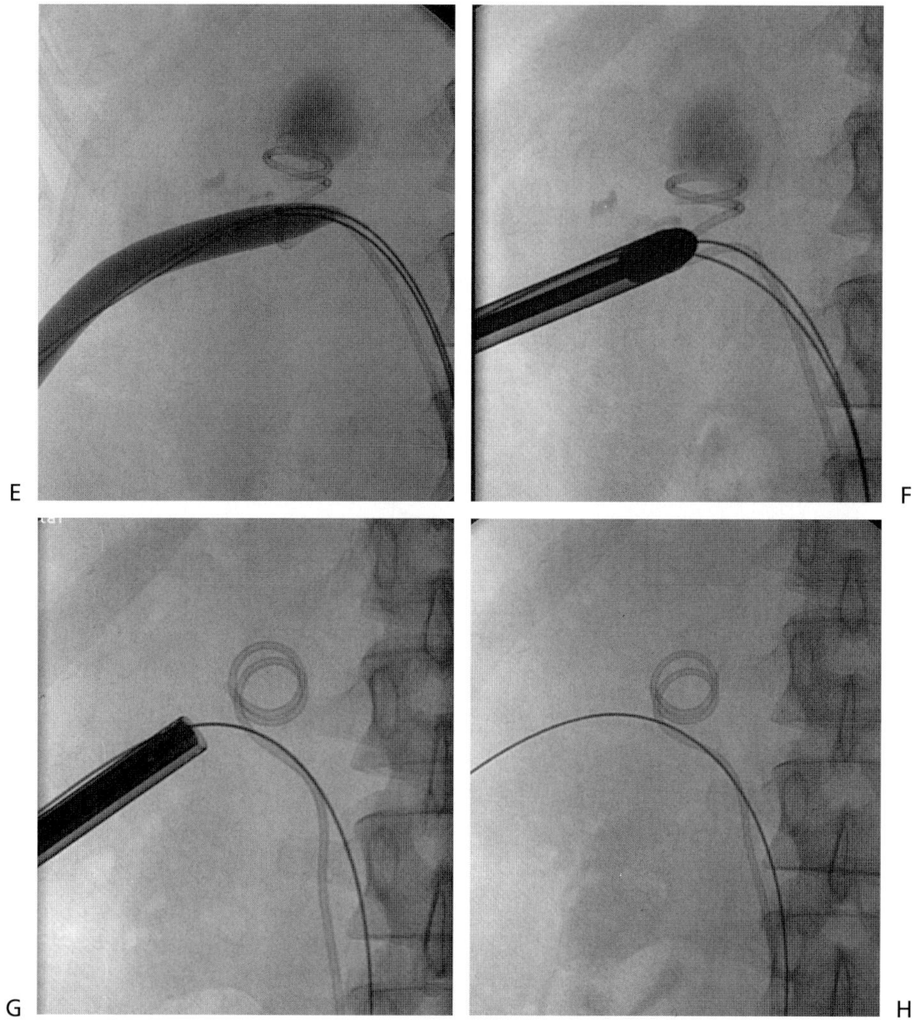

Figure 13.3.2 *(continued)*

A: Percutaneous early pyelogram with a fine needle shows a mid-size stone in a lower pole calix. Note the pigtail of the ureteral stone. **B:** Following the nephrostogram, an 18-gauge needle was introduced in the fornix of the calix for catheterization of the collecting system. **C:** A guidewire was introduced up to the upper calix. **D:** A 10-mm, high-pressure balloon was used to dilate the tract. Note the waist at the renal capsule and the double guidewire for safety. **E:** The balloon was fully dilated and the waist disappeared. **F:** The metal sheath system was advanced over the operational wire into the lower calix. **G:** The nephroscope was introduced within the sheath, and the stone was fragmented and retrieved. **H:** Final radiogram shows the kidney is free of stones. The safety wire is still located within the ureter.

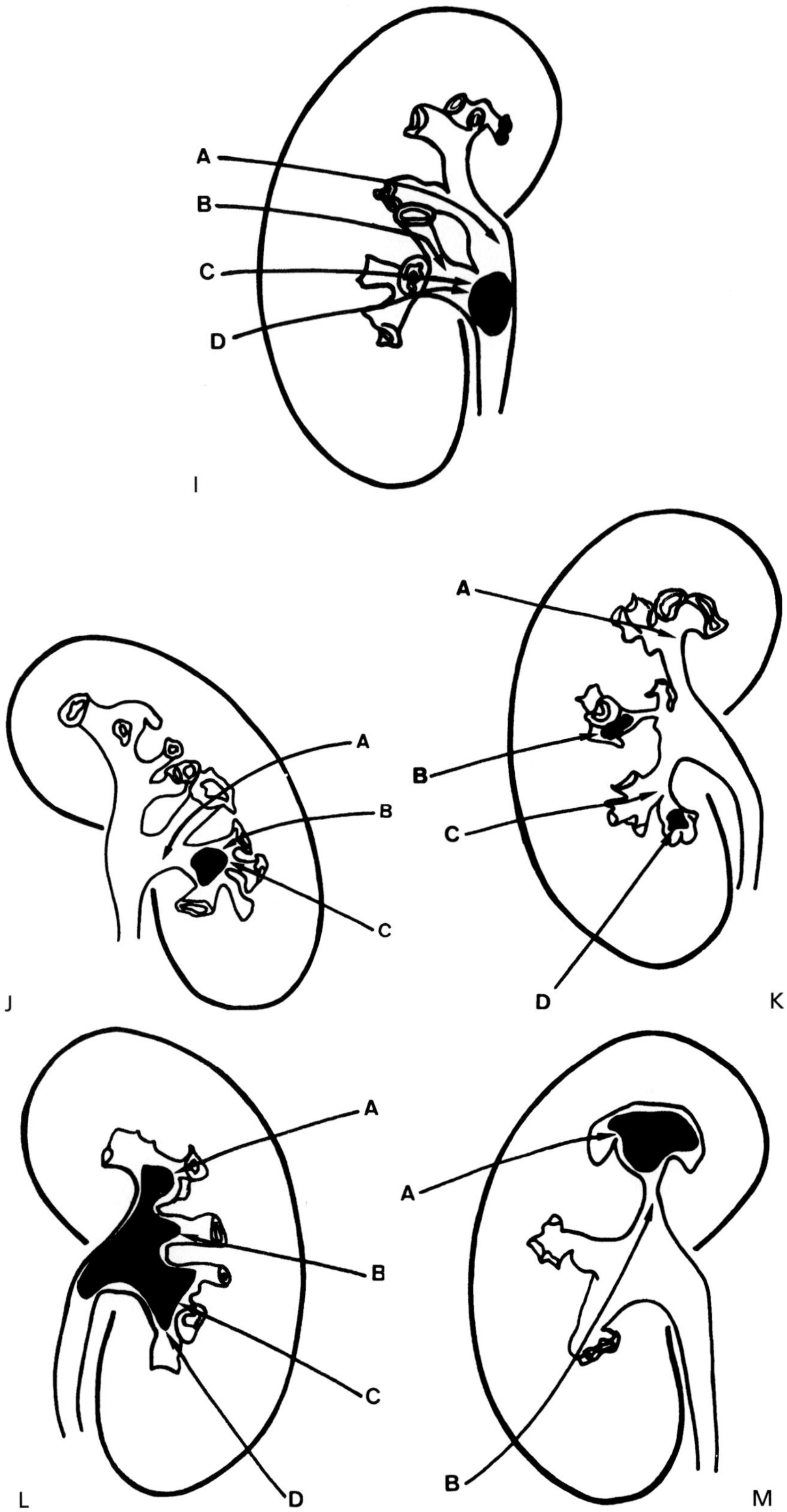

Figure 13.3.2 *(continued)*

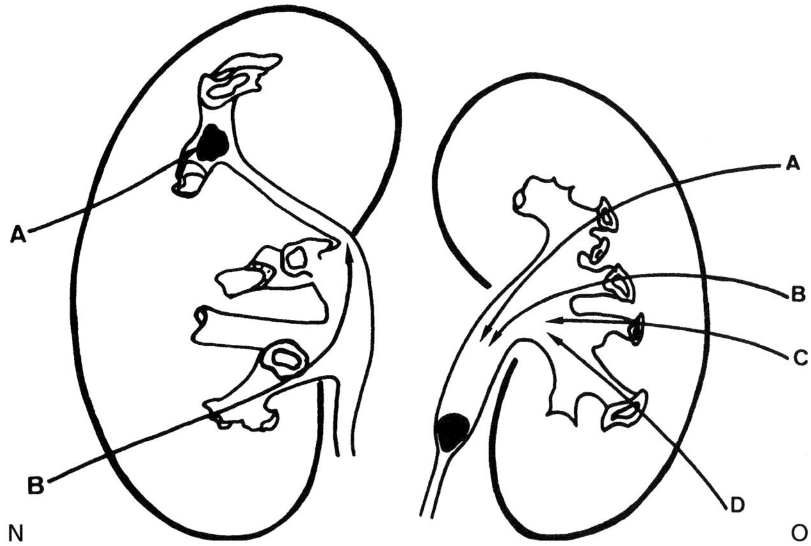

Figure 13.3.2 *(continued)*

I: Pelvic stone. Access can be approached by a middle calix *(A,B)* or a lower calix *(C,D)*. **J:** Lower calix stone. Puncture preferably should be done in the affected calix *(B,C)*, but adjacent calices may be used *(A)*. **K:** When multiple stones are encountered in middle and lower calices, the approach should be directly to the affected calices *(B,C)*. The other approaches are less desirable and should be avoided *(A,C)*. **L:** Staghorn calculi can be approached from different levels *(A–D)* and frequently require more than one approach and several lithotripsy sessions. **M:** An isolated stone in an upper pole calix with a long infundibulum should be approached directly *(A)*. Other middle or lower calix approaches are not suitable *(B)*. **N:** A large stone in an upper calix with a wide infundibulum usually can be approached by direct puncture *(A)* or from a more inferior puncture *(B)*. **O:** A smaller pelvic or proximal ureteral stone can be approached from almost any level of the caliceal system *(A–D)*; however, the upper or middle approaches are best *(A,B)*.

Comment: As with other intrarenal procedures, percutaneous nephrostomy is the initial stage. It involves the establishment of a percutaneous track to the renal collecting system, and this track can be manipulated, dilated, and maintained as long as necessary for treatment purposes. The entire procedure is dependent on the access for stone treatment. Nephrostomy is performed under fluoroscopic guidance, with previous opacification of the collecting system by intravenous contrast medium injection, percutaneous puncture, or retrograde ureteral catheterization. The straightest path to the stones is advisable to reduce trauma and procedure time and improve efficacy of the procedure. The approach can be performed in one- or two-step procedures. To reduce procedure time under general anesthesia, it is advisable to perform the procedure in two steps. Nephrostomy access is established on the afternoon of the day before the endourologic procedure. When the patient is taken to surgery the next morning, the collecting system is clean of blood and decompressed. With the patient under general anesthesia, the track is dilated and the scope is introduced for lithotripsy. It is always advantageous to have a team that includes an urologist and an interventional radiologist available. Their presence will speed up the procedure, and they can rapidly establish an additional path, if necessary. Selection of the calix to be entered depends on the location, number, and size of stones (see Fig. 13.3.2I–13.3.2O).

13.3.3 Percutaneous Lithotripsy

Case 13.3.3:

A 68-year-old male patient presented with a 6-mm pelvic stone. Percutaneous lithotripsy was planned.

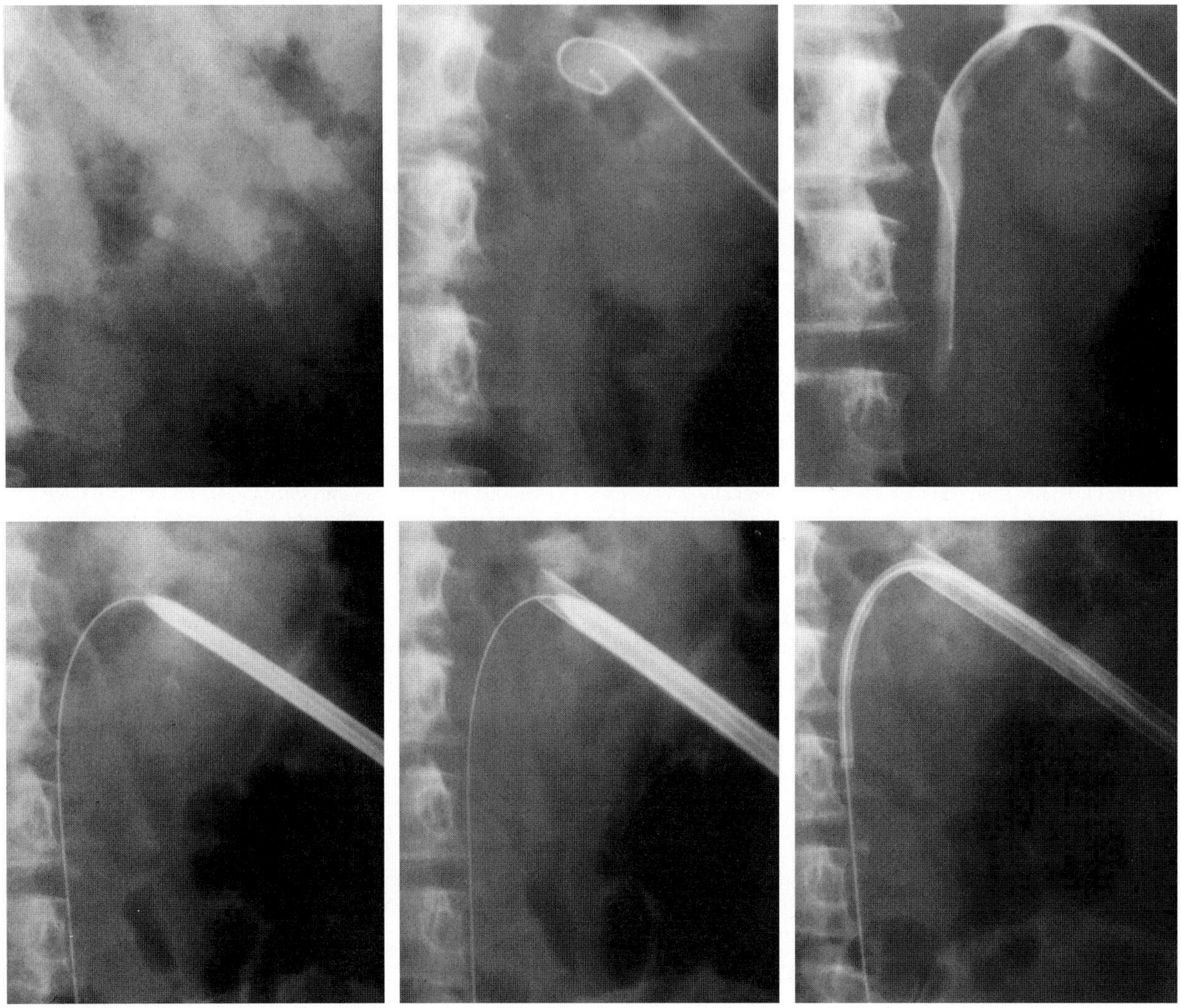

A, B C D, E F

Figure 13.3.3

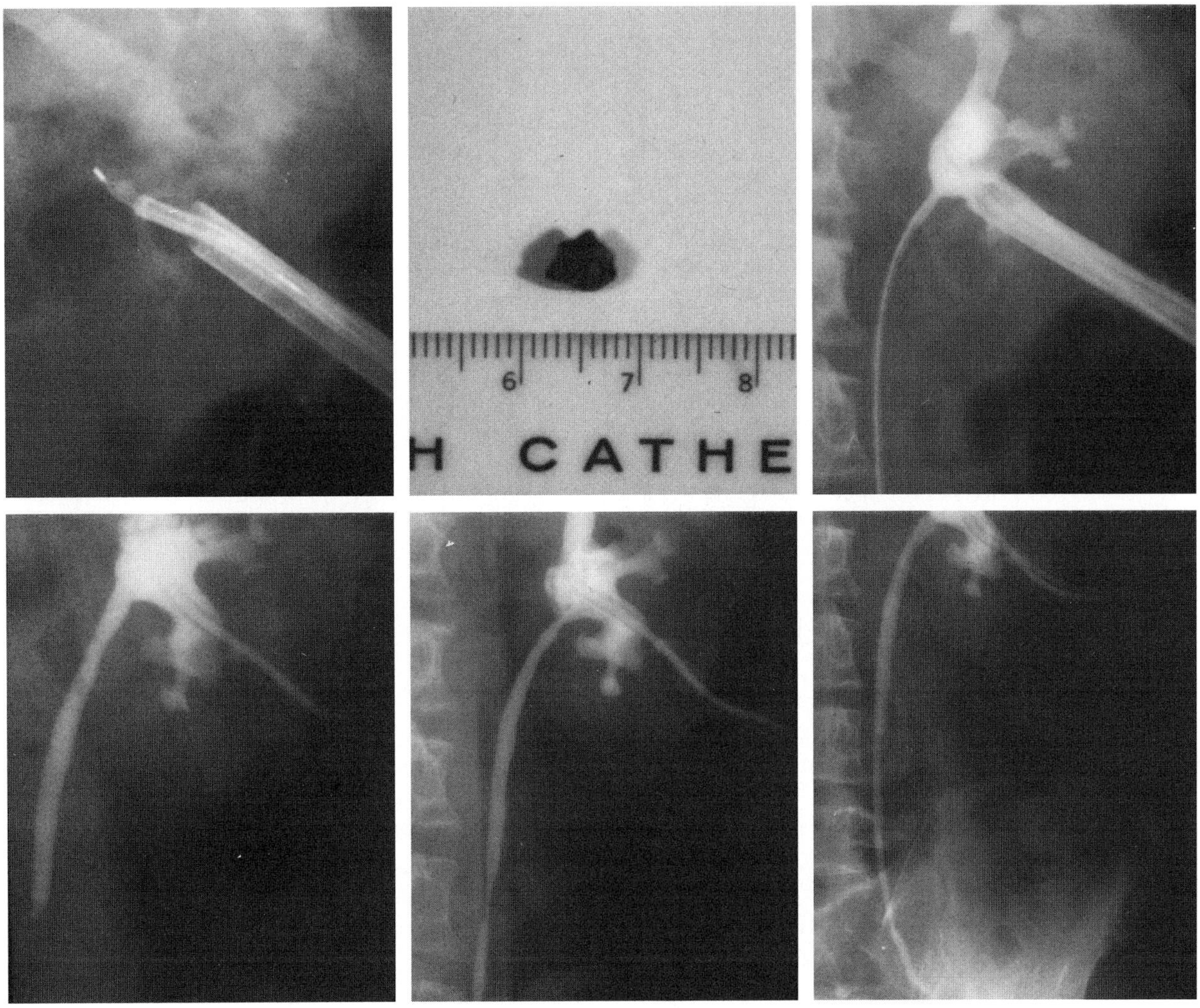

G H, I J K, L

Figure 13.3.3 *(continued)*

A: Plain film of the left kidney obtained before IVP shows a 6-mm stone in the pelvis. **B:** On the day of the access procedure, the stone had migrated to the proximal ureter, with obstruction. Percutaneous access was obtained. **C:** The ureter was catheterized, and injection of contrast shows ureteral occlusion. **D:** A guidewire was advanced across the obstruction into the distal ureter. **E:** The tract was dilated to 24F and a sheath was placed. **F:** A steerable catheter was advanced over the wire, and a Dormia basket was used to capture the ureteral stone. **G:** The stone was retrieved through the sheath. Note the stone trapped by the basket. **H:** The stone was removed and measured about 6 mm in the larger diameter. **I:** A Malecot nephrostomy catheter was placed within the pelvis. No catheter was left within the ureter. **J:** Two weeks later, nephrostogram shows occlusion of the ureter by adhesions. **K:** The obstruction was traversed and dilated with a 10F catheter. **L:** An 8F ureteral stent was left in place for 3 more weeks, and the ureter remained patent.

Comment: Standard treatment of upper ureteral calculi has been surgical removal through a ureterostomy via a flank or dorsal lumbotomy incision, because retrograde endoscopic basketing, which is effective in the lower ureter, is associated with trauma and avulsion of the ureter. The percutaneous technique can be applied easily to the proximal ureter, using the percutaneous nephrostomy tract. Percutaneous extraction is 94% successful in the upper ureter. It is always easier to bypass a stone or obstruction with a guidewire or catheter from above than retrograde from below, because the proximal ureter supports the catheter and guidewire. The frustrating problem of ureter spasm and the inability of stone baskets to open fully in nondilated ureters are the primary reasons for the lower success rate of removing ureteral stones compared with pelvic stones. Flushing the stones and using the newly designed slicker stone baskets may help the procedure. Ureteral stones frequently are embedded within the walls of the ureteral mucosa, making retrieval of ureteral stones extremely difficult. Adhesions and synechiae are frequent causes of occlusion of the ureter following stone removal, as demonstrated in the presented case.

13.3.4 Percutaneous Lithotripsy

Case 13.3.4:

A 56-year-old male patient with cadaveric renal transplant presented with hematuria and pain. US study showed a questionable stone. Percutaneous pyelogram was planned.

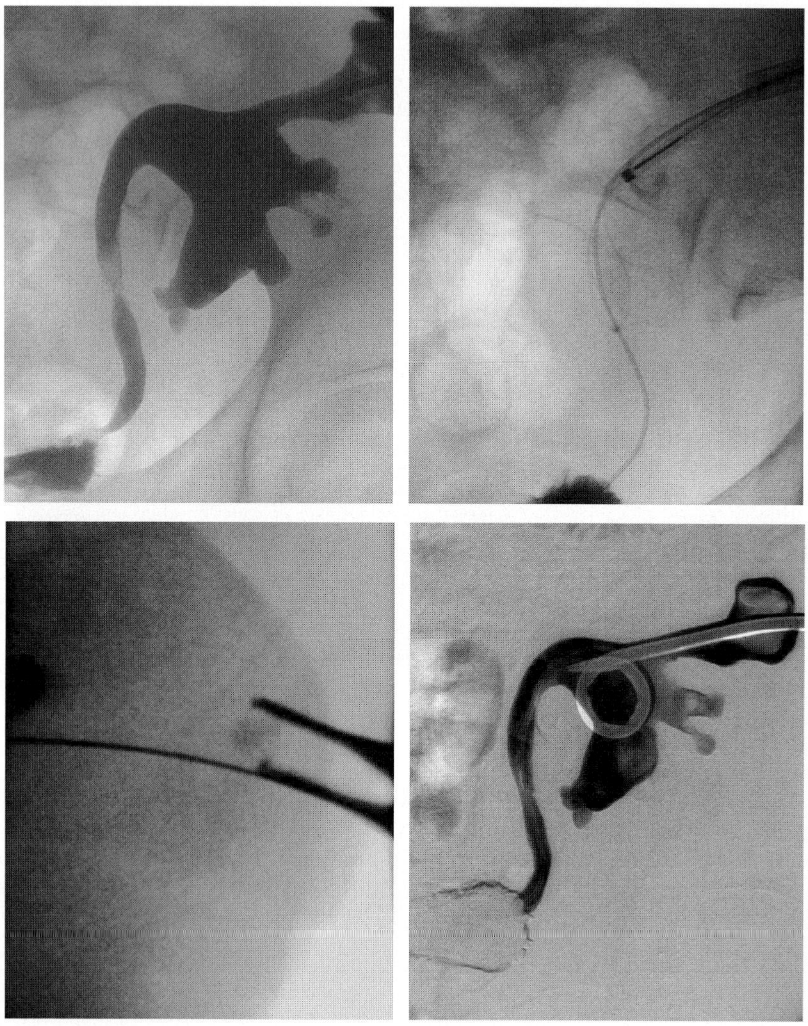

A B C D

Figure 13.3.4

A: Initial pyelogram shows moderate hydronephrosis with a stricture in the mid-ureter and a filling defect suggestive of a stone within the dilated ureter. Access was obtained from an upper pole calix, followed by catheterization of the ureter. **B:** A guidewire was passed along the stone, into the bladder. A Hawkins stone basket was used to catch the stone in the ureter and retrieve it. **C:** The stone was lost in the subcutaneous tissues but was removed using forceps. **D:** Balloon plasty of the ureteral stricture was performed with a 5-mm balloon. A nephrostomy catheter was introduced into the collecting system. Contrast material injection shows the ureter is patent and free of stones. A short 6F ureteral stent was left in place for 3 weeks.

Comment: Stone removal from the ureter may be tricky. The stones frequently are embedded in the ureteral wall, and laceration or adhesions can result from percutaneous lithotomy. In the reported case, the cause of the ureteral stricture was not clearly established; however, ischemia is always an etiologic possibility, especially in transplanted kidneys. Balloon angioplasty is useful to remodel the ureter and reestablish flow. A ureteral stent is always necessary to reduce chances of stricture recurrence and synechiae. The transplanted kidney is very accessible from the percutaneous approach, and dilation of the tract can be accomplished rapidly without many problems. The transplanted kidney may be mobile, and dilation using larger dilators may be more difficult and may require only the use of a large balloon, instead of the progressive Amplatz dilators. Use of the safer stone basket is strongly advised, because lesions on the ureter are not desirable and may worsen the situation. A Hawkins basket is adequate, but a helical Rutner-type basket, mounted on a wire, also is safe and useful. Post-lithotripsy care should include a ureteral stent for 3 to 6 weeks and a temporary nephrostomy catheter.

13.4.1 Transplanted Kidney

Case 13.4.1:

A 63-year-old diabetic black female received a cadaveric pediatric *en bloc* kidney double transplant in the right pelvis. The lateral kidney, which was hydronephrotic, was treated with a cystoscopic double J ureteral stent. The medial kidney also was dilated, and retrograde catheterization was unsuccessful. Percutaneous nephrostomy was requested.

A, B

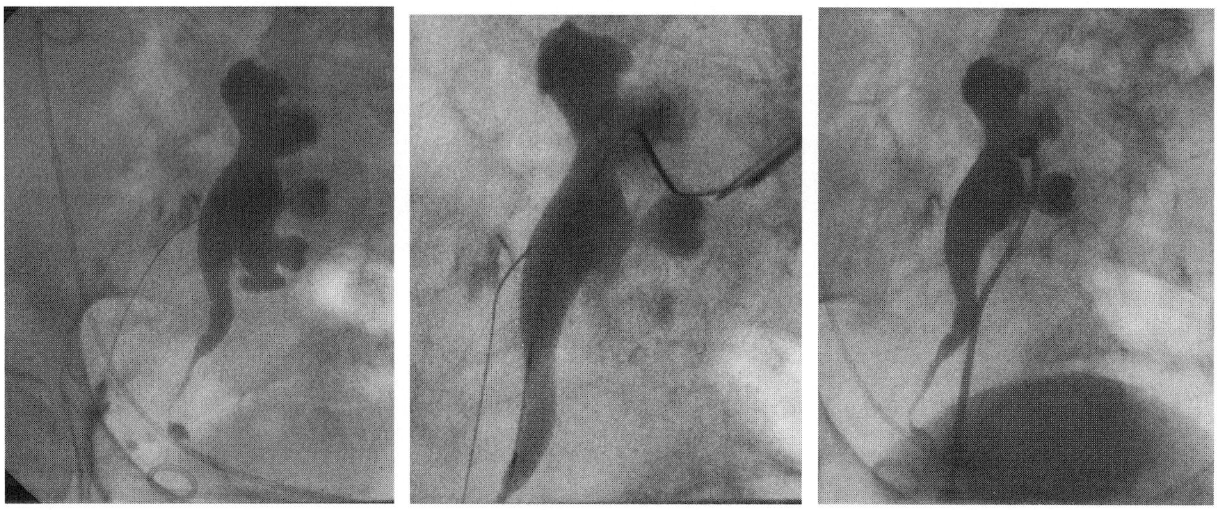

C

Figure 13.4.1

A: Percutaneous nephrostogram with a 23-gauge Chiba needle shows a moderately dilated collecting system of the medial kidney, due to distal ureteral obstruction. Note the right double J ureteral stent, placed by cystoscopy in the lateral kidney. **B:** Puncture of an anterior superior calix with an 18-gauge needle allowed access to the collecting system. Note the 0.035-inch guidewire within the collecting system. **C:** An 8F nephrostomy catheter was placed for external drainage. A ureteral stent was placed at a later date. Despite improvement in renal function, the patient developed rejection and untreatable urinary infection, despite massive antibiotic therapy and exchanges of catheters and stents, aggravated by chronic cytomegalovirus infection. Surgical revision of the ureterovesical anastomosis was performed, without significant improvement of infection. The patient eventually required transplant nephrectomy to stop immunosuppression completely and treat the infection. The patient subsequently developed a pelvic hematoma that required percutaneous drainage. Hemodialysis was resumed.

Comment: Urologic complications occur in approximately 10% of all renal allograft recipients. The complications can be early or late in the evolution of condition. The most common complications are urine leak (early) and ureteric obstruction (early or late). Diagnosis of fluid collection around the transplant kidney or hydronephrosis can be made easily with US or CT scans. Percutaneous antegrade pyelogram provides quick assessment of the problem, revealing the site of urine leak or location of the stenosis. Percutaneous pyelogram also is the first step for treatment of the problem. Urologic complications are related to increased morbidity and mortality in the renal transplant population. The most challenging differential diagnosis is between rejection and obstruction. Obstructions are related to surgical problems and are not related to immunologic problems. The most common site of obstruction is the ureterovesical junction. Obstruction can be related to kinks, fibrosis following inflammation, or ischemia. Calculi, external compression by fluid collections, tumors, and overdistended bladder are less frequent causes. Cadaveric pediatric kidney allografts are more complex to deal with and are subject to increased risk of urologic complications, such as ischemia and stenosis of the small ureteral structures. In addition to being small structures, the kidneys are involved in different anatomic situations and may have bowel loops interposed between the kidney and the abdominal wall. The presence of bowel loops in the path of the puncture for a nephrostomy is critical, because the bowel may not be appreciated under fluoroscopic or US guidance. CT scan of the pelvis, prior to the nephrostomy puncture, is useful, mainly when oral contrast is given to the patient before the procedure.

13.4.2 Transplanted Kidney

Case 13.4.2:

A 54-year-old diabetic male patient with chronic renal failure received a cadaveric kidney transplant into the left pelvic fossa. Ten years after the renal transplant, the patient developed an unresectable rectal carcinoma that was treated by radiation therapy. Stenosis of the transplanted kidney ureter developed, with worsening of renal function. Percutaneous nephrostomy was requested.

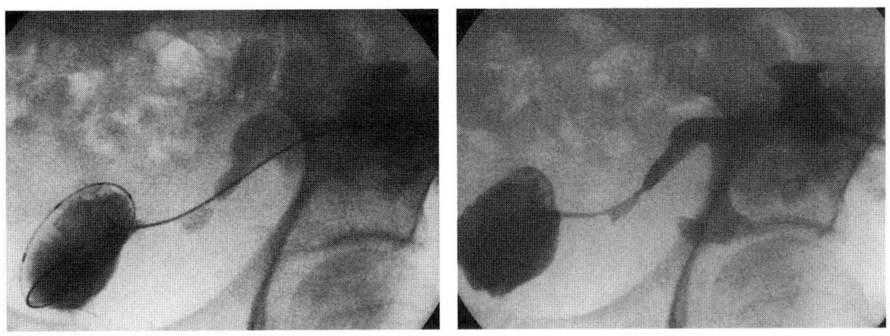

A B

Figure 13.4.2

A: Percutaneous puncture of an upper calix was performed with catheterization of the ureter. There was a distal ureteral obstruction. Balloon dilation was performed with a 5-mm balloon. **B:** A nephroureterostomy catheter was placed. Nephrostogram shows adequate placement of the catheter. The catheter was maintained externally clamped until the patient died 8 months later, with one interval exchange.

Comment: Ureteral strictures secondary to periureteral fibrosis, anastomotic fibrotic strictures, and ischemic strictures can be dilated. Radiation therapy injury to the ureter can be dilated, but the long-term chances of success are less than with other causes of strictures. Diffuse strictures secondary to rejection or necrosis cannot be properly dilated. Dilators should be used before balloon angioplasty to facilitate the crossing capability of the balloon and to reduce the chances of ureteral rupture. Balloon angioplasty should be followed by placement of a double J stent or nephroureterostomy catheter. The stent should remain in place for 3 to 4 months to increase the chances of long-term success. The combined internal-external catheter has the advantage of allowing a two-step pullback removal to the renal pelvis before final removal of the stent. External catheters carry a higher risk of infection due to continuous exposure of the catheter to the external environment.

13.4.3 Transplanted Kidney

Case 13.4.3:

A 71-year-old diabetic black female patient with chronic renal failure received a cadaveric kidney transplant into the right pelvic fossa. Worsening of renal function developed, and US and CT of the abdomen showed hydronephrosis. Stenosis of the ureter developed and caused worsening of renal function. Percutaneous nephrostomy was requested.

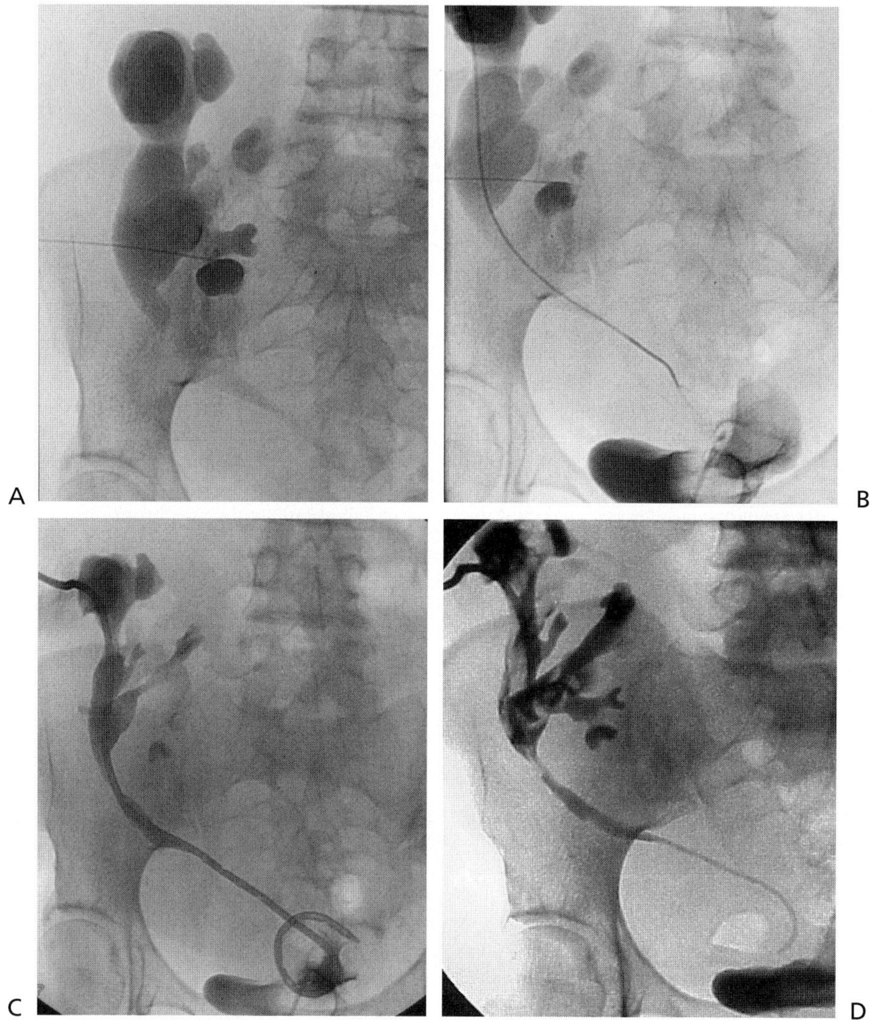

Figure 13.4.3

A: Percutaneous nephrostogram with a fine needle shows a moderately dilated collecting system due to a distal ureteral stenosis. The transplanted kidney is reversed and the pelvis faces the pelvic fossa. **B:** Puncture of the uppermost calix was used for access to the collecting system. Catheterization of the ureter was performed. **C:** After tract dilation, an internal-external drainage catheter was placed and resulted in significant improvement of renal function. Chronic rejection subsequently was diagnosed. **D:** Three weeks after successful nephrostomy, an internal ureteral stent was placed. The distal end of the stent recoiled inside the distal ureter and never functioned adequately. The nephrostomy catheter was accidentally removed at home, and a few days later the patient was readmitted with worsening renal function. A new emergency nephrostomy was placed. Cystoscopy eventually was performed, with placement of another ureteral stent under general anesthesia. The stent has been in for 8 months and has been exchanged.

Comment: Some transplanted kidneys are placed in very awkward positions within the pelvis, including 180 degrees lateral rotation and upside down. When the kidney is rotated, the most superficial calix should be punctured, always bearing in mind that the fornix of the calix should be punctured and not the pelvis or the infundibulum. Complications of percutaneous access for kidney allografts are relatively rare; however, infection almost always is present if the procedure is performed without antibiotic coverage. Recurrent intercurrent infection is present in the majority of patients when antibiotic therapy is stopped. Hemorrhage within the collecting system usually is mild and subsides within 24 to 48 hours. When more significant hemorrhage develops, larger-bore catheters should be used to reduce the risk of stent occlusion. Urine leaks following catheter removal are more common in patients with rejection and may be a problem until the rejection is controlled and the drugs are reduced. Persistent pulsatile bleedings should be considered arterial until proved otherwise. An angiogram with contemplation of embolization should be performed. Renal function may be impaired by the bleeding and by the entire angiography and embolization procedure. Urinary leaks are likely to resolve after percutaneous nephrostomy drainage, with or without stent placement within the ureter. Very often, leaks are related to strictures, and the leaks will not subside if the strictures are not treated properly or decompressed. Large urinomas may compress the kidney and ureter and cause additional impairment of renal function.

Suggested Reading

Austin PF, Cain MP, Rink RC. Nephrostomy tube drainage with pyeloplasty: is it necessarily a choice. *J Urol* 2000;163:1528–1530.

Badlani G, Eshghi M, Smith AD. Percutaneous surgery for ureteropelvic junction obstruction (endopyelotomy): technique and early results. *J Urol* 1986;135:26–28.

Bannen MP, Pollack HM. Fluoroscopically guided percutaneous extraction of upper urinary tract calculi. *Radiol Clin North Am* 1984;22:415–426.

Brannen GE, Bush WH, Correa RJ, et al. Kidney stone removal: percutaneous versus surgical lithotomy. *J Urol* 1985;133:6–12.

Castaneda-Zuniga WR. Percutaneous nephrolithotomy: removal techniques under fluoroscopic control. In: Amplatz K, Lange PH, eds. *Atlas of endourology.* Chicago: Year Book Medical Publishers, 1986:165–184.

Coleman CC. Percutaneous nephrolithotomy: approach. In: Amplatz K, Lange PH, eds. *Atlas of endourology.* Chicago: Year Book Medical Publishers, 1986:115–129.

Coleman CC. Percutaneous nephrolithotomy: dilation techniques. In: Amplatz K, Lange PH, eds. *Atlas of endourology.* Chicago: Year Book Medical Publishers, 1986:131–148.

Debbagh A, Dassouli B, Hafiani M, et al. Acute renal insufficiency due to hydronephrosis. *Ann Urol* 2001;35:26–29.

El Khader K, Karmouri T, Tazi K, et al. Our results with percutaneous nephrolithotomy. Report of 61 cases. *Ann Urol* 2000;34:398–401.

Finlayson B, Ackerman D. Overview of surgical treatment of urolithiasis with special reference to lithotripsy. *J Urol* 1989;141:778–779.

Gunther RW, Alken P. Percutaneous litholapaxy and extraction of renal calculi. In: Lang EK, ed. *Percutaneous and interventional urology and radiology.* New York: Springer-Verlag, 1986:55–74.

Gupta DK, Chandrasekharam VV, Srinivas M, et al. Percutaneous nephrostomy in children with ureteropelvic junction obstruction and poor renal function. *Urology* 2001;57:547–550.

Hogan MJ, Coley BK, Jayanthi VR, et al. Percutaneous nephrostomy in children and adolescents: outpatient management. *Radiology* 2001;218:207–210.

Hopper KD, Sherman JL, Luethke JM et al. The variable anteroposterior position of the retroperitoneal colon to the kidney. *Invest Radiol* 1978;22:298–302.

Lee WJ, Badlani GH, Karlin GS, et al. Treatment of ureteropelvic strictures with percutaneous pyelotomy: experience in 62 patients. *AJR* 1988;151:515–518.

Lee WJ, Smith AD, Cubelli V, et al. Complications of percutaneous nephrolithotomy. *AJR* 1987;148:177–180.

LeRoy AJ, May GR, Segura JW, et al. Percutaneous ultrasonic lithotripsy. *Radiol Clin North Am* 1984;22:427–432.

Mokhmalji H, Braun PM, Martinez Portillo FJ, et al. Percutaneous versus ureteral stents for diversion hydronephrosis caused by stones: a prospective, randomized clinical trial. *J Urol* 2001;165:1088–1092.

Pfister RC. Percutaneous nephrostomy. In: Lang EK, ed. *Percutaneous and interventional urology and radiology.* New York: Springer-Verlag, 1986:1–27.

Poulakis V, Witzsch U, de Vries R, et al. Antegrade percutaneous endoluminal treatment of non-malignant ureterointestinal anastomotic strictures following urinary diversion. *Eur Urol* 2001;39:308–315.

Reznek RH, Talner LB. Percutaneous nephrostomy. *Radiol Clin North Am* 1984;22:393–406.

Sampaio FJB, Aragao AHM. Anatomical relationship between the intrarenal arteries and the kidney collecting system. *J Urol* 1990;143:679–681.

Sampaio FJB, Mandarin-de-Lacerda CA. 3-Dimensional and radiological pelviocaliceal anatomy for endourology. *J Urol* 1988;140:1352–1355.

Sampaior FJB, Zanier JFC, Aragao AHM, et al. Three dimensional anatomical study for the intrarenal access. *J Urol* 1991;145:422A.

Stables DP, Ginsbert NJ, Johnson ML. Percutaneous nephrostomy: a series and review of the literature. *AJR* 1978;130:75–82.

Tazi K, Moudouni SM, Nouri M, et al. Percutaneous nephrostomy: indications, techniques and results. Retrospective study of 81 cases. *Ann Urol* 2000;34:391–397.

Uflacker R. Uroradiologic procedures: ureteral procedure. In: Uflacker R, Wholey MH, eds. *Interventional radiology.* New York: McGraw-Hill, 1991:540–552.

Uflacker R, Paolini RM, Lima S. Management of traumatic hematuria by selective renal artery embolization. *J Urol* 1984;132:662–667.

Watson GM, Patel U. Primary antegrade ureteric stenting: prospective experience and cost-effectiveness analysis in 50 ureters. *Clin Radiol* 2001;56:568–574.

Wickham JEA, Millar RA. *Percutaneous renal surgery.* New York: Churchill Livingstone, 1983:148–154.

Wicknam JEA, Keller MJ. Percutaneous pyelolysis. *Eur Urol* 1983;9:122–124.

Yoder IC, Lindfors KK, Pfister RC. Diagnosis and treatment of pyonephrosis. *Radiol Clin North Am* 1984;22:407–414.

CHAPTER 14

Interventional Procedures In The Liver, Biliary Tract, And Pancreas

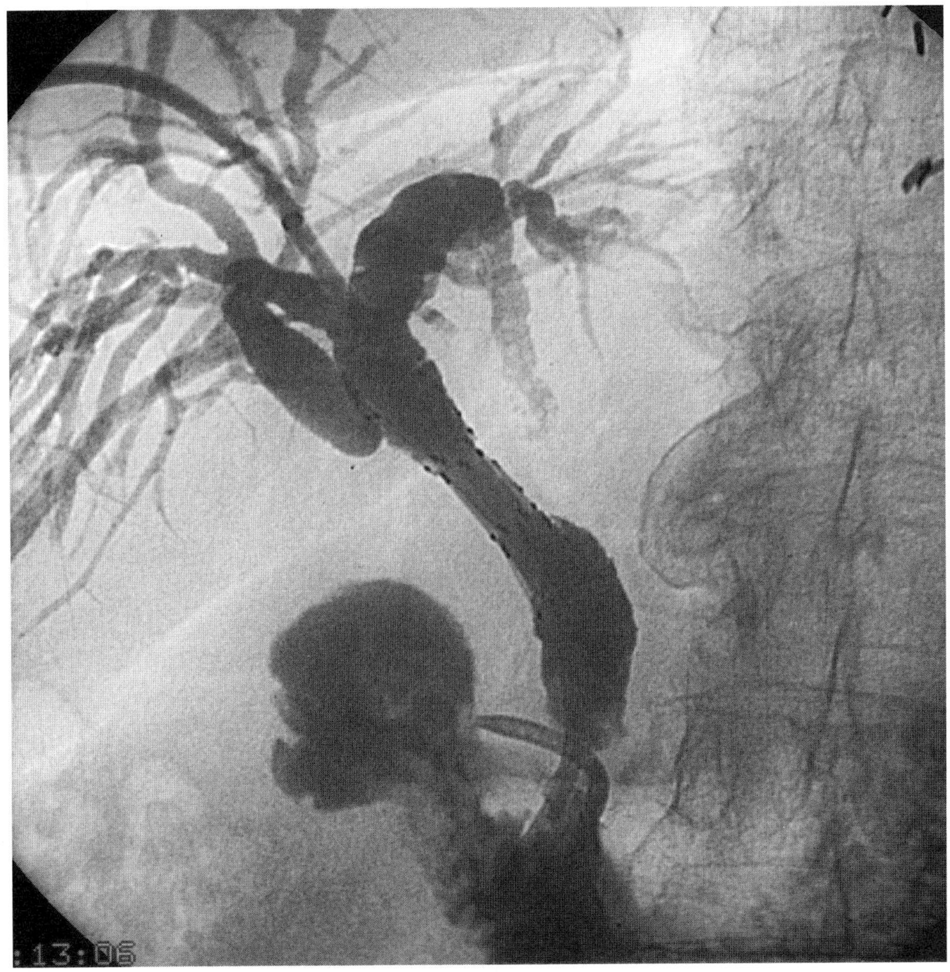

14.1.1 Interventional Procedures In Benign Diseases Of The Biliary Tract

Case 14.1.1:

A 37-year-old woman who underwent cholecystectomy developed a biliary duct stricture following surgery. Choledochojejunostomy was performed with resection of the strictured segment. Stricture of the anastomoses developed about 1 year after the choledochojejunostomy. Because endoscopic retrograde cholangiopancreatography (ERCP) was not feasible, a percutaneous transhepatic approach was requested.

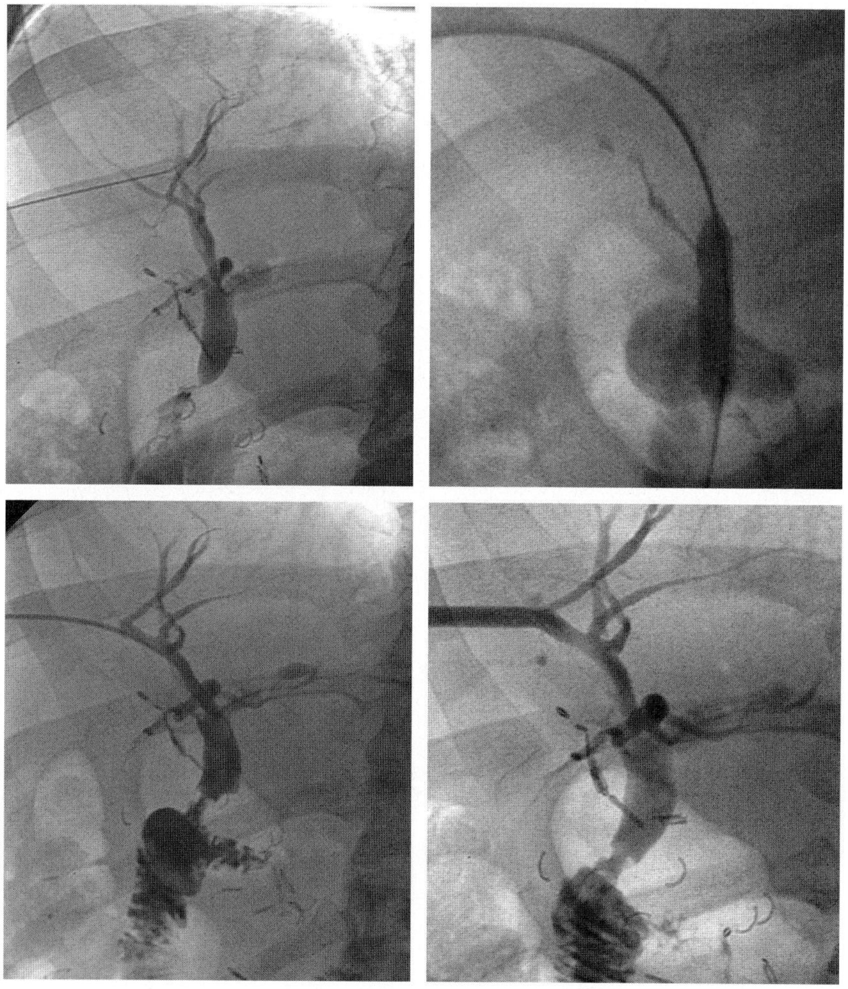

A B C D

Figure 14.1.1

A: Transhepatic percutaneous cholangiogram with a Chiba needle shows moderate dilation of the bile ducts with a severe stricture of the choledochojejunostomy anastomoses. **B:** The stricture was passed, and an 8-mm balloon catheter was used to dilate the stricture. A 10F catheter was placed for internal-external biliary drainage. **C:** The patient returned every 4 weeks for balloon dilation and catheter exchange. Catheter size was progressively enlarged to 14F. Three-month follow-up cholangiogram shows improvement of the stricture, but not enough for catheter removal. **D:** Five-month follow-up cholangiogram shows marked improvement; therefore, the drainage catheter was pulled out. The patient was doing well 12 months after catheter removal, without evidence of jaundice, cholangitis, or changes in liver function.

Comment: Surgical treatment of biliary strictures or lacerations is primarily successful in 62% to 92% of cases. Recurrence rates may be high, ranging from 15% to 30%. Multiple surgeries often are necessary to fix the problem, but the success rate decreases as the number of operations increases, leading to a lower 61% success rate after the third operation. Choledochojejunostomies and hepaticojejunostomies may be subject to recurrent cholangitis, due to either subclinical strictures or reflux of bowel contents into the bile ducts when the anastomosis is wide open. Cholangioplasty is successful in 67% to 86% of cases. More than 90% of patients can have the catheter removed successfully after some time. Patency after 3 to 5 years is around 70%. The best response to percutaneous balloon dilation is in patients with a dominant single or central obstruction. The primary morbidity and mortality of the procedure typically is related to the initial percutaneous biliary drainage and not the actual dilation procedure. The rate of major complications, which involve sepsis and bleeding, ranges from 5% to 12%. This patient responded well to balloon dilation and large-bore catheter drainage.

14.1.2 Interventional Procedures In Benign Diseases Of The Biliary Tract

Case 14.1.2:

A 37-year-old man with a history of biliary atresia treated with a Kasai procedure when he was 7 years old and then placement of a large-bore (19F) Silastic catheter at another institution presented to our institution for catheter exchange. Catheter cholangiogram was performed.

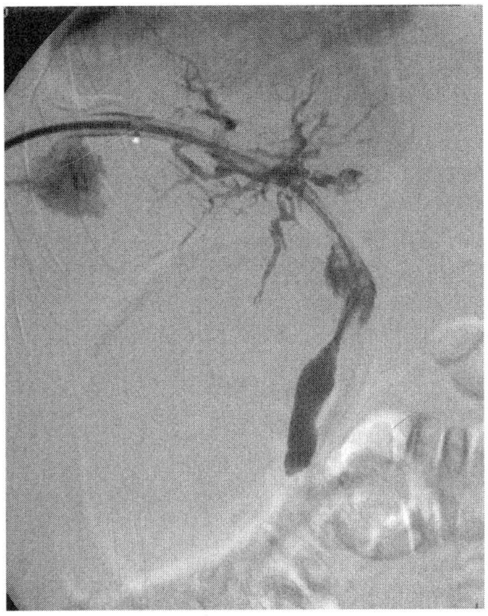

Figure 14.1.2

Catheter cholangiogram demonstrates irregular but nondilated intrahepatic bile ducts. What appeared to be a choledochojejunostomy was patent. The large-bore catheter, which was in place for 30 years, maintained the anastomosis open. Despite the patency, the patient suffered recurrent cholangitis requiring antibiotic treatment. The patient refused to have the catheter removed. The catheter was exchanged several times, and eventually the patient was referred to the hepatology service for counseling and follow-up. The catheter is still in place.

Comment: The diagnosis of biliary atresia in this patient is not definitive. A liver biopsy is planned for the near future. It is unusual to see a patient with biliary atresia who was treated by a Kasai procedure at 7 years of age and with large-bore catheter placement. The anastomosis is open and the catheter should be removed, after 30 years of drainage.

14.1.3 Interventional Procedures In Benign Diseases Of The Biliary Tract

Case 14.1.3:

A 51-year-old male patient underwent a Whipple procedure for pancreatitis with untreatable biliary stenoses and chronic pain. Choledochojejunostomy was performed with resection of the strictured segment. The patient developed a biliary duct stricture at the level of the anastomosis about 6 months after the choledochojejunostomy. Percutaneous transhepatic treatment was requested.

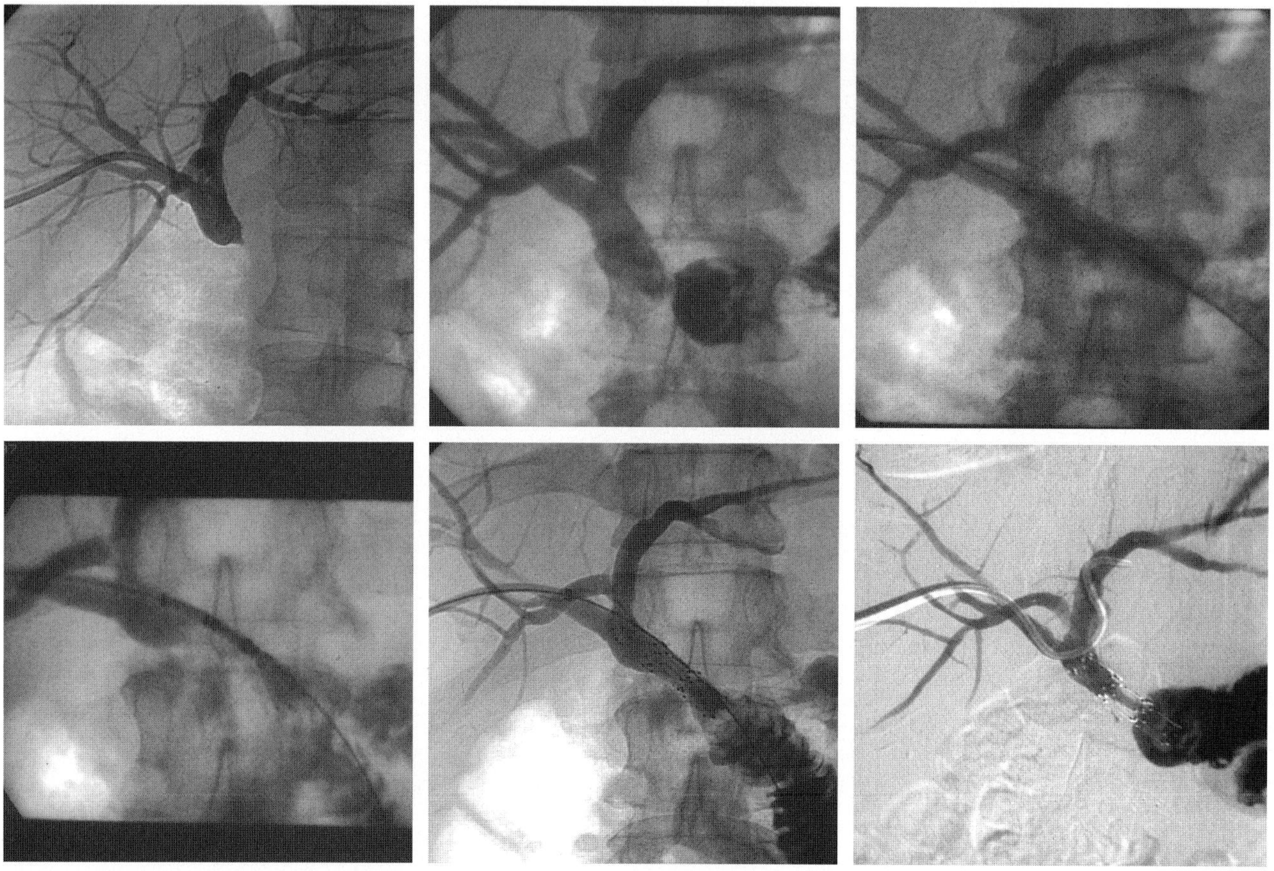

Figure 14.1.3

A: Percutaneous transhepatic cholangiogram (PTC) through the percutaneously placed catheter shows total occlusion of the anastomosis. The first attempt at crossing the stenosis was not successful. **B:** A new attempt at crossing the obstruction was successful following decompression for 48 hours. Note contrast passing through the stenosis. **C:** An 8-mm balloon was used over the wire to dilate the stenosis. Reoperation was not an option in this patient due to the changes related to pancreatitis. **D:** A Z-stent with three bodies was placed across the obstruction. Note the stent partially open during delivery. **E:** Cholangiogram obtained after stent placement shows patency of the anastomosis. The guidewire is still in place. **F:** An external drainage catheter was placed for 24 hours and eventually removed. Note patency of the stent but the much smaller diameter within the stent due to edema of the tissues through the stent struts.

Comment: Ninety-seven percent of all benign biliary obstructions are iatrogenic in nature and usually related to conventional or laparoscopic cholecystectomy. Internal-external percutaneous biliary drainage is successful in about 70% to 100% of attempts. Sometimes only external drainage is achieved initially, but a new attempt after 24 to 48 hours of external drainage usually allows for crossing of the obstruction in most cases (more than 95%). Once the obstruction is crossed, internal drainage can be performed using a catheter following balloon dilation in the case of a benign obstruction. Pancreatitis-related stenoses are very resilient and do not respond very well to balloon plasty; however, choledochojejunostomy performed for pancreatitis has the same risk of stenosis as the biliary-enteric anastomosis performed for surgical trauma. When the surgical risk is excessive, as in this case, there is indication for percutaneous treatment. Because there was excessive fibrosis in the hepatic hilum, a Z-stent was primarily placed to reduce chances of restenosis.

14.1.4 Interventional Procedures In Benign Diseases Of The Biliary Tract

Case 14.1.4:

A 55-year-old female patient underwent a Whipple procedure for pancreatitis with chronic pain. Choledochojejunostomy was performed with resection of the strictured segment. The patient developed a biliary duct stricture at the level of the anastomosis about 2.5 years after the choledochojejunostomy. Percutaneous transhepatic treatment was requested.

A

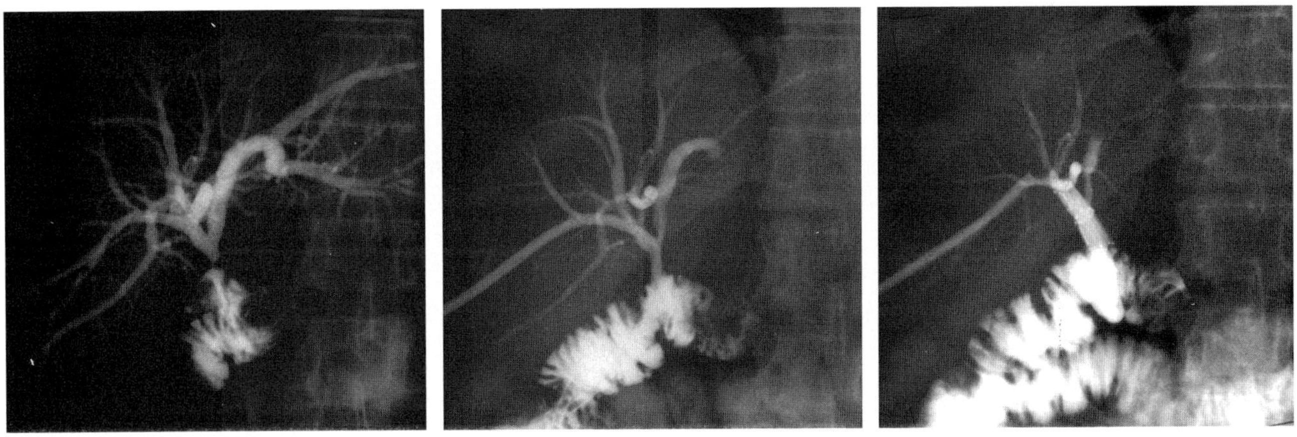

B, C

Figure 14.1.4

A: Cholangiogram after catheter placement shows moderate dilation of the bile ducts with a very tight stenosis at the level of the anastomosis. **B:** After 3 days of internal-external drainage, the anastomosis was dilated with a 10-mm balloon. **C:** A 10-mm, two-body Z-stent was placed through the balloon-dilated anastomosis. Cholangiogram through the catheter shows patency of the stent, with excellent flow into the anastomotic bowel loop. The patient has been doing well for more than 3 years.

Comment: Broad-spectrum antibiotics, including cephalosporin, are administered intravenously 30 to 60 minutes before the procedure begins until the patient is discharged. Initial percutaneous cholangiography is performed with a 23-gauge fine needle. A peripheral bile duct is selected, allowing the straightest path to the common bile duct or to the confluence of the right and left ducts. A Lunderquist needle is used for puncture and cannulation of the biliary tree. A steerable wire is used to negotiate the curves and bends of the bile ducts. When the wire reaches the level of the obstruction, the needle sheath is advanced and attempts to cross the obstruction are made. The obstruction may be totally occluded, or a small tract may be visible. Careful and precise steering of the wire may allow the wire to pass right through the obstruction, but sometimes multiple attempts are necessary and some degree of force may be necessary to overcome a very stiff and resistant stenosis. Perforation of the adjacent bile duct wall is a constant risk, but small holes can be treated by adequate internal or external drainage. Use of a stent to support the dilated stricture provided long-term patency for this patient.

14.1.5 Interventional Procedures In Benign Diseases Of The Biliary Tract

Case 14.1.5:

A 43-year-old male patient developed severe chronic recurrent pancreatitis that caused extensive stenosis of the common bile duct. Initial percutaneous catheter biliary drainage was performed, followed by several balloon dilations and long-term catheter placement, without much success.

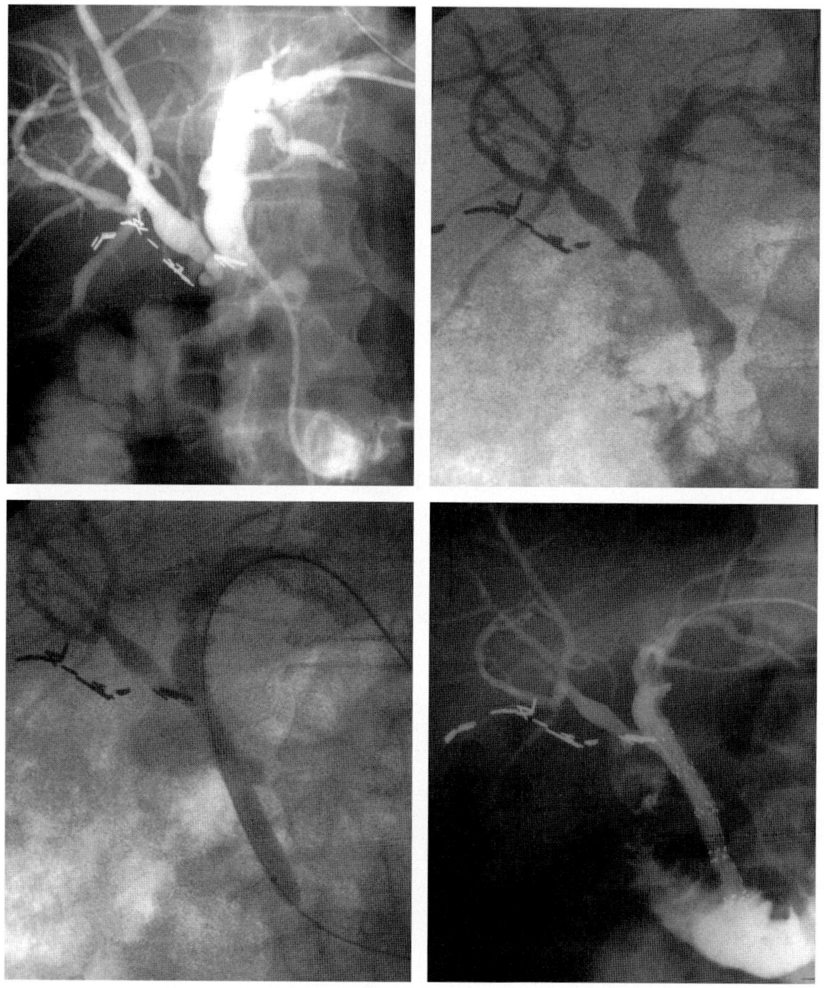
A B C D

Figure 14.1.5

A: Initial left biliary drainage was performed with a 10F catheter. Note extension of the stenosis around the catheter and the intrahepatic dilation of the bile ducts. Multiple dilations with balloon catheter were performed every 4 or 6 weeks for 8 months. The catheter was maintained in place for 8 months. **B:** The stenosis was challenged after pulling out the drainage catheter from the obstruction. Severe stricture was still observed. **C:** The stenosis was dilated again with an 8-mm balloon. **D:** A 10-mm, five-body Z-stent was placed across the obstruction to reach the duodenum. Final cholangiogram shows adequate patency of the stent with decompression of the bile ducts. Follow-up is about 5 years.

Comment: This case demonstrates how difficult it is to treat a bile duct stenosis related to pancreatitis. In the 8-month time period of catheter treatment, there was some improvement in the degree and extension of the stenosis, but persistent narrowing was observed. The fibrotic and scar tissue component of a pancreatitic stenosis usually is extensive, and recurrence or persistence of the stricture is frequent. Balloon dilation and long-term catheter placement were not adequate to control the lesion. In this case, there was a clear indication to use metal stents to prevent stenosis recurrence. Long-term clinical follow-up showed good patency of the stent. Although the literature is scanty, there is evidence supporting use of elective metal mesh self-expandable stents for biliary strictures in chronic pancreatitis, with a success rate of 90% at more than 3 years. Metal stents in benign disease are indicated mainly when catheter drainage and balloon plasty fail to keep the duct open. The metal stents require maintenance. Younger patients should be fully aware of the risks of recurrent obstruction and the need for multiple treatments to keep the stents open.

14.1.6 Interventional Procedures In Benign Diseases Of The Biliary Tract

Case 14.1.6:

A 67-year-old male patient underwent a Billroth II procedure followed by cholecystectomy. After surgery, the patient developed perforation of the common bile duct during ERCP when a stent was lost. The ERCP complication was treated by surgery with T-tube placement through the cystic duct. The T-tube became dislodged, and new surgery was undertaken. Following surgery, the patient developed a biliary fistula, the T-tube became dislodged again, and sepsis ensued. Percutaneous biliary drainage management was requested.

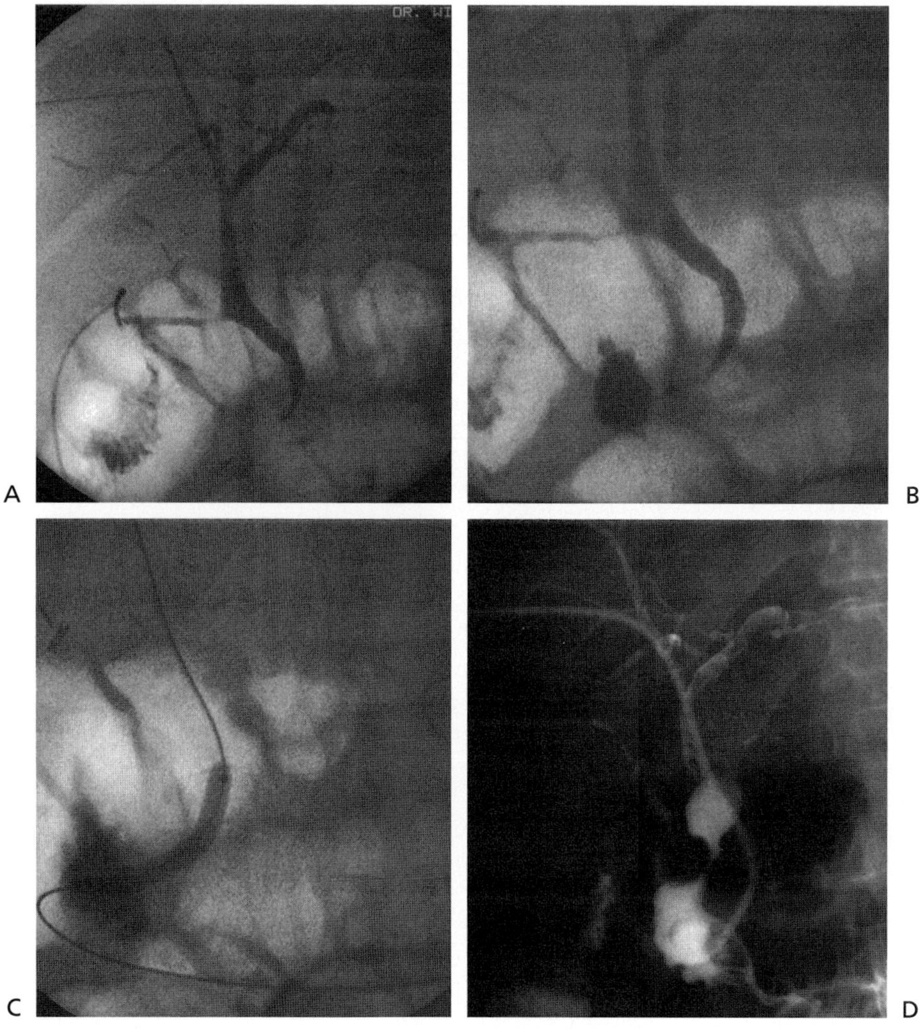

Figure 14.1.6

A: T-tube cholangiogram demonstrates a fistulous tract connecting to the common bile duct. Due to inadequate filling of the biliary tree, PTC with a Chiba needle was performed to enhance visibility of the bile ducts. The distal common bile duct was thin and occluded at the sphincter level. **B:** The bile duct was catheterized, and a wedged injection at the level of the papilla shows a small amount of contrast passing the sphincter at least partially into the duodenal lumen. **C:** After catheterization across the papilla, an 8-mm balloon catheter was used to dilate the stenosis. Note extravasation of contrast. **D:** After balloon plasty, a 10F catheter was placed for internal-external drainage. The catheter was kept in place for 5 months, and all fistulas were sealed off. The catheter eventually was removed, and the patient did well.

Comment: Percutaneous transhepatic biliary drainage may be the only alternative for helping patients who underwent multiple unsuccessful surgeries of the bile ducts. This case is a clear demonstration of the potential of the percutaneous procedure to control leaks and reverse critical situations of biliary stenosis and sepsis. Although these patients are at risk for complications related to worsening of sepsis and perforation of the biliary strictures, the percutaneous approach, when carefully performed, is safe and effective. A small extravasation of contrast was caused by manipulation of the guidewire at the level of the papilla, but adequate drainage resolves the problem in most cases. Clearly this patient would require another surgery for treatment, and the drainage was an excellent solution.

14.1.7 Interventional Procedures In Benign Diseases Of The Biliary Tract

Case 14.1.7:

A 63-year-old male patient presented with biliary obstruction and sepsis. The patient had undergone periampullary neoplasm resection and a Whipple procedure 2 years earlier. The bile ducts were dilated, and percutaneous drainage was requested after starting intravenous antibiotics.

A 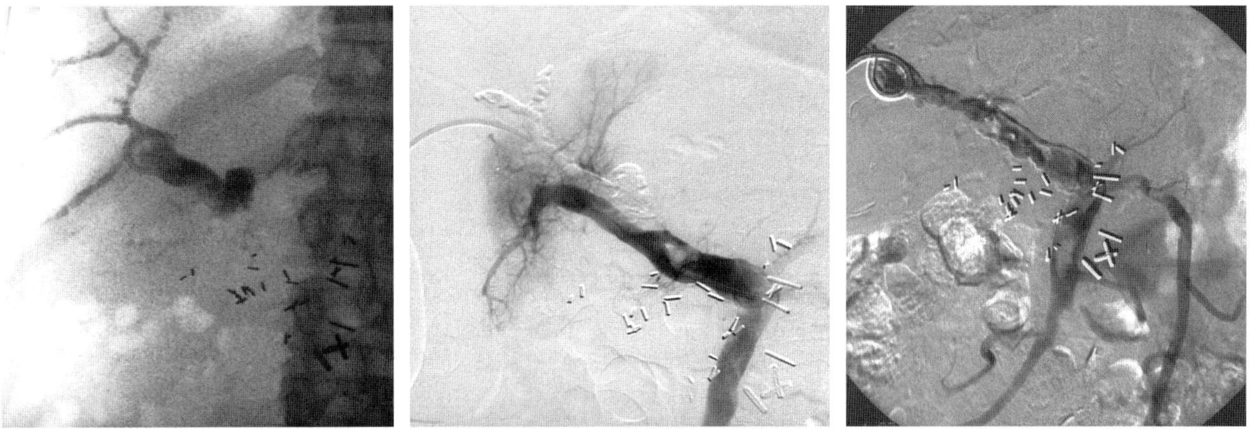 B, C

Figure 14.1.7

A: Percutaneous cholangiogram with a fine needle shows obstruction of the main bile duct, dilation, and irregularities in the peripheral bile ducts consistent with cholangitis. An external biliary drainage catheter was placed for 3 days to control the infection. **B:** Follow-up cholangiogram 3 days later shows communication of the main bile duct with the portal vein. The catheter was exchanged, but it was not possible to pass the obstruction. At the attempt to pass the obstruction, the catheter easily passed into the portal vein. The drainage catheter was left in place within the bile duct, and no significant bleeding developed. **C:** One week later, the patient returned for follow-up cholangiogram, which demonstrates that communication again was visualized. The portal vein presented extensive thrombosis. The infection was controlled.

Comment: Chronic recurrent pancreatitis sometimes requires surgical treatment with pancreatic resection and biliary-enteric anastomosis. The possibility of infection is always present in cases of benign biliary obstruction. This is an extreme example of biliary sepsis followed by a dreadful complication related to the portal vein. When thrombophlebitis develops, portal obstruction follows and variceal bleeding complications may occur. This patient is still alive and well 5 years after the procedure. No other surgical treatment could be offered. As it was never possible to cross the obstruction, external drainage alleviated the problem and the catheter was removed.

14.1.8 Interventional Procedures In Benign Diseases Of The Biliary Tract

Case 14.1.8:

A 22-year-old female patient had a history of recurrent cholangitis since she was born. Repeated bouts of jaundice and cholangitis prompted diagnosis of a choledochal cyst, which was treated several years earlier by choledochocystoduodenostomy and revision choledochojejunostomy. Repeated episodes of cholangitis and jaundice required percutaneous cholangiography for diagnosis and treatment. A diagnosis of sclerosing cholangitis was tentatively established.

A, B

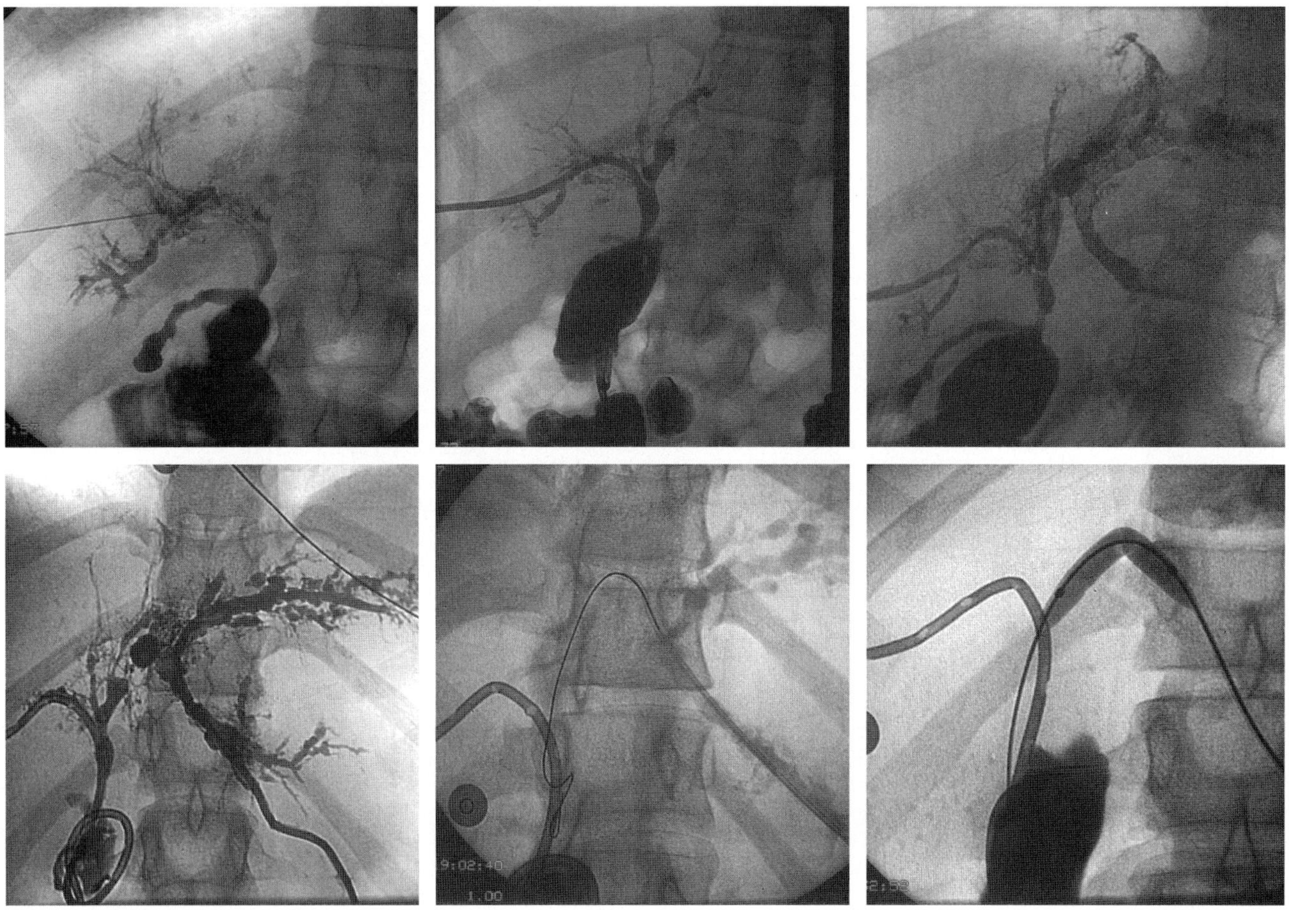

C

D, E

F

Figure 14.1.8

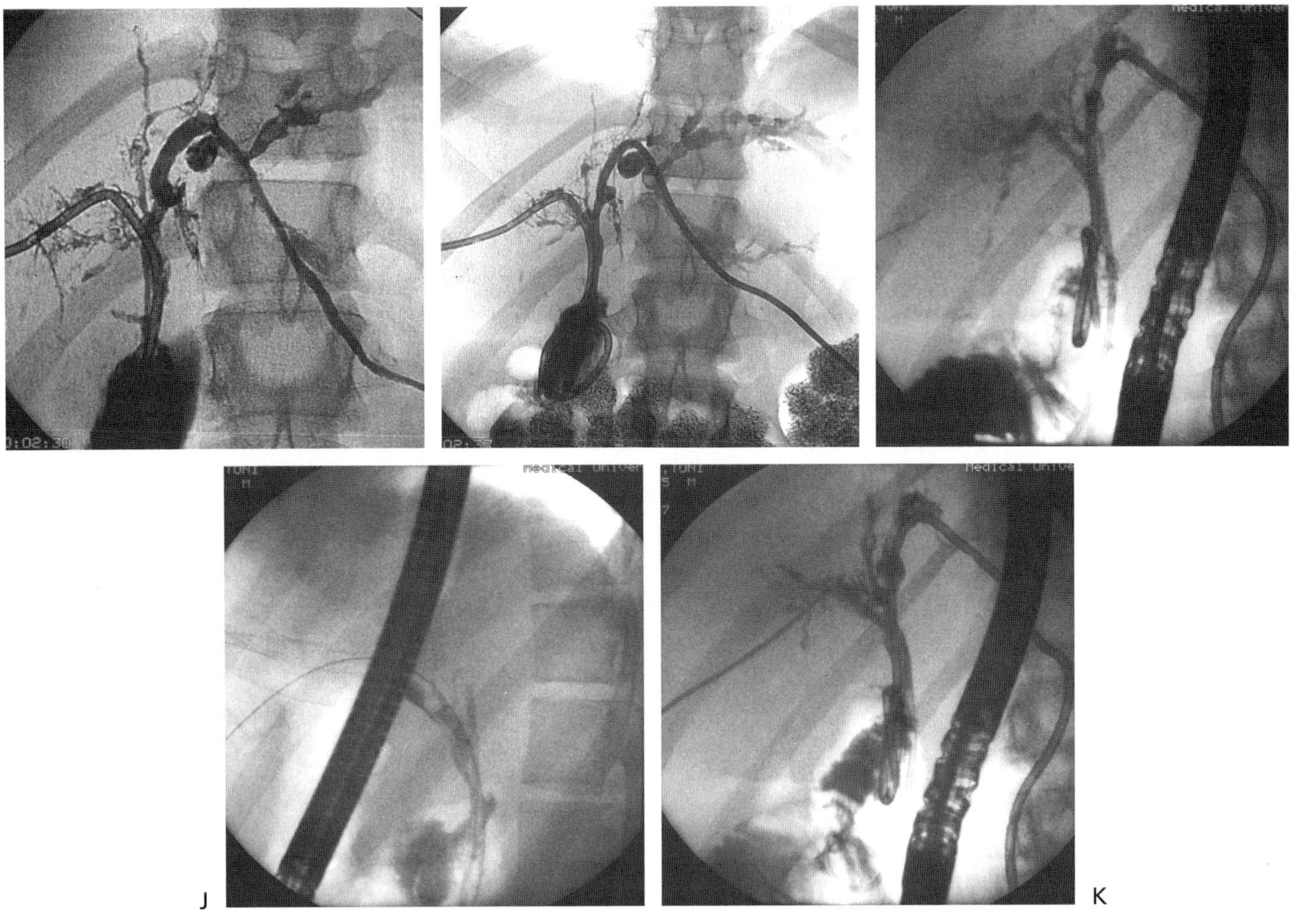

G H, I J K

Figure 14.1.8 *(continued)*

A: PTC with a fine needle shows a severely diseased biliary tree with irregularities, stenosis, and stones. **B:** An internal-external drainage biliary catheter was placed across the cystoduodenostomy. There was some improvement of the jaundice and cholangitis, but the left bile duct was occluded. **C:** A KMP catheter was advanced from the right side into the left bile duct. Injection of contrast into the left duct shows multiple stenosis and the ducts full of stones. **D:** Five days after drainage, left-side drainage was performed and shows severe areas of stenosis in the left bile duct. **E:** A small 0.018-inch steerable guidewire was passed though the obstruction and reached the main bile duct. **F:** Balloon plasty of the stenosis was performed with a 6-mm balloon catheter. **G:** An occlusion balloon catheter was used to push some stones into the main bile duct, and a drainage catheter was placed from the left side. **H:** Follow-up cholangiogram a few days later shows decompression of the left side associated with marked clinical improvement. **I,J:** Because the patient was young and there was need for long-term drainage, endoscopic stents were placed. **K:** Final cholangiogram shows the right-side stent and left-side drainage catheter. Five months after drainage, hepaticojejunostomy was performed with intrahepatic stone extraction, with an uneventful course. The patient is doing well for about 2 years.

Comment: This complex case demonstrates the severity of problems related to a choledochal cyst aggravated by possible, but unconfirmed, sclerosing cholangitis. The surgical biopsy was negative for primary sclerosing cholangitis (PSC). Percutaneous biliary drainage improved the patient's condition, which allowed her to undergo surgery. Percutaneous access was difficult due to the presence of multiple stenoses and stones. The left-side stenosis was the most difficult to treat, and patency of the left side likely improved the surgical result. Intrabiliary calculi occur relatively frequently in patients with PSC and have a unique imaging appearance. The stones are seen as a cast on ultrasound, completely filling the bile ducts. The cholangiographic appearance was of rounded or oval filling defects within the dilated or saccular bile ducts. Intrahepatic and nonanastomotic extrahepatic biliary strictures are significantly more common in patients who undergo liver transplantation for PSC than in patients who undergo liver transplantation for other diseases.

14.1.9 Interventional Procedures In Benign Diseases Of The Biliary Tract

Case 14.1.9:

A 60-year-old male patient with PSC and recurrent bouts of jaundice and infection previously treated by choledochojejunostomy was rapidly deteriorating. Percutaneous balloon plasty was used to gain time while the patient was put on the liver transplant list.

A, B

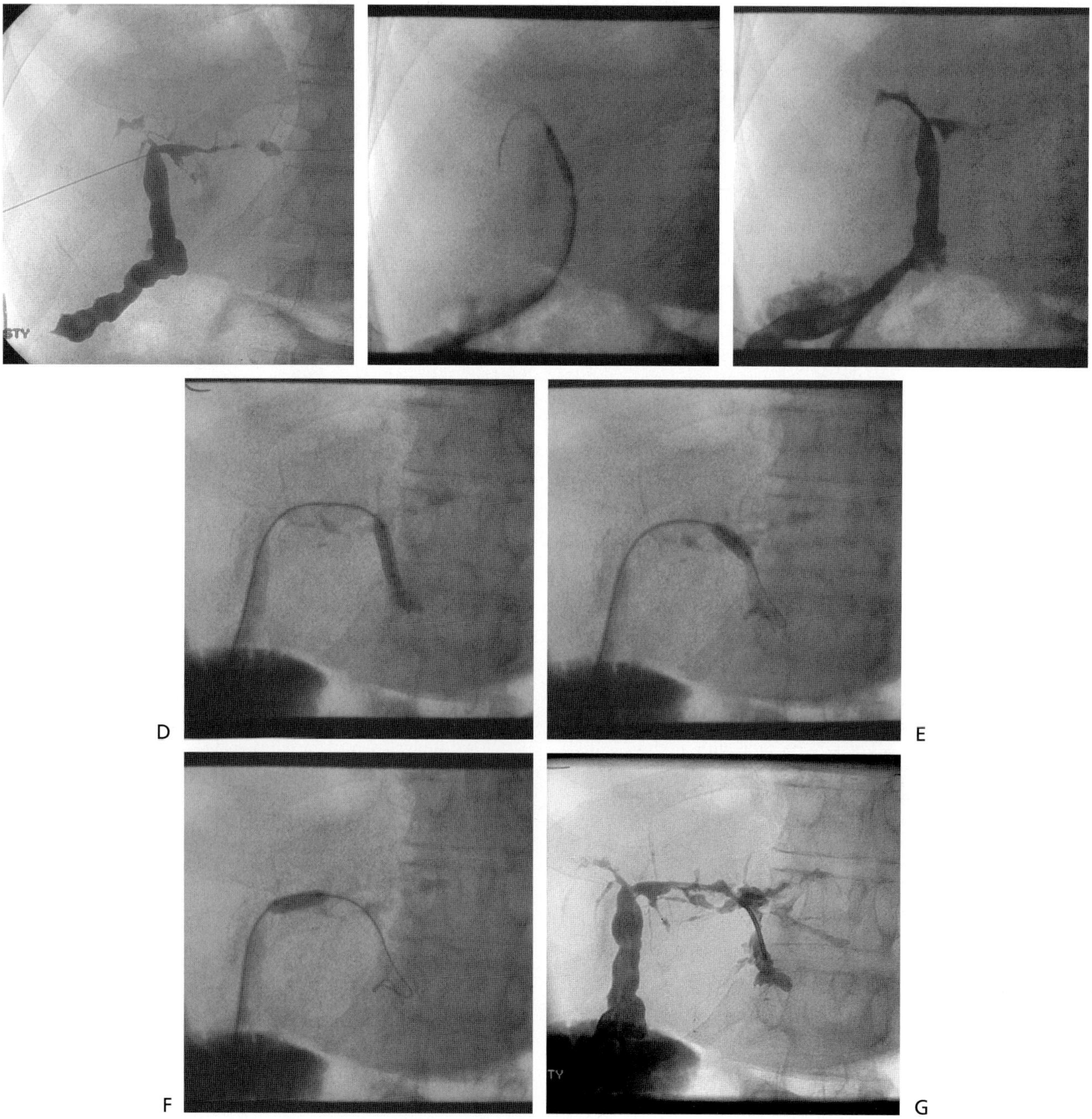

C

D E

F G

Figure 14.1.9

A: Percutaneous cholangiogram with a fine needle shows severe diffuse stenosis of the intrahepatic bile ducts and free flow of contrast into the common bile duct through the choledochojejunostomy. **B:** Because the intrahepatic bile ducts were small and irregular, puncture of the antecolic jejunal loop was performed to approach the bile ducts from below. Plasty with a 4-mm balloon was performed on the right side. **C:** Cholangiogram after plasty shows slight improvement. **D–F:** Balloon plasty with a 6-mm balloon was performed in the left duct. **G:** Final cholangiogram demonstrates some improvement in the left bile duct.

Comment: The transjejunal approach is an effective and safe route for percutaneous biliary procedures in patients with biliary-enteric anastomoses. The transjejunal approach is facilitated by surgical landmarks placed for fluoroscopic guidance. Although the marks were not present in this case, the bowel loop puncture was easy, following identification of the contrast-filled loop. It is important to maintain a route for repeated access to the biliary tree in patients in whom recurrent disease is expected, such as patients with sclerosing cholangitis. Balloon plasty of the intrahepatic bile ducts usually improves liver function, but the effect is only temporary because of the progressive nature of the disease. Strictures and diverticulum-like outpouchings, findings suggestive of PSC, are encountered in up to 47% of PSC liver grafts compared to 13% in control groups, which suggests that PSC may recur in liver transplantation.

14.1.10 Interventional Procedures In Benign Diseases Of The Biliary Tract

Case 14.1.10:

A 60-year-old female patient underwent laparoscopic cholecystectomy, which was followed by a stenosis of the common bile duct a few days after surgery. The bile duct stenosis was treated by side-to-side choledochojejunostomy. The postsurgical course was complicated by sepsis, cholangitis, jaundice, and biliary fistula draining through the surgical incision, despite the presence of a Foley catheter placed near the anastomosis. The patient was transferred to our institution for further treatment. Percutaneous biliary drainage was performed, followed by a joint procedure with the endoscopy service.

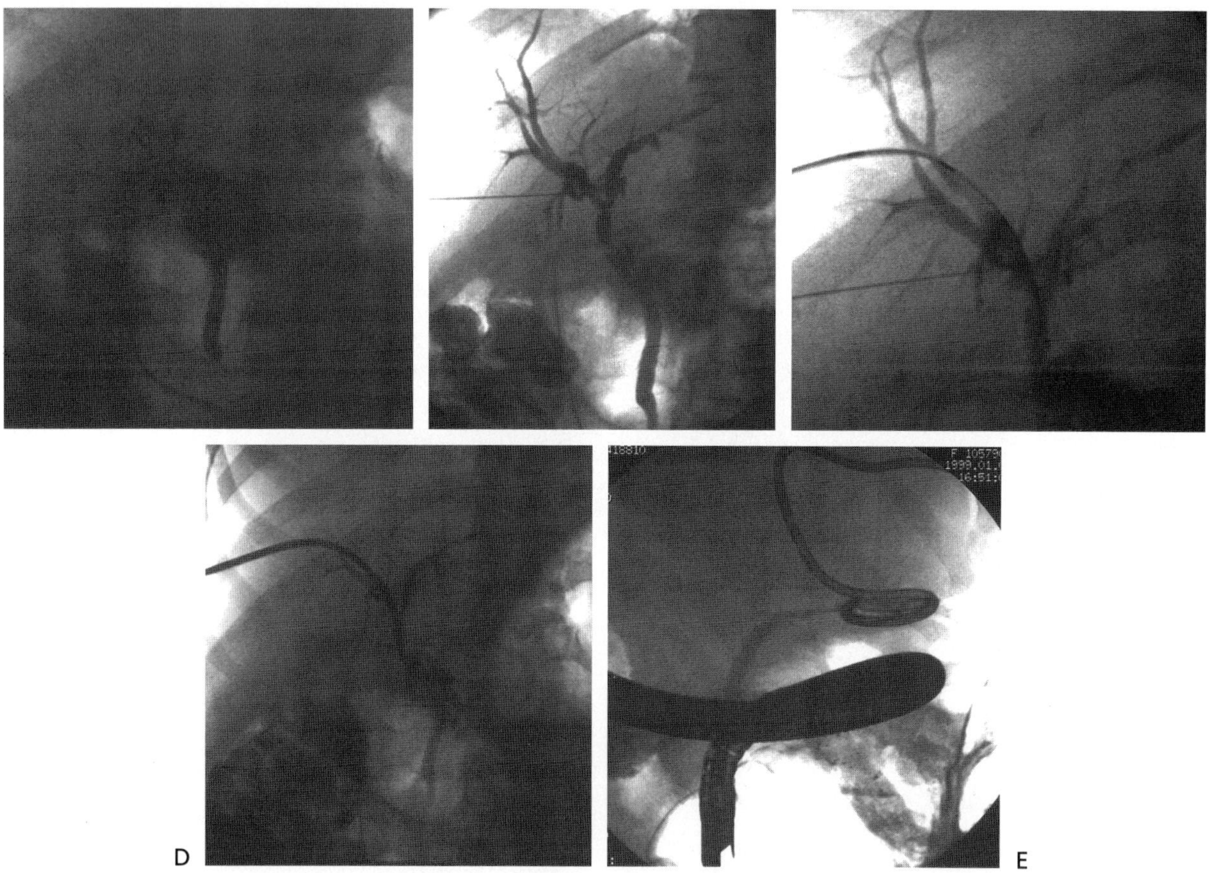

A, B C D E

Figure 14.1.10

A: Initial injection through the surgical drain shows a cavity, close to the anastomosis, with flow into the distal bile duct, and partial filling of the proximal intrahepatic bile duct. **B:** PTC shows a mildly dilated intrahepatic biliary tree and a stenosis in the main bile duct at the level of the anastomosis. **C:** Access was obtained from a higher duct, and catheterization of the bile ducts was performed. It was not possible to pass the stenosis; however, it was possible to reach through the anastomosis and into the anastomotic bowel loop. **D:** Catheter cholangiogram shows filling of the anastomotic bowel loop and the distal bile duct. **E:** After 1 week of external drainage, there was improvement of the sepsis and bile leak through the fistulous tract. A joint procedure with the endoscopy service was scheduled to try to cross the obstruction. Endoscopic cholangiogram shows the stenosis in the distal bile duct, near the side-to-side choledochojejunostomy. **F:** An ERCP catheter and guidewire were advanced into the anastomotic bowel loop. **G:** The ERCP wire was kept inside the bowel loop, but the percutaneous catheter was exchanged for a sheath and loop snare. **H–J:** The ERCP wire was snared from the percutaneous approach and exteriorized through the skin, creating a "body floss guidewire." **K:** The stricture was percutaneously dilated with a 6-mm balloon. **L,M:** A 10F internal-external biliary catheter was introduced and set for external drainage. Cholangiogram shows good flow into the duodenum and anastomotic loop. The fistula was sealed off and the sepsis improved. Two weeks later, the catheter was exchanged for a larger 12F size. When the patient resumed oral feeding, symptoms of

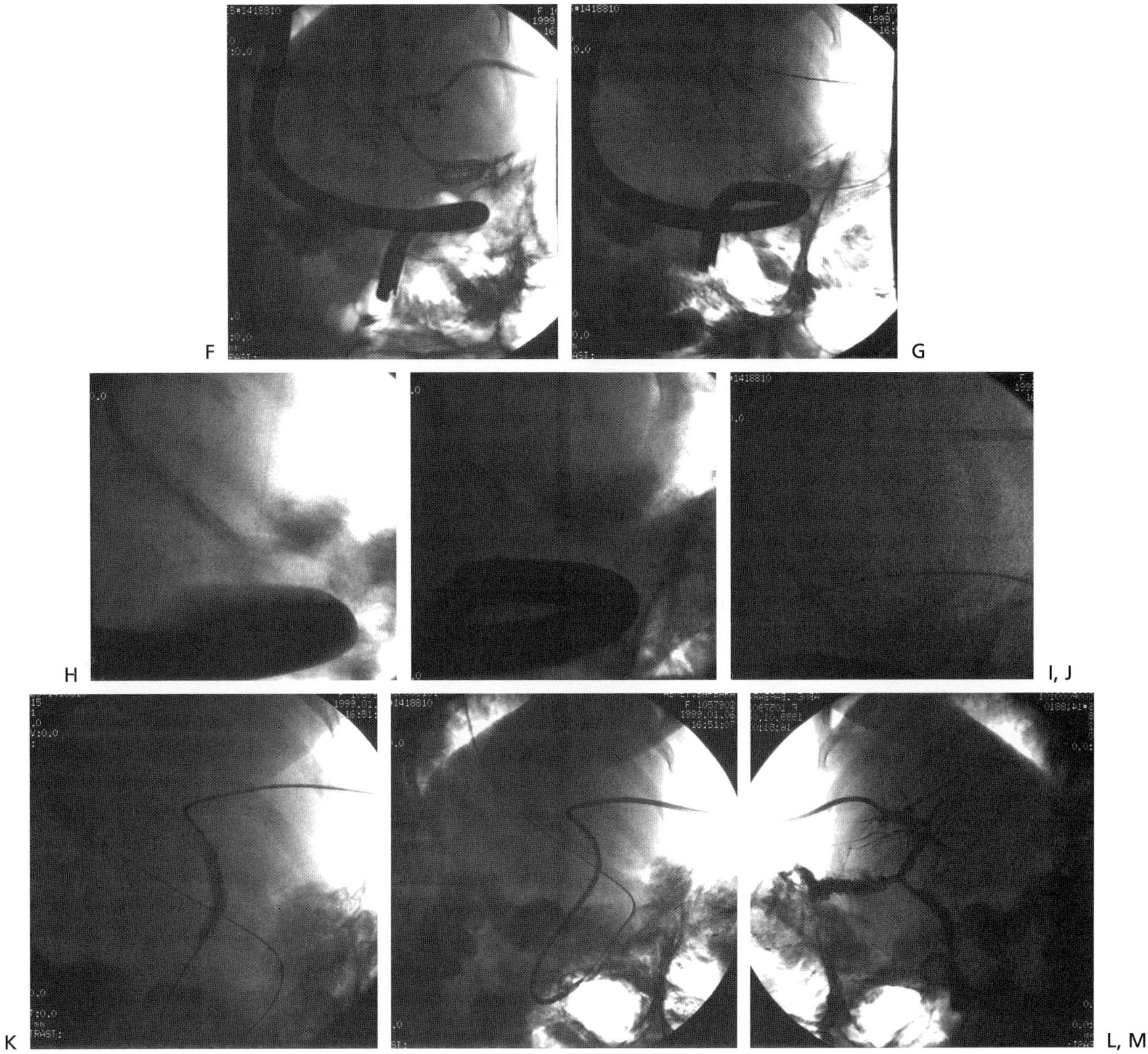

Figure 14.1.10 *(continued)*

pancreatitis developed. Reduction of catheter size to 8F and a sphincterotomy improved the patient's clinical status, which allowed her to be discharged with the catheter in place.

Comment: A multidisciplinary approach is needed if we are to provide the best care for patients. Endoscopy and interventional radiology often play complementary roles in the management of patients with benign biliary diseases. The joint procedure performed in this patient allowed for optimal treatment of the complications that ensued after laparoscopic cholecystectomy and the subsequent side-to-side choledochojejunostomy. In some benign strictures, the approach from above may not be able to cross the obstruction, thus requiring a simultaneous approach from below for a rendezvous procedure. A loop snare or stone basket may be used to capture and pull out the endoscopic guidewire or catheter placed in the bile duct from below. Once the stricture is crossed and the guidewire is exteriorized, the access may be used for balloon plasty and biliary catheter/stent placement. Percutaneous/endoscopic treatment of the complications may improve the patient's clinical condition and allow additional surgical treatment, if necessary.

14.1.11 Interventional Procedures In Benign Diseases Of The Biliary Tract

Case 14.1.11:

A 34-year-old female patient underwent laparoscopic cholecystectomy, which was followed by jaundice and pain. The patient was transferred to our institution for treatment, and PTC was requested.

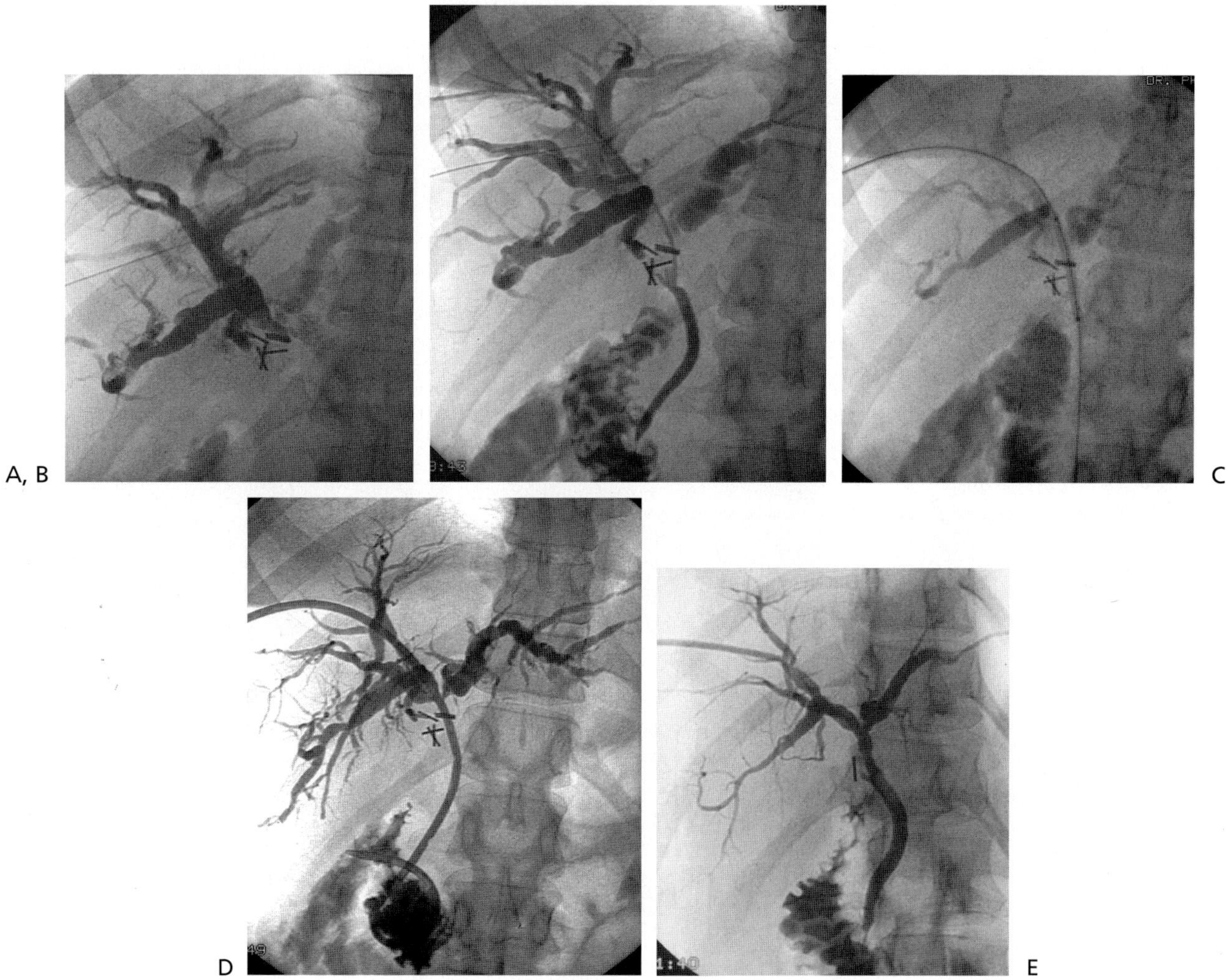

Figure 14.1.11

A: Initial PTC shows moderately dilated intrahepatic bile ducts with total obstruction at the level of the common bile duct, ending in a surgical metallic clip (type 2). **B:** A small peripheral bile duct was catheterized, and the guidewire was advanced to the level of the obstruction. Multiple attempts to cross the obstruction were made. At that time, it was not known if there was connection between the two parts of the bile duct, above and below the clip. Eventually the guidewire and the Lunderquist needle catheter were advanced through the stricture, proving that the common bile duct had been clipped during surgery but fortunately had not been sectioned. **C:** The metal clip (and the stricture) was dilated with a 4-mm balloon, and an 8F catheter was advanced for internal-external drainage. **D:** Catheter cholangiography demonstrated good biliary patency. Note that the catheter is passing through the metal clip arms. A few days later, the patient underwent laparoscopic surgery to remove the clip used to ligate the main bile duct. The drainage catheter was left in place to mold the duct. **E:** Final cholangiogram shows patency of the main bile duct at the level of the clip, despite some irregularities in the walls. Monthly follow-up cholangiograms were performed, as were balloon dilations and catheter exchange. The catheter was maintained for 4 months and then removed successfully. The patient is doing well for about 1 year.

Comment: Thorough knowledge of anatomy is necessary to perform laparoscopic cholecystectomy. Recognition of normal anatomic relationships is more difficult with laparoscopic operations, despite the excellent imaging quality of current systems. Failures and complications in laparoscopic cholecystectomies are mostly related to anatomic variations and technical problems. Injuries can be graded according to the level of the trauma in relation to the confluence of the hepatic ducts, described in the Bismuth classification for bile duct injury. A type 1 injury is a lesion of the main bile duct, located more than 2 cm distal of the bifurcation. A type 2 injury is a lesion of the main bile duct, located less than 2 cm distal of the bifurcation. A type 3 injury completely destroys the hepatic stump distal to the bifurcation but leaves the bifurcation intact. A type 4 injury partially or completely obliterates the bifurcation. A type 5 injury involves an injury of a variant right hepatic branch or of the main bile duct at its junction with the variant duct. Minor injuries are mostly related to bile leaks through the cystic duct, following gallbladder resection or common bile duct fistula. Major injuries include partial or total transection of the common bile duct with or without disconnection, strictures, and clipped ducts. Association of one or more of these problems may be found. Other lesions, such as liver lobe necrosis, may be related to inadvertent clipping of the arterial pedicle. It is rare for the interventional radiologist to be called to intervene with a patient before there is a surgical attempt to resolve the problem, as occurred in this case. It is very rare that a clipped bile duct can be treated successfully by percutaneous and laparoscopic means.

14.1.12 Interventional Procedures In Benign Diseases Of The Biliary Tract

Case 14.1.12:

A 72-year-old female patient underwent laparoscopic cholecystectomy, which was followed by a stenosis of the common bile duct several weeks after surgery. Due to other clinical problems that placed the patient at high surgical risk, percutaneous transhepatic biliary drainage was requested to minimize surgical trauma.

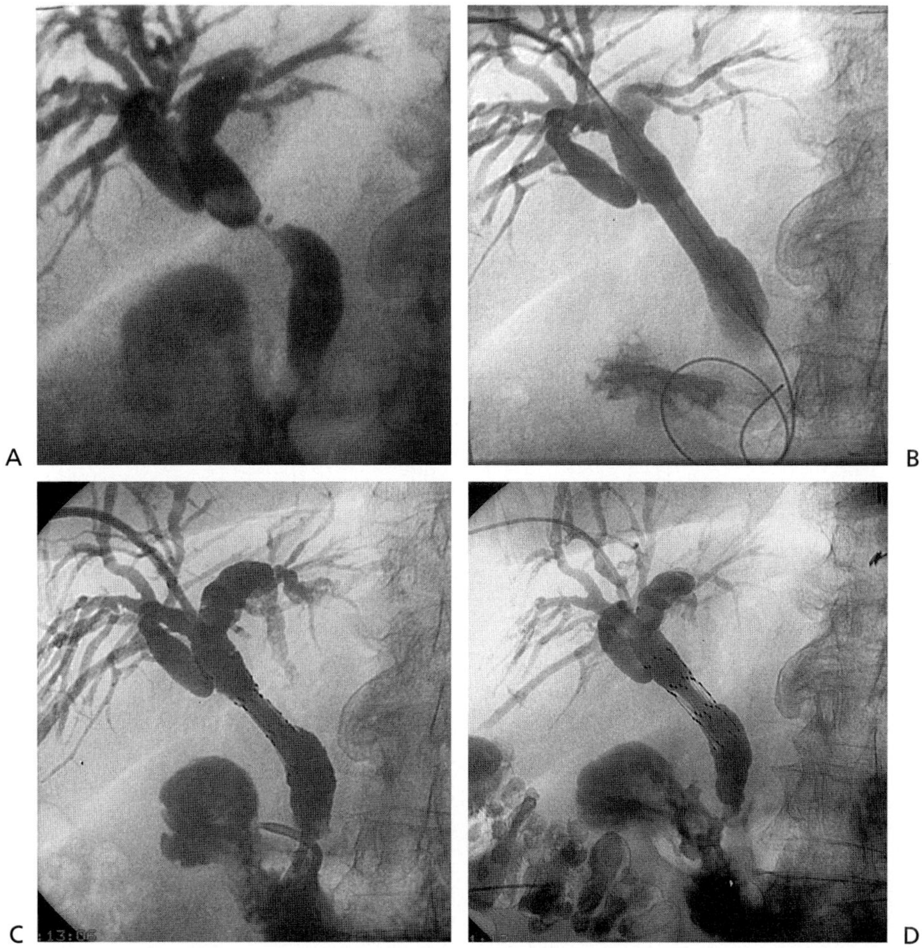

Figure 14.1.12

A: PTC shows dilated intrahepatic bile ducts and a severe type 1 stricture in the common bile duct. Note the stone within the proximal common bile duct. The stricture was dilated with a 10-mm balloon. The stone was pushed into the duodenum. **C:** Following plasty, a three-body Z-stent was placed within the stricture, and an 8F catheter was left in place for 24 hours for internal-external drainage. **D:** Follow-up cholangiogram shows some degree of stenosis within the stent, probably due to edema of the mucosa through the stent struts. Despite the stenosis within the stent, drainage was free flowing, and the catheter was pulled out. The patient did well, and the stent has been open for 3 years.

Comment: Primary repair of the main bile duct using a percutaneous technique is an alternative to surgical treatment when there is a contraindication to conventional surgery. The overall complication rate of laparoscopic cholecystectomy is about 5% to 12%. Bile duct injuries range from 0.1% to 2.2%, but the rate decreases as the learning curve improves. Strictures usually are related to direct mechanical injury to the duct and scar tissue formation, inadvertent clipping of the duct, and thermal injury when the electrocautery or laser dissection is used in the Calot triangle. Metallic biliary stents may be indicated in such cases, when the patient is older and the long-term catheterization technique is not desirable. Stenting in this case worked well. Very strict cooperation of the patient is necessary for success with this kind of treatment. The patient receiving the metal stent to treat benign bile duct disease must be aware of the possible recurrence of stenosis and the potential need for multiple follow-up procedures.

14.1.13 Interventional Procedures In Benign Diseases Of The Biliary Tract

Case 14.1.13:

A 66-year-old male patient underwent laparoscopic cholecystectomy, which was followed by infection, biliary fistula, and biloma related to transection and detachment of the right bile duct segment from the main bile duct. The patient was septic and required emergent biliary drainage.

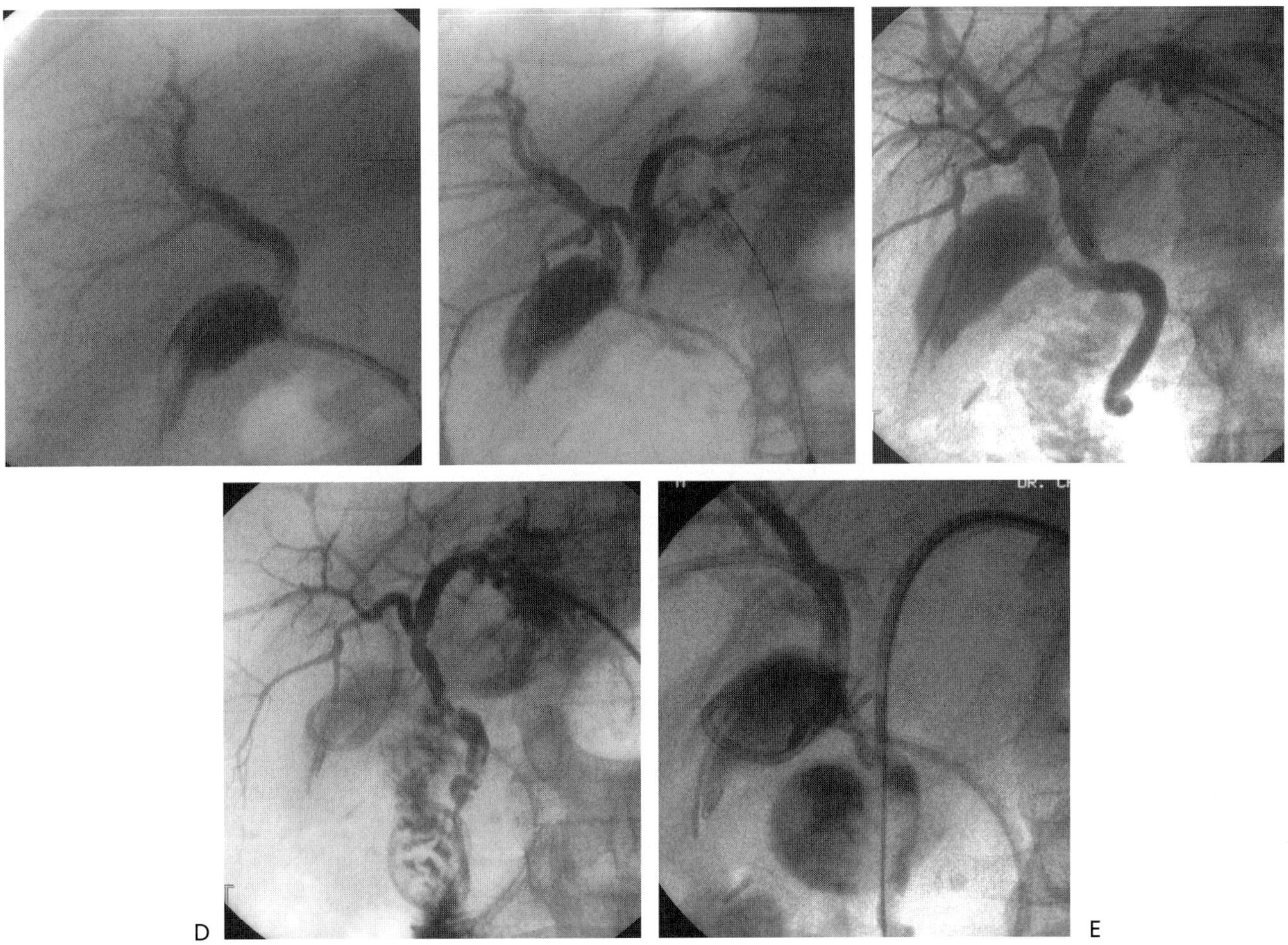

A B, C D E

Figure 14.1.13

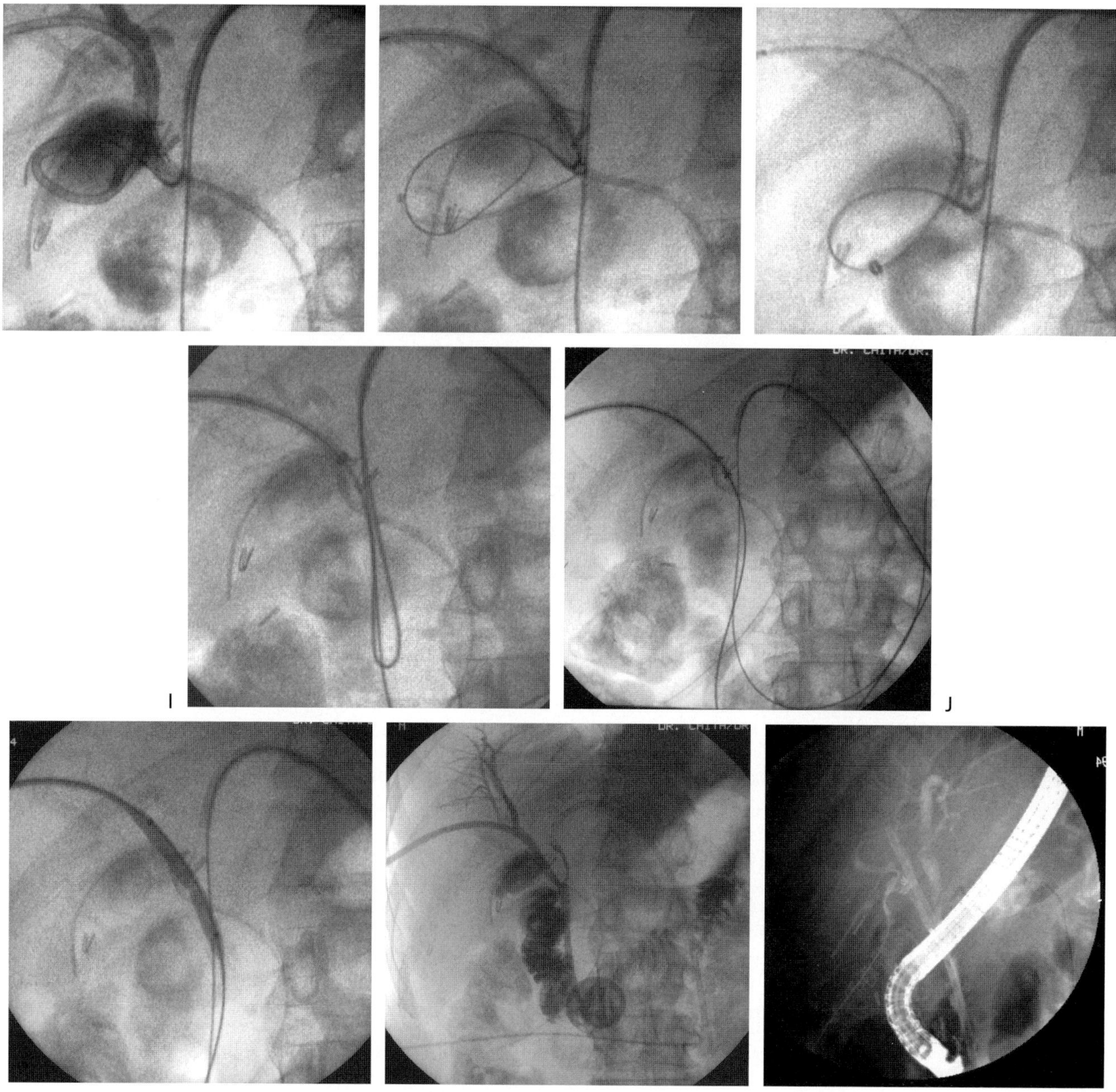

F, G H I J K, L M

Figure 14.1.13 *(continued)*

A: Injection in the subhepatic surgical drain shows filling of a biloma and retrograde filling of the right bile duct. Percutaneous transhepatic access was established, and an external drainage catheter was placed inside the biloma through the right bile duct. **B:** PTC was performed from the left side and shows possible occlusion of the main bile duct. **C:** Subsequent filling and catheterization of the common bile duct shows no significant occlusion. **D:** The right and left drainage catheters were left in open external drainage. **E:** Follow-up cholangiogram 3 days after drainage shows improvement in the biliary leak, with a reduced biloma and visibility of the right biliary stump in connection with the biloma. There was remarkable clinical improvement. **F:** The left drainage catheter was exchanged for a guidewire, and a KMP catheter was passed through the biliary stump from the left-side bile duct, common bile duct, and into the biloma. **G:** A guidewire was advanced into the biloma. **H:** The right drain was replaced by a sheath, and a loop snare was advanced into the biloma to capture the guidewire introduced from the left side. **I:** The guidewire was pulled out all the way through the sheath, exited through the skin, and buckled back into the main bile duct to reconstitute continuity with the main bile duct. **J:** The guidewire was placed from the right approach into the duodenum, creating a connection from the main bile duct, through the biloma, to the right duct segment. **K:** A 6-mm balloon was passed over the wire, and plasty of the stricture was performed. **L:** A 10F internal-external biliary catheter was placed across the lesion and open into a bag. **M:** Approximately 1 month after percutaneous drainage, an endoscopic plastic stent was placed into the right duct and exchanged for several months, which allowed the laceration to heal around the stent.

Comment: Misidentification of the common bile duct or common hepatic duct as the cystic duct during dissection for laparoscopic cholecystectomy is a classic mechanism of injury. Delayed biliary strictures usually result from thermal ischemic injury. Bilomas, transections, and leaks usually present in the immediate postoperative period. In this case, infection and leak did develop shortly after surgery. The level of biliary duct injury usually is higher and more selective in laparoscopic cholecystectomy than in conventional cholecystectomy. This increases the difficulties of surgical repair and opens a window of opportunity for interventional treatment. The aberrant union of the cystic duct with the right hepatic duct may lead to transection and separation of the right hepatic duct from the main bile duct during dissection. As occurred in the presented case, leakage and bilomas usually develop after such a complication. The bilateral approach with catheterization of the right and left bile ducts has been developed to reconstruct the connection of the detached right biliary duct to the main bile duct. The same technique has been used in several cases in our own experience.

14.1.14 Interventional Procedures In Benign Diseases Of The Biliary Tract

Case 14.1.14:

A 44-year-old female patient underwent laparoscopic cholecystectomy, which was followed by infection, biliary fistula, and biloma related to transection and detachment of the right bile duct segment from the main bile duct. The patient was septic, and biloma and biliary drainage was requested. Previous hepatico-jejunostomy was attempted, but failed.

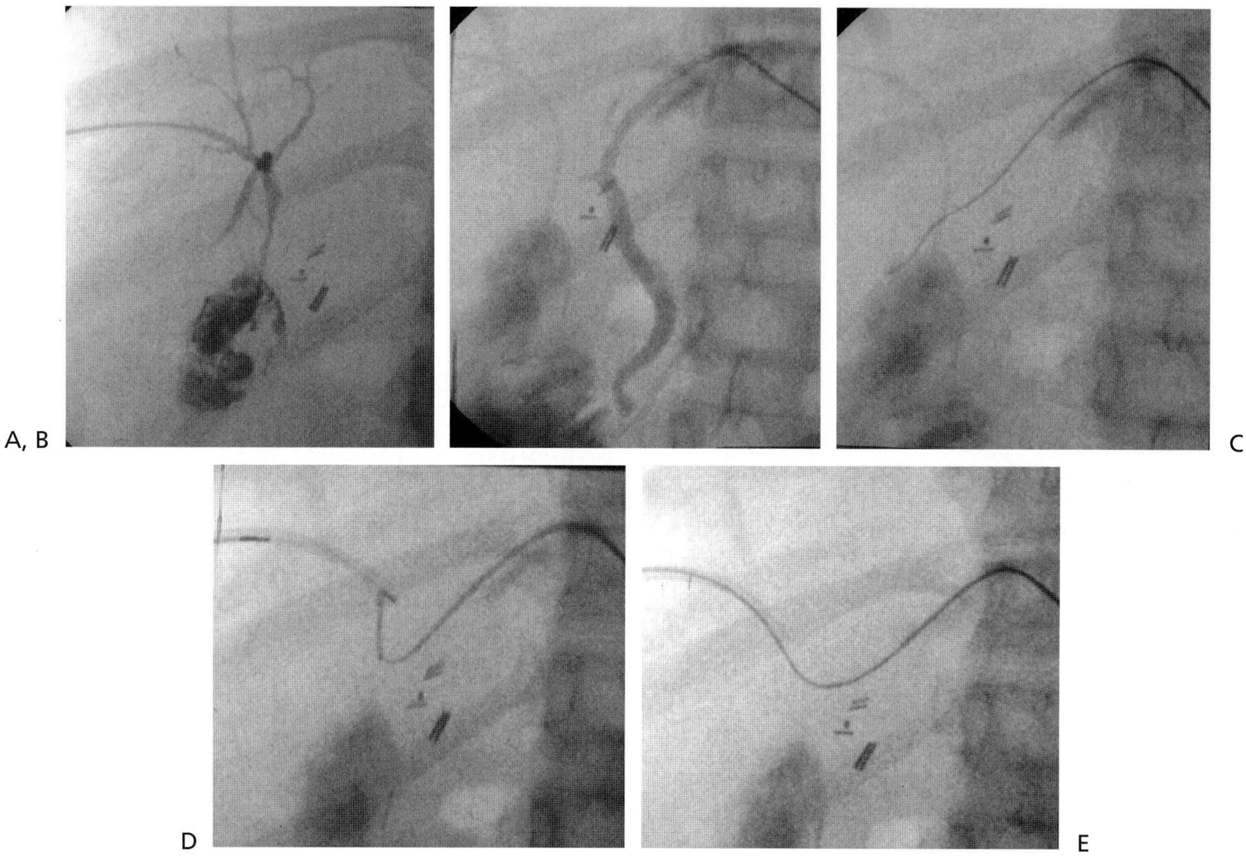

Figure 14.1.14

F

G, H

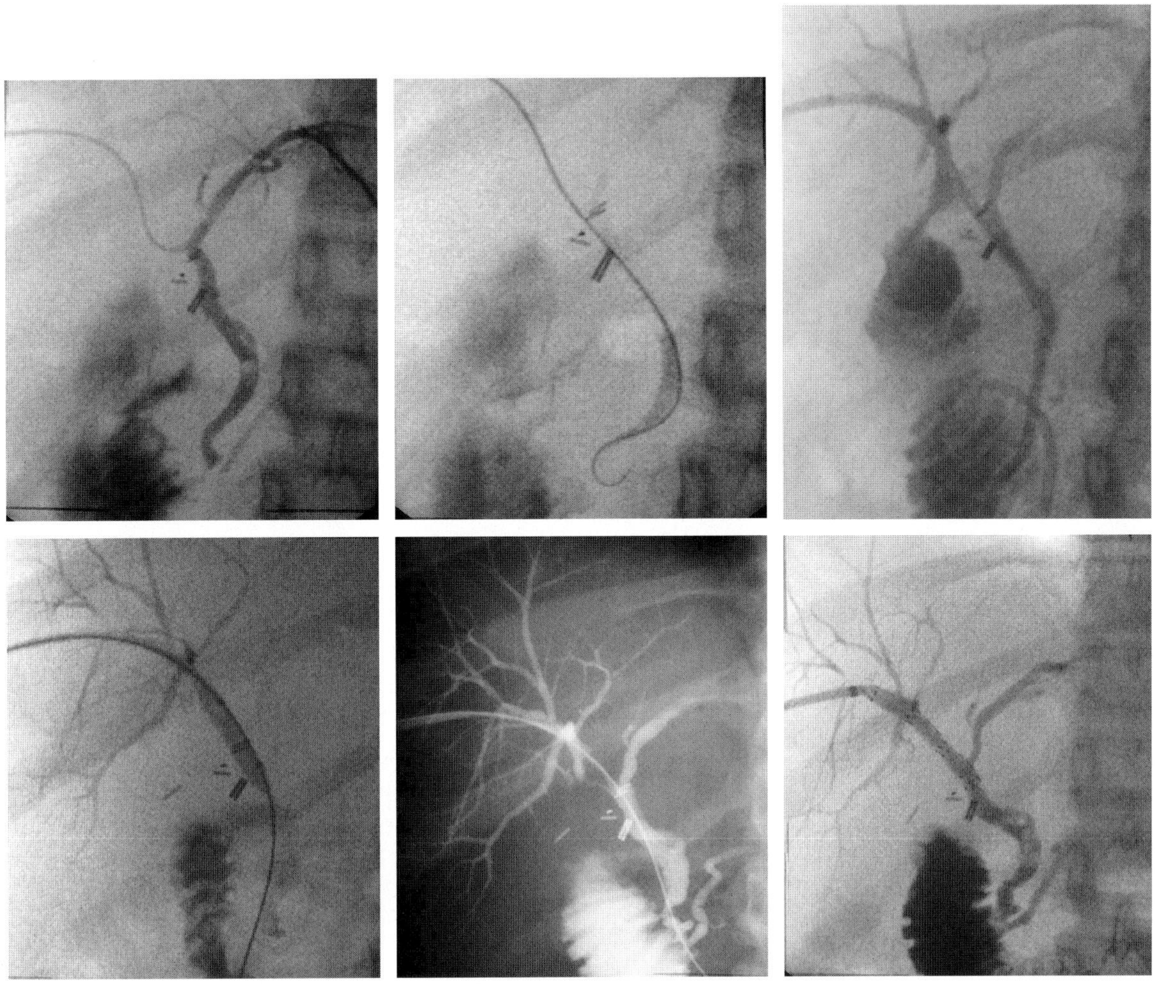

I

J, K

Figure 14.1.14 *(continued)*

A: Percutaneous transhepatic catheterization of the excluded right biliary duct with a 5F catheter was performed. The biliary fistula drains into the biloma. Note the metal clips at the liver hilum. **B:** Percutaneous access of the left bile duct with the catheter allows visualization of the unchanged common bile duct and the stump of the right bile duct, which was shattered during surgery. The catheter in the right bile duct enters the biloma. **C:** Using the left lobe approach, a steerable guidewire was manipulated through the right bile duct stump into the biloma and was in contact with the catheter introduced from the right side. **D:** The guidewire from the left was snared into the biloma using a Dormia basket and retrieved through the right bile duct into a sheath. **E:** Final position of the guidewire through and through from the epigastric puncture to the puncture on the right side, reconnecting the right bile duct with the main bile duct and passing into the sheath. **F:** Cholangiogram obtained with injection from the left-side catheter shows the normal common bile duct, the catheter reconnecting the right bile duct to the common bile duct, and the biloma and duodenum full of contrast. **G:** Catheterization of the main bile duct with a catheter and guidewire that reaches the papilla and reconnects the right bile duct with the main duct. **H:** Cholangiogram obtained after introducing an internal-external catheter from the right hepatic duct, through the transected bile duct, and into the main bile duct, reconnecting both systems. Note the normal common bile duct. The biliary fistula is still open into the biloma. Contrast flows into the duodenum. **I:** Cholangioplasty with a 6-mm balloon catheter 6 weeks after percutaneous biliary drainage. The biloma was not visible. **J:** Cholangiogram shows the stump of the occluded biliary fistula through the right percutaneous access. The biloma resolved. **K:** Final transcatheter cholangiogram after a three-body Z-stent (8 mm) was placed, bypassing the stenosis and narrowed segment at the level of the transection and reconstituting the continuity of the two biliary systems.

Comment: This case is an interesting example of a biliary laceration with detachment of the right biliary duct from the main bile duct. The through-and-through technique is the ideal approach for this type of problem. Catheterization of the biloma through the duct stump probably is the only option in this situation. In some cases, the endoscopist has the opportunity to catheterize in a retrograde fashion and achieve the same result. However, when the detachment is complete, as in this case, it is almost impossible to catheterize retrogradely without using the simultaneous percutaneous approach to snare or basket the guidewire for exteriorization through the skin. Once the straight path is achieved, balloon plasty and biliary catheter placement are straightforward. In this case, a persistent stenosis did not improve with multiple balloon plasties. This was an indication for bare stent placement to maintain the stricture open. This patient presented with two episodes of serious cholangitis in a 8-year period, which required retrograde cholangiography and brushing of the lumen of the stent to successfully clear the sludge. The patient is doing well for the last 8 years.

14.1.15 Interventional Procedures In Benign Diseases Of The Biliary Tract

Case 14.1.15:

A 33-year-old female patient underwent laparoscopic cholecystectomy followed by occlusion of the main bile duct by metal clips, requiring choledochojejunostomy. After the second surgery, the patient developed a biliary fistula, large biloma, and sepsis. The patient was septic and required emergent biliary drainage.

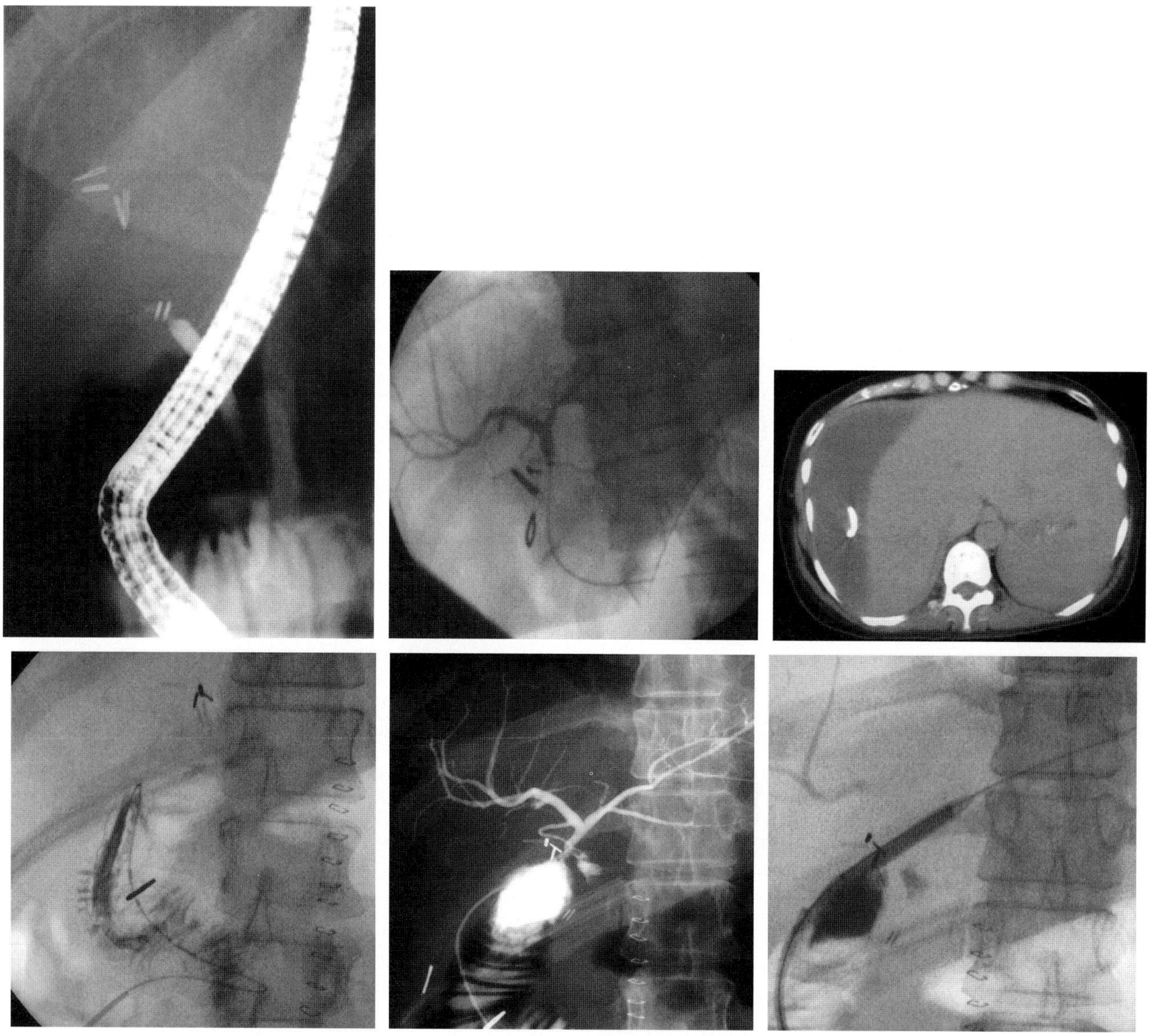

A, B C D, E F

Figure 14.1.15

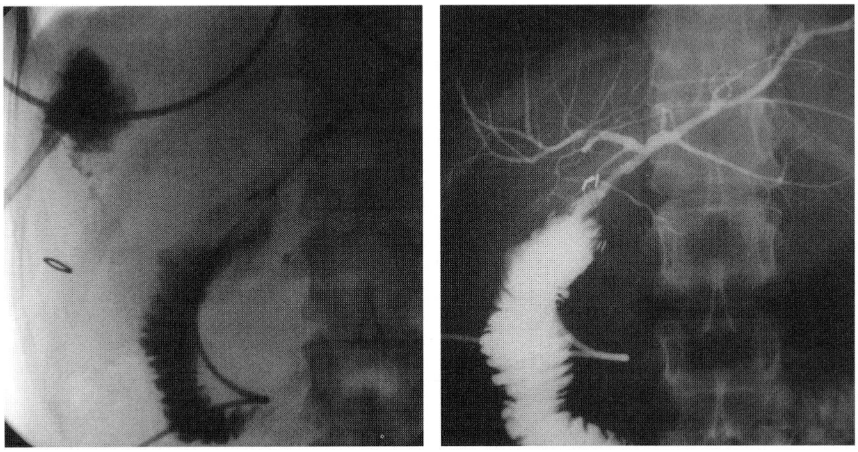

G H

Figure 14.1.15 *(continued)*

A: ERCP 2 days after surgery shows total occlusion of the main bile duct by two metal clips. **B:** Intraoperative cholangiogram shows patency of the intrahepatic bile duct and a stent into the bowel loop. **C:** Following the surgery, a biloma that developed due to a biliary fistula required CT-guided drainage. **D:** Percutaneous transjejunal approach to the biliary system was performed. It was difficult to enter the orifice because of the stenosis. **E:** After multiple attempts, biliary catheterization was performed, which demonstrated the orifice with the fistula. **F:** Balloon plasty with a 6-mm catheter was performed. **G:** Two months after drainage, there was free flow through the stenosis. Note the small size of the residual cavity of the biloma. **H:** Five-month follow-up cholangiogram shows no residual stenosis, and the catheter was removed.

Comment: Puncture of the Roux-en-Y jejunal limb can be achieved blindly or with contrast material injected transhepatically. When the stenosis is tight, it may be difficult to retrogradely catheterize the bile ducts; thus, a steerable catheter and guidewire are necessary. Balloon dilation resolves the stricture. Once the bile duct is adequately drained, the fistula usually subsides; however, in selected cases embolization of the biliary leak may be necessary. It is generally agreed that symptomatic bilomas require treatment, especially if there is evidence of continuous bile leak. Postoperative biliary leaks are difficult to manage; reexploration is difficult in the majority of cases and requires percutaneous drainage. Occasionally, a covered stent may be required to treat a biliary fistula; however, simple catheter drainage is efficient in the majority of cases. The strictures are treated successfully by cholangioplasty in about 67% to 86% of cases; 91% of patients may have all catheters removed. Success is predictable in about 75% of cases with biliary-enteric anastomosis. Restenosis may occur in about 29% of cases. The complications rate after the procedure ranges from 0% to 24.3%. Fever and sepsis may follow the procedure in 47% of cases in some series.

14.2.1 Interventional Procedures In Malignant Obstruction Of The Biliary Tract

Case 14.2.1:

A 67-year-old man with colon cancer resected 7 years earlier developed obstructed jaundice. CT scan of the abdomen, endoscopic US, and biopsy showed the cause of biliary obstruction was hilar metastatic disease. ERCP failed to properly catheterize the bile ducts, and the patient was sent for percutaneous treatment.

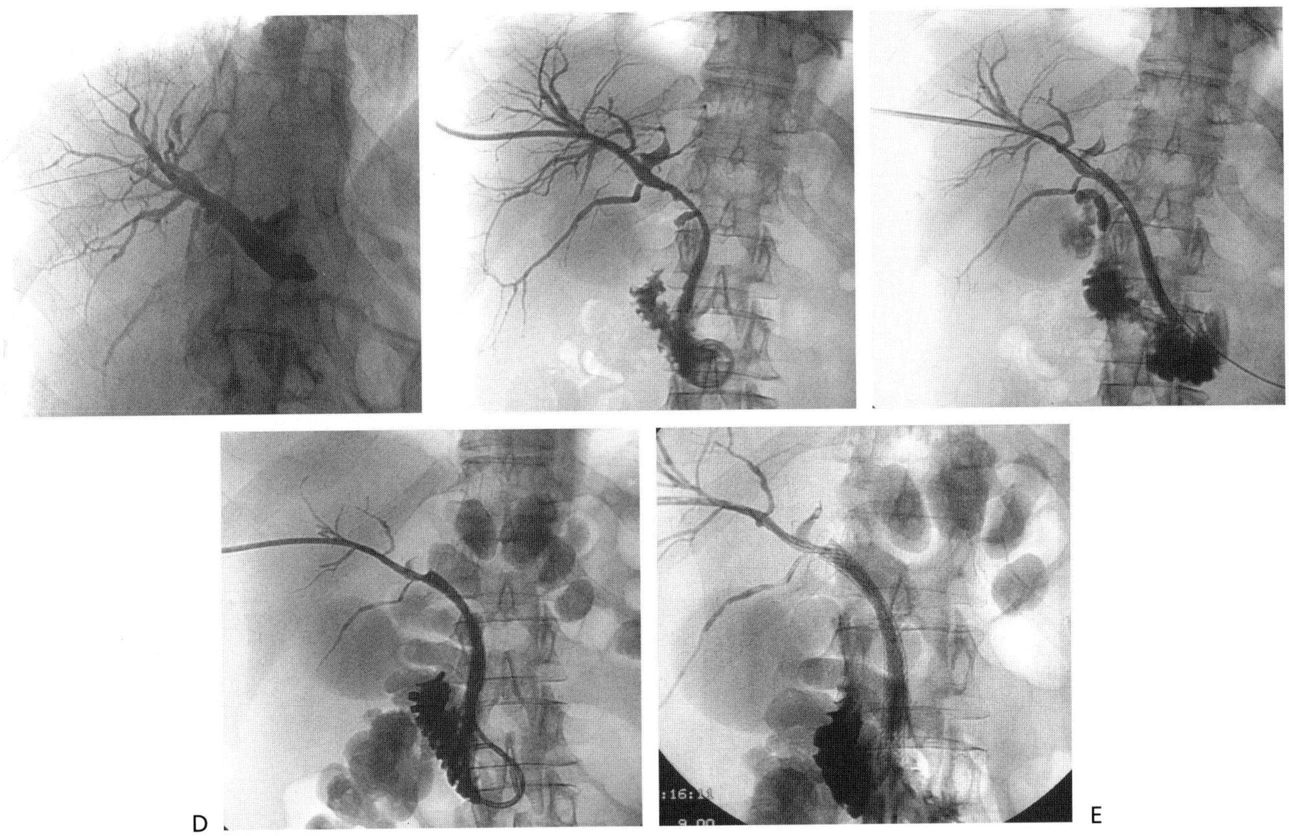

A B, C D E

Figure 14.2.1

A: PTC with a fine needle shows moderately dilated intrahepatic bile ducts with obstruction of the common bile duct. **B:** Percutaneous catheterization and drainage of the intrahepatic bile ducts was performed with an 8F catheter after crossing the obstruction and reaching the duodenum. No balloon dilation was necessary. Some degree of intrabiliary bleeding was observed. Cholangiogram obtained after 48 hours shows decompression of the intrahepatic bile ducts and free flow of contrast into the duodenum. Note the relatively long stricture in the common bile duct. **C:** A 10 × 68-mm Wallstent was placed and dilated to 6 mm only. Injection of contrast shows free flow into the duodenum. An internal-external drainage catheter was placed for another 24 hours. **D:** Catheter cholangiogram obtained the next day shows further expansion and patency of the stent. **E:** The catheter subsequently was removed. Challenge cholangiogram shows adequate patency of the stent.

Comment: Malignant biliary obstruction is a common cause of jaundice and cholestasis. Surgical biliary decompression and transhepatic biliary drainage are palliative treatments for advanced nonresectable malignant biliary obstruction. Metastatic biliary liver hilum obstruction is considered nonsurgical, and palliative treatment is indicated. ERCP with biliary stent placement is a good alternative, but if it is unavailable or unsuccessful, the percutaneous approach is an adequate alternative. In this case, the initial drainage was performed with an internal-external catheter to decompress the bile ducts and reduce potential infection before metallic stent placement. Metastatic periportal lymphadenopathy may be more indolent than pancreatic cancer. With adjuvant therapies, such as chemotherapy and radiation therapy, longer survivals may be expected. Catheter drainage is indicated more for patients with longer survival because access is maintained.

14.2.2 Interventional Procedures In Malignant Obstruction Of The Biliary Tract

Case 14.2.2:

A 67-year-old man with colon cancer resected 2 years earlier developed obstructed jaundice. US of the abdomen and ERCP showed the biliary ducts were obstructed by periportal metastatic disease. The patient was sent for percutaneous treatment.

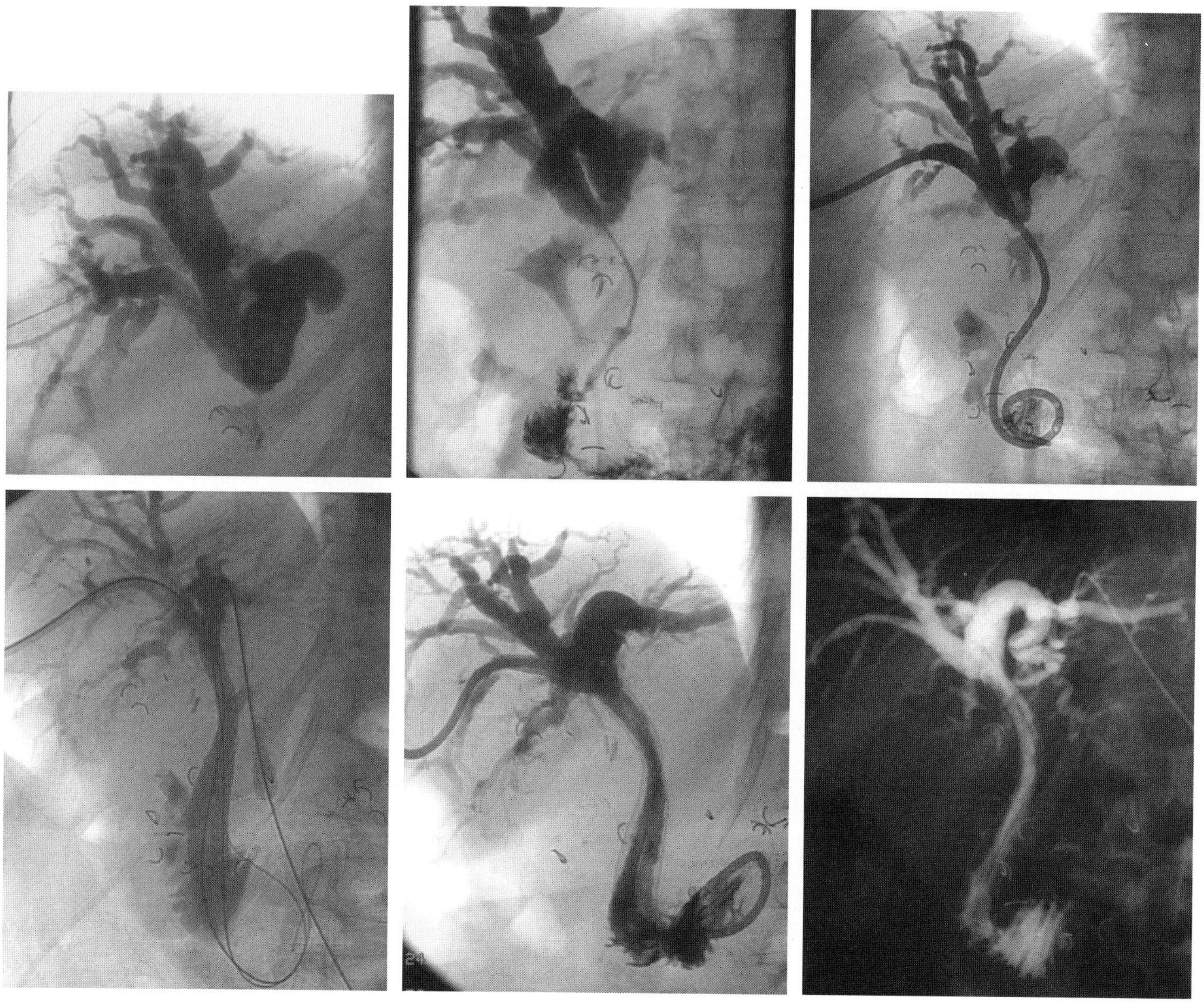

A, B C
D, E F

Figure 14.2.2

A: PTC shows dilated intrahepatic bile ducts with high common bile obstruction. **B:** Percutaneous catheterization allowed passing of the extensive obstruction. Note the small distal bile duct draining into the duodenum. **C:** A 10F biliary catheter was used for internal-external biliary drainage. **D:** After a few days, bilateral biliary access was obtained for placement of bilateral stents, which were placed because of the high level of obstruction, which could progress to total occlusion due to proximal extension of the lesion. **E:** A drainage catheter was kept through the stent for 48 hours. Cholangiogram through the catheter shows patency of the stents. **F:** Cholangiogram obtained after removal of the catheter shows stent patency. Survival of this patient was short, only 6 months.

Comment: Periportal metastatic disease is a good application for metallic stents because the obstructive lesion is generally noninfiltrative and there is no tumor growth into the stent. Although endoscopic plastic stents also can be used for palliation, they require multiple endoscopic procedures for stent exchange. Metallic stents also are preferred for endoscopic drainage. Although they are an important refinement in the technique, metallic stents cannot be replaced, and restenting or catheter drainage may be necessary for long-term survival.

14.2.3 Interventional Procedures In Malignant Obstruction Of The Biliary Tract

Case 14.2.3:

A 67-year-old man with colon cancer resected 7 years earlier developed obstructed jaundice. CT scan of the abdomen, endoscopic US, and biopsy showed the cause of biliary obstruction was hilar metastatic disease. ERCP failed to properly catheterize the bile ducts, and the patient was sent for percutaneous treatment.

A, B

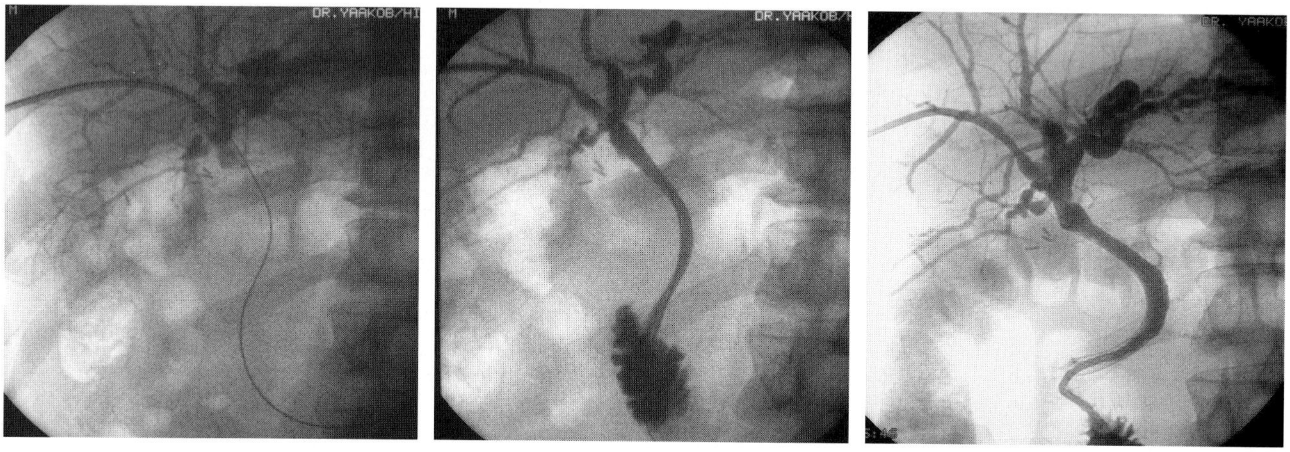

C

Figure 14.2.3

A: Percutaneous cholangiography shows dilated intrahepatic bile ducts and obstruction of the common bile duct. After catheterization of the bile duct, a guidewire was introduced through the obstruction and reached the duodenum. **B:** A 10 × 90-mm Wallstent was placed, and the balloon was dilated to 6 mm to achieve patency of the bile duct in the cholangiogram. **C:** An 8F catheter was placed for temporary internal-external drainage for 48 hours and subsequently removed. The final cholangiogram is not shown.

Comment: The metal stent initially was placed for internal drainage, instead of a catheter. In general, it is preferable to begin drainage using a catheter and then exchange the catheter for a metallic stent after infection and bleeding are controlled and clinical improvement is achieved. In this case, there was no significant bleeding or infection, and a decision was made to place the stent immediately. A catheter was kept in place for 2 days and then removed successfully.

14.2.4 Interventional Procedures In Malignant Obstruction Of The Biliary Tract

Case 14.2.4:

A 50-year-old man with a large nonfunctioning islet cell tumor of the pancreas that had been resected presented with recurrent biliary obstruction and jaundice. Percutaneous drainage was requested.

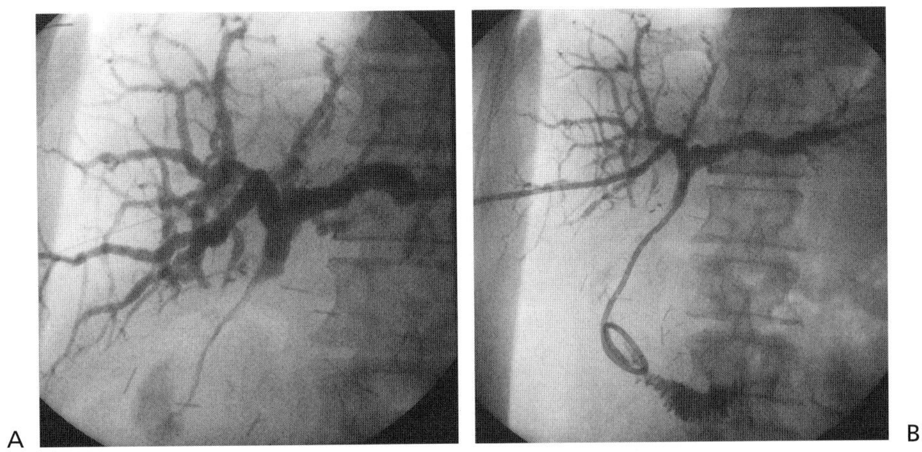

Figure 14.2.4

A: PTC shows a long stenosis in the common bile duct. **B:** A 10F catheter was placed for internal-external drainage. Following clinical improvement, the patient was taken to surgery for choledochojejunostomy.

Comment: Fine-needle cholangiogram and percutaneous internal-external biliary drainage can be used as a temporary measure for recurrent biliary obstruction. In this case, the obstruction was not related to tumor recurrence but to scar tissue. Biliary drainage can result in clinical improvement of the patient until surgery can be performed. If the lesion is untreatable by surgery, a metal stent can be placed.

14.2.5 Interventional Procedures In Malignant Obstruction Of The Biliary Tract

Case 14.2.5:

A 44-year-old woman presented with pancreatic cancer and biliary obstruction. ERCP showed the obstruction but did not allow placement of a stent for adequate drainage. Percutaneous biliary drainage was requested for palliation.

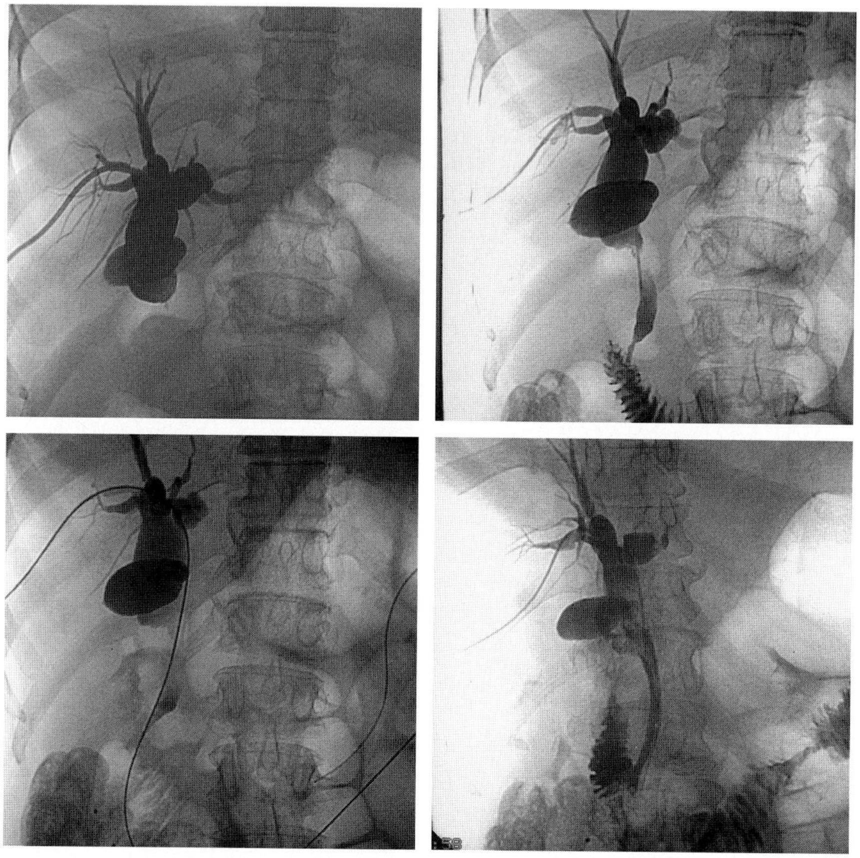

A B C D

Figure 14.2.5

A: PTC shows dilated intrahepatic bile ducts with abrupt occlusion of the common bile duct. Note the cystic duct and gallbladder overlapping the bile duct. It was not possible to pass the obstruction. Temporary external drainage for 48 hours was achieved using an 8F catheter. **B:** Catheterization through the obstruction with a Lunderquist guidewire allowed injection into the distal nondilated bile duct draining into the duodenum through the papilla. Note the relatively small segment of occlusion. The tumor was inoperable. **C:** Following catheterization of the distal bile duct, a guidewire was passed into the duodenum and the tract was dilated. **D:** A 10 × 68-mm Wallstent was placed into the bile duct to overcome the tumoral obstruction. Note adequate initial patency of the stent.

Comment: Metallic biliary stents are used in patients with a malignant biliary stricture who are not surgical candidates. One of the most common causes of malignant biliary strictures is pancreatic cancer causing a middle or distal obstruction. Stent length may vary according to the length of the lesion to be treated. Usually, a 68-mm-long stent should be used for common bile duct obstruction. Most common stent diameters needed to drain an occluded bile duct range from 8 to 10 mm. Stent deployment is generally successful and results in relief of jaundice. Displacement of the Wallstent is rare but may occur, especially if the stent is introduced inside the duodenum through the papilla. Thirty-day mortality in patients with pancreatic cancer may be as high as 20%. Median survival time is about 3 months, despite initial clinical improvement. Recurrent occlusion is more common in patients with tumor growth into the bile duct lumen and may occur in as many as 30% to 40% of patients 2 to 6 months after drainage. Causes of occlusion include tumor ingrowth, tumor overgrowth, and granulation tissue.

14.2.6 Interventional Procedures In Malignant Obstruction Of The Biliary Tract

Case 14.2.6:

A 61-year-old man with pancreatic cancer had a tumor resection and a Whipple procedure, including choledochojejunostomy. About 1 year after surgery, jaundice developed due to tumor recurrence. Percutaneous biliary drainage was requested for palliation.

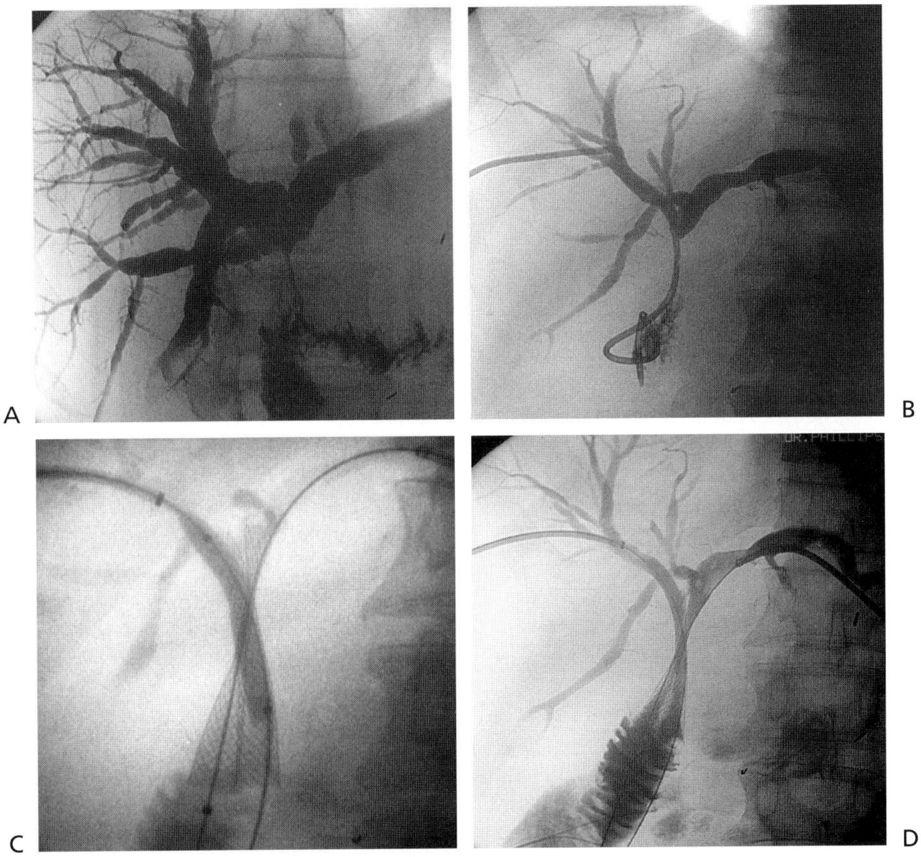

Figure 14.2.6

A: Percutaneous cholangiogram shows dilated intrahepatic bile ducts. Note the relatively long stricture and filling of the bowel loop with contrast. **B:** Following catheterization of the stricture and balloon dilation, an internal-external drainage catheter was placed. **C:** After 2 days of external drainage, the left side was accessed and bilateral Wallstent placement was performed. **D:** Cholangiogram obtained after stent placement shows adequate internal drainage. The introducer sheaths were removed.

Comment: Metallic biliary endoprostheses have been widely accepted in clinical practice, due to patient comfort compared to that of an internal-external catheter. Metallic stents achieve large diameters and theoretically last longer than plastic endoprostheses. Because metallic stents are introduced in a collapsed form, an additional benefit of the technique is the reduced introductory tract compared to larger-diameter catheters or plastic stents. However, there still is some controversy regarding the clinical efficacy of metallic stents compared to plastic stents.

In this particular case, a bilateral approach with simultaneous Wallstent placement was used due to the high level of the obstruction. If only one stent were used, there would have been an increased risk of early occlusion of the unstented side. In this case, a self-expandable, flexible stent was selected due to the length of the obstruction and tortuosity of the tract. Technically, implantation of a metallic stent is similar to implantation of a plastic stent. Although these stents can be placed endoscopically, in this case it was not possible due to the nature of the previous surgical procedure.

14.2.7 Interventional Procedures In Malignant Obstruction Of The Biliary Tract

Case 14.2.7:

A 42-year-old woman presented with cholangiocarcinoma and obstruction of the common bile duct. ERCP showed the obstruction, and a nasobiliary tube was placed for initial drainage. Permanent percutaneous biliary drainage with stent placement was requested for palliation.

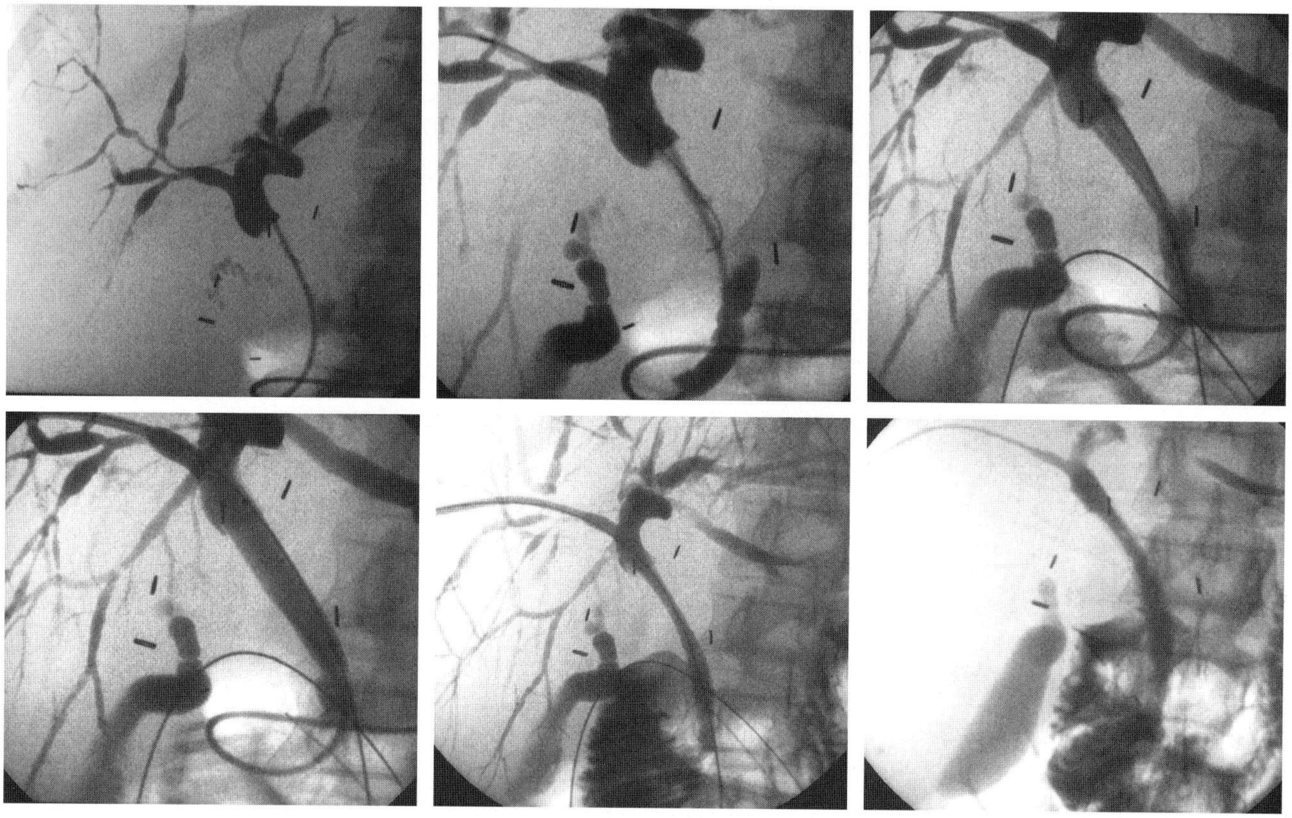

A, B C

D, E F

Figure 14.2.7

A: Initial cholangiogram performed through the nasobiliary tube shows dilated intrahepatic bile ducts. **B:** The right biliary duct was catheterized, and a steerable guidewire was advanced through the occlusion. **C:** A catheter was advanced through the stenosis. **D:** Plasty was performed with a 6-mm balloon. **E:** A 10 × 68-mm Wallstent was placed for internal drainage. **F:** Final cholangiogram control, obtained 24 hours later, shows patency of the stent. The percutaneous catheter was removed.

Comment: Metallic stents provide good palliative drainage and are well tolerated by patients. It is simple and safe to use and may reduce hospital stay. Migration problems are minimal. Proximal and distal overgrowth of the tumor is possible, but ingrowth through the wall into the spaces between struts probably is a more common cause of occlusion. In general, bare stents are sufficient to maintain the bile ducts open for long periods of time. Intraluminal tumors, such as cholangiocarcinomas, probably are more prone to grow within a stent than pancreatic carcinomas, which only invade or compress the bile ducts. In this case, only one stent was believed to be necessary; however, if the lesion had been higher, bilateral stenting possibly would be needed. In this case, the stent was deployed above the papilla and the sphincter mechanism was preserved. In some cases where the stent is above the papilla, spasm of the sphincter or kinking of the distal bile duct may develop and cause secondary obstruction. Deployment of the stent through the papilla, inside the duodenum, does not preserve the sphincteric mechanism, and the bile duct is always open to the duodenal lumen. Although the secondary causes of obstruction are avoided, reflux of duodenal content into the stent may cause mechanical obstruction of bile flow and recurrent cholangitis. Antibiotic prophylaxis should be given before treatment if cholangitis is clinically detected and continued for at least 5 to 7 days. In some cases, erosion of the duodenal wall may be caused by the sharp end of the stent, and GI bleeding may be a serious complication.

14.2.8 Interventional Procedures In Malignant Obstruction Of The Biliary Tract

Case 14.2.8:

A 51-year-old man with cholangiocarcinoma was treated endoscopically with one Wallstent, which subsequently occluded. A plastic stent was placed within the metal stent. Cholangitis developed due to obstruction of the left side, and percutaneous drainage was necessary.

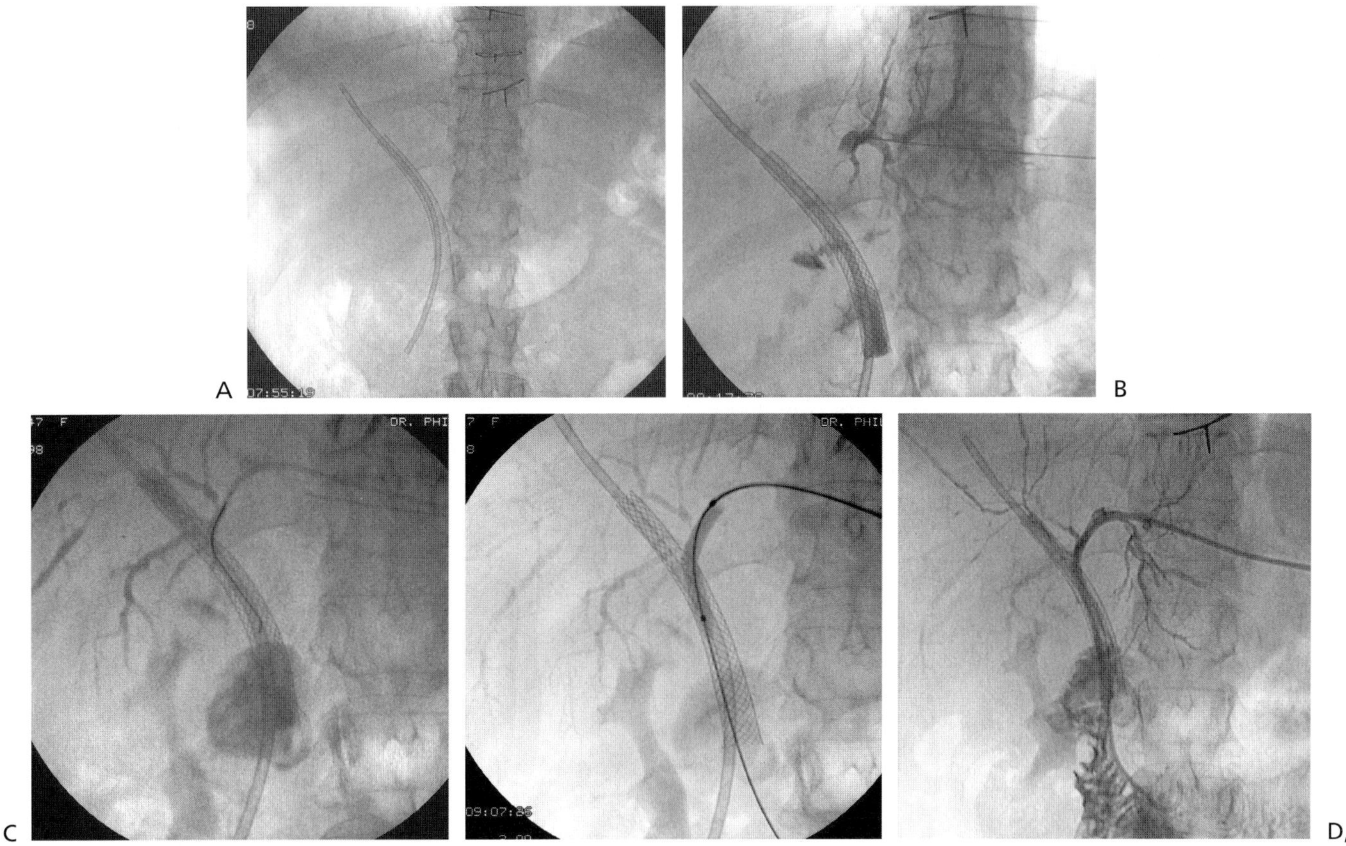

Figure 14.2.8

A: Plain film of the abdomen shows the Wallstent and the plastic stent within the metal stent. **B:** Left-side PTC shows occlusion extending into the left bile duct. **C:** After careful manipulation, a guidewire was advanced into the obstruction, through the stent mesh, and into the main lumen of the stent. **D:** Dilation of the stent mesh was performed with a balloon catheter to allow for left-side internal-external drainage. **E:** An internal-external drainage catheter was advanced to drain the left bile duct and reduce the infection.

Comment: It usually is difficult to anticipate which patient will survive longer and, thus, decide the correct type of drainage for that specific patient. Some patients with cholangiocarcinoma may have a significantly longer survival than others, and metallic stents will not stay open for the entire survival period. Endoscopic restenting usually will resolve the obstruction. Placement of bilateral metallic stents by endoscopic technique is more difficult. When one of the bile ducts is excluded by a single stent, as demonstrated in this case, catheterization of the occluded side is nearly impossible by ERCP. Percutaneous catheterization and stenting of the occluded side are necessary for access and infection control. To cross the stent mesh, a small steerable wire is necessary, followed by progressive balloon dilation and catheterization or stenting across the wall. To overcome the flexibility and recoil of the stent wall, a balloon-expandable stent may be necessary. Biliary decompression usually is considered successful when the levels of serum bilirubin drop by more than 30%. In a recent publication, the use of metallic stents was compared with plastic stents for malignant biliary obstructions. The metallic self-expanding stents appeared to provide substantial benefits to patients. The 30-day mortality rate was lower with metal stents (10% vs. 24%). The obstruction rate was 19% versus 27%, with a better median patency. Hospital stay also was shorter (10 vs. 21 days).

14.2.9 Interventional Procedures In Malignant Obstruction Of The Biliary Tract

Case 14.2.9:

A 79-year-old woman presented with cholangiocarcinoma and biliary obstruction. Percutaneous biliary drainage was requested for palliation.

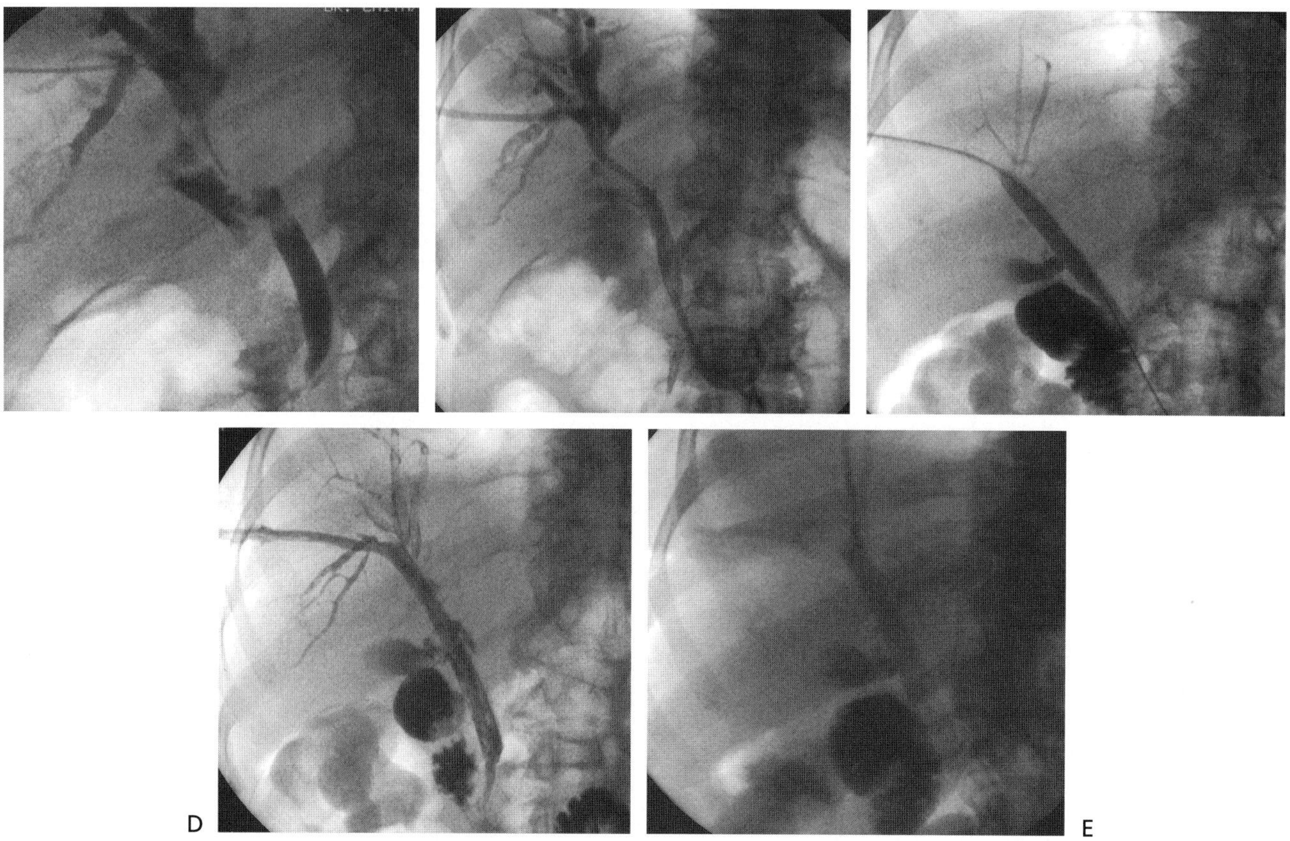

A, B C D E

Figure 14.2.9

A: Percutaneous cholangiogram shows a proximal obstruction by tumor growth 2 cm from the biliary confluence. Note filling of the distal common bile duct after the obstruction was crossed with a small catheter. **B:** An internal-external catheter was placed for external drainage for a few days. **C:** Follow-up procedure included balloon dilation and replacement of the catheter for a Wallstent. **D:** Cholangiogram performed just after stent placement shows multiple filling defects resulting from intrabiliary bleeding. Despite the bleeding, drainage into the duodenum was adequate. The catheter was pulled out. **E:** Final cholangiogram shows patency. The intraparenchymatous tract was embolized with a VasoSeal plug.

Comment: One of the complications related to percutaneous biliary drainage is intrabiliary bleeding. Usually the bleeding is of venous origin and self-limited. Occasionally, bleedings may originate from an artery and generally requires more aggressive treatment. It usually is sufficient to keep the catheter draining open in a bag. The bleeding will stop and the bile will clear. However, when there is a side hole of the catheter inside a branch of the portal vein or hepatic vein, repositioning of the catheter will be necessary. When the tract traverses a venous structure, bleeding may occur upon retrieval of the catheter, with temporary occlusion of the stent. Embolization of the tract with cyanoacrylate or a VasoSeal plug is a fast and reliable way to seal off the tract and control bleeding. Care should be exercised to avoid embolization of the bile ducts or the stent.

14.2.10 Interventional Procedures In Malignant Obstruction Of The Biliary Tract

Case 14.2.10:

A 42-year-old man presented with cholangiocarcinoma and biliary obstruction. Percutaneous biliary drainage for palliation and brachytherapy with iridium seeds was requested.

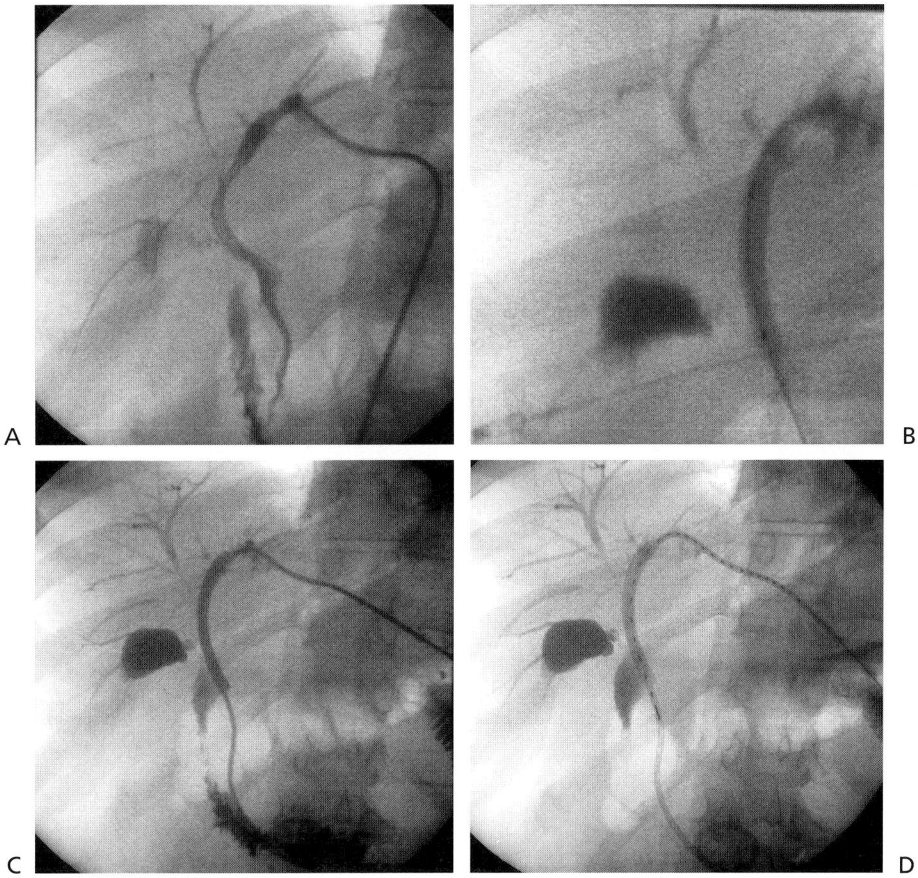

Figure 14.2.10

A: Cholangiogram following catheterization of the bile ducts shows a long occlusion of the common bile duct. **B:** After catheterization, balloon plasty with a 6-mm catheter was performed. **C:** A 10 × 40-mm Wallstent was placed to traverse the obstruction, and a 10F catheter was placed to guide the brachytherapy radiopaque wire marker. The right bile duct was not drained. **D:** Photograph with the brachytherapy marker obtained for guidance.

Comment: Percutaneous drainage provides easy access for insertion of iridium seeds for brachytherapy, which is used to improve local control of the malignancy. The results of brachytherapy are not well established. Some patients respond well with control of tumor growth, whereas other patients do not respond at all. It appears that brachytherapy may reduce tumor growth into the stent and extends stent patency in patients with cholangiocarcinoma. Survival is extended in this group of patients compared with other groups of patients treated with stents alone. Intraluminal iridium-192 therapy for other extrahepatic bile duct malignant diseases is not as effective. Following treatment, the catheter can be removed and the patient can undergo other adjuvant therapies, if necessary.

14.2.11 Interventional Procedures In Malignant Obstruction Of The Biliary Tract

Case 14.2.11:

A 61-year-old man with inoperable extensive cholangiocarcinoma and biliary obstruction was referred for endoscopic treatment. ERCP showed the biliary occlusion at the level of the confluence. Acute massive hemorrhage ensued, with hemodynamic instability, decreased hematocrit, and hypotension. At that time, the endoscopist requested an emergency hepatic arteriogram and possible embolization to control the bleeding. Biliary drainage was performed 5 days later when the patient was more stable.

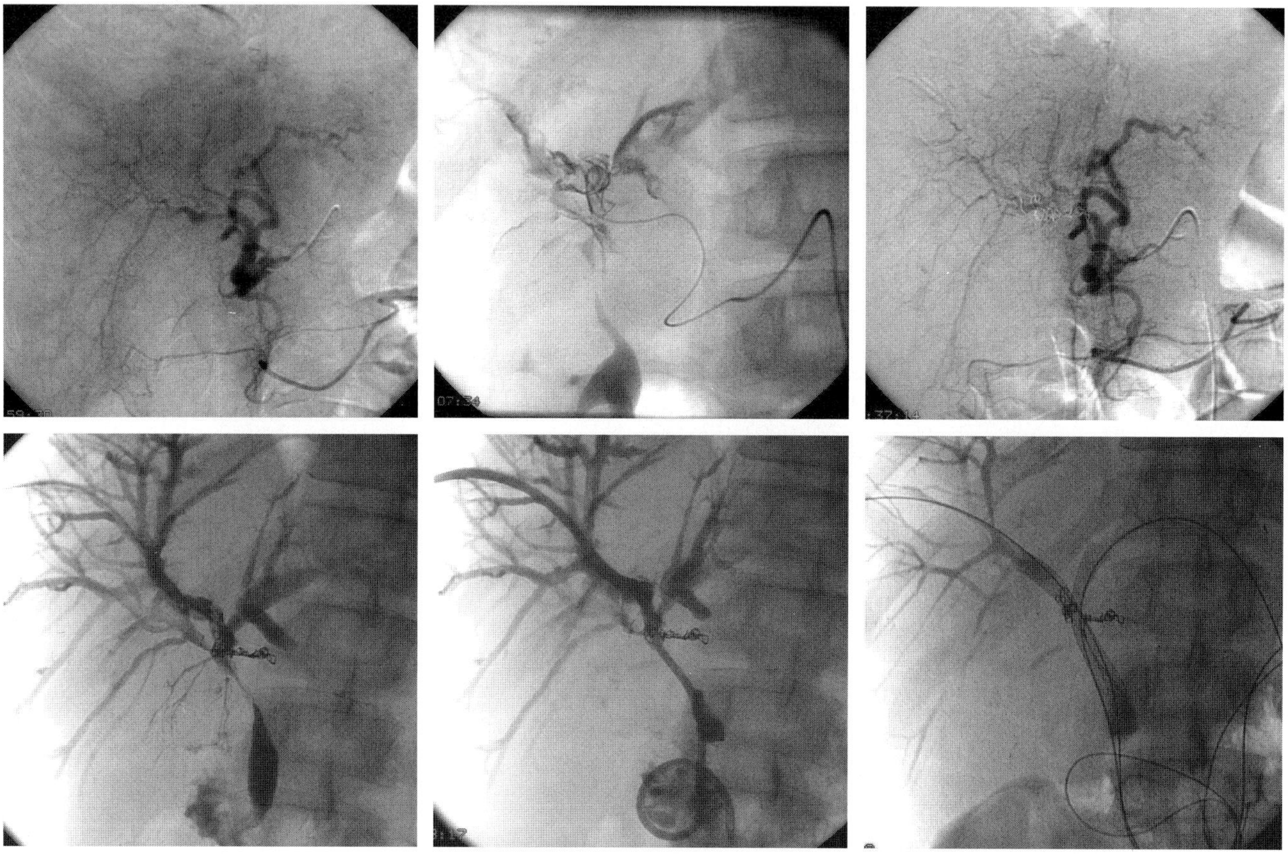

Figure 14.2.11

A: Hepatic arteriogram shows a fusiform pseudoaneurysm in the right hepatic artery. **B:** A microcatheter was advanced to the level of the pseudoaneurysm. A hand injection produced opacification of the bile ducts, which are full of clots. Note the filling defects within the bile ducts. **C:** Embolization with microcoils was performed. Postembolization hepatic angiography shows occlusion of the aneurysm, and the bleeding was controlled. **D:** Five days after bleeding control, percutaneous biliary drainage was performed. PTC shows bile ducts dilation. The right bile duct was catheterized. Injection at the level of the obstruction shows the relationship of the bile duct with the coils. **E:** An 8F catheter was placed across the obstruction and internal-external drainage was obtained. Cholangiogram shows catheter patency. **F:** Forty-eight hours later, left-side access was obtained and two Wallstents were placed side by side. **G:** Injection through the catheters shows adequate patency of the stents. The catheters were removed. **H:** A late picture shows adequate emptying of the bile ducts and verifies patency of the stents. **I:** Five months after stent placement, the patient developed mild jaundice and cholangitis, suggesting stent occlusion. Left percutaneous cholangiography shows patency of the left-side stent. **J:** Right PTC shows occlusion of the stent and multiple small peripheral abscesses. **K,L:** Intraluminal ultrasound shows the stent full of material (tumor?) and the coils. **M:** An internal-external drainage catheter was placed to treat the infection. The patient died 2 months after catheter drainage.

Comment: Complications related to biliary stent placement range from 14% to 20%. Hemorrhagic complications of biliary drainage occur in fewer than 5% to 7% of cases and usually are related to parenchymatous

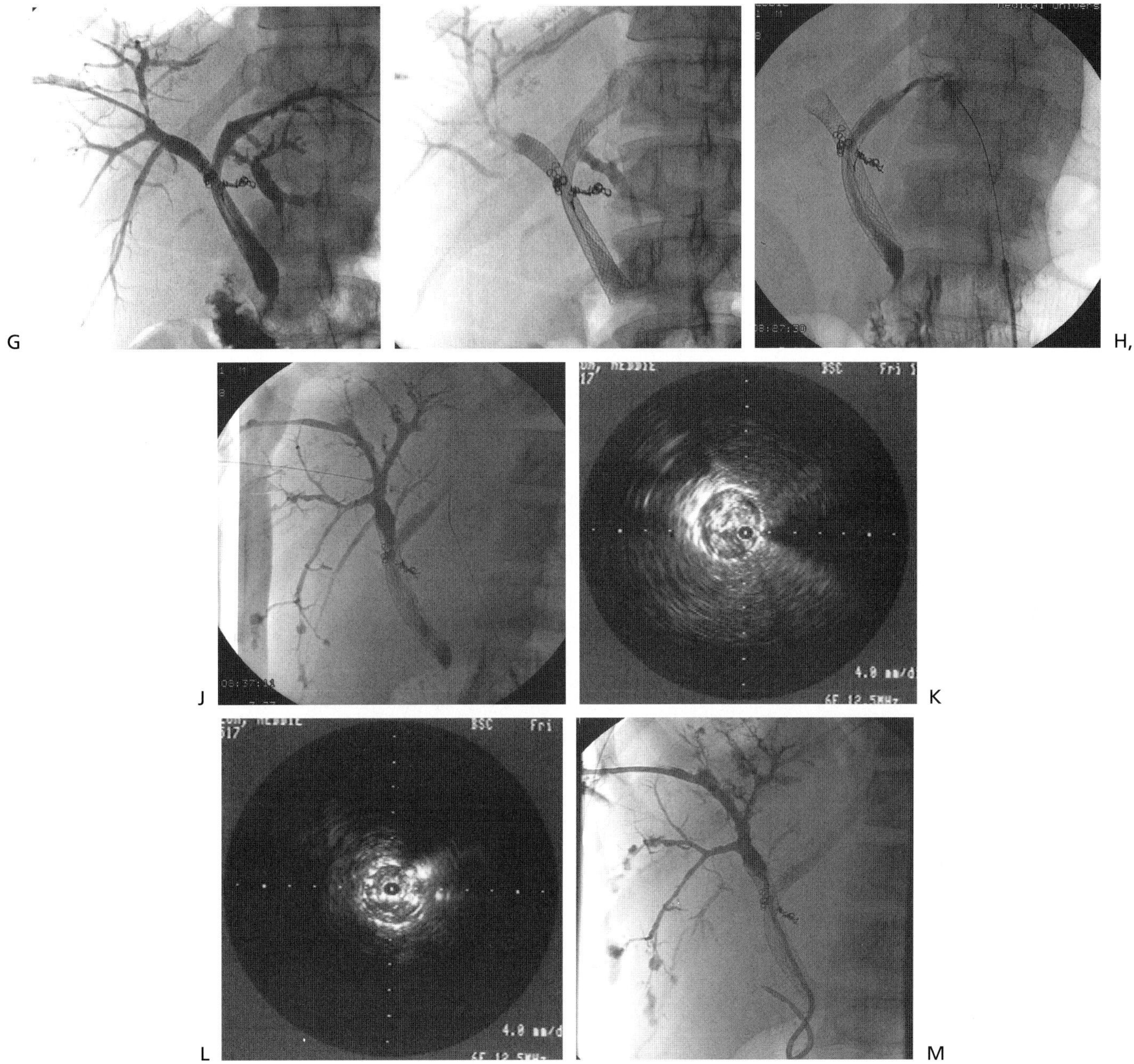

Figure 14.2.11 *(continued)*

tract trauma, with venous or arterial perforation/laceration. Spontaneous bleeding by tumor invasion is relatively rare, but cholangiocarcinomas and hepatocellular carcinomas may invade the bile ducts and actively bleed. The bleeding usually is diffuse. On most cases, one single artery cannot be identified as the cause of bleeding. The arteriogram performed in the case reported here showed a pseudoaneurysm in the right hepatic artery, which was the cause of bleeding. Bile duct erosion and bleeding were related to the pseudoaneurysm. Endoscopic manipulation may have been the traumatic starting factor for the bleeding, but probably not related to pseudoaneurysm formation. The bleeding was massive, and an emergency arteriogram was indicated. Embolization with microcoils was a life-saving procedure, and the patient recovered rapidly. Unfortunately, the stents did not stay open long enough and had to be redrained. However, hemorrhage was permanently controlled.

14.2.12 Interventional Procedures In Malignant Obstruction Of The Biliary Tract

Case 14.2.12:

A 64-year-old woman with resected pancreatic carcinoma presented with recurrent jaundice, white stools, and pain. A Whipple procedure was performed with choledocho-jejunostomy. Recurrent disease was suspected. Percutaneous biliary drainage was requested.

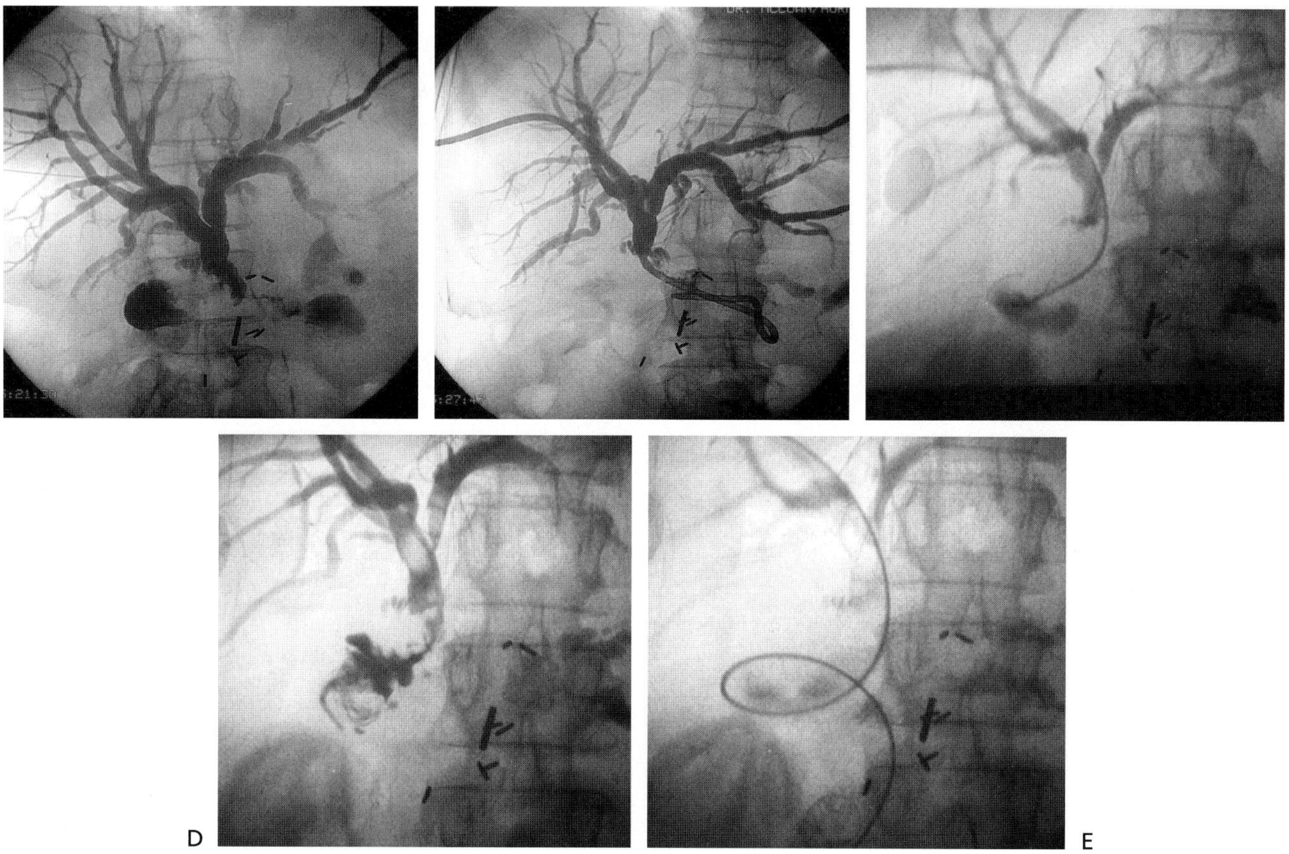

A, B C D E

Figure 14.2.12

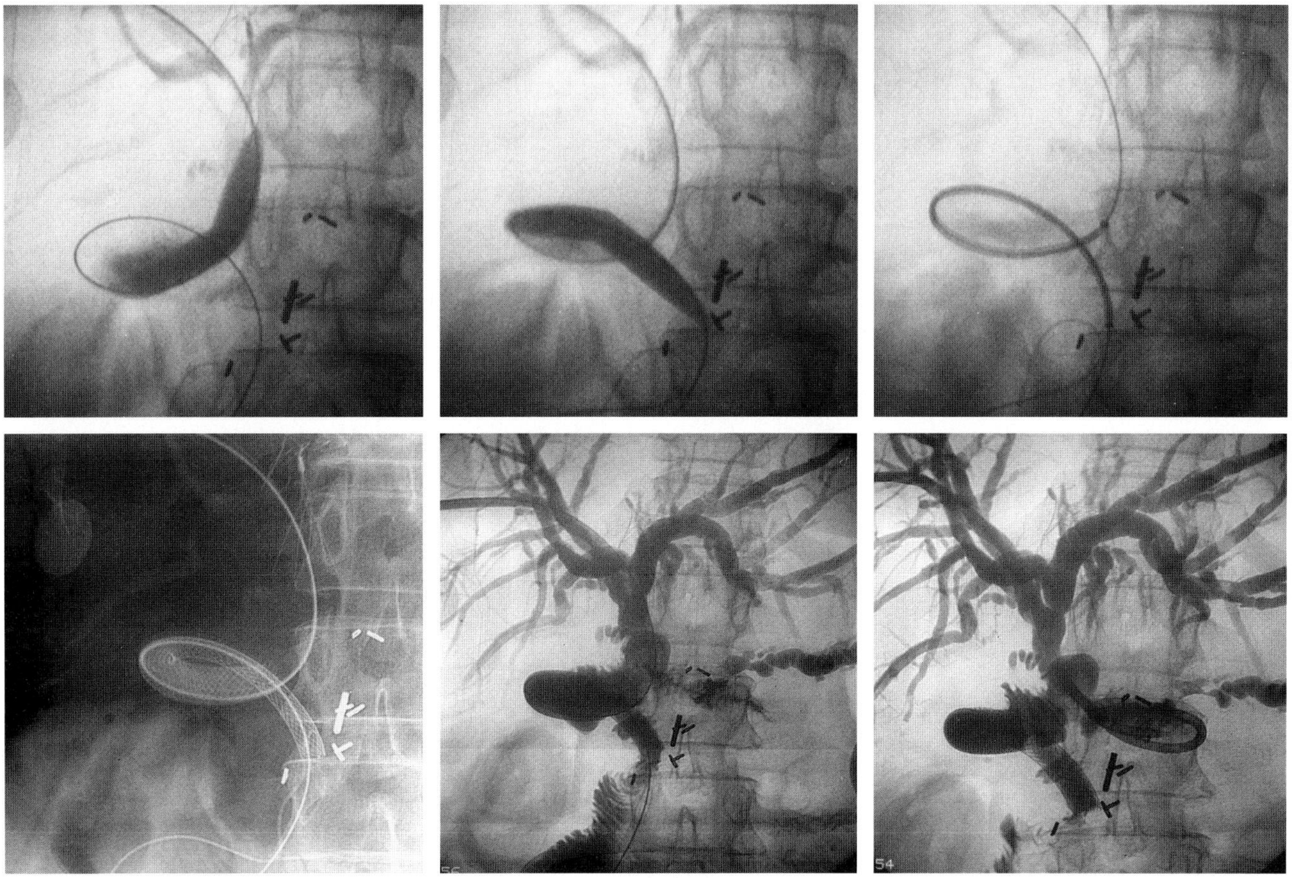

F G, H I J, K

Figure 14.2.12 *(continued)*

A: PTC demonstrates dilated intrahepatic bile ducts with irregularities at the level of the choledochojejunostomy but no significant stenosis. **B:** The bile duct was catheterized, the tract dilated, and choledochojejunostomy dilated with an 8-mm balloon, followed by placement of a 10F internal-external drainage catheter. Stenosis and occlusion of the bowel loop were evidenced by the lack of contrast flow. In this case, the jaundice was related to bowel loop stricture and not occlusion of the bile duct. **C–E:** Three days later, catheterization of the stenotic bowel loop was performed, with advancement of the heavy-duty guidewire beyond the stenosis. **F,G:** Balloon dilation of the stenosis was performed. **H,I:** A 12 × 90-mm Wallstent was placed. **J:** Cholangiogram with the guidewire still in place shows patent stent and bowel loop. **K:** A 10F catheter was placed for internal drainage. The catheter subsequently was removed, and the patient survived for 6 months.

Comment: Recurrent tumor may not only obstruct the bile duct but also infiltrate the bowel loop used for choledochojejunostomy. Even if the anastomosis is treated, the bowel loop will require some type of decompression. In this case, the bowel loop occlusion was causing the biliary outlet obstruction and jaundice. Although the biliary anastomosis was irregular, there was no significant obstruction. Balloon plasty alone is not sufficient to treat bowel stricture; a stent is necessary for decompression. In this case, a long Wallstent was selected because of the need for flexibility to overcome the tortuosity of the bowel loop. Decompression within the stent lasted for the remaining 6-month survival of the patient. There was only one episode of jaundice, which was related to cholangitis.

14.2.13 Interventional Procedures In Malignant Obstruction Of The Biliary Tract

Case 14.2.13:

A 59-year-old woman presented with jaundice and a previous history of a choledochal cyst 37 years before, when she was 22 years old, which was treated by duodenal-cystic anastomosis. Biopsy demonstrated advanced cholangiocarcinoma of the walls of the choledochal cyst extending into the intrahepatic bile ducts and duodenum. Initial percutaneous biliary drainage was performed. A percutaneous approach in conjunction with endoscopy was later performed. Endoscopy revealed a hole in the wall of the duodenum above the papilla.

A, B

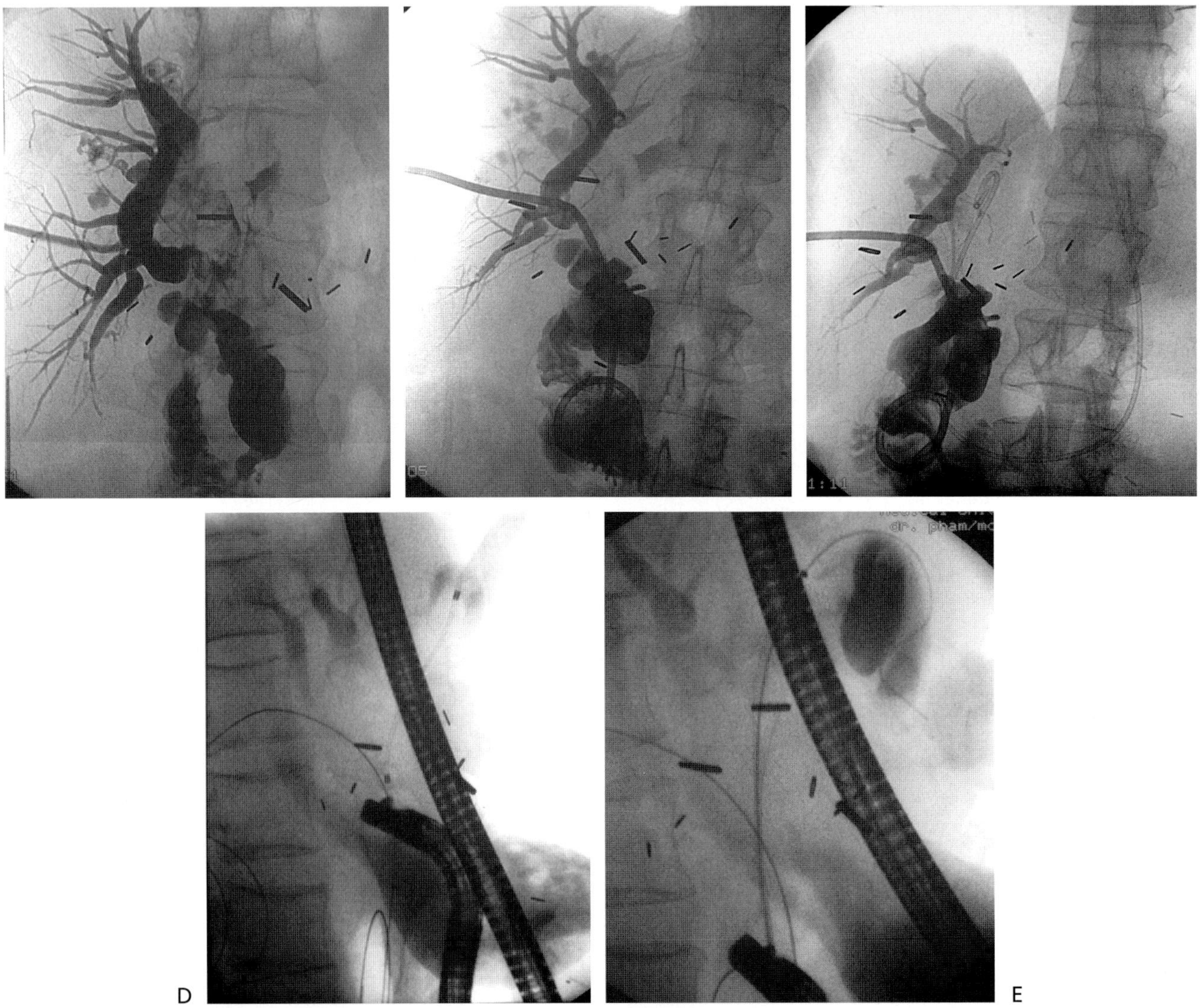

C

D

E

Figure 14.2.13

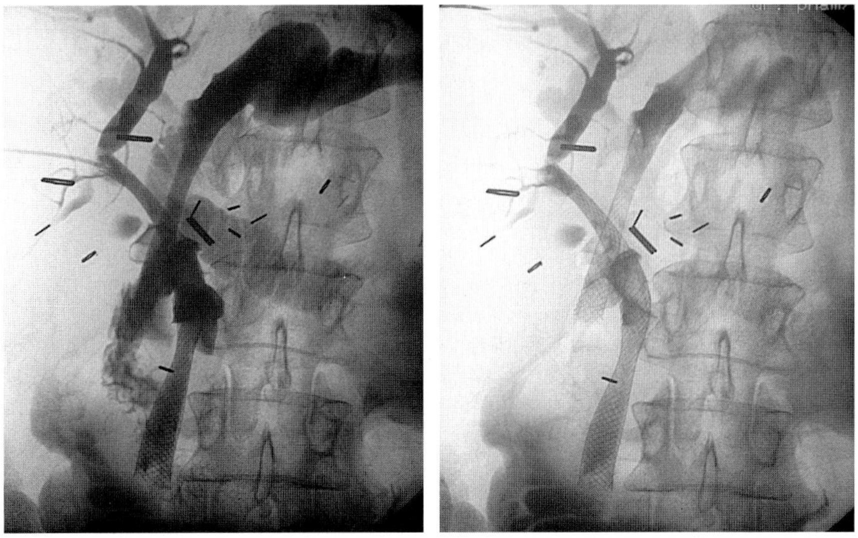

F G

Figure 14.2.13 *(continued)*

A: PTC shows biliary dilation and massive filling defects inside the bile ducts and choledochal cyst that were causing biliary obstruction. **B:** An internal-external catheter was placed in the bile ducts, through the cyst (tumor), and into the duodenum. **C:** Cholangiogram performed about 1 week after the initial procedure and after a nasobiliary tube was placed into the left duct, through the duodenal-cystic anastomosis, shows partial decompression of the intrahepatic bile ducts. **D:** The right biliary catheter was removed, and endoscopic selective catheterization of the left duct was performed for stent placement. **E:** A Wallstent was placed through the anastomosis into the left bile duct. **F:** Two long Wallstents were placed for internal drainage of the right bile duct into the common bile duct and through the papilla. **G:** Late picture shows efficient drainage of the right and left bile ducts through the stents.

Comment: Cystic dilation may involve the free portion of the common bile duct, i.e., choledochal cyst, or may be present as diverticulum formation in the intraduodenal segment. In the latter situation, chronic reflux of pancreatic juice into the biliary tree can produce inflammation and stenosis of the extrahepatic bile ducts, leading to cholangitis or biliary obstruction. Because the process may be gradual, approximately 50% of patients present with onset of symptoms after age 10 years. The classic triad of abdominal pain, jaundice, and abdominal mass should lead to the diagnosis in a young patient. Surgical treatment should include excision of the cyst and biliary-enteric anastomosis. Patients with choledochal cysts are at increased risk for development of cholangiocarcinoma. This case is an example of what may happen if the cyst is not resected. Percutaneous drainage may be extremely complex in patients with an enormous intracystic mass. Long and large-diameter stents probably are the best choice in such cases. Endoscopic drainage also was helpful for access through the duodenal-cystic anastomoses.

14.2.14 Interventional Procedures In Malignant Obstruction Of The Biliary Tract

Case 14.2.14:

A 59-year-old woman presented with jaundice and abdominal pain due to an aggressive unresectable gallbladder carcinoma invading the common biliary duct and duodenum. Bilateral percutaneous biliary drainage was performed. A large Wallstent was endoscopically placed in the duodenum to relieve severe stenosis. Two months after biliary drainage, hemobilia developed with intraduodenal bleeding and through the catheters, requiring 2 units of blood transfusion. Emergency arteriography was requested for diagnosis and treatment.

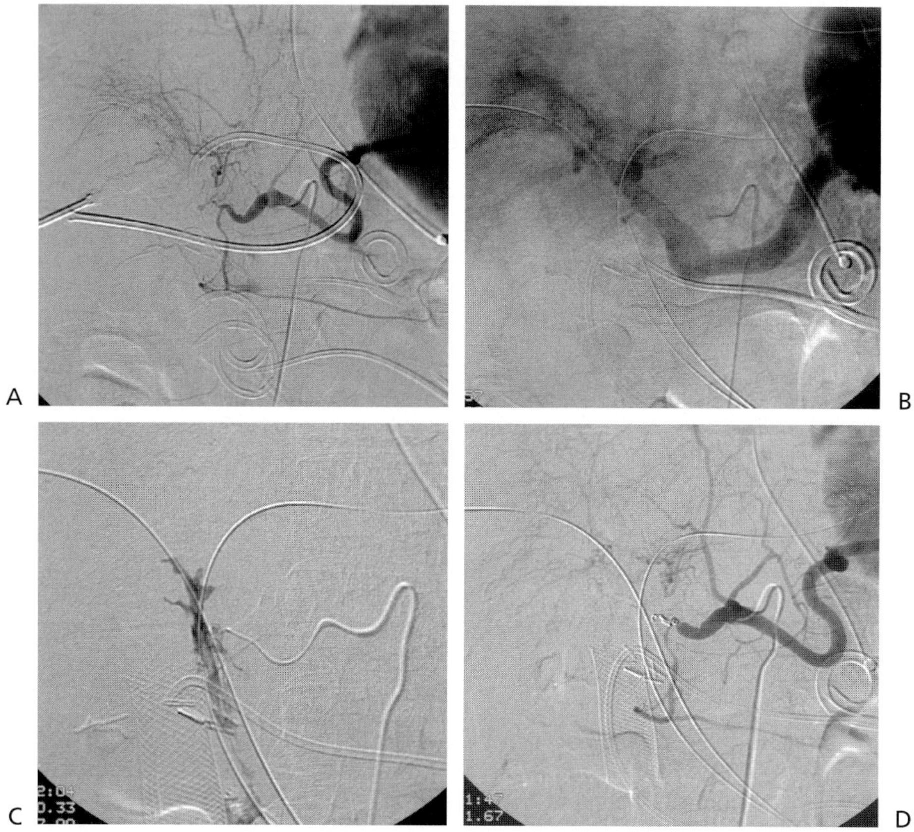

Figure 14.2.14

A: Selective celiac arteriography demonstrates the hepatic artery is occluded by tumoral invasion, with partial intrahepatic reconstitution. A small pseudoaneurysm is seen in close proximity to the main bile duct (overlapping one of the draining catheters). **B:** Late-phase arteriogram shows contrast stasis within the pseudoaneurysm. The portal vein is patent but slightly bowed by the tumor. **C:** Selective injection of contrast within the branch feeding the pseudoaneurysm shows abundant intrabiliary extravasation of contrast. **D:** Embolization with small microcoils occluded the pseudoaneurysm and the feeding artery. Selective celiac arteriography demonstrates occlusion of the pseudoaneurysm, which was followed by control of the bleeding. Twenty-four hours after embolization, the patient was transferred from the intensive care unit to a regular bed. Note that there is partial filling of the intrahepatic arteries.

Comment: Intrabiliary bleeding from tumor invasion is not very unusual; however, development of a hepatic artery pseudoaneurysm is more rarely seen. Tumoral bleeding usually is more diffuse, and it is difficult to determine a single bleeder vessel. In this case, the tumor infiltrated and occluded the bile duct and hepatic artery. It is not known if the presence of the catheter inside the bile duct, in close contact with the tumor, was responsible for the pseudoaneurysm formation. Embolization is the best option to treat this kind of bleeding and was very effective in this case. Surgical treatment carries a high morbidity, and gaining access to the bleeding point would be very complex. Diagnostic angiography provided precise information regarding the location of the lesion and the cause of bleeding. Embolization was a continuation of the diagnostic procedure.

14.3.1 Percutaneous Cholecystostomy And Stone Manipulation

Case 14.3.1:

A 60-year-old male patient recovering from miocardial infarction presented with acute cholecystitis manifested by fever, pain, and right upper quadrant tenderness. Due to the high surgical risk, emergency percutaneous cholecystectomy was requested.

A

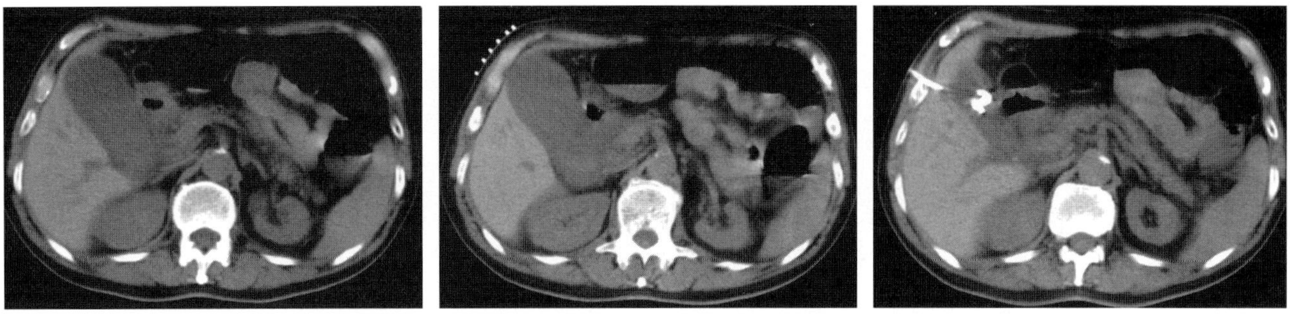

B, C

Figure 14.3.1

A: CT of the abdomen shows a distended gallbladder, without evidence of stones. **B:** A radiopaque marker was placed on the skin and the best window for puncture was selected. An 18-gauge needle was used for access, and a short 0.035-inch guidewire was used to advance a dilator and a drain. **C:** An 8F catheter was used for drainage and kept open in a bag for 7 days, when it was pulled out. Postdrainage CT scan shows decompression of the gallbladder.

Comment: Percutaneous gallbladder interventions yield good clinical efficacy and have a low complication rate. The gallbladder usually is superficially located and easily localized by ultrasonography or CT for percutaneous puncture and drainage. The main indications for percutaneous access to the gallbladder are acute calculous or acalculous cholecystitis, empyema, pericholecystic abscess, decompression of obstructive jaundice, and, more recently, as an access route to perform percutaneous endoscopy, dissolution of gallstones, and/or mechanical lithotripsy. We usually prefer the percutaneous approach with the Seldinger technique using US or CT guidance, and pigtail catheter drainage. Introduction of the guidewire should be very gentle to reduce the risks of perforating the gallbladder wall. Contrast material injection should be performed cautiously, following drainage, or not at all, to reduce the risk or worsening of sepsis. It usually is beneficial to delay the cholecystogram for 24 or 48 hours. Eventually it will be necessary to inject contrast material to identify stones or biliary strictures that may have caused the acute cholecystitis in most of patients. Visualization of the bile duct usually is quite adequate 1 or 2 days after decompression.

14.3.2 Percutaneous Cholecystostomy And Stone Manipulation

Case 14.3.2:

An 81-year-old female nursing home patient who had pancreatic cancer treated palliatively with a endoscopic biliary stent presented with signs and symptoms of acute cholecystitis. Emergency percutaneous cholecystectomy was requested.

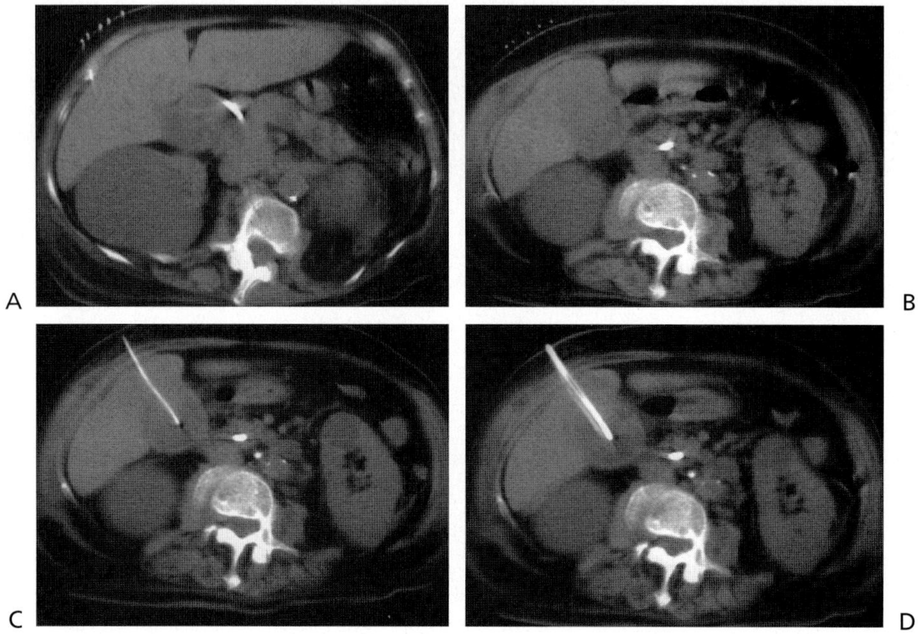

Figure 14.3.2

A: CT scan of the abdomen shows a mass in the head of the pancreas and the biliary stent. Note the small amount of air in the left bile duct and the large renal cyst. The radiopaque marker is visualized in the skin. **B:** A lower CT slice shows the dilated bile duct with thickening of the gallbladder wall. **C:** An 18-gauge needle was used for puncture and the guidewire was introduced. **D:** An 8F catheter was placed for external drainage.

Comment: Extensive experience is available for review in the literature. Successful cholecystostomy is the rule in dilated, infected gallbladder, with relief of symptoms in a few hours. This case presents a situation of acute acalculous cholecystitis. Septic, immunocompromised, diabetic, and multiorgan system failure patients may have mortality rates as high as 20% with emergency surgical cholecystectomy. Percutaneous cholecystostomy temporizes and stabilizes the high-risk patient in preparation for later surgery. In a recent publication, emergency percutaneous cholecystostomy was successful in up to 98% of cases, with 63% clinical improvement, 12% complication rate, and no deaths related to the procedure. However, 51% of the patients in this high-risk population died during the prolonged hospitalization.

14.3.3 Percutaneous Cholecystostomy And Stone Manipulation

Case 14.3.3:

An 83-year-old female nursing home patient with Alzheimer disease developed acute abdomen and fever. Ultrasound was consistent with cholecystitis. Due to the high surgical risks, emergency percutaneous cholecystectomy was requested.

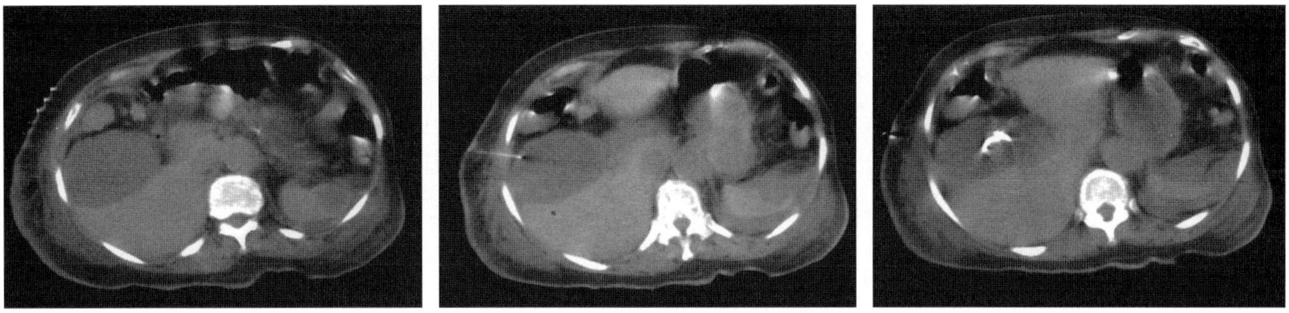

A B, C

Figure 14.3.3

A: CT of the abdomen shows a dilated gallbladder. Note the radiopaque markers on the wall. US demonstrated thicker walls (not shown). **B:** An 18-gauge trocar was used for access to the gallbladder. **C:** An 8F pigtail drainage catheter was positioned within the gallbladder for external drainage. The catheter was pulled out 6 weeks later.

Comment: Bile leakage is the most common complication of cholecystostomy. Removal of the catheter should be performed after the tract develops because, even in decompressed systems, premature removal of the catheter can cause leakage from the gallbladder. Sepsis is not a significant complication of the procedure; however, long and abrupt manipulation carries a higher risk. Intraperitoneal puncture of the gallbladder may cause leakage; in such cases, an anchorage device is advisable. Vagal reactions are expected and may be severe. Minimizing the amount of manipulation and the use of intravenous atropine should reduce the incidence of vagal reactions. Percutaneous cholecystostomy was very effective in treating this frail woman.

14.3.4 Percutaneous Cholecystostomy And Stone Manipulation

Case 14.3.4:

A 71-year-old female patient presented with acute cholecystitis manifested by fever and right upper quadrant pain. Due to the high surgical risks, emergency percutaneous cholecystectomy was requested.

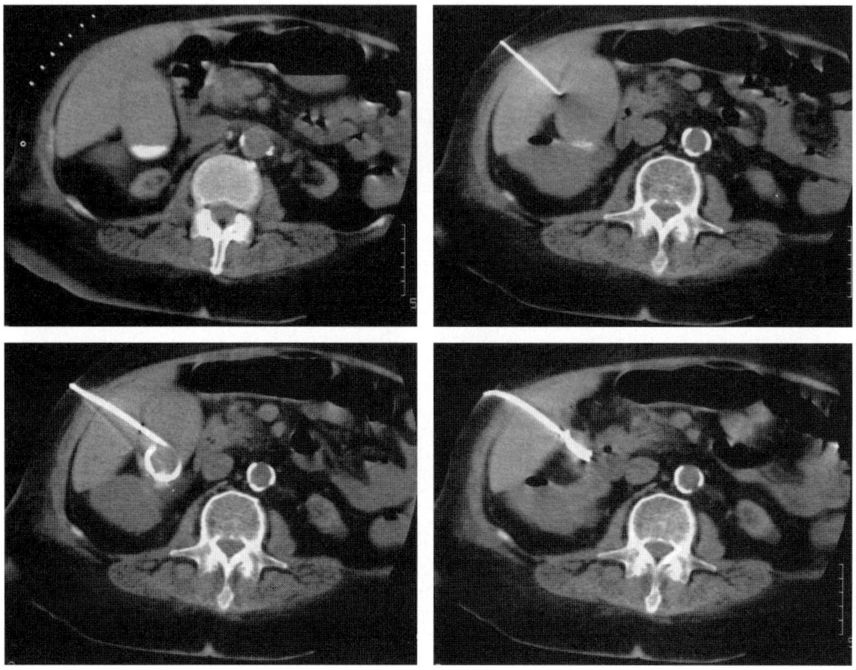

A B C D

Figure 14.3.4

A: CT-guided cholecystostomy was started by marking the skin with a radiopaque grid. Axial view of the abdomen shows a dilated gallbladder with stones in the fundus. **B:** An 18-gauge needle was used for percutaneous puncture and access to the gallbladder. **C:** An 8F pigtail drainage catheter was used to drain the gallbladder. **D:** Total emptying of the gallbladder was achieved following drainage. There was excellent clinical improvement after treatment.

Comment: Calculous cholecystitis is a relatively common cause of clinical worsening during the course of other diseases. If there is excessive clinical risks for surgery, percutaneous cholecystostomy is an effective temporizing measure until a more definitive treatment can be undertaken. Control of infection includes drainage and antibiotic therapy. The stones can be treated by laparoscopic cholecystectomy after reducing the inflammation or by percutaneous extraction of the stones through a larger percutaneous sheath, using a basket or cholangioscopy with lithotripsy.

14.3.5 Percutaneous Cholecystostomy And Stone Manipulation

Case 14.3.5:

A 57-year-old male patient presented with acute cholecystitis, and a surgical cholecystectomy was performed. For some reason, there was a residual gallbladder and cystic duct remnant with stones. A catheter was left in place. Because the patient's clinical condition deteriorated, manifested by sepsis and pain, new surgery was contraindicated. Percutaneous treatment was requested.

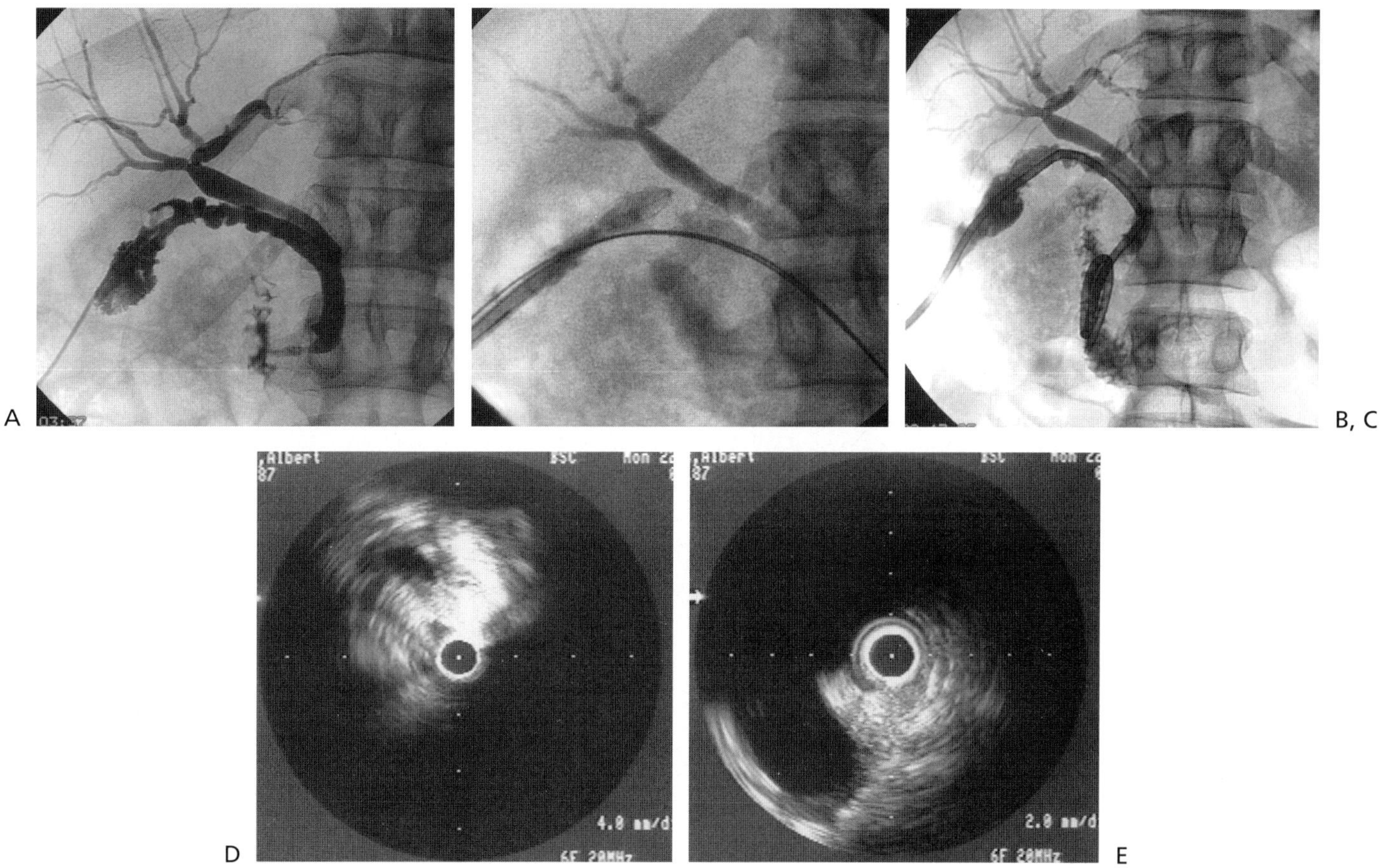

Figure 14.3.5

A: Cholangiography performed through the surgical cholecystostomy catheter shows a small gallbladder and cystic duct remnant with filling defects, consistent with residual stones. The common duct is large but does not show any stones. **B:** After catheterization of the main bile duct, a larger introducer sheath was introduced and a nitinol snare was used to retrieve the stones. **C:** Catheter cholangiogram following stone treatment shows no residual stones. **D:** Intrabiliary ultrasound (IBUS) shows echogenic images within the gallbladder remnant, consistent with the stones. **E:** IBUS after stone treatment does not show residual stones.

Comment: In addition to its therapeutic value, percutaneous cholecystostomy yields important diagnostic and prognostic information. Gram stains and cultures of obtained bile are useful in determining the cause of cholecystitis. By providing direct access to the gallbladder lumen, the percutaneous approach complements surgery for treatment of gallstones. Fragments of stones or smaller-size stones can be extracted, suctioned, or flushed out of the gallbladder. Snaring of the stones is probably the most common technique used to extract stones. In this case, multiple residual stones were identified within the remnant gallbladder and cystic duct, and percutaneous basketing of the stones spared the patient a new surgery. The optimal entry technique, with a trocar or Seldinger technique, is still controversial. Multiple punctures may be necessary using the trocar technique, whereas the Seldinger technique may cause intraperitoneal bile leak.

14.3.6 Percutaneous Cholecystostomy And Stone Manipulation

Case 14.3.6:

A 71-year-old female patient presented with acute cholecystitis manifested by fever and right upper quadrant pain. Due to the high surgical risks, emergency percutaneous cholecystectomy was requested.

A, B

C

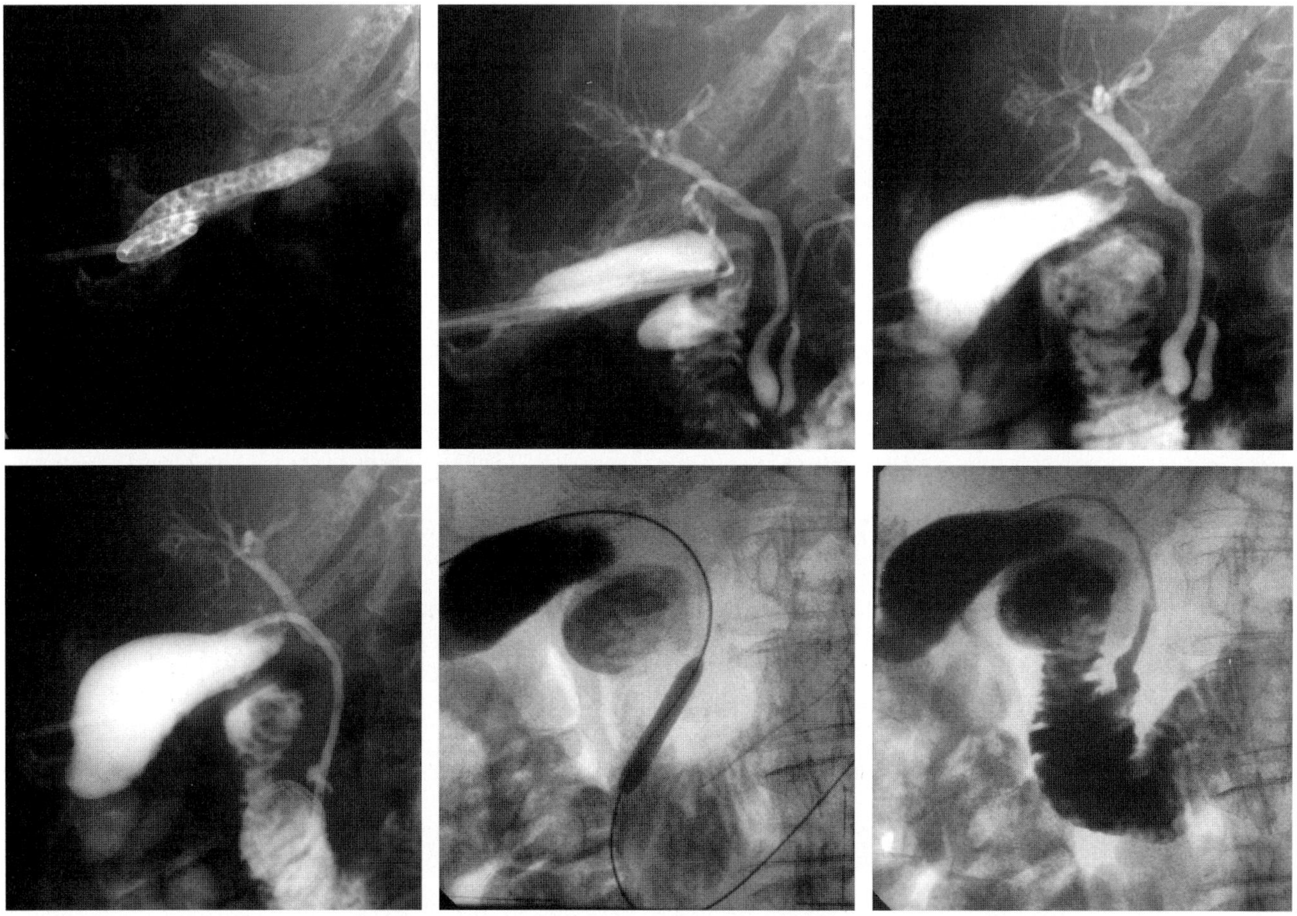

D, E

F

Figure 14.3.6

A: Transcatheter cholecystogram shows multiple small gallstones with obstruction of the cystic duct. **B:** Cholecystogram after stone removal shows a clean gallbladder. Note the large size of the introducer sheath. A KMP catheter was used to catheterize the cystic duct and common bile duct. Most of the stones were simply flushed with saline. **C:** An 8F catheter was placed through the gallbladder, common bile duct, and sphincter. **D:** Balloon plasty of the sphincter was performed. **E:** Cholangiogram following plasty shows patency of the sphincter. **F:** Final cholangiogram following stone removal and balloon plasty of the sphincter shows patent bile ducts and gallbladder.

Comment: Cross-section imaging is critical for successful access to the gallbladder. To avoid leakage, an anterior or anterolateral transhepatic approach to the gallbladder has been used by most investigators. Puncture into the upper third of the gallbladder near its attachment to the liver has the advantage of reducing the risk of bile leakage into the peritoneal cavity. However, in another report, the transhepatic approach did not effectively allow puncture of the bare area of the gallbladder in 58% of patients. In about 13% of patients, the bowel may be interposed between the gallbladder fundus and the skin entry site. In most individuals, the shortest route between the skin and the gallbladder is via the transhepatic approach. The direct gallbladder fundal approach eliminates the hepatic trauma associated with the large sheaths required for percutaneous stone removal. The fundal approach may require the use of removable anchoring devices to fasten the gallbladder to the anterior abdominal wall and reduce the chances of bile leakage. One puzzling aspect of the treatment of acute cholecystitis with percutaneous cholecystostomy is the progression of gallbladder wall necrosis following effective catheter treatment with rupture, which requires surgical cholecystectomy.

14.4.1 Interventional Procedures In The Pancreatic Duct

Case 14.4.1:

A 43-year-old female patient presented with pancreatitis, abdominal pain, and a pseudocyst. CT-guided percutaneous pseudocyst drainage was performed. The internal pancreatic fistula produced continuous drainage of more than 100 mL of pancreatic fluid per day. After a failed attempt at endoscopic catheterization of the papilla, a combined percutaneous and endoscopic treatment was planned.

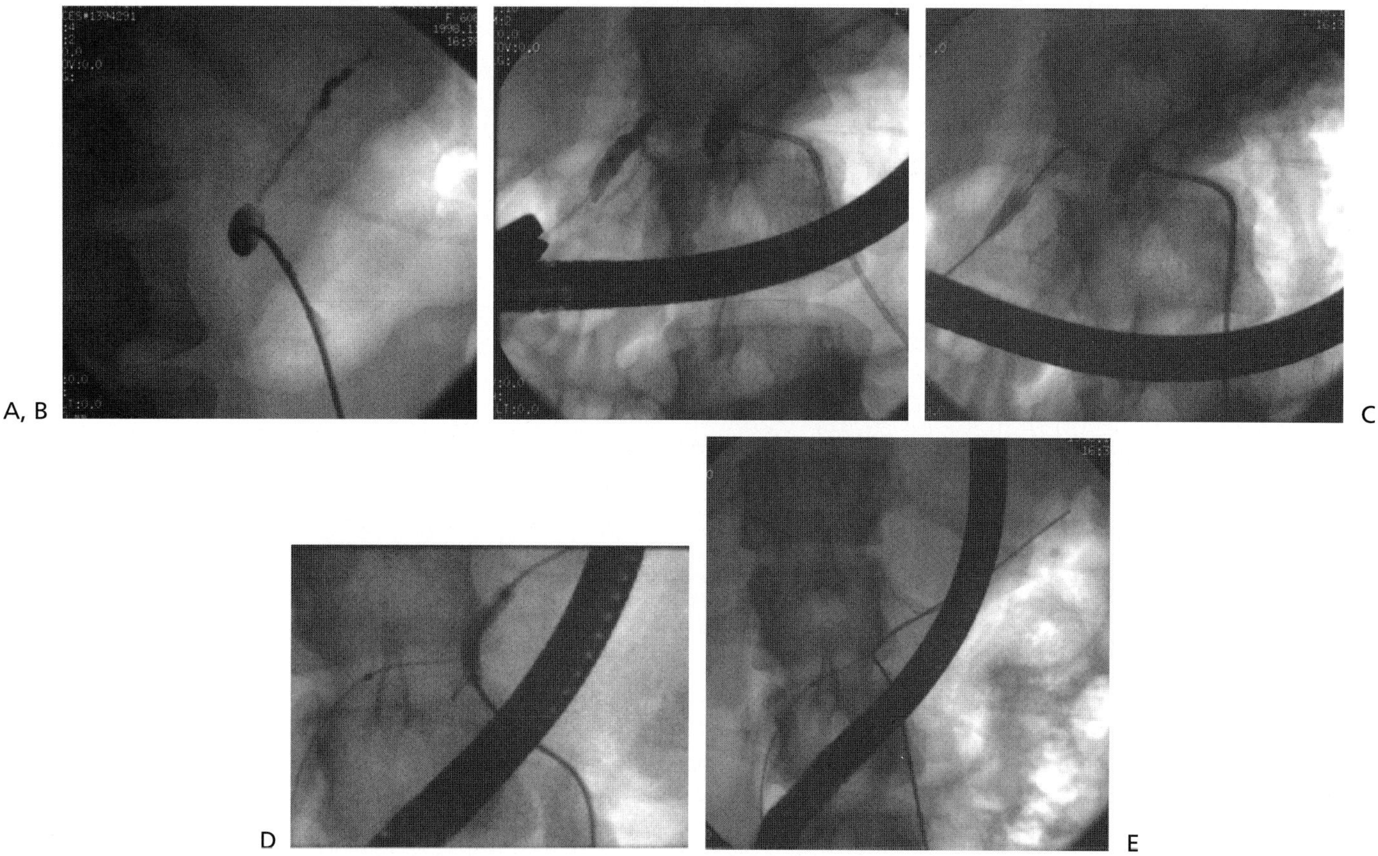

Figure 14.4.1

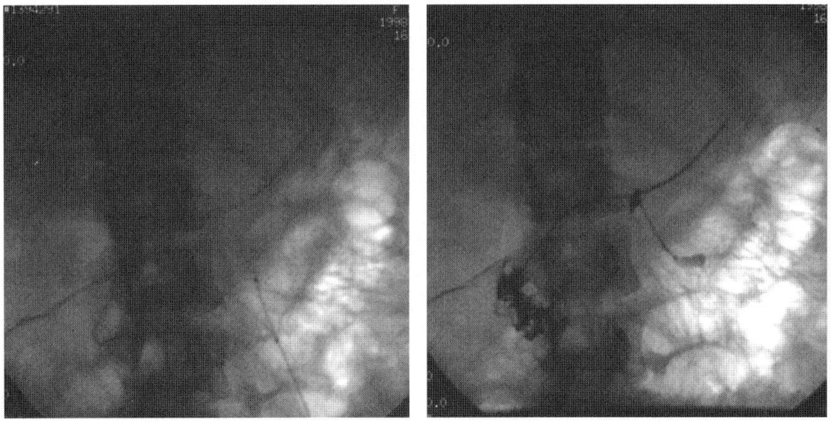

F G

Figure 14.4.1 *(continued)*

A: Injection into the drainage catheter 30 days after the initial drainage shows a small cavity around the tip of the catheter and filling of the distal pancreatic duct. **B:** Simultaneous ERCP shows a short segment of pancreatic duct with distal occlusion close to the pseudocyst. **C:** An endoscopic guidewire was advanced into the cavity. **D:** The distal pancreatic duct was catheterized, and 5-mm balloon plasty was performed in the transition between the pseudocyst and the distal duct. **E:** The distal pancreatic duct was percutaneously catheterized, and the endoscopic wire was advanced into the distal duct. **F:** An endoscopic stent was placed for drainage of the pancreatic duct and reconstitution of the duct. **G:** Injection into the percutaneous tract shows good patency of the pancreatic duct and the functional stent draining into the duodenum.

Comment: Internal pancreatic fistula is a complication of pancreatitis and pancreatic surgery, with a reported incidence of 4% to 6%. Traditional treatment has been conservative medical therapy and surgery. Conservative therapy fails in 20% to 50% of cases, and surgery is associated with significant morbidity of about 13% and mortality of 8%. Endoscopic stents are well established as treatment for pancreatic duct fistulas; however, stent insertion may not be possible in the presence of a pancreatic duct stricture. When there is a percutaneous access to the pancreatic duct through a preexisting drainage catheter in the peripancreatic fluid collection, percutaneous balloon plasty may be used to facilitate endoscopic catheterization and stenting. The presence of the stent reduces resistance to flow into the duodenum and may bridge the leak. There are little data on the optimum period of treatment by pancreatic stents, but 6 to 8 weeks probably is sufficient, particularly if imaging confirms resolution of fluid collections.

14.4.2 Interventional Procedures In The Pancreatic Duct

Case 14.4.2:

A 22-year-old male patient presented with pancreatitis and a pseudocyst due to pancreas divisum. CT-guided percutaneous pseudocyst drainage was performed. The internal pancreatic fistula produced continuous drainage of more than 80 mL of pancreatic fluid per day. After a failed attempt of endoscopic catheterization of the pancreatic duct, a combined percutaneous and endoscopic treatment was planned.

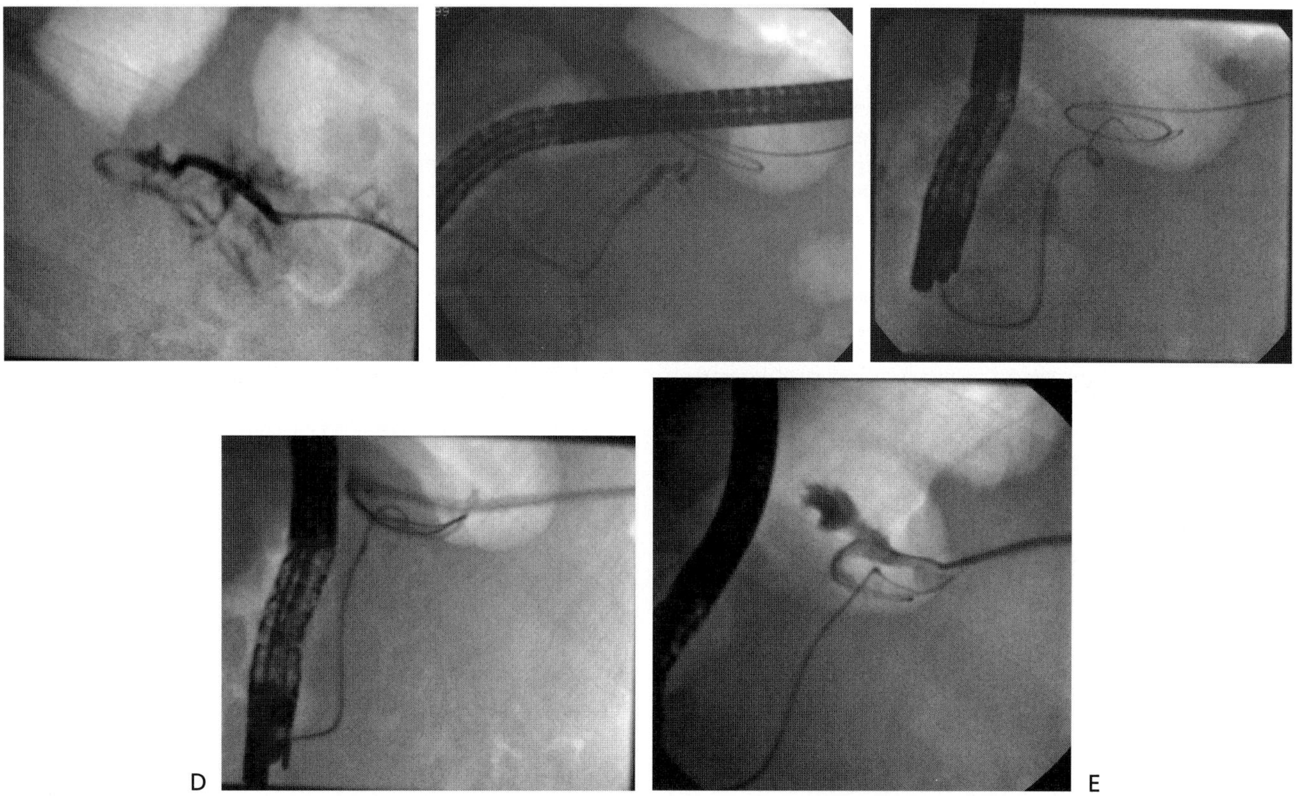

A, B C

D E

Figure 14.4.2

F 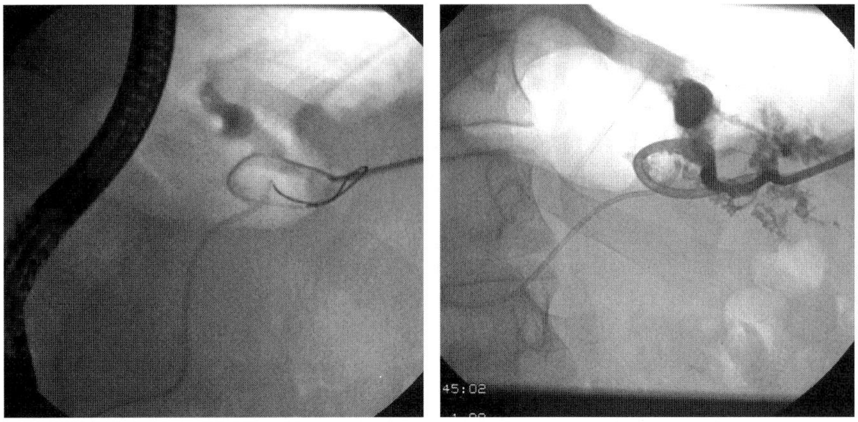 G

Figure 14.4.2 *(continued)*

A: Injection through the drain catheter shows filling of the distal pancreatic duct, which is highly irregular and contains multiple branches. **B:** Retrograde endoscopic injection through the papilla shows occlusion of the duct close to the pseudocyst. **C:** The endoscopic guidewire was advanced into the cavity. **D:** A loop snare was placed percutaneously to capture the endoscopic wire and allow for introduction of a pancreatic stent. **E:** Filling of the percutaneous tract, which was occluded with a balloon, shows filling of a lateral cavity related to the pseudocyst. **F:** While holding the wire, a pancreatic stent was advanced into the cavity and attempted to be advanced into the distal pancreatic duct. **G:** A drainage catheter was repositioned into the percutaneous tract. Contrast injection does not show drainage through the pancreatic stent.

Comment: Long-term drainage failed to close the internal pancreatic fistula in this case. Although it was possible to fill and percutaneously catheterize the distal pancreatic duct, it was not possible to properly catheterize the distal pancreatic duct from the endoscopic approach. Failure of catheterization required the lesion to be treated by surgery, with resection of the distal pancreatic tail. Percutaneous catheterization of the pancreatic duct is a good method to resolve this difficult problem; however, when endoscopic complementation is not feasible, as in the present case, the only alternative is surgical treatment.

14.4.3 Interventional Procedures In The Pancreatic Duct

Case 14.4.3:

A 54-year-old male patient with chronic pancreatitis and a pseudocyst that was drained under CT guidance. The drainage catheter was maintained for several weeks. The internal pancreatic fistula produced continuous drainage of more than 100 mL of pancreatic fluid per day. After a failed attempt at endoscopic catheterization of the pancreatic duct, a combined percutaneous treatment was planned.

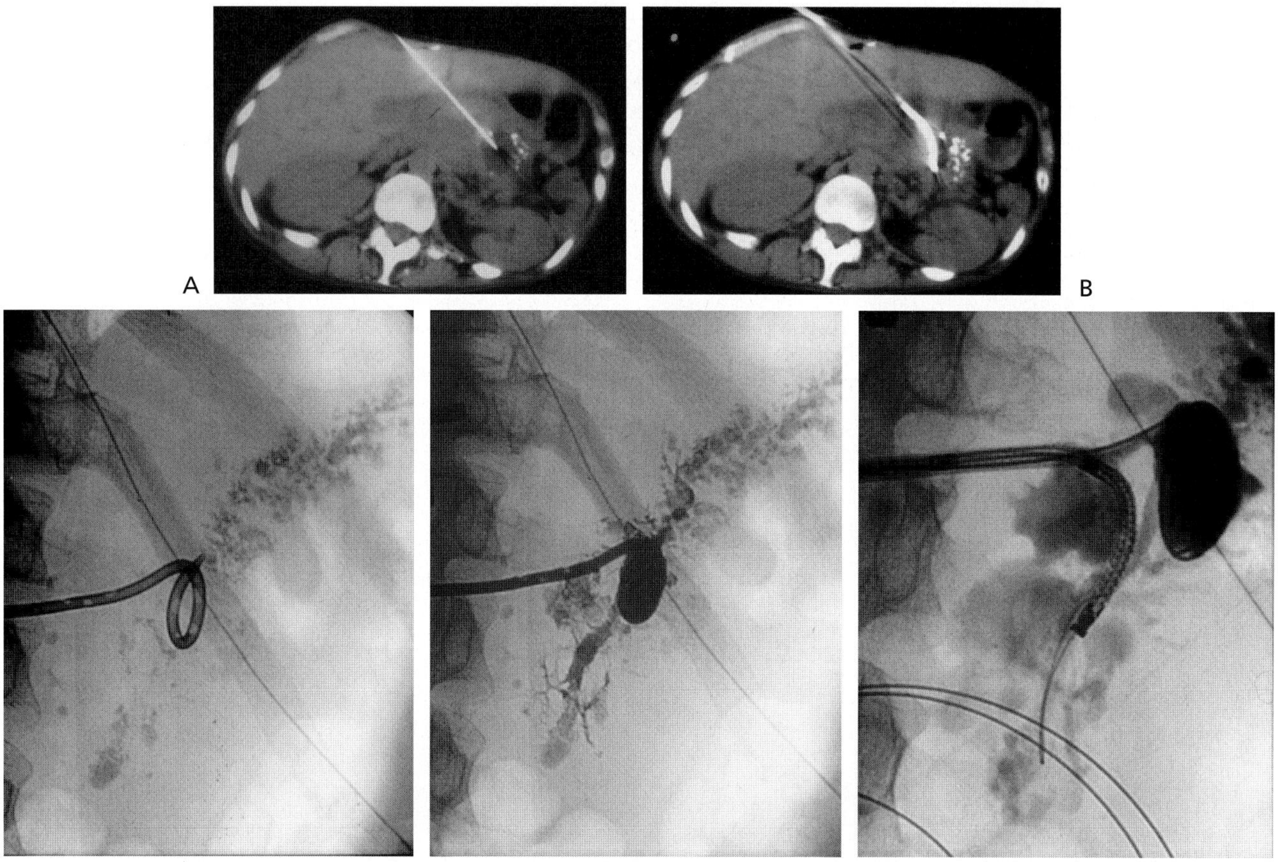

A B

C, D E

Figure 14.4.3

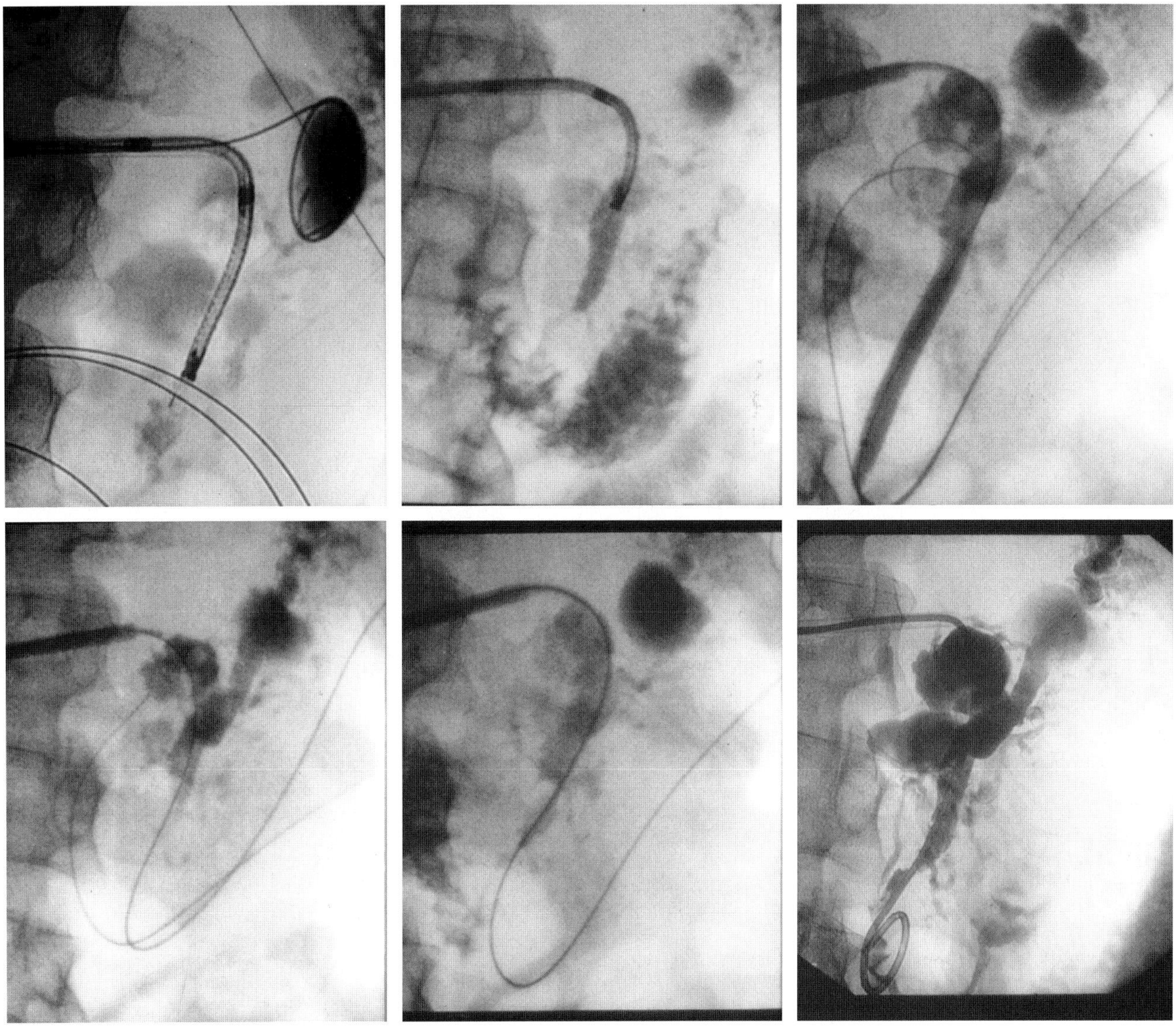

Figure 14.4.3 *(continued)*

L, M

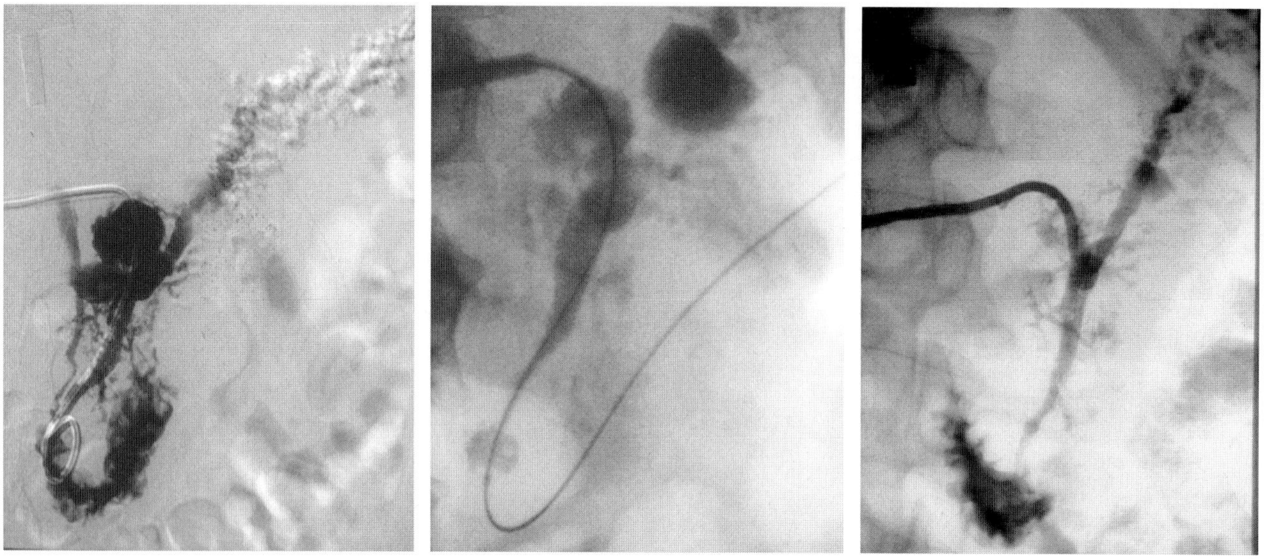

N

Figure 14.4.3 *(continued)*

A: CT of the abdomen shows two pancreatic pseudocysts in the body of the pancreas. A transhepatic approach was used. Note the needle passing through the liver and into the pancreatic pseudocysts. **B:** A 10F catheter was used for external drainage. Extensive calcifications in the pancreas are seen. **C:** Plain film of the abdomen shows extensive calcifications along the pancreas and occlusion of the main duct by a larger stone. **D:** Injection of contrast media shows occlusion of the pancreatic duct at the level of the papilla and severe disruption and irregularities all along the pancreatic duct. **E:** A guidewire was advanced into the pancreatic pseudocyst. Through an introducer sheath, the proximal pancreatic duct was retrogradely catheterized percutaneously and the cholangioscope was advanced over the wire. **F:** The cholangioscope was advanced into the pancreatic duct, and electrohydraulic lithotripsy was performed to break down the pancreatic duct stones. **G:** Following lithotripsy of the pancreatic duct stones, the duct was injected and considered to be free of major stones. **H:** Balloon dilation of the papilla was performed over the wire, to 6 mm. **I:** The guidewire was maintained through the papilla, and an occlusion balloon was advanced to push the stones into the duodenum. **J:** An occlusion balloon was effectively advanced through the papilla. **K:** An internal-external drainage catheter was placed, and external drainage was achieved. Note the remaining pseudocysts **L:** Injection through the catheter shows patency of the duct, in antegrade and retrograde segments. Note filling of the pseudocysts and severe irregularities in the distal duct. The bile duct also is opacified. **M:** An occlusion balloon was passed through the papilla to further push stones into the duodenum. **N:** Several weeks after the procedure, the catheter was pulled back into the fistula. Injection of contrast material shows remarkable improvement of the pancreatic duct irregularities, resolution of the pseudocysts, and patency of the papilla. The catheter was removed shortly thereafter.

Comment: Chronic pancreatitis is very disruptive of the pancreatic duct and may lead to stenosis and rupture of the pancreatic duct, with pseudocyst formation and fistulization. Severe spread calcifications usually are present, which worsen the obstructive pattern. In this case, percutaneous drainage of the pseudocysts provided adequate access to the pancreatic duct, which allowed for lithotripsy of the intraductal stones and balloon plasty of the sphincter stenoses. After treatment of the stone obstruction, adequate catheter decompression improved the drainage and the anatomic abnormalities resulting from chronic pancreatitis.

14.5.1 Intraluminal Ultrasound In The Bile Ducts

Case 14.5.1:

A 55-year-old male patient with pancreatitis developed pancreatic pseudocyst and obstructive jaundice. ERCP and stent placement were not possible, and percutaneous cholangiogram and catheter drainage were requested.

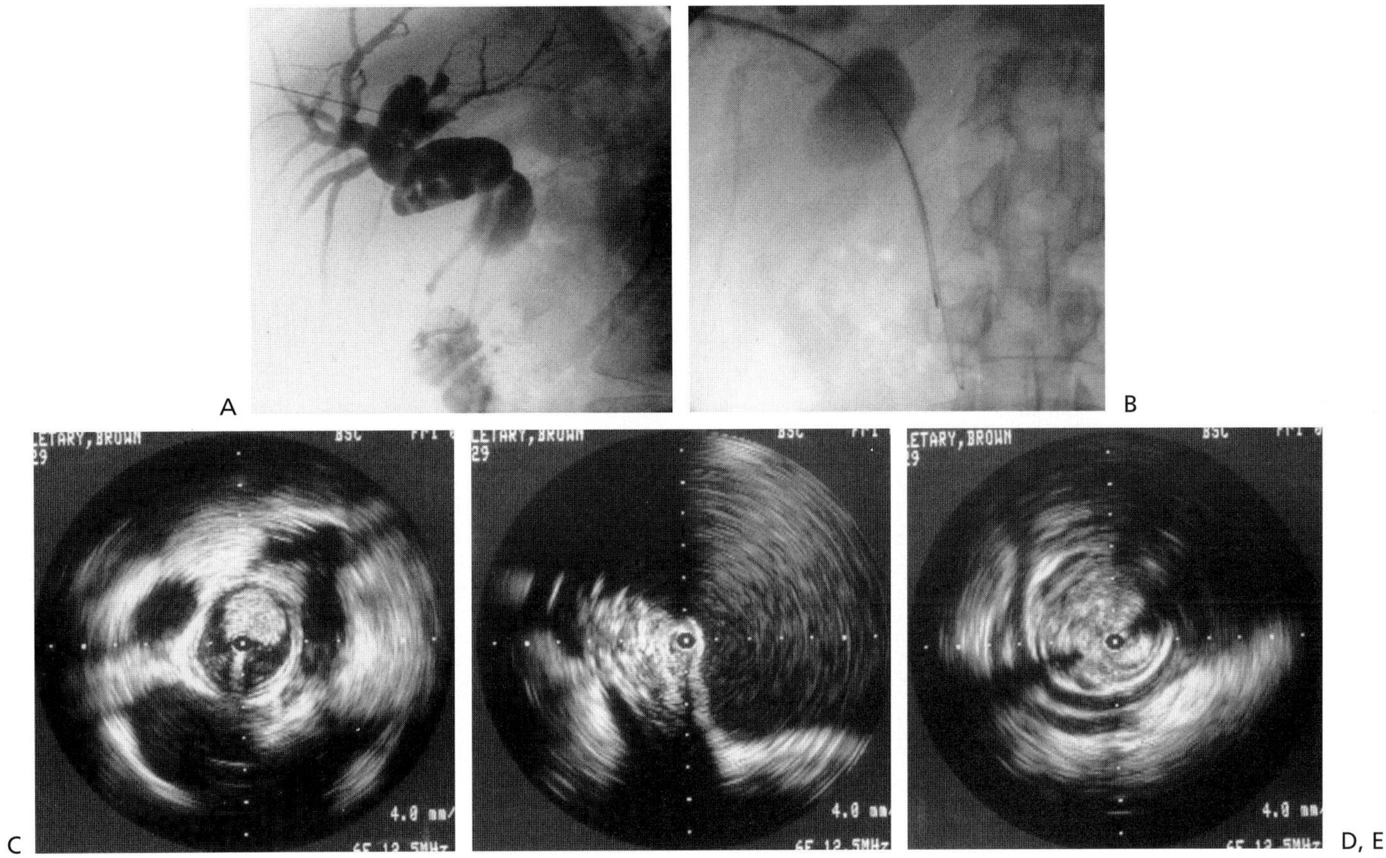

Figure 14.5.1

A: PTC shows the intrahepatic bile ducts are dilated and severe stricture of the distal common bile duct. **B:** After a guidewire was passed into the duodenum and through the papilla, a 6F (12.5-MHz) ultrasound probe was passed through the stenosis for intrabiliary ultrasound (IBUS). **C:** IBUS at the level of the proximal dilated common bile duct shows a filling defect (most likely a blood clot) within the large duct (about 12 mm). Note the hyperechoic tissues around the bile duct most likely due to fibrosis and inflammatory process related to pancreatitis. The hepatic artery is at 10 o'clock and the portal vein at 6 to 7 o'clock. The cystic duct is visualized on the right side of the duct. **D:** IBUS at the level of the stricture shows the duct is not well defined and the large pseudocyst adjacent to the bile duct. **E:** Distal to the stricture, IBUS shows the sonographic image of the sphincter of Oddi. The ultrasound catheter is within the common bile duct. The hypoechoic bands represent the muscle layers (ML) of the sphincter of Oddi. A, adventitia; M, mucosa; SM, submucosa.

Comment: Normal bile duct appearance on IBUS is a two- or three-layered wall, with an inner echogenic layer, a middle hypoechoic layer, and an outer echogenic layer. Histopathologic correlation revealed a mucosal layer, a fibromucosal/submucosal layer, and an outer adventitial layer. Normal pancreas is seen as a fine reticular pattern surrounding the bile duct. The IBUS aspect of chronic pancreatitis reveals an inhomogeneous echo-poor pancreatic parenchyma with a fine reticular pattern (not demonstrated in this case). Echogenic calcifications may be visible. The pancreatic pseudocyst is seen as a large homogeneous hypoechoic cystic structure with thick hyperechoic walls. The thickness of the duct wall is not well visualized at the level of the stricture.

14.5.2 Intraluminal Ultrasound In The Bile Ducts

Case 14.5.2:

A 45-year-old male patient with pancreatitis was treated with a Whipple procedure. Three months after surgery, he developed stricture of the anastomosis, which was treated by balloon cholangioplasty and ultimately by Z-stent placement. The stents occluded after several weeks, and a new percutaneous biliary drainage was placed. The balloon plasty failed, and a new stent was placed.

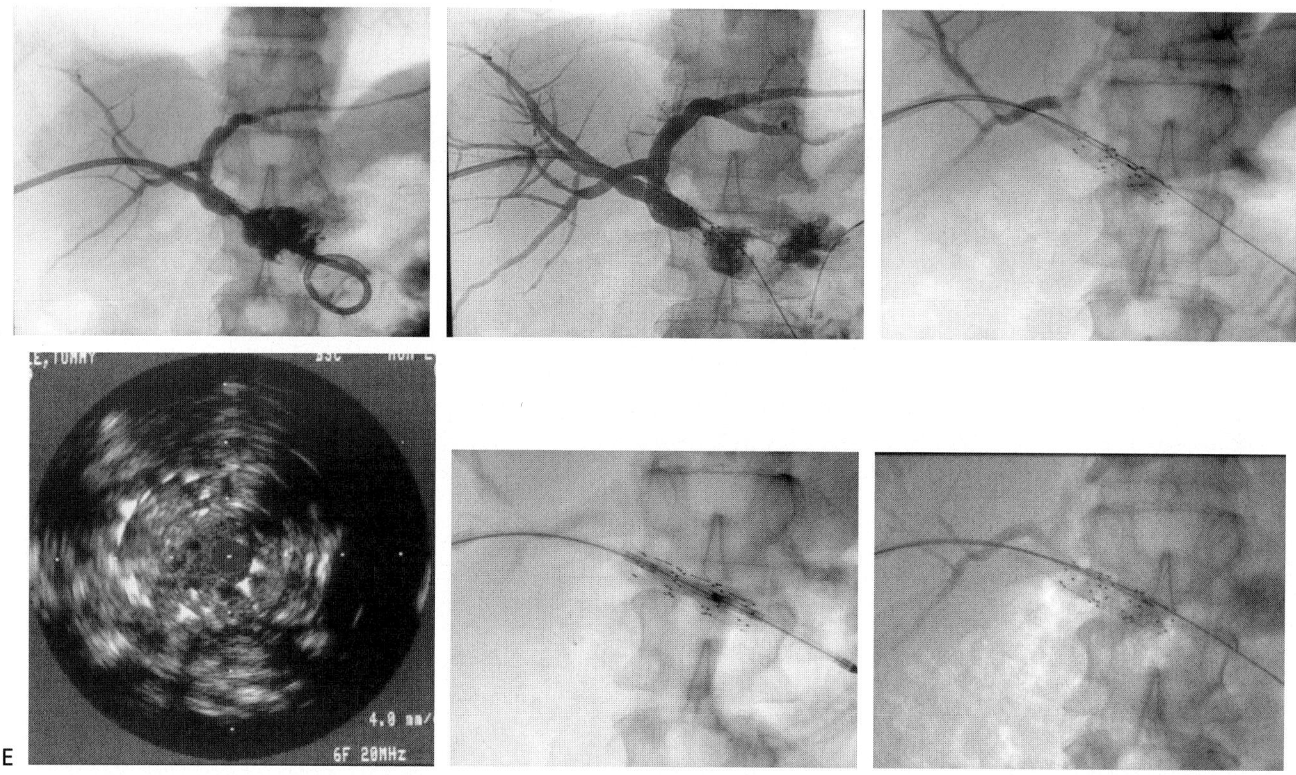

A, B C D, E F

Figure 14.5.2

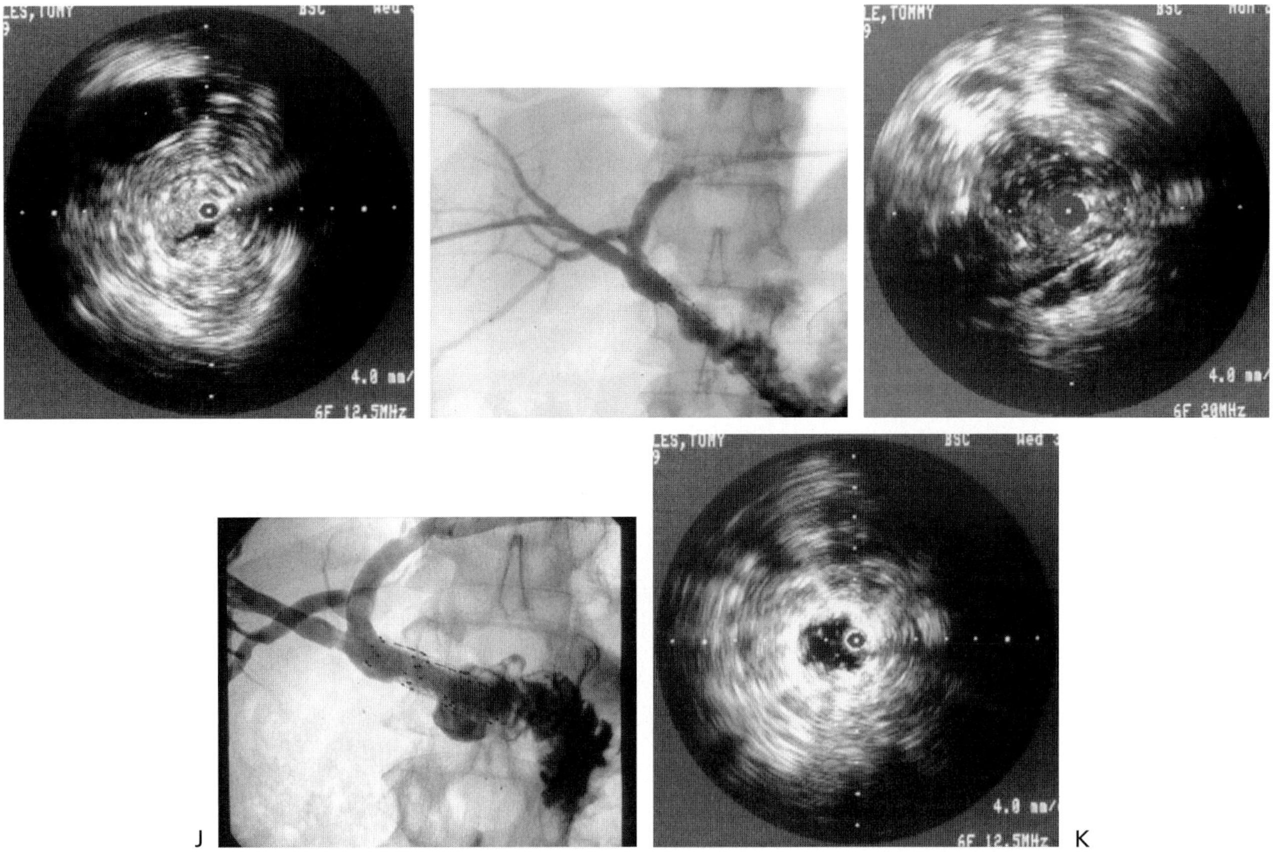

G H, I J K

Figure 14.5.2 *(continued)*

A: Catheter cholangiogram shows a stricture in the middle of the stent. **B:** After the catheter was removed but the guidewire maintained through the stenosis, persistent occlusion is seen. **C:** Note the ultrasound catheter probe within the stent. **D:** IBUS shows total occlusion of the lumen of the stents by an amorphous material. **E:** A directional atherectomy device was used to debulk the material within the stent. Pathologic analysis shows it was edematous intestinal mucosa. **F,G:** After debulking, IBUS shows improvement in patency of the stent lumen, around the probe. Note probe in **(F)**. **H:** Cholangiogram after debulking shows improvement in lumen size. **I:** Another IBUS shows the lumen is still full of material. **J:** A 394 Palmaz stent was placed within the stent lumen, and good patency was achieved. **K:** IBUS after Palmaz stent placement shows greatly improved patency of the choledochojejunostomy, which resolved the patient's problem in follow-up of more than 2 years.

Comment: Benign biliary strictures are readily identified by IBUS. The bile duct wall is thickened and may be difficult to differentiate from cholangiocarcinoma. IBUS assessment before and after balloon plasty is useful, and recoil of the bile duct wall is visible. Laceration and dissection of the bile duct mucosa also are identifiable. The presence of bile sludge is visualized as a heterogeneous, moderately hyperechoic substance within the duct without significant acoustic shadow. Stones are hyperechoic structures with typical radial acoustic shadowing. Bile duct mucosal hyperplasia or bowel mucosa within the stent is seen as heterogeneous structures with air shadowing within. Prestent and poststent placement control is possible with IBUS, which depicts improvement of the bile duct lumen within the stent. Evaluation of the metallic stent demonstrates strong circumferential echogenicity.

14.5.3 Intraluminal Ultrasound In The Bile Ducts

Case 14.5.3:

A 50-year-old male patient with bilateral hepaticojejunostomies developed strictures of the anastomosis. Because endoscopic treatment was not possible, the percutaneous approach was attempted.

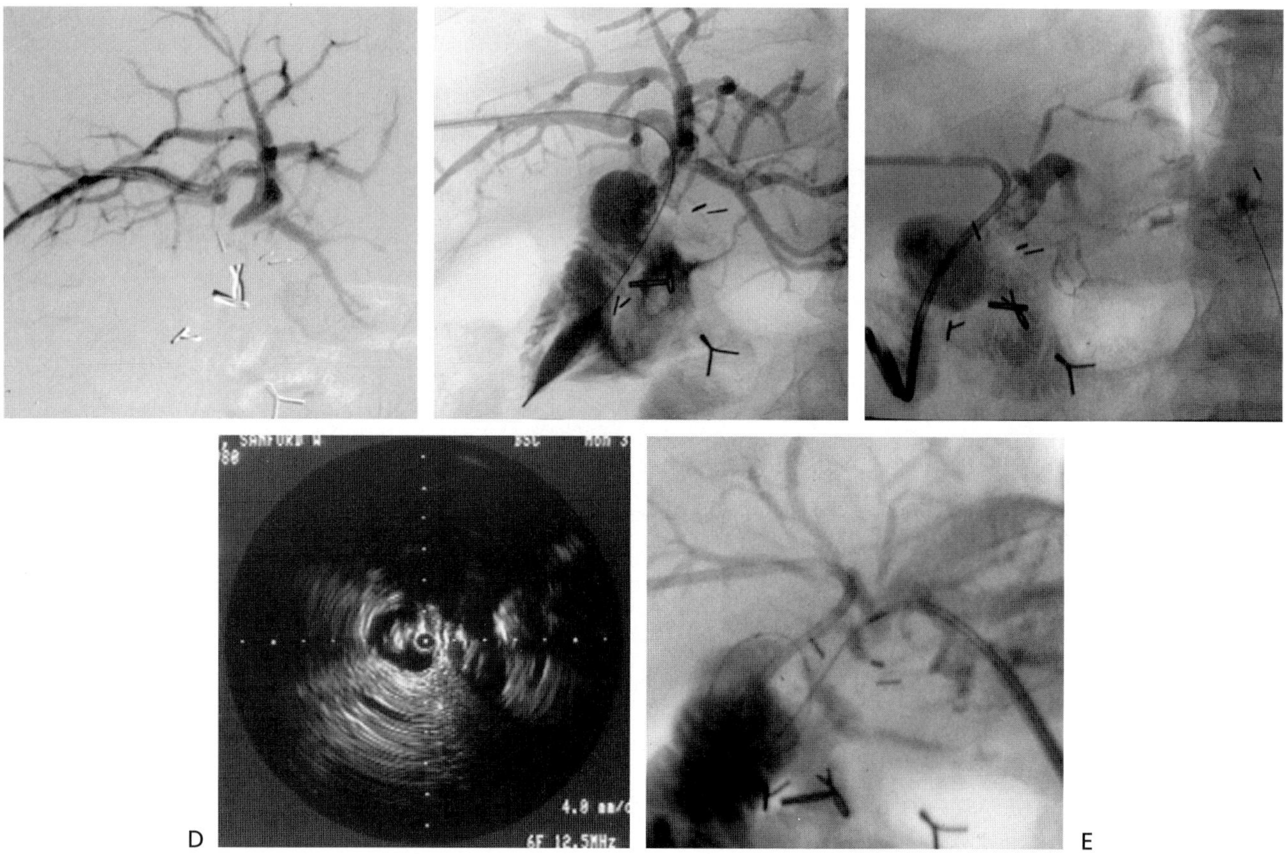

Figure 14.5.3

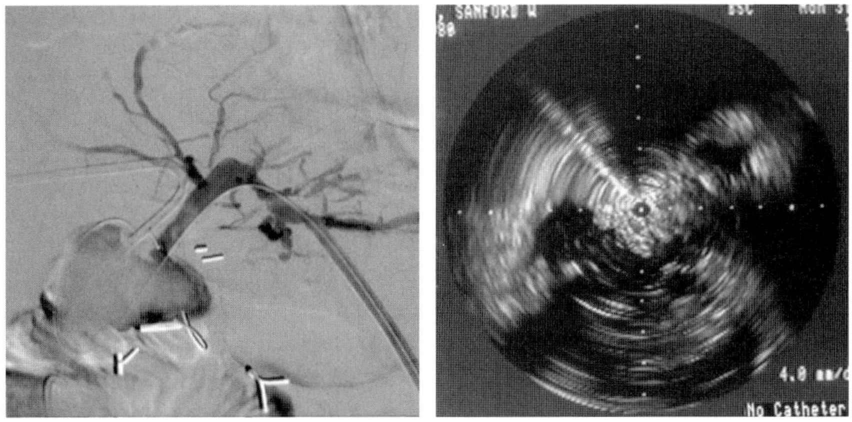

F G

Figure 14.5.3 *(continued)*

A: Right PTC shows obstruction of the anastomoses. **B:** The occlusion was traversed and dilated. Cholangiogram shows patency of the anastomoses. **C:** After draining the right bile duct, left PTC shows moderate bile duct dilation with filling defects suggesting stones. **D:** An ultrasound catheter probe was placed for IBUS and shows duct enlargement and a hyperechoic filling defect, consistent with a small stone within the duct. Note the acoustic shadow of the stone. **E:** The IBUS probe was advanced over the wire to the stricture. IBUS at the level of the stricture demonstrated no lumen and thick walls, with poor definition of the structures. **F:** Postplasty cholangiogram shows patency of the anastomosis. **G:** After dilation, IBUS did not show much improvement, despite cholangiographic patency.

Comment: In the case presented here, the biliary sludge is seen as hyperechoic structures with shadowing. The bile duct stricture is visible, but the bile duct wall at the level of the stricture is not well identified, but there is definitely thickening of the duct wall. Postplasty IBUS did not show much improvement despite improved cholangiographic appearances.

14.5.4 Intraluminal Ultrasound In The Bile Ducts

Case 14.5.4:

A 65-year-old male patient with obstructive jaundice due to sclerosing cholangitis or cholangiocarcinoma was referred for percutaneous treatment and biopsy. Multiple brushing biopsies obtained endoscopically failed to provide the diagnosis.

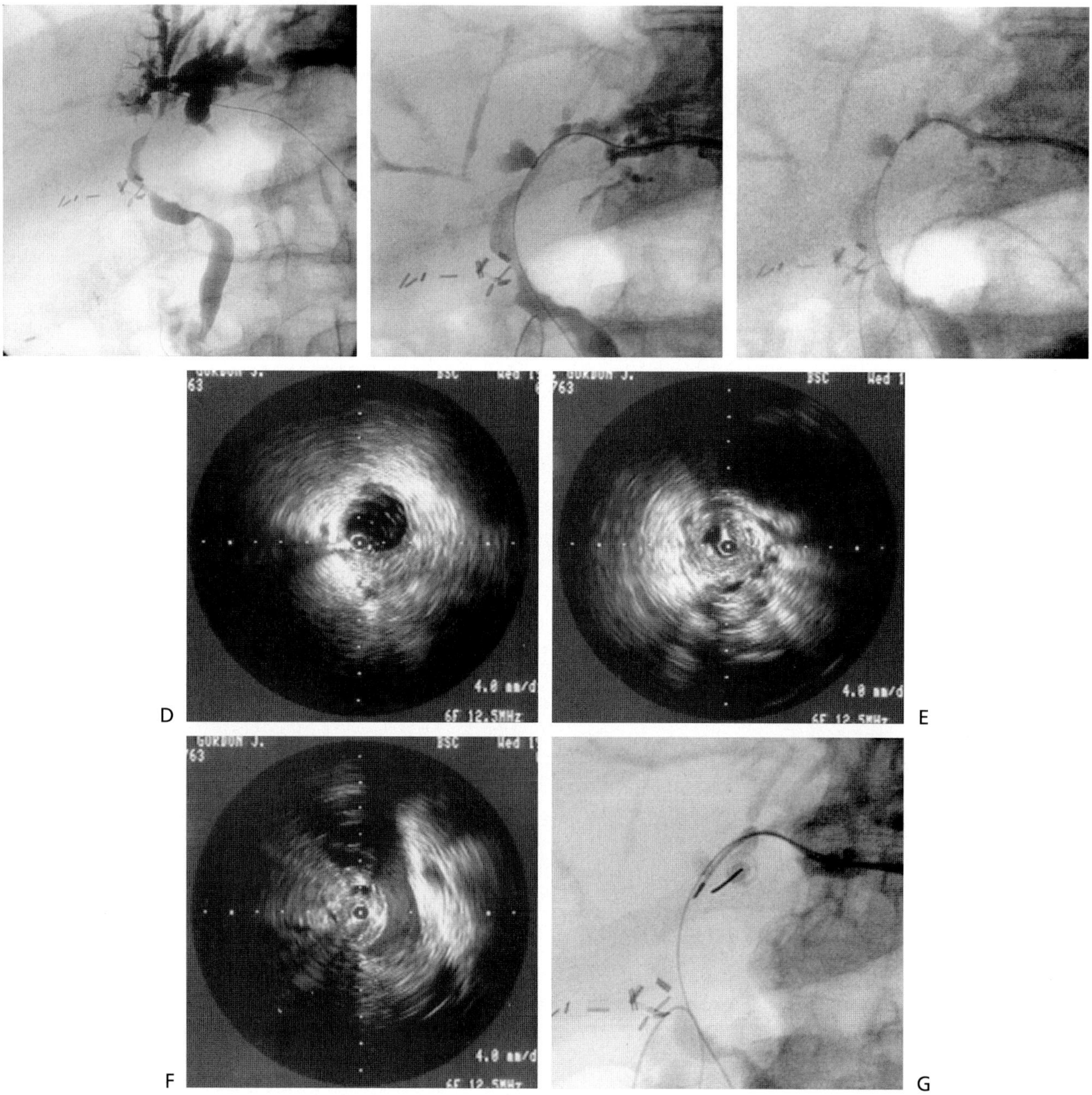

A, B C D E F G

Figure 14.5.4

A: PTC of the left bile duct shows dilation of the intrahepatic bile ducts and at least three segments of stenosis: one at the confluence, one at the proximal common bile duct, and one at the middle level of the common bile duct. The right bile duct was not yet opacified (not shown). **B:** The IBUS probe was introduced into the left dilated duct. **C:** IBUS probe shows the dilated duct with normal walls. **D:** IBUS image shows dilated duct with normal walls. **E:** IBUS at the level of the obstruction shows obstruction of the duct lumen, with thickening of the duct wall and disappearance of the normal wall configuration. **F:** Intrahepatic view of the needle shows the acoustic shadows of the needle in movement near the bile duct. Note the mass around and inside the bile duct lumen. The biopsy was positive for cholangiocarcinoma. **G:** Percutaneous fine-needle aspiration biopsy was performed under fluoroscopic and IBUS guidance. Note the proximity of the needle to the ultrasound probe. **H:** Note the acoustic shadow of the needle near the bile duct.

Comment: Cholangiocarcinoma presents as a mass effect and wall thickening. There is obstruction of the bile duct, surrounded by a hypoechoic mass. The mass is located within and, in most cases, also outside the bile duct. The bile duct wall is not very well defined, and the three-layer appearance is lost. When the tumor extends proximal or distally, it is possible to evaluate the extension of the mass. It may be possible to identify infiltration of adjacent vascular structures, such as the portal vein. Lymph nodes surrounding the tumor were detected by some authors, but we were unable to detect enlarged lymph nodes in our cases. IBUS also can be used to guide percutaneous needle biopsies in association with fluoroscopy, as demonstrated.

14.5.5 Intraluminal Ultrasound In The Bile Ducts

Case 14.5.5:

A 60-year-old male patient presented with obstructive jaundice due to cholangiocarcinoma. Percutaneous drainage was requested because endoscopic access was not possible.

A, B

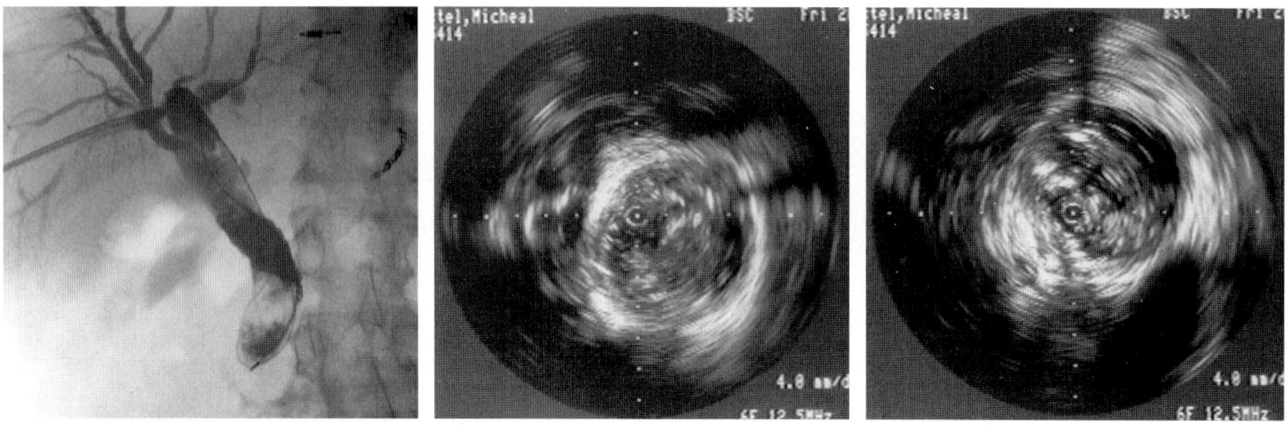

C

Figure 14.5.5

A: Percutaneous cholangiogram was performed after the bile duct was catheterized. The intrahepatic and extrahepatic bile ducts are dilated, and there is a large filling defect obstructing the distal bile duct, consistent with cholangiocarcinoma. **B:** IBUS of the distal choledochal lesion shows a dilated segment of bile duct with certain areas of an undefined parietal structure and a hypoechoic heterogeneous mass occupying the center of the bile duct, but significant extension of the tumor beyond the ductal wall. **C:** IBUS of the cholangiocarcinoma closer to the level of the papilla shows a small amount of tumor beyond the ductal wall. The portal vein is observed nearby and is not encased by the tumor. Due to the high surgical risk, surgical removal of the tumor was not proposed.

Comment: Intralaminar cholangiocarcinomas are readily identified by IBUS. The mass is seen as heterogenous and predominantly hypoechoic, with areas of increased echogenicity within the mass. The three-layered appearance of the bile duct wall is lost or very difficult to identify. The attachment of the tumor to the wall may be encountered and suggested by infiltration of the wall by the tumor.

14.5.6 Intraluminal Ultrasound In The Bile Ducts

Case 14.5.6:

A 57-year-old female patient presented with obstructive jaundice due to a cholangiocarcinoma at the confluence. Percutaneous treatment with metal stent placement was requested.

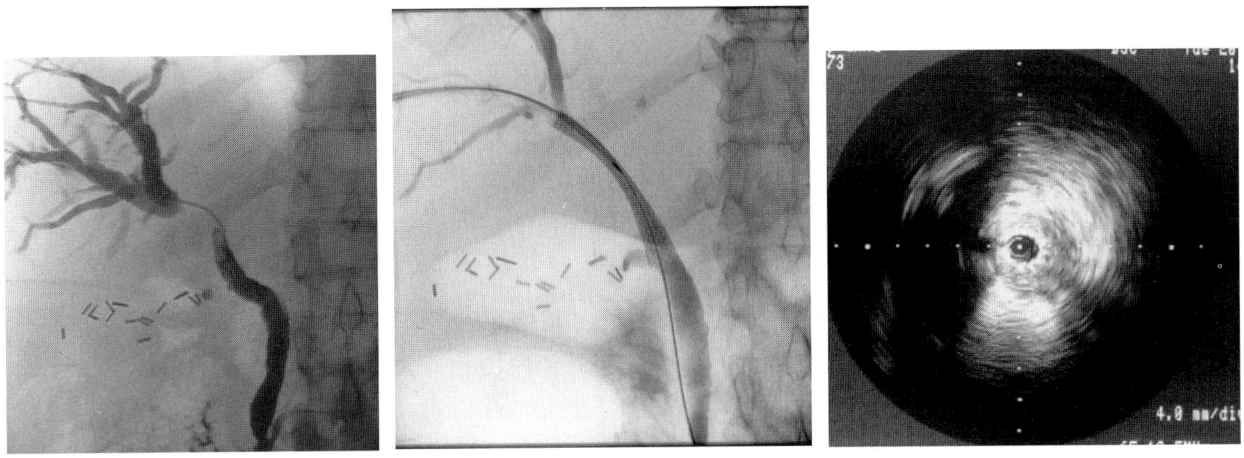

A B, C

Figure 14.5.6

A: Cholangiogram performed after catheterization of the intrahepatic bile ducts crossing the obstruction at the hepatic duct confluence. Note the gap between the right bile duct and the hepatic bile duct. The distal common bile duct is of normal caliber. A needle biopsy was performed using the cholangiogram and fluoroscopy as guidance. **B:** Cholangiogram after placement of a Wallstent across the obstruction shows patency through a partially expanded stent. Note the ultrasound probe within the stent. **C:** IBUS shows the partially expanded stent within a hypoechoic mass extending from the wall of the bile duct. Due to the presence of the stent and tumor infiltration, the duct wall was not readily appreciated.

Comment: Cholangiocarcinomas are presented as hypoechoic masses in close relationship with the bile duct wall. The layers of the duct are not visible. Stent placement impairs visibility of the tumor, which is visualized as a dense circumferential echogenic structure. The IBUS probe can be used to help guide biopsy.

14.5.7 Intraluminal Ultrasound In The Bile Ducts

Case 14.5.7:

A 70-year-old male patient presented with obstructive jaundice, due to pancreatic cancer, which could not be drained endoscopically. Percutaneous drainage was requested.

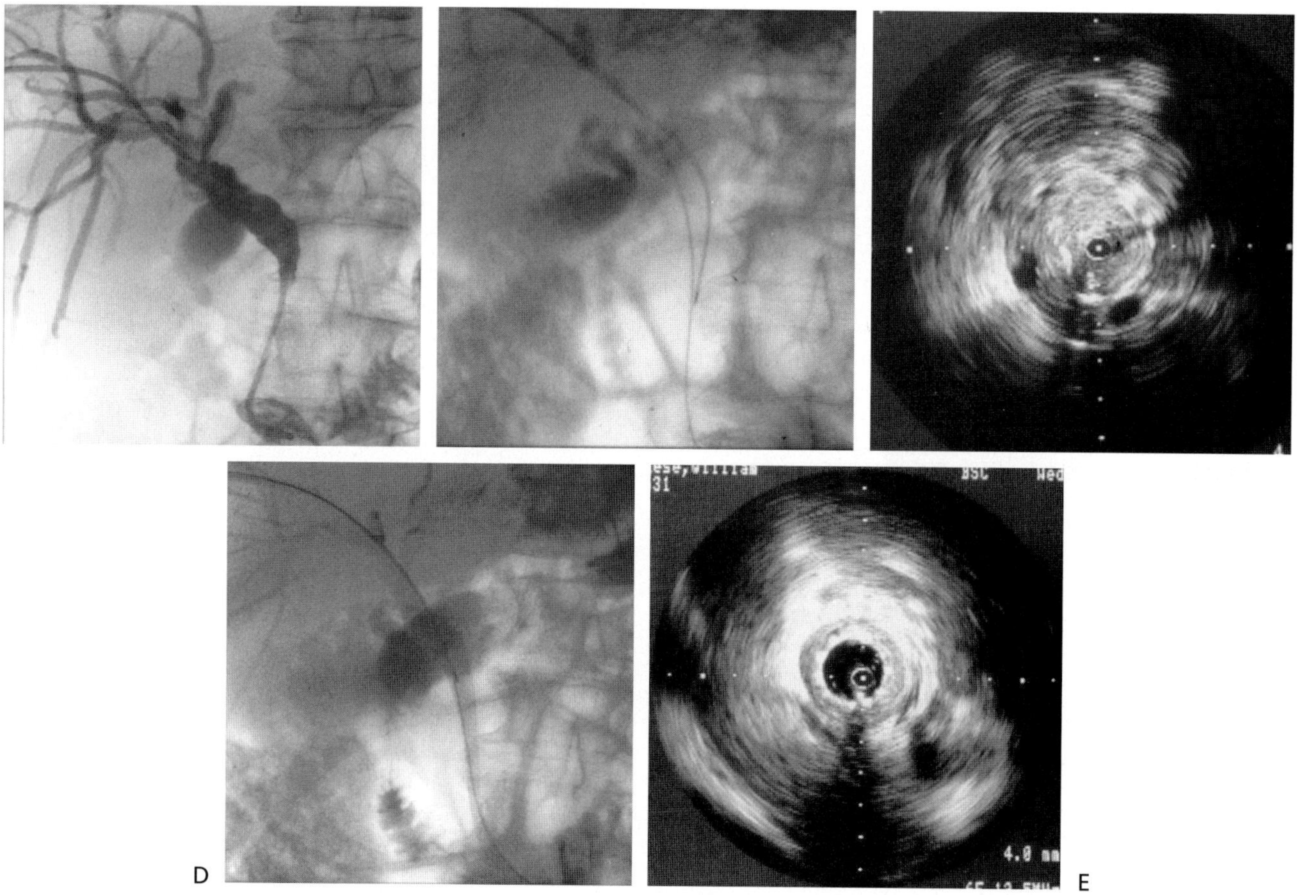

A, B C D E

Figure 14.5.7

F 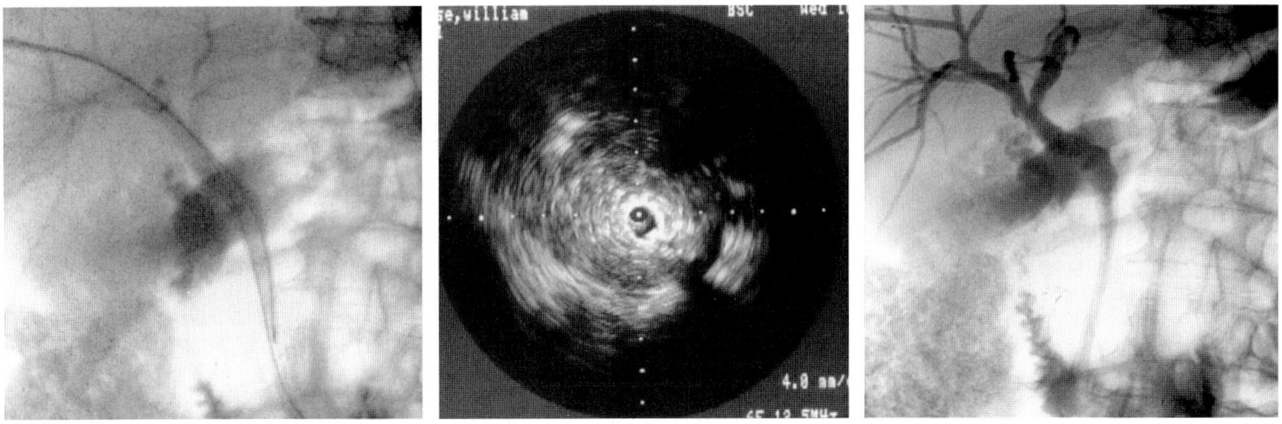 G, H

Figure 14.5.7 *(continued)*

A: Catheter cholangiogram following drainage with a 10F catheter was performed. Note the long stricture. There is partial filling of the gallbladder and duodenum. **B:** The ultrasound catheter was advanced over the wire for IBUS. **C:** IBUS shows a large complex mass with areas of hyperechogenicity and hypoechogenicity, surrounding the bile duct and invading and filling the main bile duct. The tumor extends from the head of the pancreas. The borders of the tumor are not visible due to the limited range of the ultrasound probe. The portal vein is not readily appreciated in this view but there is an artery parallel to the occluded bile duct. **D:** Following Wallstent placement the catheter/transducer was used for evaluation. **E:** IBUS post stent placement shows the open lumen and a thickened bile duct wall. **F:** The probe was advanced down into the stent in an area not totally expanded within the tumor. **G:** IBUS within the main tumor level shows the constricted stent walls and the large tumor within the head of the pancreas surrounding the bile duct. **H:** Final cholangiogram after stent placement shows adequate drainage into the duodenum.

Comment: Pancreatic tumors are observed on IBUS as hypoechoic masses surrounding the bile ducts and extending into the pancreas. It is difficult to identify the intrapancreatic boundaries of the tumor, because the penetration depth of ultrasound waves in the available catheters/probes is limited. Axial resolution of the image is limited to a few millimeters. The biliary wall structure is lost. Irregularities and ulcerations in the mucosa and tumor may be seen within the bile duct. Invasion of the portal vein may be identified. We were not able to identify lymph nodes around the bile duct or pancreatic tumor.

14.6.1 Percutaneous Management Of Biliary Duct Stones

Case 14.6.1:

A 50-year-old male patient presented with stenosis of the sphincter, recurrent obstructive jaundice, and a single large stone. Repeated attempts at endoscopic stone removal were not successful, due to the size of the stone and the stenosis. A percutaneous approach was requested to obtain access for lithotripsy.

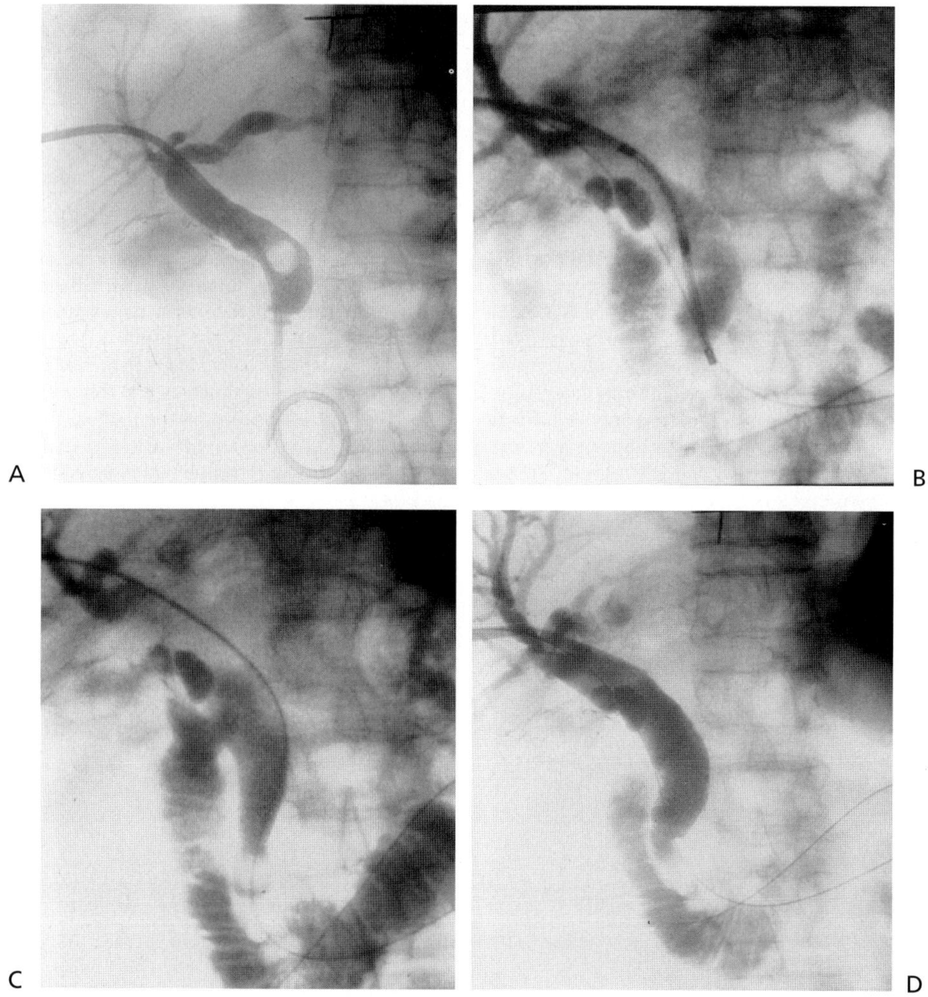

Figure 14.6.1

A: Catheter cholangiography shows a dilated bile duct, large stone, and sphincteric stenosis. An internal-external drainage catheter was placed for 2 weeks. **B:** Following percutaneous tract dilation, a 12F introducer sheath was placed to provide access for the cholangioscope and the lithotriptor. **C:** An occlusion balloon catheter was passed several times over the wire to push the stones into the duodenum. Note the balloon at the level of the papilla. **D:** Catheter cholangiogram shows patent bile duct without residual stones.

Comment: A significant number of patients with biliary strictures develop intrahepatic stones, which may be associated with recurrent cholangitis. The long-term presence of intrahepatic stones and frequent recurrence of stones after treatment ultimately may progress to secondary biliary cirrhosis and portal hypertension. Percutaneous treatment of stones in cases with strictures requires balloon cholangioplasty of the strictures, basket extraction of stones, and/or electrohydraulic lithotripsy using cholangioscopy. A percutaneous transhepatic approach usually is best, allowing access to the right and left ducts. When a T-tube has been in place for 5 to 6 weeks, the mature tract can be used for stone treatment as initially described in the literature. In patients with choledochojejunostomy or hepaticojejunostomy, when access from above is difficult or impossible, the retrograde approach can be used through percutaneous transjejunal puncture and balloon dilation of the stricture and stone extraction.

14.6.2 Percutaneous Management Of Biliary Duct Stones

Case 14.6.2:

A 49-year-old female patient with a postcholecystectomy stenosis of the common bile duct underwent three surgeries and eventually a right and left hepaticojejunostomy. Three years after the last surgery, the patient developed cholangitis and jaundice. Percutaneous cholangiogram showed stenosis of the hepaticojejunostomy and stones.

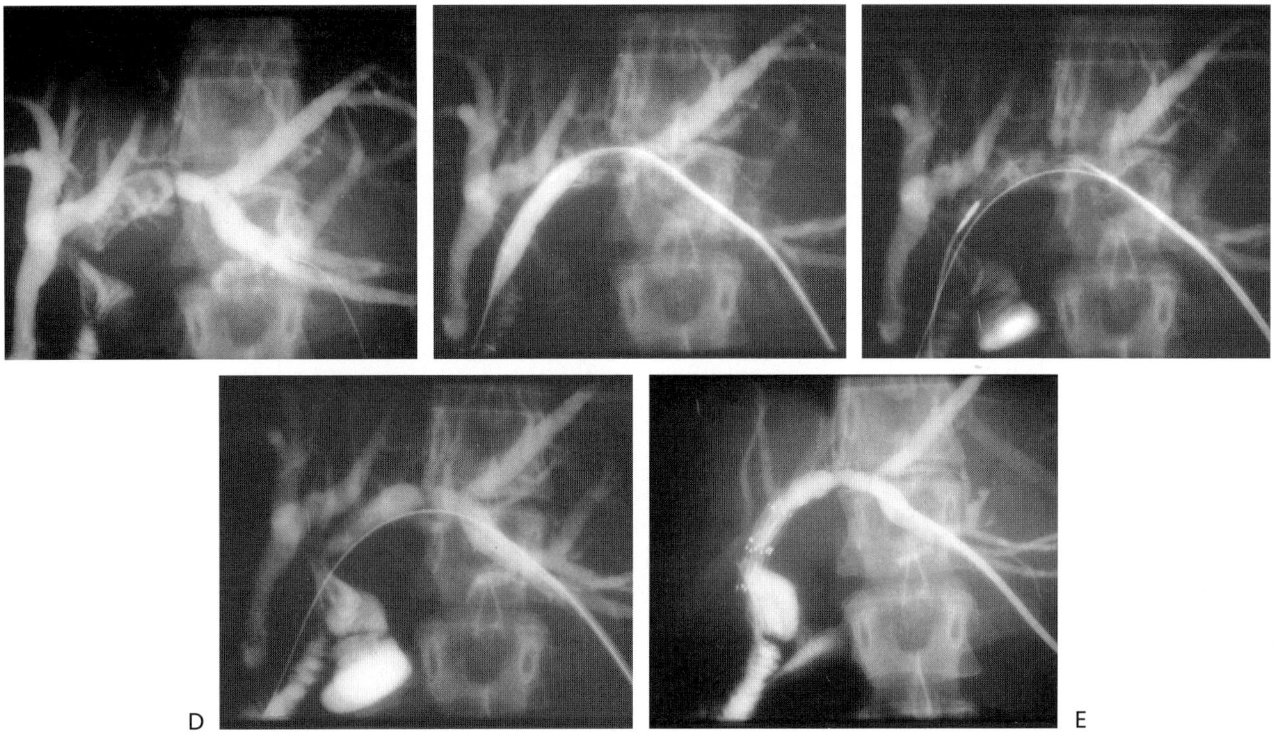

Figure 14.6.2

A: PTC with a fine needle shows dilated intrahepatic bile ducts, particularly on the left side, which shows a stenosis of the anastomosis and large stones impacted at the stricture. **B:** Percutaneous catheterization of the left duct was performed and a guidewire was passed through the stenosis, followed by placement of an 8-mm balloon to dilate the stricture. **C:** Through a introducer sheath, a basket was used to fragment and pass the stones through the anastomosis and into the bowel loop. **D:** Follow-up cholangiogram shows the bile ducts are clear of stones and of residual stenosis. **E:** A double-body, 8-mm Z-stent was placed across the stenosis to allow for better drainage. The patient did well, and the catheter was pulled out 2 days later. The patient had a recurrence of stones with one episode of cholangitis, which again was treated percutaneously with balloon dilation. Follow-up is now more than 5 years, without recurrence of symptoms.

Comment: Percutaneous treatment spared this patient a difficult surgery. The anastomosis was very high after the last surgery, and a new surgery would have been quite difficult. Percutaneous catheterization allowed subsequent adequate treatment. The stent was placed because the stricture recoiled. In an attempt to keep the stricture open, a decision was made to expand it with a stent. Despite one recurrence of stricture and stones, follow-up is long and the patient is doing well. The overall success rate of dilation of strictures is almost 90%, and the complete stone extraction rate is about 80%. Stone impaction may be a preclude to successful catheterization and dilation. Clinical symptoms improve in almost all patients shortly after stone extraction and dilation of the strictures.

14.6.3 Percutaneous Management Of Biliary Duct Stones

Case 14.6.3:

A 71-year-old male patient presented with a single large common duct stone and jaundice. Due to a stenosis in the papilla, endoscopic treatment was not successful. A percutaneous approach was requested for biliary drainage and access for lithotripsy.

A 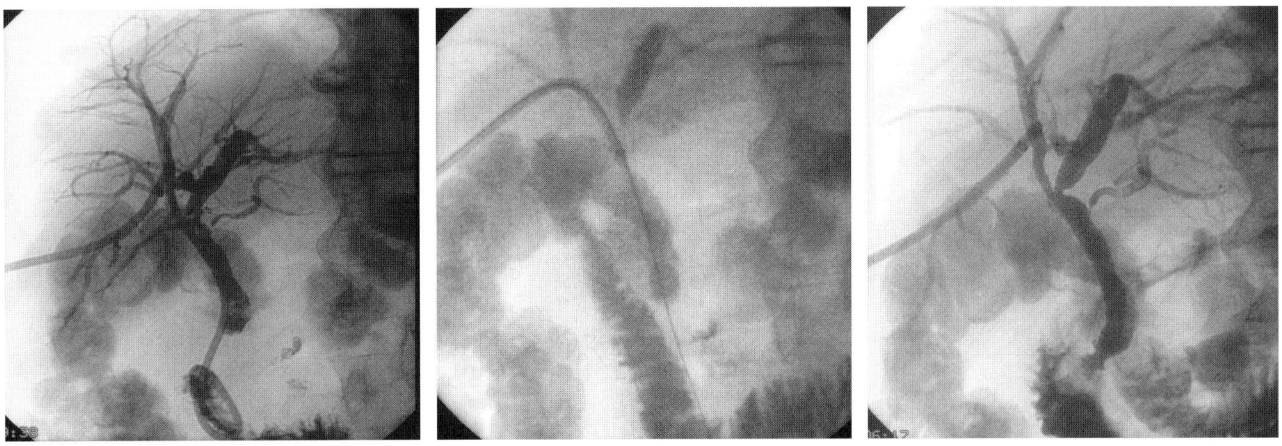 B, C

Figure 14.6.3

A: Percutaneous catheterization of the bile duct was performed. A few days later, catheter cholangiogram shows moderately dilated bile ducts and a large stone in the distal common bile duct. **B:** The papilla was dilated with an 8-mm balloon, and a latex occlusion balloon was advanced several times over the wire to push the stone into the duodenum. Note the inflated balloon in the middle of the common bile duct. An 8F Flexor sheath was used to provide access. **C:** Final cholangiogram shows patency of the bile duct with free flow of contrast media into the duodenum. The catheter subsequently was pulled out.

Comment: Single common bile duct stones can be treated by balloon extraction if the size of the stone is suitable to pass through the papilla. In case of larger stones, fragmentation may be required. Basket fragmentation or electrohydraulic lithotripsy may be used in such cases. It is necessary to dilate the papilla or perform a sphincterotomy to make room for the stone to be pushed through. Significant spasm of the sphincter may be caused by manipulation of the stone and balloon through the papilla, and temporary occlusion may be present. In this specific case, ERCP with papillotomy was not possible, and percutaneous access was the best alternative.

14.6.4 Percutaneous Management Of Biliary Duct Stones

Case 14.6.4:

A 33-year-old male patient was treated for gallstones by conventional cholecystectomy, followed by placement of a T-tube drain into the common bile duct. The patient was referred for treatment through the T-tube fistula after the drain was in place for 6 weeks, for residual common duct stones.

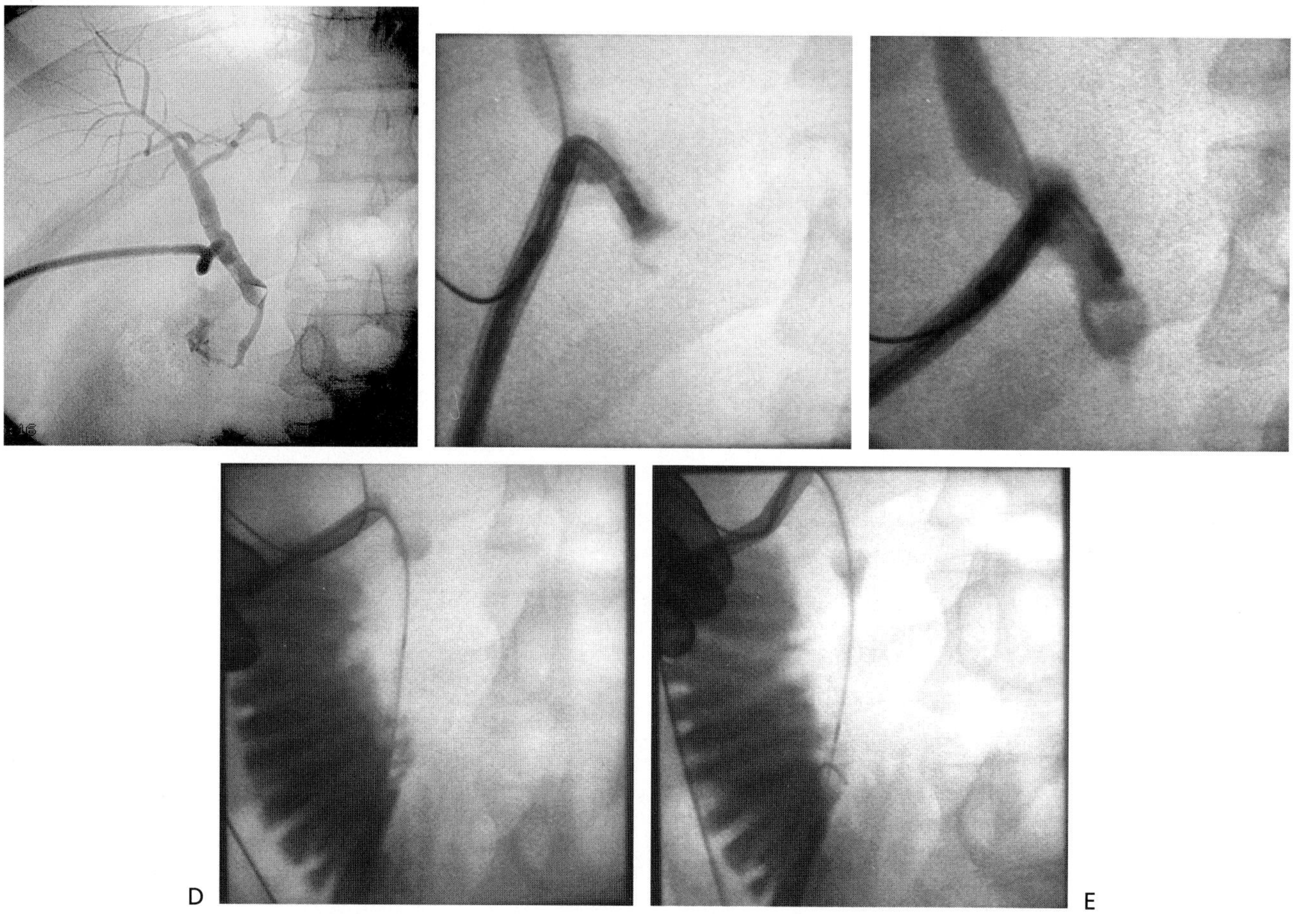

A, B C D E

Figure 14.6.4

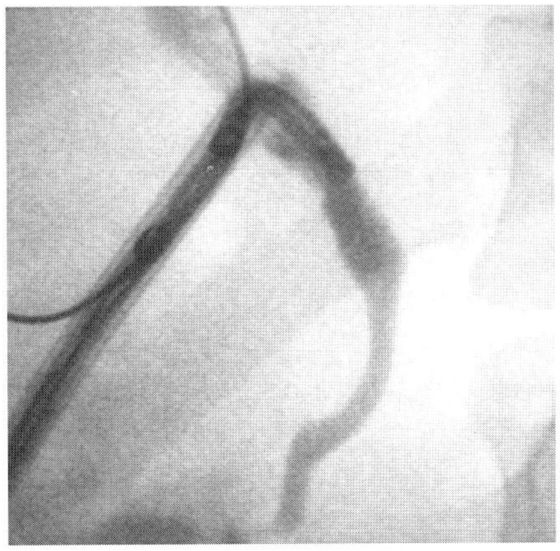

F

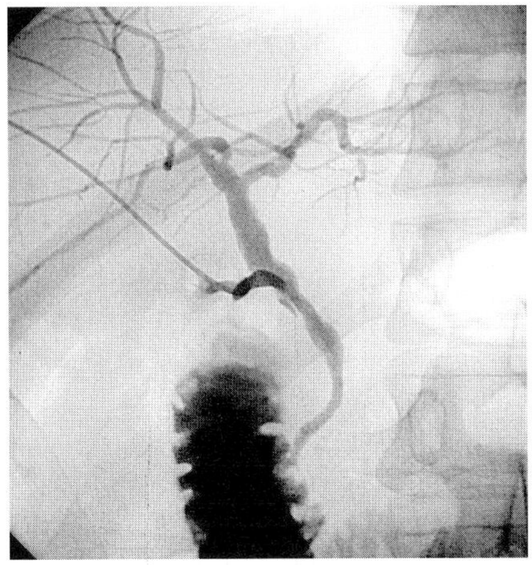

G

Figure 14.6.4 *(continued)*

A: T-tube cholangiogram shows a large stone in the distal common bile duct. Note free passage of contrast through the papilla. The T-tube was displaced and was lying partially in the tract. **B:** A safety guidewire was introduced toward the liver to maintain the access through the fistula, while the cholangioscope was introduced toward the distal common bile duct. **C:** After contact with the stone, the lithotriptor probe was advanced toward the stone for fragmentation. **D,E:** Following fragmentation, a latex balloon was pushed over the wire to expel the fragments into the duodenum. **F:** Following cholangioscopic inspection, which showed no residual stones, contrast injection was used to demonstrate that the distal common duct was clean. **G:** Final cholangiogram shows patency of the intrahepatic and extrahepatic bile ducts. The catheter was pulled and the fistula sealed off.

Comment: The best indication for percutaneous transhepatic electrohydraulic lithotripsy is failure of endoscopic treatment or in the situation of strictured hepaticojejunostomy where endoscopic treatment is not possible. It requires the placement of a percutaneous drainage catheter in the right or left bile duct, depending on the location of the stones and stricture. When a T-tube tract is available, it can be used for the access, as long as it is mature for about 6 weeks. About 92% of patients are free of stones after treatment. In patients with diffuse intrahepatic stones, only 75% of the stones can be cleared. Despite the high success rate, one large series reported severe complications, including hemobilia requiring transfusion, bile duct perforation, cholangitis, acute pulmonary edema, and hemothorax, in 22% of patients, with an 8% mortality rate using the percutaneous approach.

14.6.5 Percutaneous Management Of Biliary Duct Stones

Case 14.6.5:

A 61-year-old female patient with multiple problems was transferred for treatment of a left hepatic abscess and multiple common bile duct stones. The patient was treated for sepsis in the intensive care unit for several days. At laparotomy, a left liver abscess was drained and debrided. A splenectomy was performed, and the common bile duct was explored for extraction of multiple stones. An indeterminate amount of stones were left within the bile ducts. Multiple drains were placed, including a T-tube drain, and the abdomen was closed. About 20 days after surgery, percutaneous stone treatment was attempted through the drain tract.

A, B

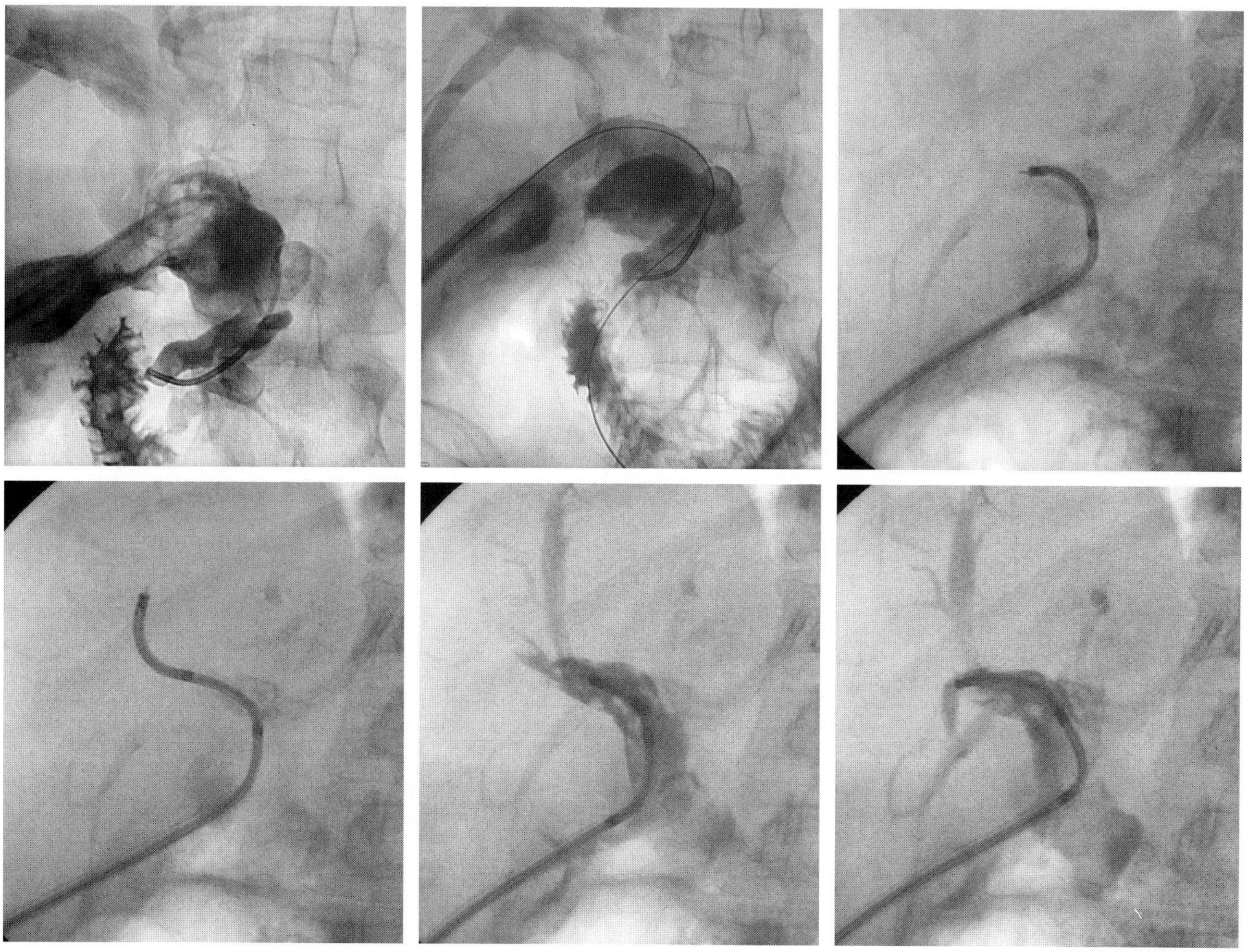

C

D, E

F

Figure 14.6.5

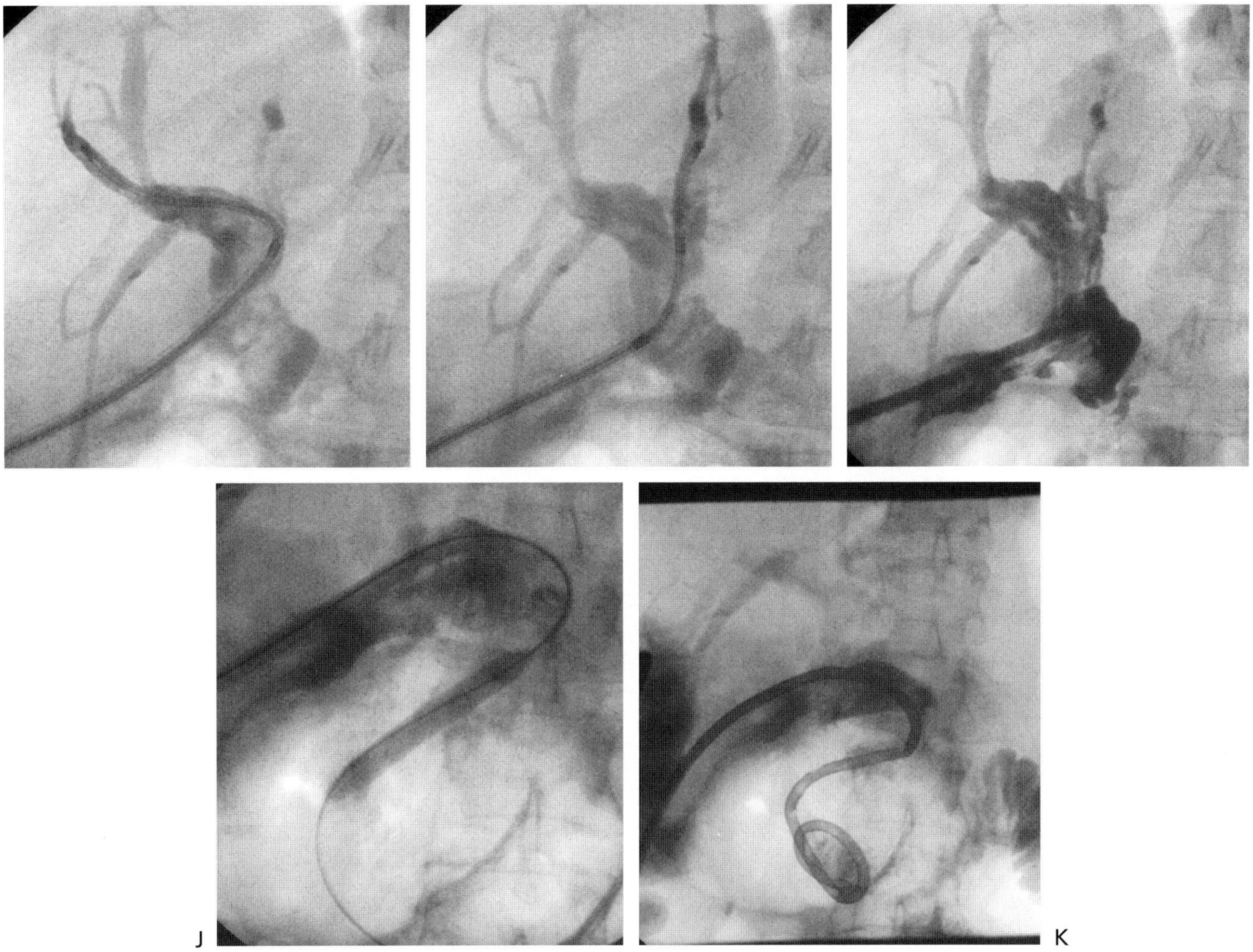

G H, I J K

Figure 14.6.5 *(continued)*

A: Catheterization through the T-tube tract was performed. Injection of contrast material demonstrates a markedly enlarged bile duct with multiple stones. Injection close to the sphincter shows stenosis of the papilla. **B:** A guidewire was passed into the duodenum. **C–H:** The cholangioscope was used for lithotripsy of the multiple biliary stones in different positions, the common bile duct, and the ducts of the right and left hepatic lobes. **I:** Cholangiogram after lithotripsy shows the bile ducts are dilated but free of major stones. **J:** An 8-mm balloon was used to dilate the papilla. **K:** A 10F internal-external biliary catheter was placed for 1 week and then removed.

Comment: Endoscopic sphincterotomy can be accomplished successfully in about 90% of patients in whom the papilla can be approached. In the remaining 10% of patients, previous conditions, such as Billroth gastric resection, intradiverticular papilla, and duodenal stenosis, make access to the papilla difficult or impossible. Percutaneous approach may permit access to the papilla from inside, and a sphincterotomy can be passed to open up the papilla. Alternatively, but not as effectively, balloon dilation can be used to enlarge the sphincter and promote the passage of stones and fragments after lithotripsy. The approach for lithotripsy and sphincter dilation also can be performed through the T-tube tract, as demonstrated in this case.

Electrohydraulic lithotripsy facilitates stone treatment and larger stones may be managed, as opposed to the Burhenne technique, where the larger stones must be removed by basket or crushed before removal.

14.6.6 Percutaneous Management Of Biliary Duct Stones

Case 14.6.6:

A 41-year-old female patient with postlaparoscopic cholecystectomy complications, followed by two surgical repairs, developed stenosis of the hepaticojejunostomy with multiple intrahepatic stones, jaundice, and recurrent cholangitis. The patient refused surgery, and an extensive percutaneous treatment was proposed.

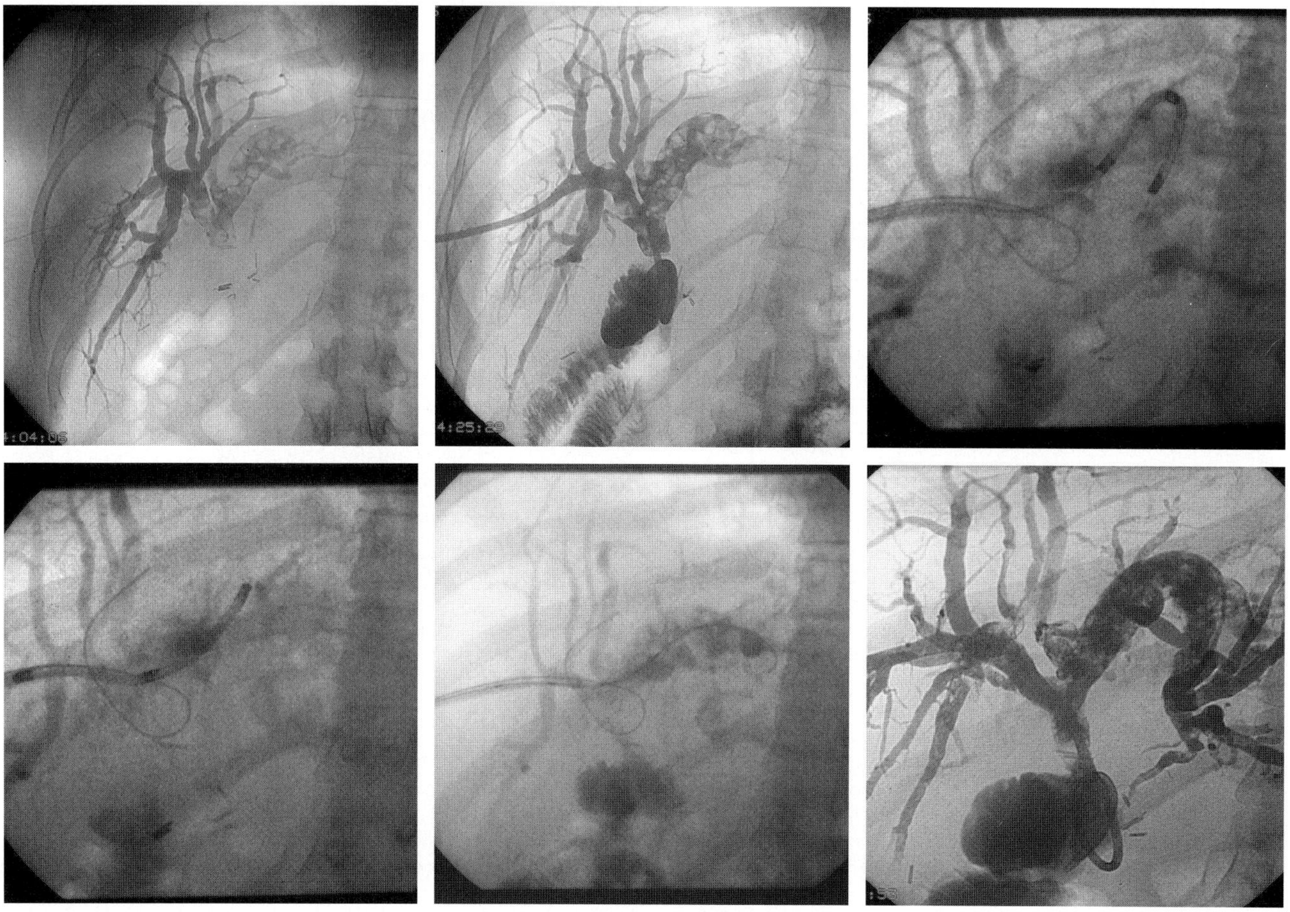

A, B C D, E F

Figure 14.6.6

A: PTC with a fine needle shows dilated intrahepatic bile ducts and innumerable stones. Note total obstruction of the hepaticojejunostomy. **B:** Following percutaneous catheterization of the bile duct, an internal-external drainage biliary catheter was passed through the occluded anastomoses after balloon dilation. **C,D:** Two days after establishing external access, electrohydraulic lithotripsy was performed. Following catheterization of the left hepatic duct, the cholangioscope was advanced over the wire in the peripheral segment of the left hepatic duct. Lithotripsy was performed in retrograde fashion down to the confluence and common hepatic duct. Note the tip of the lithotripsy probe. **E:** An occlusion balloon was passed centripetally, several times, to pull the fragments into the main bile duct. A 10F catheter was placed for internal-external drainage. **F:** Catheter cholangiogram performed 3 days after lithotripsy shows dilated bile ducts with a multitude of stone fragments and debris. **G,H:** New lithotripsy was performed through the percutaneous access. **I:** Catheter cholangiogram 2 days after the second treatment shows at least two stones in the left and common hepatic ducts, which were removed by basket and balloon retrieval. **J:** Follow-up cholangiogram shows the intrahepatic biliary tree is free of stones. The access was maintained. **K:** One week later, a new cholangiogram shows one residual stone, which was removed with an occlusion balloon. **L:** Follow-up cholangiogram shows the bile ducts are free of stones. **M:** A 10-mm Z-stent was placed at the level of the stricture. The patient has been doing well for about 3 years.

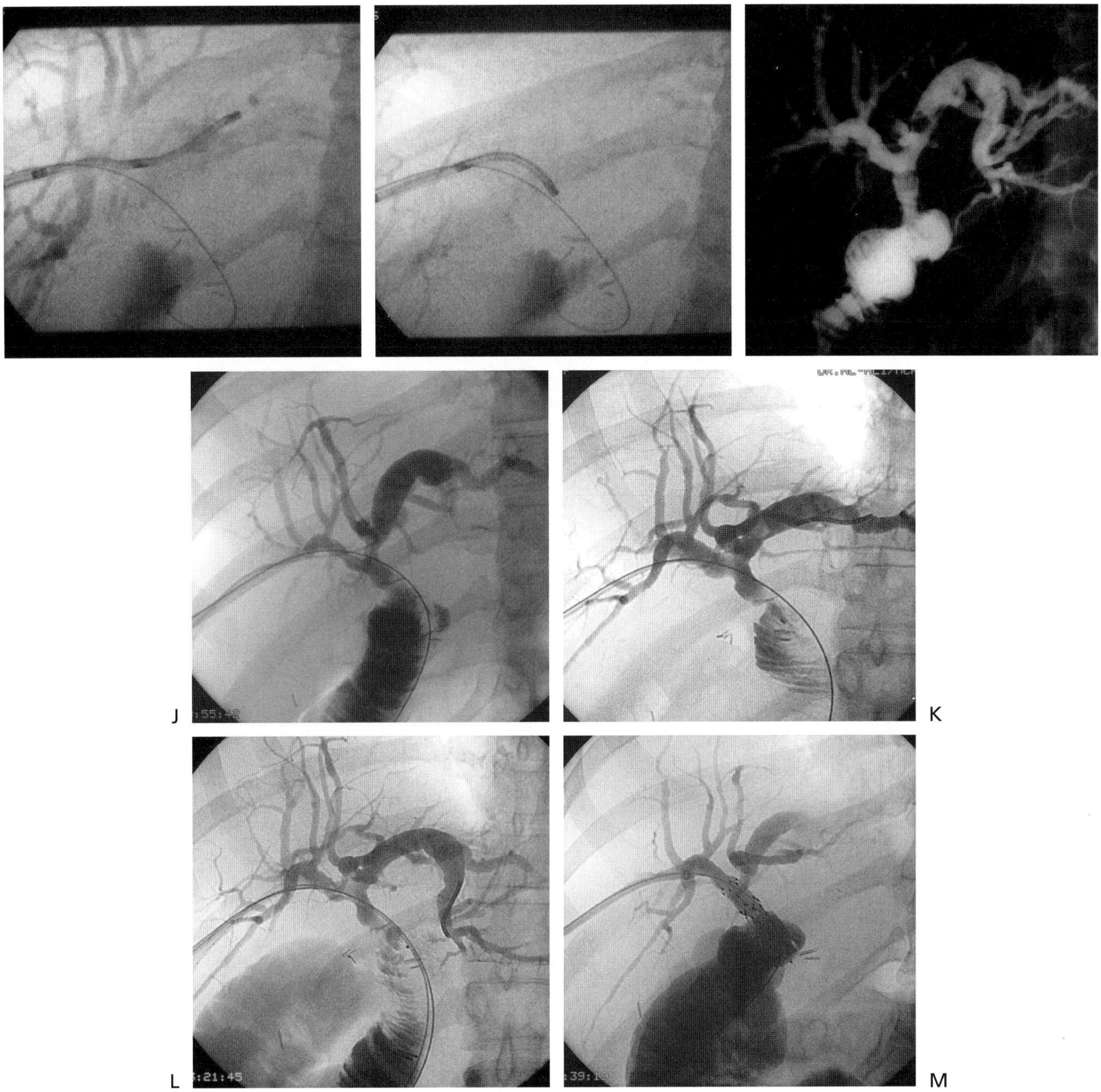

Figure 14.6.6 *(continued)*

Comment: This is a typical case where percutaneous lithotripsy could maximize benefit for a patient who had undergone three previous surgeries on the bile ducts. Although the stenosis and intrahepatic stones developed 2 years after the last surgery, the patient refused surgery and accepted the percutaneous alternative. After obtaining access, multiple procedures were necessary, and a few residual stones were noted in follow-up studies. Two electrohydraulic procedures were performed successfully, and two complementary balloon stone extractions further cleaned the bile ducts. Multiple balloon dilations of the stenosis were performed. However, persistent recoil of the stricture was seen, which led to the decision to place a Z-stent. Final cholangiogram following stent placement showed adequate patency, which allowed for long-term follow-up.

14.6.7 Percutaneous Management Of Biliary Duct Stones

Case 14.6.7:

A 73-year-old male patient presented with large stones in the common bile duct 2 years after cholecystectomy. Percutaneous biliary drainage was performed to provide decompression and access for cholangioscopic treatment.

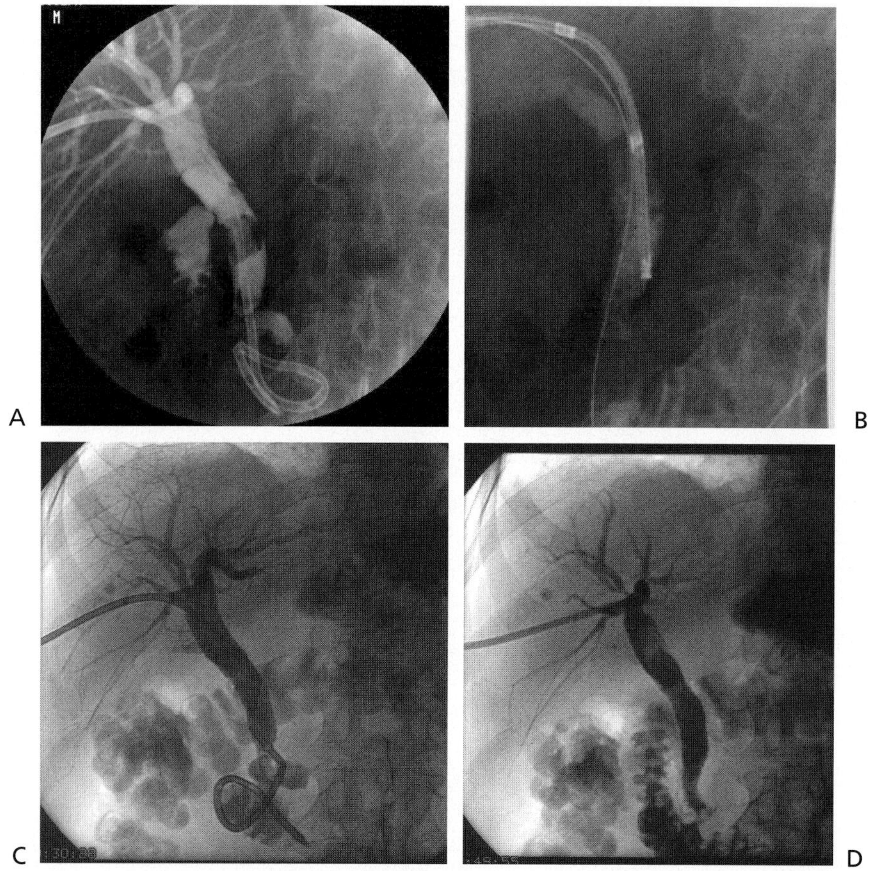

Figure 14.6.7

A: Catheter cholangiography showed one large stone and at least two smaller stones/fragments. **B:** The catheter was exchanged over the wire, the wire was kept as a safety wire, and a 12F sheath was placed for the cholangioscope. The probe broke the stones, and the debris was pushed into the duodenum by the scope and occlusion balloon. **C:** The following day, a cholangiogram was performed to search for residual stones. No fragments were identified. **D:** The catheter was removed, and a challenge cholangiogram shows the ducts are clean and the papilla is patent. No residual stones were seen on IBUS (not shown). The patient is doing well for the last 2 years.

Comment: The left lobe approach is preferred by some authors, because it provides a straighter path with direct access to the common bile duct. In addition, the left lobe approach poses no risk of crossing the pleural space. Because the tract does not pass between the ribs, there is no intercostal pain. When the initial biliary drainage is performed for cholangitis and jaundice, as in this patient, external drainage is provided until the infection resolves. If sepsis is not a concern, immediate tract dilation can follow the initial percutaneous access. The tract can be dilated by coaxial telescoping dilators or balloon dilation. A Teflon sheath should always be used to protect the liver parenchyma and avoid bleeding. The choledochoscope systems are sized between 12F and 18F. A variety of standard instruments can be used through the working channel of the choledochoscope to aid in stone removal. When the tip of the device is maximally deflected, the semirigid instruments usually do not pass through the channel. Although baskets and grasping forceps can be used for stone extraction, the most reliable technique is intracorporeal lithotripsy. Our experience is more extensive with electrohydraulic lithotripsy, but ultrasonic and laser instruments also are available. In the presented case, electrohydraulic lithotripsy was used and crushed the stones very easily. In our experience, complications directly related to percutaneous biliary endoscopy are rare and mild. Vagal reactions may occur. Transient bacteremia is unusual but may develop after manipulation. An appropriate period of external drainage should be allowed before any elective stone manipulation. Disruption of the tract may occur and can be avoided in most cases by gentle manipulation and use of a protecting sheath.

14.6.8 Percutaneous Management Of Biliary Duct Stones

Case 14.6.8:

A 32 -year-old female patient presented with sepsis and jaundice. US showed dilated bile ducts and large stones in the right and left bile ducts extending into the stump of the hepatic duct, 5 years after conventional surgical cholecystectomy. After cholecystectomy, the patient developed a stenosis that was treated by hepaticojejunostomy. Percutaneous biliary drainage was performed to provide decompression and access for treatment.

A, B

C

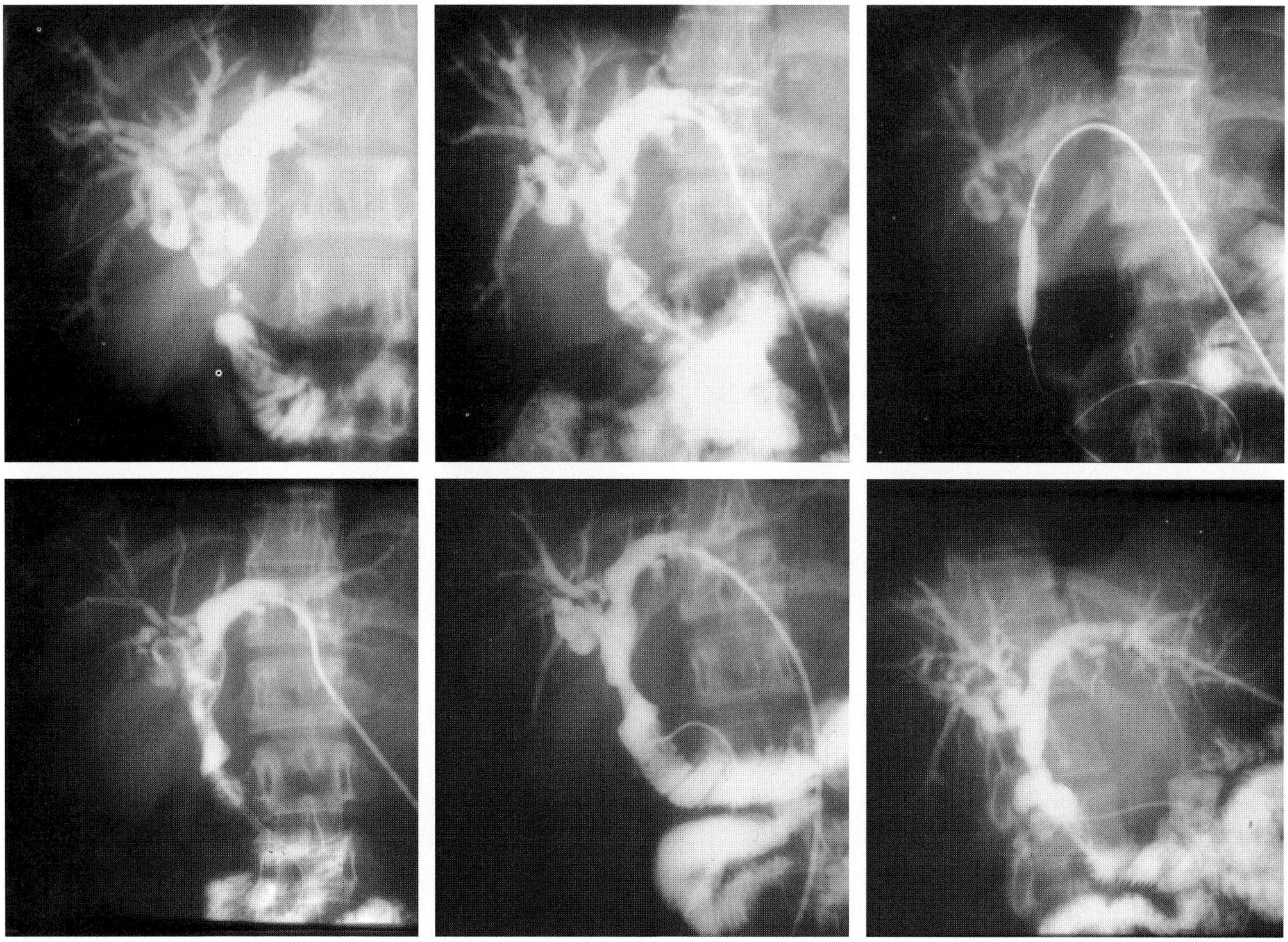

D, E

F

Figure 14.6.8

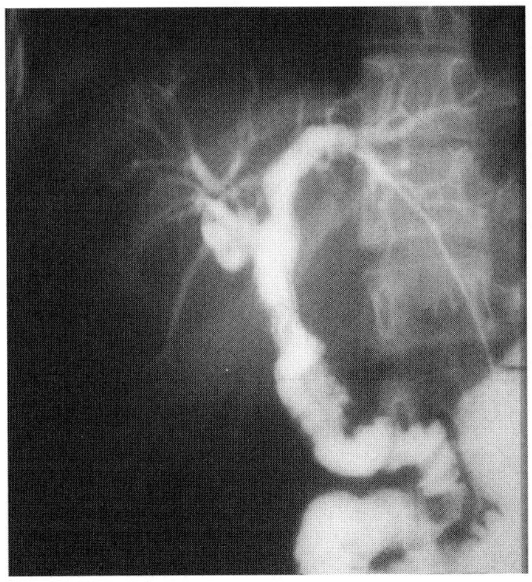
G

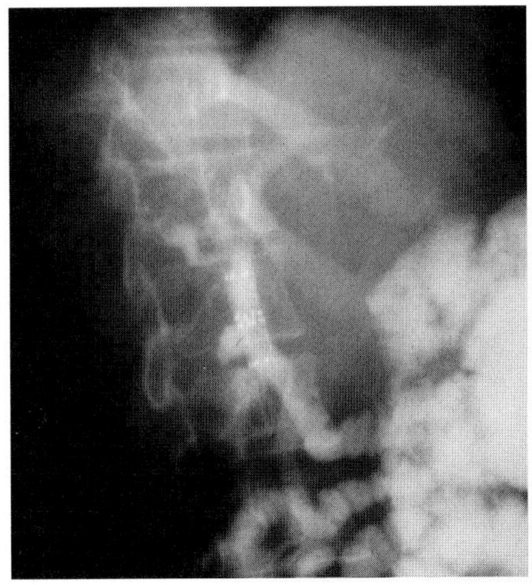
H

Figure 14.6.8 *(continued)*

A: Percutaneous cholangiogram with a fine needle showed extremely dilated intrahepatic bile ducts with impacted stones in the right and left bile ducts. There was a severe stenosis at the hepaticojejunostomy that caused infection and stone buildup. Note passage of contrast medium into the bowel loop. **B:** Percutaneous access was obtained from the left hepatic duct, due to the anatomy and disposition of the stones. **C:** A guidewire was passed through the stenosis, and a 10-mm balloon was used to dilate the stricture. **D:** After external drainage was obtained and the infection was controlled, extracorporeal shockwave lithotripsy was performed to fragment the stones and facilitate extraction. **E–G:** Three percutaneous procedures were used to pass stone fragments into the bowel loop and clean up the multiple cavities and pouchs within the bile ducts. An additional transjejunal approach was utilized to facilitate pulling of stone fragments into the bowel loop using occlusion balloons and baskets. A double body Z-stent was placed through the stenosis to improve long-term drainage. **H:** Late film shows good emptying of the contrast from the bile ducts. This patient still is doing well at more than 7 years of follow-up, without symptoms of biliary obstruction.

Comment: This case demonstrates the need to use multiple procedures and techniques to overcome the specific difficulties of overdilated ducts associated with severe stenosis. When stones are packed, it is difficult to use balloons to pull or push the stones from the bile ducts into the bowel loop. Puncture of the Roux-en-Y jejunal limb can be performed easily when contrast material is injected into the bile duct and readily passes into the jejunal loop. When the stenosis is tight, it may be difficult to pass the stricture; however balloon dilation made the task easier in this case. Extracorporeal shockwave lithotripsy was used to break the stones into smaller fragments, as electrohydraulic lithotripsy was not yet available at that time. Multiple procedures were necessary to clean up the bile ducts. The metal stent kept the anastomosis open and produced good long-term results.

Suggested Reading

Benign Diseases

Amor A, Chapoutot C, Michel J, et al. Secondary sclerosing cholangitis. *Presse Med* 1995;24:948–952.

Boland GW, Mueller Peter R, et al. Laparoscopic cholecystectomy with bile duct injury: percutaneous management of biliary stricture and associated complications. *AJR* 1996;166:603–607.

Citron SJ, Martin LG. Benign biliary strictures: treatment with percutaneous cholangioplasty. *Radiology* 1991;178:339–341.

Dodd GD, Niedzwiecki GA, Campbell WL, et al. Bile duct calculi in patients with primary sclerosing cholangitis. *Radiology* 1997;203:443–447.

Hausegger KA, Kluger C, Uggowitzer M, et al. Benign biliary obstruction: is treatment with the Wallstent advisable? *Radiology* 1996;200:437–441.

Maccioni F, Rossi M, Salvatori FM, et al. Metallic stents in benign biliary strictures: three year follow-up. *Cardiovasc Intervent Radiol* 1992;15:360–366.

Morgan RA, van Sonnenberg E, Wittich GR, et al. Percutaneous management of bile duct injury after laparoscopic cholecystectomy. *AJR* 1996;165:985–990.

Mueller PR, van Sonnenberg E, Ferrucci JT, et al. Biliary stricture dilatation: multicenter review of clinical management in 73 patients. *Radiology* 1986;160:17–22.

Perry LJ, Stokes KR, Lewis WD, et al. Biliary intervention by means of percutaneous puncture of the antecolic jejunal loop. *Radiology* 1995;195:163–167.

Soulez G, Therasse E, Oliva VL, et al. Left hepaticogastrostomy for biliary obstruction: long-term results. *Radiology* 1997;204:780–786.

Tarnasky PR, Cunningham JT, Hawes RH, et al. Transpapillary stenting of proximal biliary strictures: does biliary sphincterotomy reduce the risk of postprocedure pancreatitis? *Gastrointest Endosc* 1997;45:46–51

Uflacker R, Mourao GS, Piske RL, et al. Percutaneous transhepatic biliary drainage: alternatives in left hepatic duct obstruction. *Gastrointest Radiol* 1989;14:137–142.

Uflacker R, Wholey MH, Amaral NM, et al. Parasitic and mycotic causes of biliary obstruction. *Gastrointest Radiol* 1982;7:173–179.

Uflacker R. Percutaneous biliary procedures. *Gastrointest Endosc Clin N Am* 1996;6:177–215.

Vorwerk D, Kissinger G, Handt S, et al. Long-term patency of Wallstent endoprosthesis in benign biliary obstructions: experimental results. *J Vasc Interv Radiol* 1993;4:625–634.

Malignant Diseases

Boguth L, Tatalovic S, Antonucci F, et al. Malignant biliary obstructions: clinical and histopathologic correlation after treatment with self-expanding metal prostheses. *Radiology* 1994;192:669–674.

Eschelman DJ, Shapiro MJ, Bonn J, et al. Malignant biliary duct obstruction: long-term experience with Gianturco stents and combined-modality radiation therapy. *Radiology* 1996:200:717–724.

Gillams A, Dick R, Dooley JS, et al. Self-expandable stainless steel braided endoprosthesis for biliary strictures. *Radiology* 1990;174: 137–140.

Gordon RL, Ring EJ, LaBerge JM, et al. Malignant biliary obstruction: treatment with expandable metallic stents. Follow-up of 50 consecutive patients. *Radiology* 1992;182:697–701.

Hausegger KA, Kleiner R, Lammer J, et al. Malignant biliary obstruction: histologic findings after treatment with self-expandable stents. *Radiology* 1992;185:461–464.

Lammer J, Hausegger KA. Flückiger F, et al. Common bile duct obstruction due to malignancy: treatment with plastic versus metal stents. *Radiology* 1996;201:167–172.

Rossi P, Bezzi M, Rossi M, et al. Metallic stents in malignant biliary obstruction: results of a multicenter European study of 240 patients. *J Vasc Interv Radiol* 1994;5:279–285.

Uflacker R, Mourão GS, Piske RL, et al. Hemobilia: transcatheter occlusive therapy and long-term follow-up. *Cardiovasc Intervent Radiol* 1989;14:136–141.

Uflacker R, Mourão GS, Piske RL, et al. Percutaneous transhepatic biliary drainage: alternatives in left hepatic duct obstruction. *Gastrointest Radiol* 1989;14:137–142.

Uflacker R. Percutaneous biliary procedures. *Gastrointest Endosc Clin N Am* 1996;6:177–215.

Percutaneous Cholecystostomy And Stone Manipulation

Browning PD, Mcgahan JP, Gerscovich EO. Percutaneous cholecystostomy for suspected acute cholecystitis in the hospitalized patient. *J Vasc Interv Radiol* 1993;4:531–538.

LaBerge JM, Gordon RL, Kertan RK, et al. Delayed gallbladder rupture following percutaneous cholecystostomy. Delayed gallbladder rupture following percutaneous cholecystostomy. *J Vasc Interv Radiol* 1991;2:539–541.

Lindeman SR, Tung G, Silverman SG, et al. Percutaneous cholecystostomy: a review. *Semin Interv Radiol* 1988;5:179–185.

Nemcek AA, Bernstein JE, Vogelzang RL. Percutaneous cholecystostomy: does transhepatic puncture preclude a transperitoneal catheter route? *J Vasc Interv Radiol* 1991;2:543–547.

Pearse DM, Hawkins IF, Shaver R, et al. Percutaneous cholecystostomy in acute cholecystitis and common duct obstruction. *Radiology* 1984;152:365–367.

Uflacker R. Percutaneous biliary procedures. *Gastrointest Endosc Clin N Am* 1996;6:177–215.

Van Sonnenberg E, Wittich GR, Casola G, et al. Diagnostic and therapeutic percutaneous gallbladder procedures. *Radiology* 1986;160: 23–26.

Management Of Bile Duct Stones

Angelini G, Mansueto G, Giacomin D, et al. Percutaneous transhepatic sphincterotomy of the major papilla and stone extraction without endoscopic control. *Cardiovasc Intervent Radiol* 1997;20:213–215.

Clouse ME, Stokes KR, Lee RGL, et al. Bile duct stone: percutaneous transhepatic removal. *Radiology* 1986;160:525–529.

Han JK, Choi BI, Chung J-W, et al. Cholecystocholedochostomy with use of a self-expandable metallic stent: treatment method for nonfunctioning cholecystojejunostomy. *J Vasc Interv Radiol* 1996;7:757–760.

Harris VJ, Sherman S, Trerotola SO, et al. Complex biliary stones: treatment with a small choledoscope and laser lithotripsy. *Radiology* 1996:199:71–77.

Jan YY, Chen MF. Percutaneous transhepatic cholangioscopic lithotomy for hepatolithiasis: long-term results. *Gastrointest Radiol* 1995;42:1–5.

Picus D, Weyman PJ, Marx MV. Role of percutaneous intracorporeal electrohydraulic lithotripsy in the treatment of biliary tract calculi. *Radiology* 1989;170:989–993.

Sheng R, Ramirez CB, Zajko AB, et al. Biliary stones and sludge in liver transplant patients: a 13-year experience. *Radiology* 1996;198: 243–247.

Sherman S, Hawes RH, Lehman GA. Management of bile duct stones. *Semin Liver Dis* 1990;10:205:221.

Wu SM, Marchant LK, Haskal ZJ. Percutaneous interventions in the biliary tree. *Semin Roentgenol* 1997;3:228–245.

Intraluminal Ultrasound In The Bile Ducts

Engstron CF, Wiechel KL. Endoluminal ultrasound of the bile ducts. *Surg Endosc* 1990;4:187–190.

Furukawa T, Naitoh Y, Tsukamoto Y, et al. New technique using intraductal ultrasonography for the diagnosis of diseases of the pancreatobiliary system. *J Ultrasound Med* 1992;11:607–612.

Kaufman AR, Sivak MV Jr. Endoscopic ultrasonography in the differential diagnosis of pancreatic disease. *Gastrointest Endosc* 1989;35:214–219.

Kuroiwa M, Tsukamoto Y, Naitoh Y, et al. New technique using intraductal ultrasonography for the diagnosis of bile duct cancer. *J Ultrasound Med* 1994;13:189–195.

Miller LS, Scciano TD, Liu J-B. Pancreaticobiliary tract. In: Liu J-B, Goldberg BB, eds. *Endoluminal ultrasound: vascular and nonvascular applications.* London: Martin Dunitz, 1998:229–250.

Shapiro MJ, Bonn J, Sullivan KL et al. Endoluminal biliary ultrasound: initial clinical experience. *J Vasc Interv Radiol* 1991;2:11–12.

Tamada K, Ido K, Ueno N, et al. Preoperative staging of extrahepatic bile duct cancer with intraductal ultrasonography. *Am J Gastroenterol* 1995;90:239–246.

van Sonnenberg E, D'Agostino HB, Sanchez RL, et al. Percutaneous intraluminal US in the gallbladder and bile ducts. *Radiology* 1992;182:693–696.

Yasuda K. Ultrasonic probes for pancreaticobiliary strictures. *Gastrointest Endosc* 1996;43:S35–S38.

CHAPTER 15

Percutaneous Management Of Fluid Collections, Cysts, And Fistulas

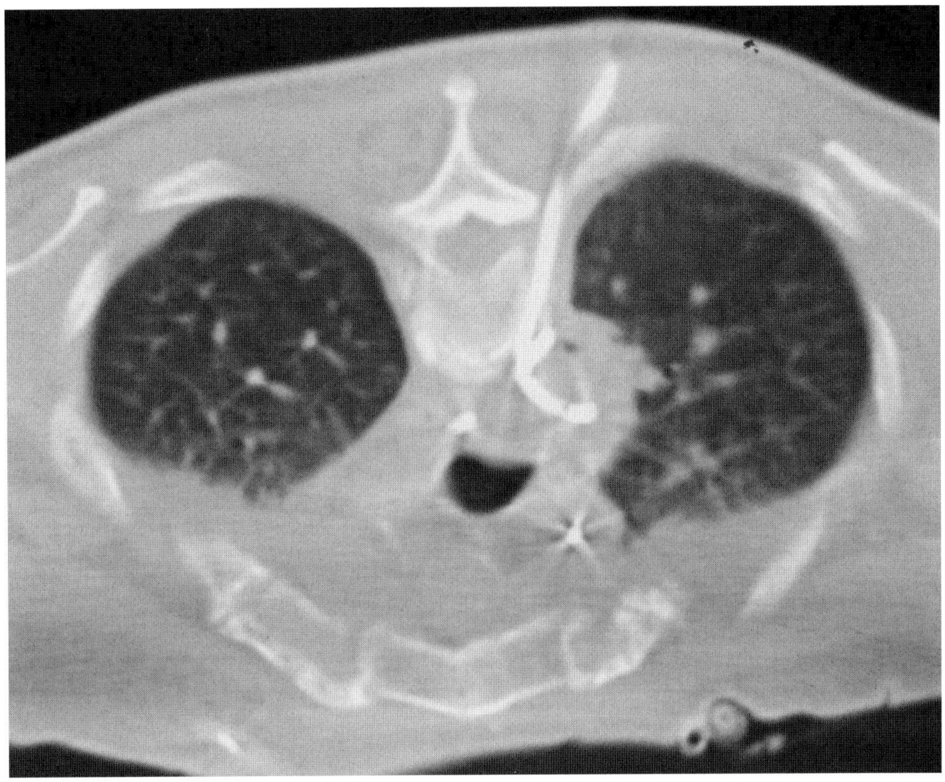

15.1.1 Drainage Of The Chest

Case 15.1.1:

A 43-year-old alcoholic male involved in a motor vehicle accident suffered severe abdominal trauma that required nephrectomy and pancreatectomy. Postoperative course was plagued by intrathoracic infection with loculated thoracic empyema. Percutaneous drainage was requested.

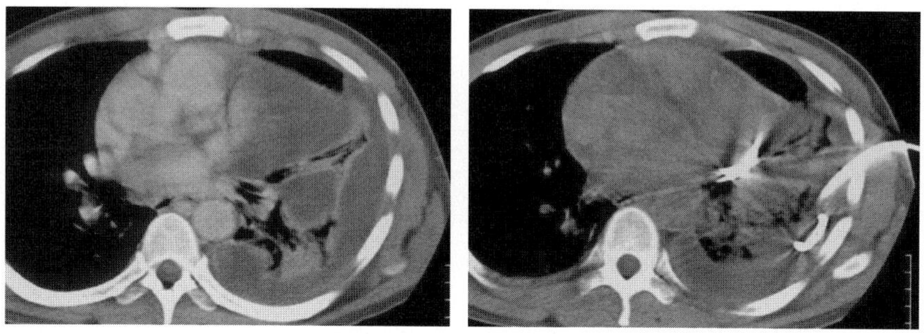

A B

Figure 15.1.1

A: Computed tomographic (CT) scan of the chest shows multiple loculated empyemas at the base of the left chest. **B:** Two 12F catheters were placed within the intrathoracic fluid cavities and connected to a water seal with negative pressure. The infection gradually improved with drainage and antibiotics. The drains were removed in 1 week. One year later, the patient was involved in a second motor vehicle accident and suffered head trauma, which required surgical drainage of a subdural hematoma.

Comment: The role of interventional radiology in the management of intrapulmonary and intrapleural air and fluid collections is becoming more important. Improvements in percutaneous techniques now allow percutaneous access to closed fluid collections, with less morbidity and mortality than surgical open treatment. CT largely replaced chest radiography in the assessment of intrathoracic fluid collections. Not only is the diagnosis more detailed, but CT allows precise guidance for percutaneous drainage. On CT, intrapleural or pulmonary fluid appears as a homogenous density that may be surrounded by an enhanced rim. Mediastinal fluid collections also are readily depicted by CT scan. Major indications for percutaneous drainage in the chest are (i) empyema and parapneumonic effusions, (ii) other pleural effusions, (iii) refractory lung abscesses, and (iv) mediastinal collections. Pleural effusions are classified as transudate or exudate, depending on fluid characteristics. This distinction is important in suggesting the appropriate differential diagnosis and determining treatment options. Criteria used to diagnose an exudative effusion include pleural fluid to serum protein ratio >0.5, pleural fluid lactic dehydrogenase (LDH) >200, and pleural fluid to serum LDH ratio >0.6. Other parameters, including protein level 3 g/dL, pH >7.3, and specific gravity >1.016, also have been used to diagnose exudative effusions.

The choice of imaging used to detect thoracic fluid collections and guide drainage depends on the availability of the modalities, location of the collection, and expertise of the operator. Ultrasound (US) can be used to treat more peripheral chest collections, but CT is more precise. Diagnostic thoracentesis is a common procedure guided by US. More involved drainages of complex collections are performed more precisely with CT guidance.

The patient may be positioned prone or supine on the CT table. The lateral decubitus position may be necessary in some cases. Once a diagnostic study is performed, the windows for puncture are determined. With conventional CT guidance, a radiopaque localization grid is taped to the patient's skin and the site is rescanned. Once an optimal trajectory for the needle is found, the skin site is indicated with an ink marker. More recently, CT fluoroscopy has become available. The skin site can be identified in real time under direct fluoroscopic observation. The optimal needle trajectory selected should avoid transgression into normal lung parenchyma, avoid injury to vital structures, and provide access to the main portion of the collection. The skin is prepared and draped. Under local anesthesia, the needle is introduced through a small nick in the skin. An 18-gauge needle is advanced to a predetermined depth. The stylet is removed, a small amount of fluid is aspirated, and a sample is sent for grain stain and cultures. A guidewire is advanced within the fluid collection, the tract is dilated, and the catheter is introduced over the wire. Catheter size depends on the viscosity of the fluid collection; sizes 10F to 14F are advisable for most collections. The pigtail-tipped catheter is the most useful for chest drainage because the snare is less traumatic and stable. The catheter must be sutured directly to the skin. Use of Vaseline gauze to seal the entry site is not necessary in most cases. The catheter should be connected to a water seal, and application of negative pressure may be necessary in the most resilient fluid collections. Multiple unconnected cavities will require multiple catheters.

Malignant pleural effusions can be managed traditionally by doxycycline pleurodesis or, more recently, with an indwelling tunneled pleural drain (Pleurx) connected to a vacuum bottle for relief of dyspnea. A randomized study comparing the two techniques showed reduced hospitalization time in the group treated with the indwelling pleural catheter, but improvements in dyspnea and quality of life were comparable: 21% of patients treated with doxycycline had late recurrence of pleural effusion, and 13% of patients treated with the indwelling catheter had recurrence or blockage of the catheter after initial successful treatment.

15.1.2 Drainage Of The Chest

Case 15.1.2:

A 73-year-old man with esophageal squamous cell cancer presented with severe dysphagia and regurgitation. Esophageal resection was performed, followed by esophageal bypass with colon, in a second procedure. Right chest pneumothorax and loculated empyema developed in the days following surgery. Percutaneous drainage was requested.

A 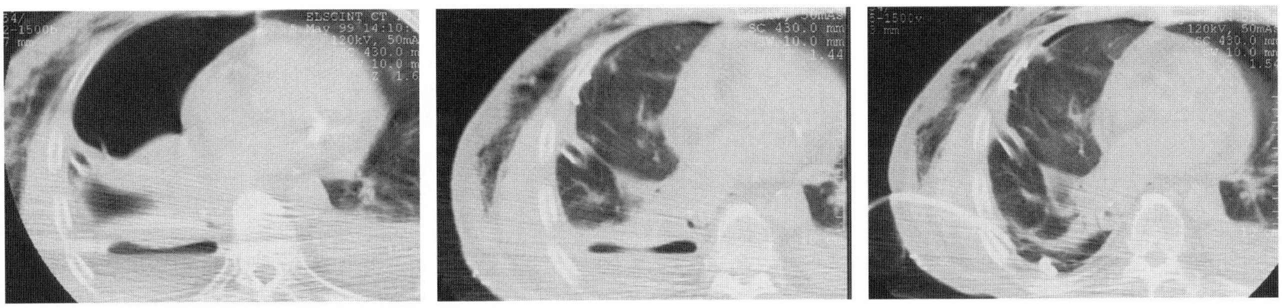 B, C

Figure 15.1.2

A: CT scan of the chest shows a large right-side pneumothorax with total lung collapse and posterior fluid collection with air-fluid level. **B:** Drainage of the pneumothorax was performed with a 10F pigtail catheter under CT guidance. Aspiration of the free air from the right pleural cavity promoted immediate expansion of the right lung. Note residual pleural thickening and the drain within the pleural space, as well as persistence of the posterior fluid collection. **C:** An additional 10F catheter was placed within the fluid collection for external drainage. The tubes were connected to a water seal with negative pressure.

Comment: Esophageal perforation most often is the result of instrumentation or surgery. The presentation may include pneumothorax, pneumomediastinum, pleural effusion, and mediastinal abscess. The problem usually is related to perforation of the esophagus or breakdown of a surgical anastomosis. Although surgical correction of the problem may be necessary, there is a place for percutaneous management in a number of cases, either before surgical correction or as the definitive treatment. The patient's condition for reoperation usually is poor, and percutaneous drainage sometimes is necessary to improve the clinical condition before surgical fix. Active suction is necessary in all cases to overcome the flow of fluids. Drainage may need to be extended for several weeks (2 to 4 weeks or more) and is very successful in the majority of cases. Catheter exchange should be performed in a timely fashion to avoid inevitable catheter blockage.

Complicated pleural effusions are those that do not resolve without drainage. They can be unilocular or multilocular. Drainage in these cases is necessary to control pleural sepsis, allow reexpansion of the underlying lung, and prevent the long-term sequelae of pleural fibrosis and lung entrapment. Two techniques have been used in an effort to improve the efficacy of closed-tube drainage: (i) image-guided placement of a drainage catheter and (ii) intracavitary fibrinolytic therapy. Image guidance improves the problems related to tube malposition; however, drainage failure due to small-diameter catheters and occlusion by fibrinous debris or clotted blood commonly may occur. Enzymatic breakdown of the fibrin sheath covering the catheter and the pleural surface with fibrinolytic therapy has been used successfully to increase the effectiveness of tube drainage. A 6-mg dose of tissue plasminogen activator is dissolved in 50 mL of normal saline. After 50 mL of the solution is instilled, the chest drain is clamped for 2 to 4 hours. The fluid then is aspirated, and a second instillation can be performed. One to four instillations can be performed in 1 day. Hemorrhagic complications are rare.

15.1.3 Drainage Of The Chest

Case 15.1.3:

A 43-year-old man with pharyngeal squamous cell cancer that extended into the jaw and who was suffering much pain presented with a lung nodule. The patient had a tracheostomy, was alcoholic, and was noncompliant with treatments. Pulmonary lung nodule biopsy demonstrated the lesion was positive. A large pneumothorax developed and caused severe dyspnea. A 24F surgical chest drain was placed, without improvement. Percutaneous CT-guided drainage was requested.

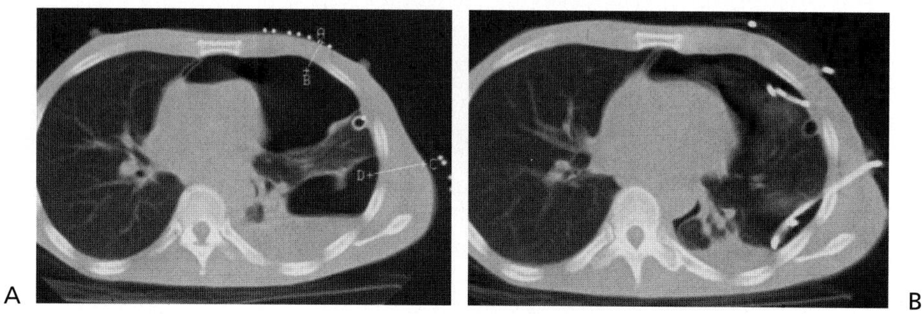

Figure 15.1.3

A: CT scan of the chest shows large, biopsy-related pneumothorax that developed after placement of the surgical drain. Note the mediastinal shift to the right due to the hypertensive pneumothorax. The surgical chest drain was ineffective due to poor positioning within the lung parenchyma. **B:** Two 10F drainage catheters were placed using CT guidance. Aspiration through both catheters significantly reduced the pneumothorax and reduced the tension. Note residual pneumothorax in both compartments. There was continued air leak that required prolonged drainage for 5 additional days. The patient died 2 years later from progression of the disease.

Comment: Clinically significant pneumothorax with collapse caused by increased pleural pressure usually results from disruption of the visceral pleura. This may occur spontaneously or as a result of chronic lung disease, trauma, or an iatrogenic cause (biopsy). The incidence of pneumothorax is 5% to 20% following thoracentesis and 10% to 50% after transthoracic needle lung biopsy. Most iatrogenic pneumothoraces can be treated by small-bore tubes with a 7F to 10F tube. Success rates are reported to be 87% to 97%; the pneumothoraces resolve 24 to 72 hours after tube placement. CT- and US-guided catheter drainage of empyemas and pneumothoraces after chest-tube failure is successful in more than 88% of cases. Malpositioning of the surgical chest tube is the most common cause of failure of this technique. Insertion of the large-bore tube in the lung parenchyma or within an interlobar fissure is a common cause of inefficacy. CT guidance correctly identifies loculations and directs the selective placement of as many catheters as necessary to treat the problem.

15.1.4 Drainage Of The Chest

Case 15.1.4:

A 26-year-old female patient with cystic fibrosis who was on home O_2, had a history of multiple hospital admissions, and currently was experiencing symptom exacerbation presented with dyspnea and signs of air leak in the pleural cavity. On admission, the patient was infected with respiratory *Pseudomonas* and *Aspergillus.* Pneumothorax was clinically diagnosed, but symptoms did not improve over a period of 24 hours. Percutaneous drainage was requested.

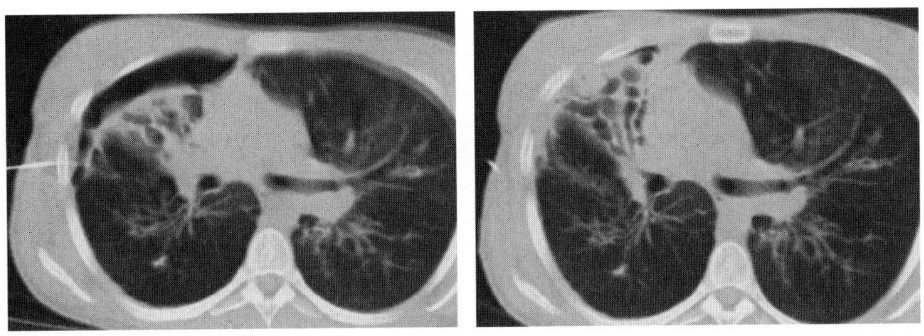

Figure 15.1.4

A: CT scan of the chest shows a moderate-size spontaneous pneumothorax in the right side of the chest. Note lung consolidation and bronchiectasias. The needle was visible in the lateral aspect of the chest. **B:** A 10F pigtail catheter was placed for drainage. Aspiration of the free air produces resolution of the pneumothorax, but no significant expansion of the diseased lung. The catheter was kept in continuous aspiration and eventually was pulled out 3 days after drainage.

Comment: Although the most common indication for radiologic drainage of pleural air is the development of postbiopsy pneumothorax, other causes are becoming more frequently encountered in clinical practice. A more recent application of CT-guided drainage of pneumothorax is in patients with chronic severe pulmonary disease who develop loculated pneumothoraces. Compromised ventilatory status in these patients suggests that evacuating dead space and improving the volume of ventilated lung may be beneficial. Small-bore catheter placement (7F to 10F) is successful in 87% to 97% of patients. The vast majority of pneumothoraces will resolve 24 to 72 hours after tube drainage. Persistence usually is due to technical factors, malposition, occlusion, or large air leak. Pneumothoraces larger than 20% to 25% of the volume of the hemithorax, progressive enlargement, or tension should be drained as soon as possible. A chest x-ray film should be obtained after 18 to 24 hours of drainage. If the pneumothorax has resolved, the catheter should be clamped for 4 or 5 hours; if the lung remains expanded, the catheter can be removed. Persistent pneumothoraces may benefit from chemical pleurodesis using sclerosing agents such as doxycycline, talc, or bleomycin.

15.1.5 Drainage Of The Chest

Case 15.1.5:

A 51-year-old male patient with pneumonia developed pericardial effusion and bilateral pleural effusion. The patient developed dyspnea and progressive constriction of the heart caused by the pericardial effusion, with increased venous pressure and tachycardia that risked acute tamponade. Emergency drainage of the pericardial and pleural effusion was requested.

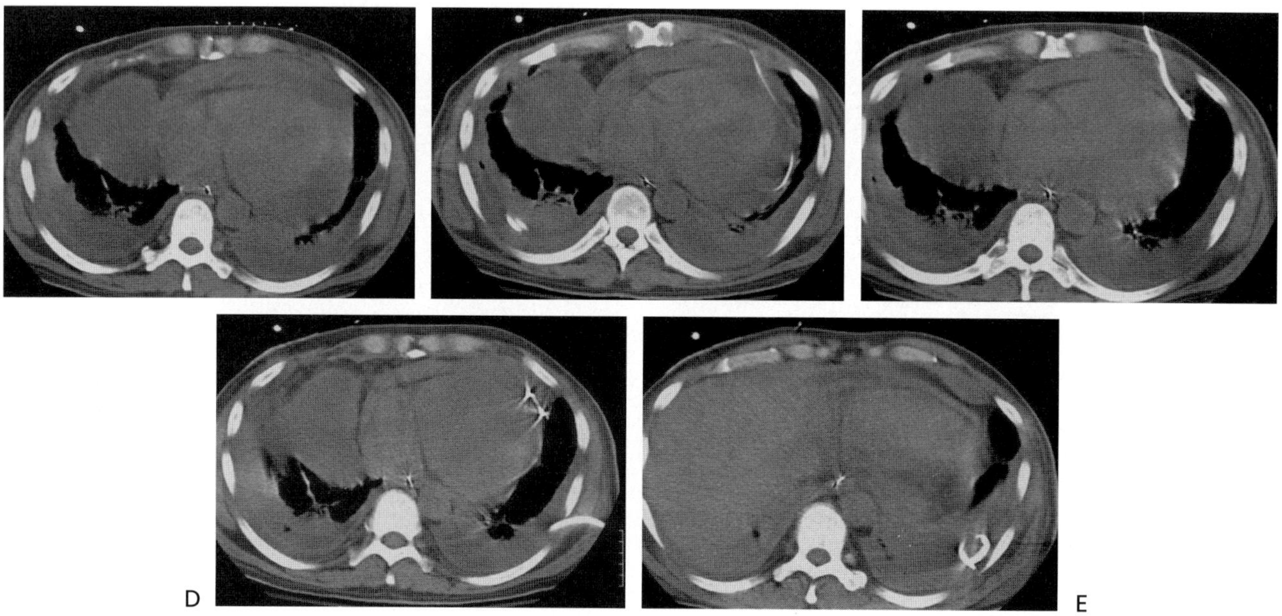

Figure 15.1.5

A: CT scan of the chest shows massive pericardial effusion and bilateral pleural effusion. Note the radiopaque grid in the anterior aspect of the chest wall. **B:** After puncture with a blunt trocar needle, a J-tip guidewire was advance within the pericardial space, around the heart. **C:** An 8F catheter was placed for drainage. About 800 mL of fluid was slowly removed from the pericardial space. **D,E:** Following the pericardial drainage, the left pleural effusion was drained with a 10F catheter to improve lung expansion.

Comment: The normal pericardial space usually contains less than 30 mL of fluid. A number of disease processes may lead to accumulation of fluid within the pericardial cavity. The clinical significance of the effusion will depend upon the total amount of fluid, rate of accumulation, pericardial compliance, and overall cardiologic status of the patient. Large effusions may be clinically silent; however, symptoms are the result of hemodynamic compromise caused by impaired filling of the heart. Echocardiography is the procedure of choice for diagnosis of pericardial effusion and cardiac tamponade. The pathophysiology of cardiac tamponade is related to restricted ventricular filling by fluid accumulation in the closed pericardial space. Increased venous pressure and tachycardia are natural compensatory mechanisms that may provide a hint to the diagnosis. In tamponade, there is equilibration of the intrapericardial right ventricular and left ventricular diastolic pressures. The presence of cardiac tamponade should prompt drainage to resolve hemodynamic compromise. Aspiration of pericardial fluid is indicated for both diagnosis and therapy. Neither surgical drainage nor percutaneous pericardiocentesis is devoid of risk. Echocardiographic and fluoroscopic guidance traditionally have been used for pericardiocentesis and drainage; however, CT scan recently has became very useful for diagnosis and drainage guidance. CT allows precise pericardial space puncture and catheter insertion for drainage, with the patient under local anesthesia. The multihole catheter should be advanced over the wire and placed within the pericardial space. The catheter then is connected to a three-way stopcock and the fluid is aspirated. Rapid decompression may cause heart failure. When dealing with large effusions, it is advisable to remove the fluid slowly (no more than 500 mL) and allow the remaining fluid to drain over time. Drainage may be prolonged for several days or even weeks, in which case the catheter needs to be maintained as a sterile system. Removal of the catheter is easily accomplished and can be painless. Complications range from 0% to 20%. Possible complications include puncture of the cardiac chambers and bleeding. Coronary artery laceration is a rare but severe and potentially lethal complication. Vagal reactions with hypotension, bradycardia, and cardiac arrest are uncommon but potentially lethal problems. Infection is rare and usually related to more prolonged drainage, especially in an immunocompromised patient.

15.1.6 Drainage Of The Chest

Case 15.1.6:

A 75-year-old male patient underwent an endoscopic procedure that resulted in esophageal perforation. The patient developed sepsis and severe chest pain. CT scan of the chest showed a large abscess causing compression of the trachea and mediastinal widening. Percutaneous abscess drainage was requested.

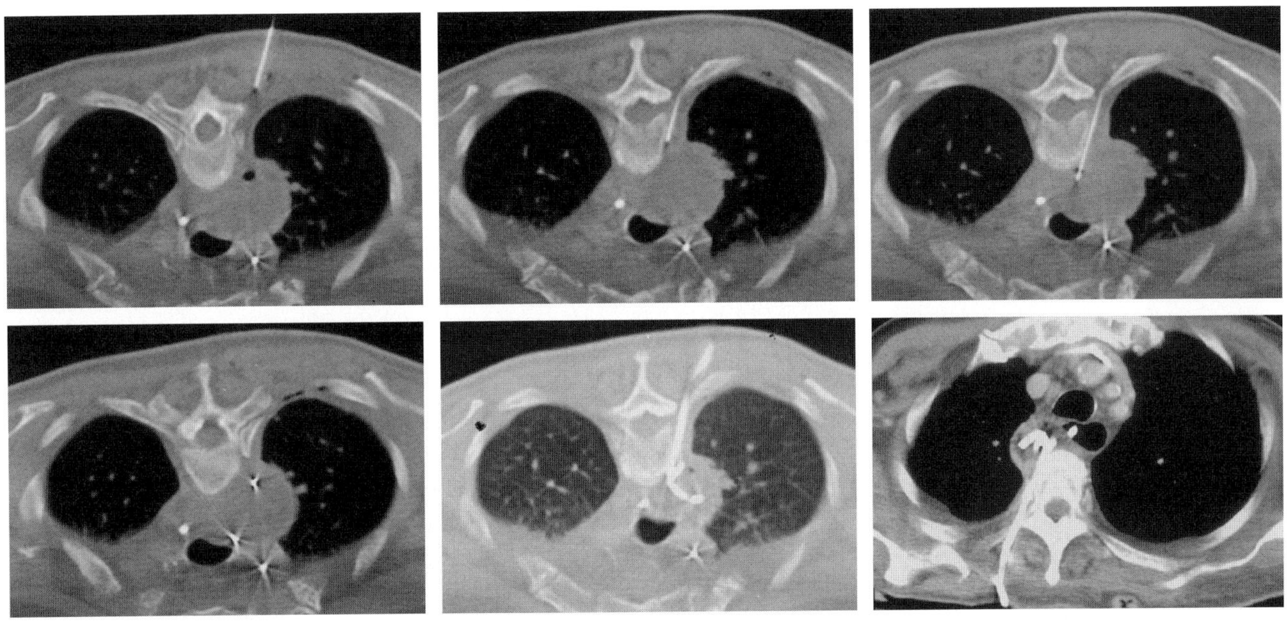

A B, C D E, F

Figure 15.1.6

A: CT of the chest shows a large mediastinal fluid collection with free air inside. **B:** A posterior, paraspinal, extrapleural needle approach was used. The patient was placed in a prone position. A fine needle was introduced in the paraspinal space and lidocaine was injected to widen the virtual space and numb the tract for drainage. **C:** As the needle touched the bone, it was slightly redirected toward the fluid collection wall. **D:** Once the needle reached the collection, a guidewire was introduced. The needle was exchanged over the wire for a dilator, and a drainage catheter was introduced. **E:** A 10F catheter was introduced for drainage, and the entire purulent collection was evacuated. **F:** Follow-up CT scan of the chest shows significant resolution of the abscess. Note the presence of a nasogastric catheter used for continuous suction. The drain was removed after 2 weeks.

Comment: Mediastinal abscess is a serious condition associated with high morbidity and mortality. Common causes are esophageal perforation, penetrating trauma, surgery breakdown, and extension of infection from contiguous areas. These collections are among the most challenging infections to treat. Patients usually are very ill and constitute poor surgical risk. Placement of a percutaneous drain is the most effective treatment. Technique of catheter placement and aftercare are approximately the same as for empyema, except a longer duration of drainage is to be expected if there is esophageal perforation. CT is used exclusively to guide drainage of mediastinal abscesses because of their deep location, their long access paths, and the intimate relationship between the adjacent structures and the fluid collection. If the lesion is anterior, a good practice is to carefully avoid the internal mammary artery and the ascending segment of the aorta. The posterior approach should always be performed from the right side, to avoid the descending aorta. The paraspinal extrapleural approach should be always used, when possible, to reach the mediastinal lesion, avoiding passing through the lung parenchyma. Potential problems related to the paraspinal approach include intercostal nerve damage, small pneumothorax, and bleeding from an intercostal vessel or azygos vein.

15.1.7 Drainage Of The Chest

Case 15.1.7:

A 31-year-old male patient with a 20-year history of chronic alcohol abuse and recurrent gastric ulcers was treated by subtotal gastrectomy, Billroth II anastomosis, and vagotomy 5 years earlier. The patient developed esophageal varices, portal hypertensive gastropathy, and signs of pancreatitis, dysphagia, and postprandial vomiting. A mediastinal cyst, which could be traced to the tail of the pancreas, was identified by endoscopic US, suggesting the diagnosis of a mediastinal pancreatic pseudocyst. Surgery was contemplated, but the patient's poor nutritional status increased the surgical risk. Percutaneous drainage was requested.

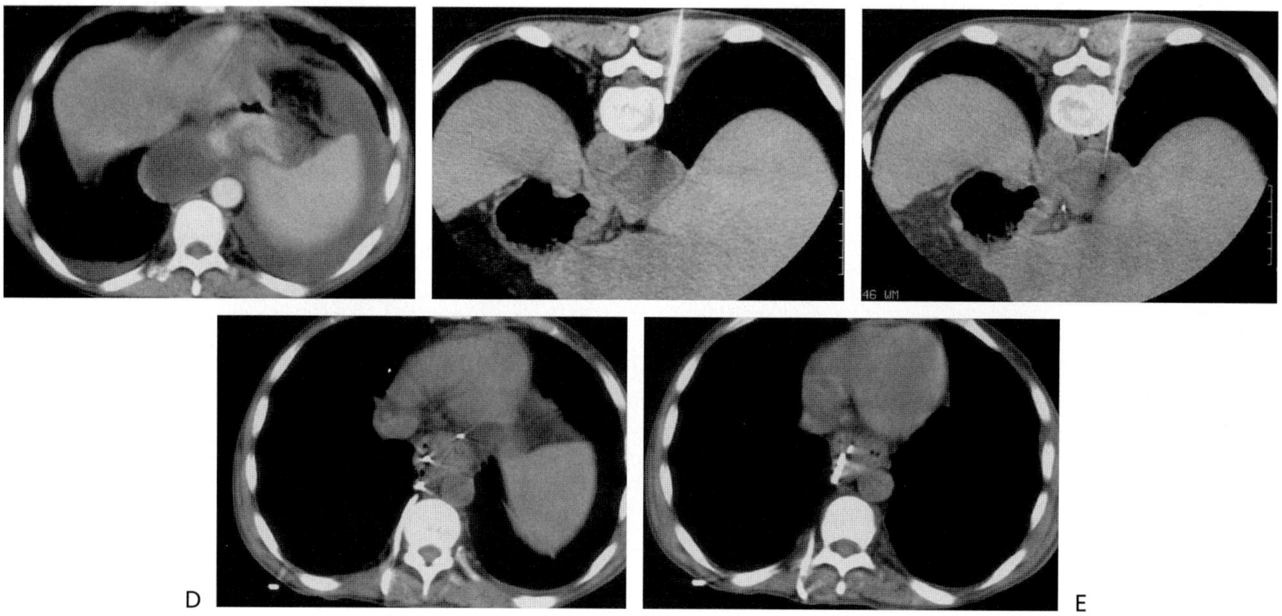

A, B C D E

Figure 15.1.7

A: Initial diagnostic CT scan demonstrates the mediastinal pseudocyst. **B:** CT scan shows the fine needle in the paraspinal extrapleural space, with the tip in the soft tissues of the paravertebral space. **C:** Fine needle was identified by CT scan within the pseudocyst. **D,E:** An 8F drainage catheter was placed within the cavity. The pseudocyst resolved, and the catheter was removed 1 week after drainage. About 1 week after the drain was removed, there was recurrence of the pseudocyst with infection by *Staphylococcus aureus.* A new drain was placed (not shown) for 6 weeks. Follow-up is more than 2 years, and the patient has not experienced recurrence of the mediastinal lesion.

Comment: Pancreatic pseudocysts are common among patients with acute chronic pancreatitis. The pseudocysts usually are located in the retroperitoneal space, pancreas, or adjacent spaces, but other locations are not unusual. Mediastinal pancreatic pseudocysts are rare, but several cases have been reported in the literature. Surgical treatment of mediastinal pancreatic pseudocysts is more complicated because of the location; percutaneous access is more desirable. Although a transabdominal approach for a low mediastinal pseudocyst has been described, the paraspinal approach has proved very useful and safe. The approach with fluoroscopic guidance used in this case was described originally by Nordenstrom in 1972. CT guidance and particularly CT fluoroscopy make this paraspinal extrapleural approach extremely useful and safe for access to the posterior mediastinum.

15.1.8 Drainage Of The Chest

Case 15.1.8:

A 67-year-old male patient with a large recurrent empyema of the right chest was referred for percutaneous drainage. Upon puncture, the material proved to be extremely viscous. A significant amount of debris were identified.

A 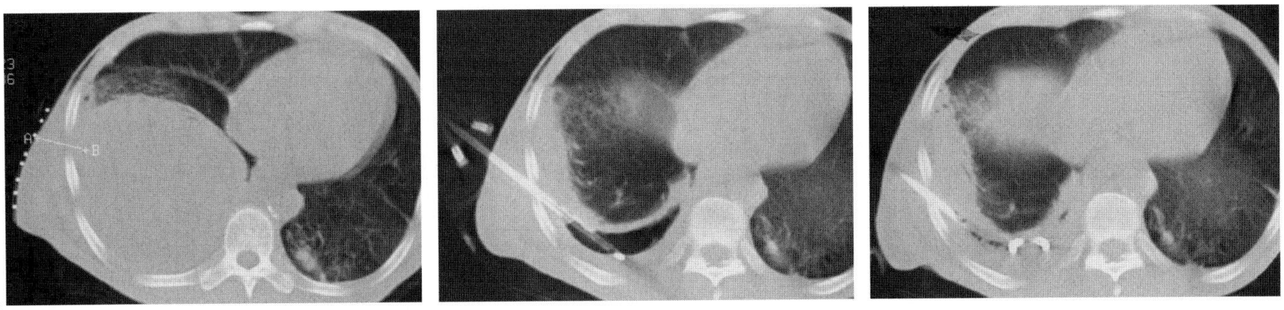 B, C

Case 15.1.8

A: CT scan of the chest shows a large empyema of the right chest. Note the marking grid on the wall of the chest and a measuring line that shows the depth distance to be used for percutaneous puncture. **B:** CT scan after using the suction catheter within the pleural empyema, shows total evacuation of the fluid and debris. Note that there is a significant amount of air within the cavity, as the sheath used was a peel-away system, with no valve. **C:** CT scan of the chest after debridement of the empyema shows significant resolution of the problem. Note residual thickening of the parietal and visceral pleura. There was partial collapse of the right lower lobe seen by air bronchogram. The 14F catheter was left within the empyema cavity for further drainage. Surgical decortication was performed a few weeks later after the infection was controlled.

Comment: A number of collections may be found in the chest. Most are amenable to percutaneous drainage, including free-flowing pleural effusions, loculated effusions, empyema, infected bronchopleural fistula, mediastinal abscess, lung abscess, pericardial empyema pneumothorax, and cystic collections. Superficial lesions may be amenable to treatment by percutaneous drainage using ultrasonography. CT scan is the best option for deeper located, loculated, multiloculated, and complex lesions. Typically when a chest drainage is requested, some form of therapy has been already attempted. Lung abscesses often are improved dramatically by drainage. Persistent sepsis rapidly responds to evacuation of the pus. For empyemas that are quite thick and do not drain well with conventional catheters, lytic agents can be used to improve treatment by allowing lysis of the thick material. Suction and debridement is an alternative option for coagulopathy in patients with contraindication to lytic therapy. The catheter suction system used in this case is described in more detail in "Drainage of Pancreatic Diseases" section.

15.2.1 Drainage Of The Peritoneal Cavity

Case 15.2.1:

A 67-year-old female patient with gallstones underwent laparoscopic cholecystectomy. The patient developed fever and abdominal pain after surgery. A large subphrenic fluid collection developed, as well as right-side pleural effusion. Endoscopic retrograde cholangiopancreatography (ERCP) showed active bile leak from the cystic duct. A biliary stent was placed, and the large fluid collection was drained using CT guidance.

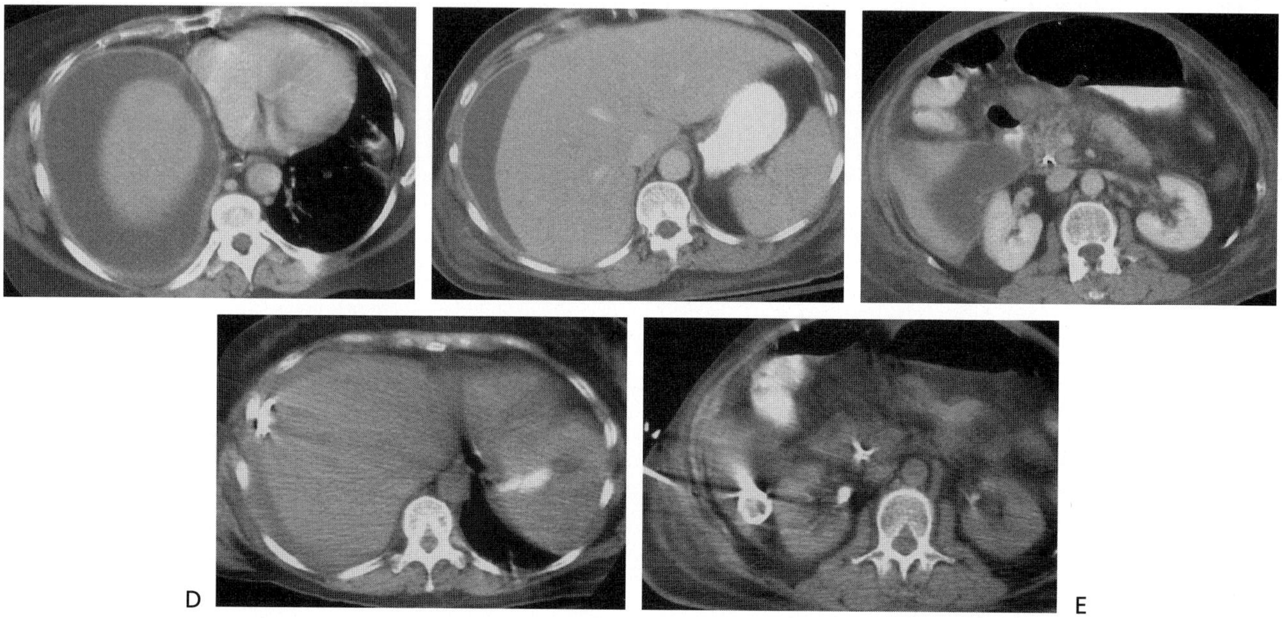

Figure 15.2.1

A: CT scan of the abdomen at the level of the diaphragm shows a large subphrenic fluid collection causing elevation of the diaphragm and medial displacement of the liver. **B:** The fluid collection extended down around the right lobe of the liver. **C:** There is a separate subhepatic fluid collection extending from the area of the cystic duct leak down to the anterior aspect of the right kidney. **D,E:** Two separate percutaneous drainage catheters were placed, one in the subphrenic space from the lateral aspect using CT guidance through a low intercostal approach.

Comment: Confirmation of the diagnosis of subphrenic collections usually is made by sonography and CT scan. Percutaneous CT- or US-guided drainage currently is one of the most important tools for management of these lesions. Common causes of subphrenic abscesses usually are related to posttraumatic and postoperative conditions. Perforated ulcers, acute cholecystitis with perforation, bile duct leaks, perforated adenocarcinoma of the colon, diffuse ascites with loculations, inflammatory disease of the colon or small bowel, liver resections, and previous splenectomy are some of the conditions related to subphrenic fluid accumulation and infection. Right-side subphrenic abscesses are more commonly reported in the literature. Technically, subphrenic abscesses need to be accessed via an anterior or lateral subcostal approach. The intercostal approach should not be used, to avoid puncturing the pleura or lung. Needle aspiration and subsequent catheter placement can be performed under US or CT guidance. Identification of the fluid collection is followed by puncture with a 20- or 18-gauge needle and confirmation of the presence of purulent material. The drainage catheter is placed by the Seldinger or the trocar method. Catheter placement is done over the wire. Catheter size is variable, but an 8F to 14F size usually is necessary. Selection of catheter size is dependent on the amount, nature, viscosity, and location of the fluid to be drained. Only local anesthesia is necessary for percutaneous catheter drainage. However, when an intercostal approach is used, care should be exercised to avoid hitting or touching the intercostal nerve with the catheter. Other related conditions may prevent that subphrenic catheter drainage alone cure the infection. Fistulas within the bile ducts, small bowel, stomach, duodenum, and colon may prolong drainage time to 10 days or longer, as opposed to other locations in the abdomen where 5 to 7 days of drainage usually is enough. Biliary leaks can be treated by decompression with endoscopic stents or percutaneous biliary catheters.

15.2.2 Drainage Of The Peritoneal Cavity

Case 15.2.2:

A 69-year-old male patient underwent partial pancreatectomy and splenectomy for chronic pancreatitis. The patient developed fever and abdominal pain after surgery. A pancreatic duct leak was identified, and an endoscopic stent was placed. A subphrenic abscess developed. Percutaneous CT-guided drainage was performed.

A

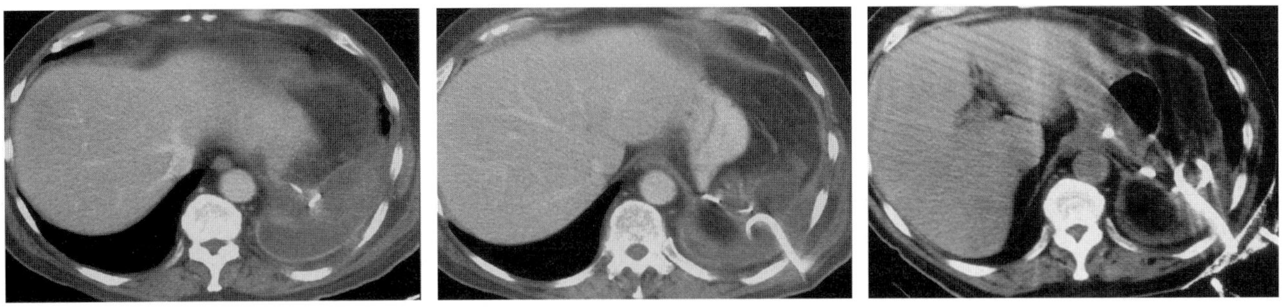

B, C

Figure 15.2.2

A: CT scan of the patient shows a left subphrenic multiloculated fluid collection. **B:** CT-guided drainage was performed with two 12F catheters. **C:** There was not immediate improvement. Urokinase infusion was used to break down the septations and fibrin within the fluid cavity. Percutaneous suction also was used and resulted in eventual resolution of the abscess.

Comment: Successful drainage of subphrenic abscesses and fluid collections is achieved in 85% to 90% of cases. Success is defined as cure with percutaneous drainage alone; failures are defined as situations where patients require additional surgical procedures. These cases usually benefit from drainage to control the infection and allow underlying problems, such as fistulas and other conditions, to be corrected safely by surgery. Fistulas often seal off just by controlling the drainage and establishing a tract that progressively closes down. About one third of subphrenic abscesses have some form of communication with the bowel or biliary tree, which considerably increases the drainage time until the fistula closes. Intraperitoneal fluid cavities heal differently than infected fluid within the liver, for example. After the intrahepatic liver abscess has been removed, normal hepatic parenchyma surrounding the collection collapses and granulates around the catheter quite readily. Good vascularization of the normal parenchyma accelerates the healing process. Subphrenic fluid collections take longer to heal and are subject to a higher rate of failure because they are not surrounded by vascularized parenchyma. The most important feature of percutaneous drainage is the immediate major therapeutic effect of the initial complete evacuation of purulent material. Critically unstable patients recover within a matter of hours.

15.2.3 Drainage Of The Peritoneal Cavity

Case 15.2.3:

A 51-year-old female patient developed an intraabdominal abscess following an episode of diverticulitis and perforation of the colon. The patient developed sepsis, chills, fever, and abdominal pain. An abscess was found on US and CT.

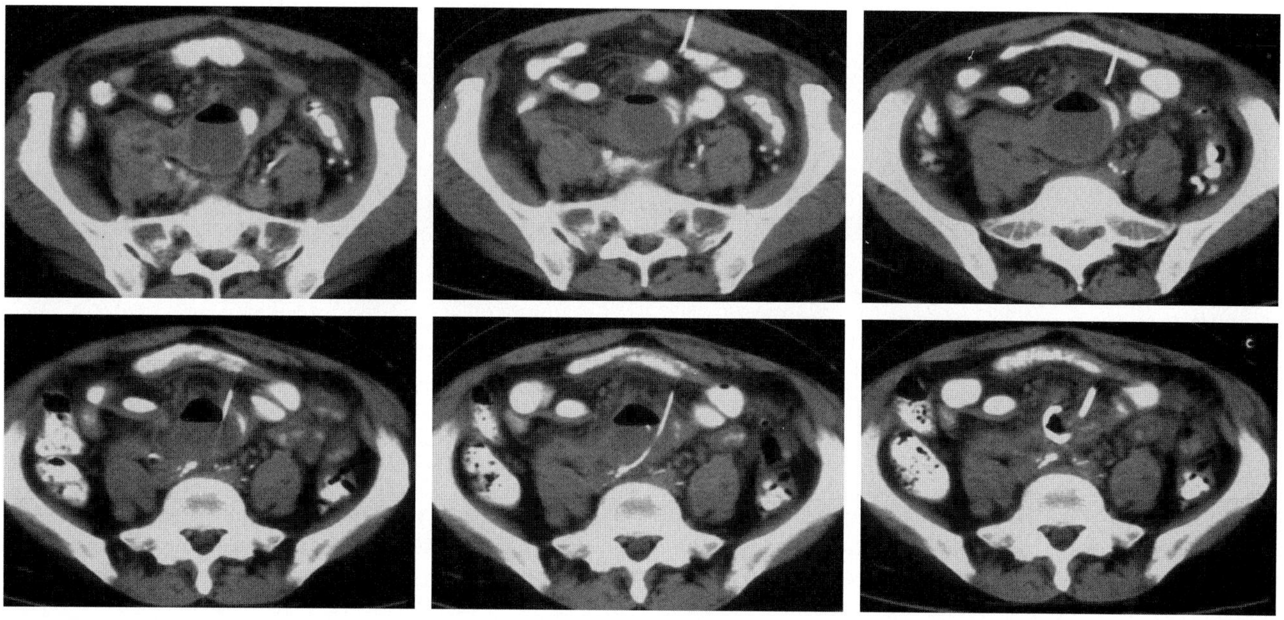

A, B C

D, E F

Figure 15.2.3

A: CT scan of the abdomen shows a mid-abdominal fluid collection with air-fluid level within. Note that the abscess is surrounded by bowel, which reduces the number of access windows. **B:** A blunt needle was used for puncture. Note that the point of entry is just at the edge of a contrast-filled bowel loop. **C:** Using the blunt stylet, the needle was advanced toward the abscess. Note that a bowel loop is adhered to the abscess wall. **D:** The needle was used to puncture the abscess with the blunt stylet and spared the bowel loop. A sample of purulent material was obtained and sent for grain stain and cultures. **E:** A guidewire was advanced inside the abscess, the tract was dilated, and a catheter was introduced over the wire. **F:** Total evacuation of the abscess was performed, with aspiration of a total of 50 mL of pus. The catheter was sewn to the skin and open to gravity drainage in a bag. The catheter was flushed daily for 4 days. The catheter was removed 7 days later, without the need for surgery.

Comment: This case demonstrates the importance of the location of the abscess/fluid collection within the abdomen and the careful selection of a window for safe access. However, fluid collection positioned in such a central location does not allow many options for safe percutaneous access. In these cases, it is important to use oral contrast for small and large bowel opacification, to avoid puncturing the bowel loops. One additional safety measure is the use of a blunt puncture needle and CT fluoroscopy for guidance. The blunt needle is used in three steps. First, a safe window with a tract selected in a space between the opacified bowel loops should be picked. Second, the abdominal wall is punctured using the sharp stylet in the needle, with the patient under local anesthesia. Third, when the needle is in the peritoneal cavity but not in contact with the bowel wall, the sharp stylet is withdrawn and the blunt stylet is used to advance the needle under CT guidance. Use of fluoroscopic CT is preferable to guide the needle, because progressive advancement can be monitored closely and the bowel wall can be avoided. Once the wall of the fluid cavity is reached, the blunt stylet can be replaced with the sharp stylet and the wall traversed. However, in most cases, the blunt stylet is able to penetrate the abscess wall without difficulty. Drainage can be performed following the regular technique.

15.2.4 Drainage Of The Peritoneal Cavity

Case 15.2.4:

A 12-year-old male patient with a large abdominal lymphangioma developed a large cystic lesion that was causing compression of the bladder and discomfort. Evacuation of the cystic lesion was requested.

A 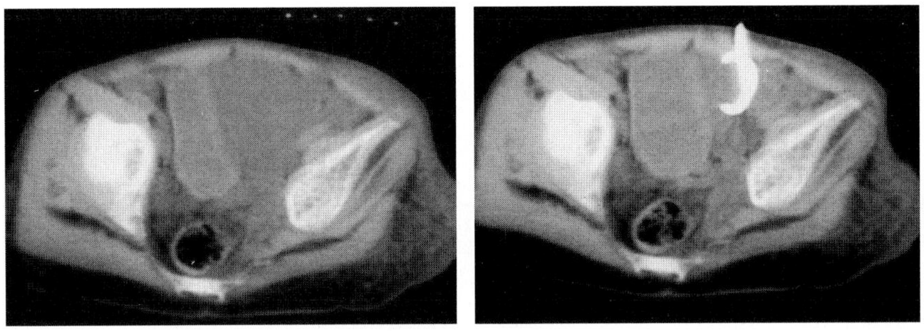 B

Figure 15.2.4

A: CT scan of the lower abdomen shows a large cystic lesion laterally displacing the bladder. **B:** Direct CT-guided drainage of the fluid collection was performed with a 12F catheter. Total evacuation was performed, with aspiration of 500 mL of lymphatic material. Absolute ethanol 20 mL was injected through a catheter.

Comment: Lymphangiomas are benign, soft tissue tumors consisting of abnormal lymphatic channels that appear most commonly in the head and neck regions in newborns or young children. Intraabdominal lymphangiomas are rare. The most common locations are the mesentery, omentum, mesocolon, and retroperitoneum. Some patients present acutely with intestinal obstruction, volvulus, infarction, bleeding, or infection, whereas others present with increasing abdominal girth, vague discomfort, and pain. Lymphangiomas should be differentiated from mesenteric cysts and other cystic lesions, which may be derived from mesothelial tissues. Mesenteric cysts usually follow a benign course, whereas lymphangiomas are larger and may follow a proliferative and invasive course. Pathologically, lymphangiomas can be classified into macrocystic, microcystic, or mixed. The macrocystic type consists of large cystic spaces, sometimes with septations. We illustrate the case of a child with a macrocystic retroperitoneal lymphangioma presenting with bladder compression, increasing abdominal girth, and chronic pain who responded well to percutaneous ablation with dehydrated alcohol. In a recent publication, intralesional injection of OK-432 was used as primary therapy for 46 lesions, with good response in 31 cases, and as second-line therapy after failure of bleomycin in a few patients. Only minor complications, including fever and a local inflammatory reaction, were reported. A successful case of radiation treatment has been reported. More recently, a report of 200 patients with various types of lymphangioma treated by injection of bleomycin-A5 showed an improvement rate of 97% and a curative rate of 86.5%, without significant complications. The sclerosing agent doxycycline has been described, with some degree of success, in a small group of patients. Ethanol is a well-known sclerosing agent used for tumor ablation and arteriovenous malformation repair. It is available, inexpensive, and easily delivered through small needles. Alcohol has been used in a small number of cases with lymphangioma and has been successful in reducing lesion size.

15.2.5 Drainage Of The Peritoneal Cavity

Case 15.2.5:

A 40-year-old male patient with Hodgkin lymphoma previously treated with radiation therapy underwent family-related bone marrow transplant about 1 year before and was placed on immunosuppression. More recently, the patient developed radiation pneumonitis, sepsis due to *Nocardia,* and prostate abscess accompanied by severe perineal pain that prevented the patient from sitting and walking adequately. Due to the patient's overall clinical situation of immunosuppression and deteriorating health, surgery was not considered an option. Percutaneous drainage was requested. Transrectal approach was considered, but a percutaneous transabdominal approach was preferred because of the immunosuppression.

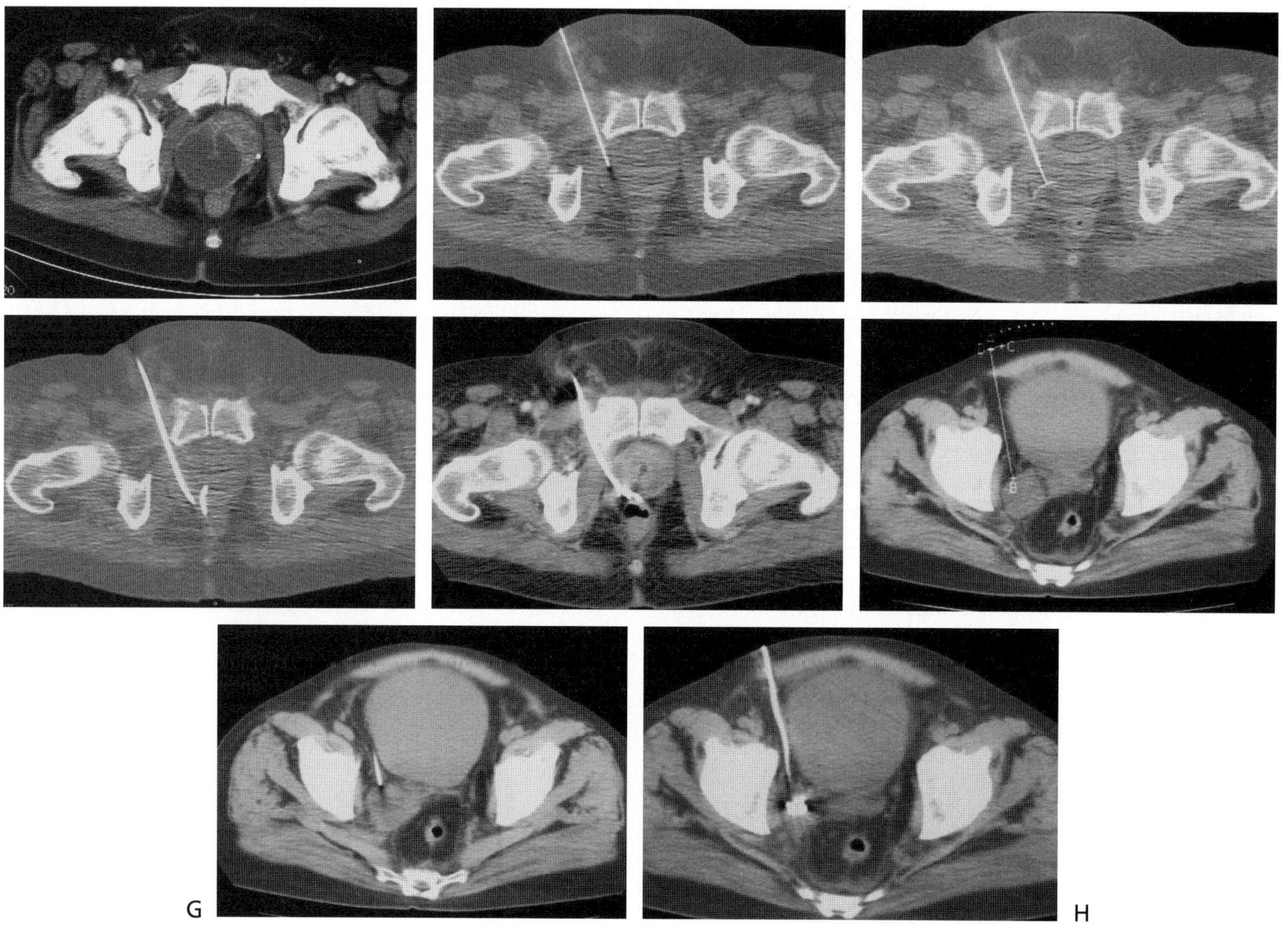

A, B C
D, E F
G H

Figure 15.2.5

A: CT scan of the perineal and prostatic areas shows a large fluid collection, consistent with a prostatic abscess. Note the closeness of the abscess to the obturator foramen, which became the natural window for drainage. **B:** Using CT fluoroscopy, an 18-gauge needle was advanced through the obturator foramen into the abscess within the prostate gland. A sample of purulent material was sent for gram stain and cultures. **C:** An Amplatz guidewire was advanced into the abscess and the tract dilated to 10F. **D:** A 10F pigtail catheter was placed within the abscess. **E:** Postdrainage CT scan shows total evacuation of the abscess. There was immediate improvement of the perineal pain but low fever persisted. **F:** About 2 weeks after prostate drainage, another intrapelvic abscess was noted to be enlarged. Due to the position of this fluid collection, an anterior approach was selected, despite the distance from the anterior abdominal wall. **G:** The needle was introduced under CT fluoroscopic guidance. Note the iliac vessels are lateral to the tract selected for puncture. **H:** A 10F catheter was introduced and the abscess was totally evacuated. The catheter was removed in about 1 week. Despite the recurrence of pelvic abscess after removal of the prostatic catheter, which was treated by new drainage using the same technique and aggressive long-term antibiotic therapy, the patient improved immediately and was doing well as of the latest follow-up at two years.

Comment: Prostatic abscesses are not seen commonly in clinical practice because antibiotic therapy has reduced the complications of prostatitis. The organisms most frequently involved are *Escherichia coli* and *Staphylococcus*; *Gonococcus* is now rarely encountered. Prostatic abscesses mainly affect diabetic and immunosuppressed patients. Immunocompromised patients and those with acquired immunodeficiency syndrome are prone to infections caused by a number of less common infectious agents. *Cryptococcus, Microsporidia, Aspergillus, Histoplasma, Tuberculosis,* and *Nocardia* are reported in the literature as causes of prostatic abscesses in this population. The case reported here is one example of an immunocompromised individual who developed systemic nocardiosis and prostate abscess with dramatic symptomatology. Current treatment of such a condition is aggressive antibiotic therapy and drainage. Multiple drainage techniques have been developed. US-guided needle aspiration is commonly used, through a transperineal, transrectal, or hypogastric approach, with a success rate of 83% to 86%. Transurethral resection of the prostate, or unroofing, has been utilized for prostatic abscess treatment. CT-guided drainage has not been widely used for prostate abscess drainage but allows precise puncture, as demonstrated in the presented case. Note that the CT image allows the operator to precisely place the needle through the obturator foramen, avoiding the spermatic cord medially and the femoral artery/vein laterally, and the obturator artery, directly into the abscess. On the follow-up CT scan, there was total resolution of the abscess.

15.2.6 Drainage Of The Peritoneal Cavity

Case 15.2.6:

A 52-year-old female patient underwent abdominal hysterectomy and salpingo-oophorectomy for a tumor 1 year before. The tumor was determined to be benign on pathologic examination. The patient recently developed low abdominal pain with a palpable pelvic mass. CT scan of the pelvis showed a round pelvic fluid collection with peripheral rim enhancement, consistent with an abscess. Percutaneous biopsy and possible drainage were requested.

A, B

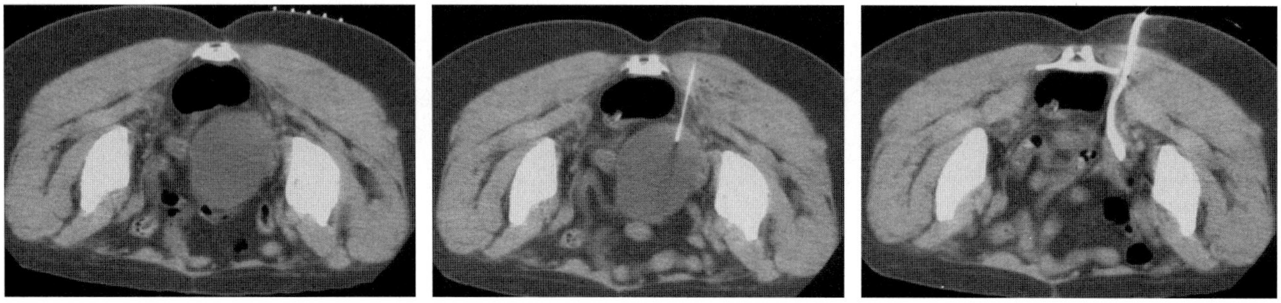

C

Figure 15.2.6

A: CT scan of the pelvis demonstrates a large round pelvic fluid collection in front of the rectum, on the left side. Note the marking grid over the left buttock. **B:** A point over the buttock was selected, as close as possible to the sacrum bone. An 18-gauge needle was used to puncture the abscess through the greater sciatic foramen through the posterior insertion of the sacrospinous ligament. If the puncture were higher, the needle would cross the piriform muscle (only partially visualized). Note that the rectum is moderately dilated with air. **C:** Final CT scan of the pelvis showing resolution of the abscess and the catheter in position.

Comment: The greater sciatic foramen is an oval space in the posterolateral aspect of the pelvis that lies just inferior to the sacroiliac articulation. The relation of the sacral plexus and the sciatic nerve to each other and to surrounding structures can be understood easily by dividing the greater sciatic foramen into a superior part that contains the piriform muscle and the sacral plexus, and an inferior part that contains the sacrospinous ligament and upper sciatic nerve. The piriform muscle and the sacrospinous ligament are reliable landmarks for identifying the superior and inferior parts of the greater sciatic foramen. Identification of the sacral plexus is somewhat less reliable, largely because of difficulty in differentiating the sacral plexus from the piriform muscle. The sacral plexus is ventral to the piriformis and is formed from branches of the ventral sacral nerves and the lumbosacral trunk, which descends from the lumbar plexus. The sacral plexus continues inferiorly as the sciatic nerve and crosses the anterior third of the foramen on the anterior surface of the piriformis, posterior to the sacrospinous ligament at its insertion into the ischial spine. The superior and inferior gluteal arteries and veins and the superior gluteal nerve also cross the foramen in the more cephalad aspect. Lesions of the sacrum are known to produce complaints referred to the sacral nerves and sacral plexus. Lesions adjacent to the sacrum, rectum, and sacral nerves within the pelvis also are potentially highly symptomatic. All perirectal fluid collections may have to be approached with the patient in a prone position to ensure adequate access through the gluteal muscles. The puncture approach is to be as close to the sacrum as possible at the level of the sacrospinous ligament, to avoid the more lateral sciatic nerve. The approach through the piriformis area may be required in some cases. In this case, entry should be planned as close as possible to the sacrum. Initial puncture may be performed with a small-gauge needle and exchanged for an introducer system that will allow use of a larger guidewire. Once the guidewire is securely within the abscess, the tract is dilated, and the catheter advanced and placed to external drainage.

15.2.7 Drainage Of The Peritoneal Cavity

Case 15.2.7:

A 37-year-old female patient with chronic pancreatitis and multiple interventions for hysterectomy and salpingectomy, as well as jejunostomy and gastrostomies, had a new surgical gastrostomy tube partially pulled out, which caused intraperitoneal leak of gastric fluids. The tube was surgically replaced, but the patient developed fever and abdominal pain. Diagnostic CT scan showed a perirectal abscess. Percutaneous CT-guided drainage was performed.

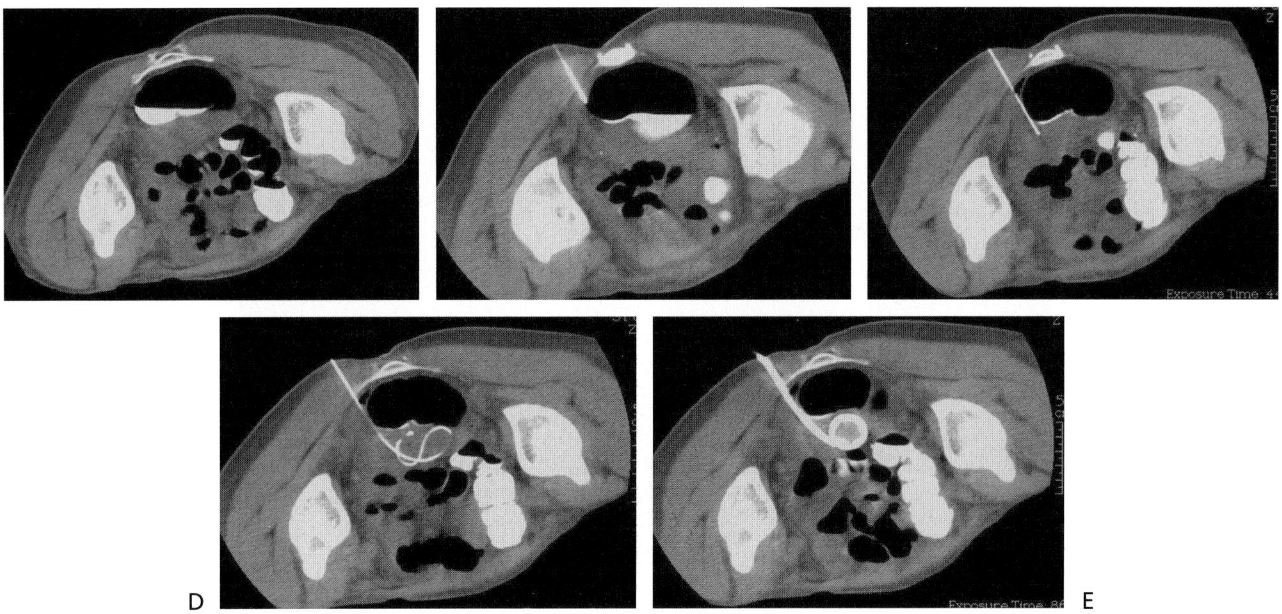

Figure 15.2.7

A: CT of the pelvis in a prone position shows a small abscess in front of the rectum. Since the diagnostic CT scan was obtained and because of the patient's prone position, the size of the rectum enlarged and the transgluteal window was not as clear. **B:** A blunt needle was used to access the lesion. Initially, the sharp stylet was used to penetrate the muscle. **C:** The blunt stylet then was used to advance the needle touching the rectum wall, until it reached the abscess. A fluid sample was obtained for cultures. **D:** An Amplatz guidewire was advanced into the abscess cavity and the tract was dilated to a 10F size. **E:** A 10F drain was placed, with total evacuation of the abscess. There was improvement of the fever and signs of infection, but the pain did not subside. The catheter was removed after 1 week, followed by improvement of the pain.

Comment: The diagnosis of a deep pelvic abscess in the perirectal area usually is made on a supine CT scan. The rectum may be empty and collapsed. Once the patient is turned to a prone position, the rectum tends to fill with gases and become dilated. In the reported case, note that the rectum is large and the abscess has been pushed forward to a prerectal position. Puncture with a blunt needle is helpful in such cases. The needle should be advanced, as close as possible to the bone, with the sharp stylet, to the vicinity of the rectum. Once in contact with the rectum wall, the stylet is exchanged for the blunt tip and the needle is pushed against the rectum wall and forward toward the fluid collection. Once the needle is in place, drainage is accomplished according to the regular technique. This type of drainage should be always performed with the patient in a prone oblique or lateral position to ensure access through the gluteal muscles. The best puncture site is as close as possible to the sacrum, at the level of the sacrospinous ligament, to avoid the more lateral sciatic nerve. The transrectal catheter technique is certainly an alternative to the transgluteal technique, but it is not as comfortable. The transgluteal approach also may be uncomfortable and painful for some patients.

15.2.8 Drainage Of The Peritoneal Cavity

Case 15.2.8:

A 21-year-old male patient with acute appendicitis underwent appendectomy. Fever developed 1 week after surgery, accompanied by abdominal pain and extreme rectal discomfort when the patient had bowel movements. Diagnostic CT scan showed a perirectal abscess. Percutaneous CT-guided drainage was performed.

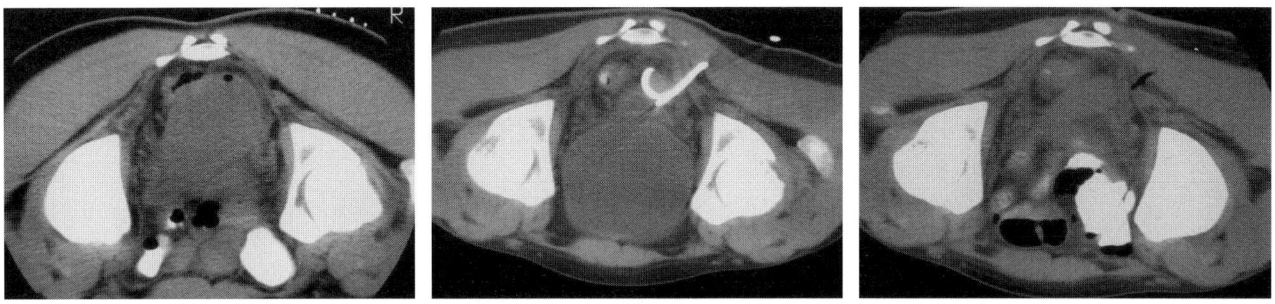

A B, C

Figure 15.2.8

A: CT scan of the pelvis performed with the patient in prone position shows a large perirectal fluid collection displacing the rectum to the right. There is a gas bubble within the fluid collection. Note the radiopaque grid on the surface of the left buttock. A puncture site was selected close to the sacral bone, and an 18-gauge needle was used to puncture the fluid collection and aspirate purulent material. **B:** A 12F catheter was placed for drainage. Acute aspiration of the pus produced immediate decompression of the pelvis with symptom improvement. Note that the cavity is totally empty after aspiration. **C:** After 1 week of drainage, the patient improved clinically and the drainage was reduced to less than 1 mL per day. The catheter was pulled out, and a final CT scan shows no significant residual fluid and a small segment of the catheter tract delineated by air.

Comment: Percutaneous drainage of intraabdominal abscesses by interventional radiologic procedures has become a well-accepted practice in both adults and children. Both CT scan and ultrasonography have been used for abscess drainage guidance. Most procedures can be performed under local anesthesia and conscious sedation, even in children. Superficial collections can be treated by anterior or lateral abdominal wall percutaneous puncture. Deep fluid collections are better treated by a transrectal or transgluteal approach. Large pelvic fluid collections that dramatically displace the rectum are accessed more easily through the transgluteal approach. Total evacuation of the fluid collection is a sign of easier resolution of the collection, if there is no intestinal fistula. Drainage should be complete at the time of the procedure. Multiple catheters may be necessary to drain multiple loculations or multiple fluid collections. Catheters are left in place for as many days as necessary and removed when there is no more drainage or there is less than 5 to 10 mL of serosanguineous fluid (range 1 to 7 days, mean 4 days). The presence of septicemia usually increases the time required for drainage and hospitalization. Antibiotic therapy should be adequate for the type of infection and response to the treatment. Almost half of patients with intraabdominal abscesses related to appendicitis will develop an intrapelvic collection. About one fourth of patients will require more than one catheter. New fluid collections or reaccumulation of pus may occur in about 15% of patients. Appendiceal rupture may perpetuate a fistula, and the patient may have to undergo surgery. Catheter drainage and antibiotic therapy are successful in about 90% of children and young patients with appendicial abscesses, with a complication rate of less than 2%. Overall success of abdominal abscess drainage procedures in adults ranges from 62% to 84% and in children from 88% to 91%.

15.2.9 Drainage Of The Peritoneal Cavity

Case 15.2.9:

An 8-year-old female patient with a history of acute appendicitis treated by surgical appendectomy presented with a pelvic abscess that was causing fever and pain. CT-guided transgluteal drainage was performed and the catheter maintained for 1 week. Massive hemorrhage followed catheter removal. Emergency arteriography was performed for hemorrhage control.

A, B

C

D, E

F

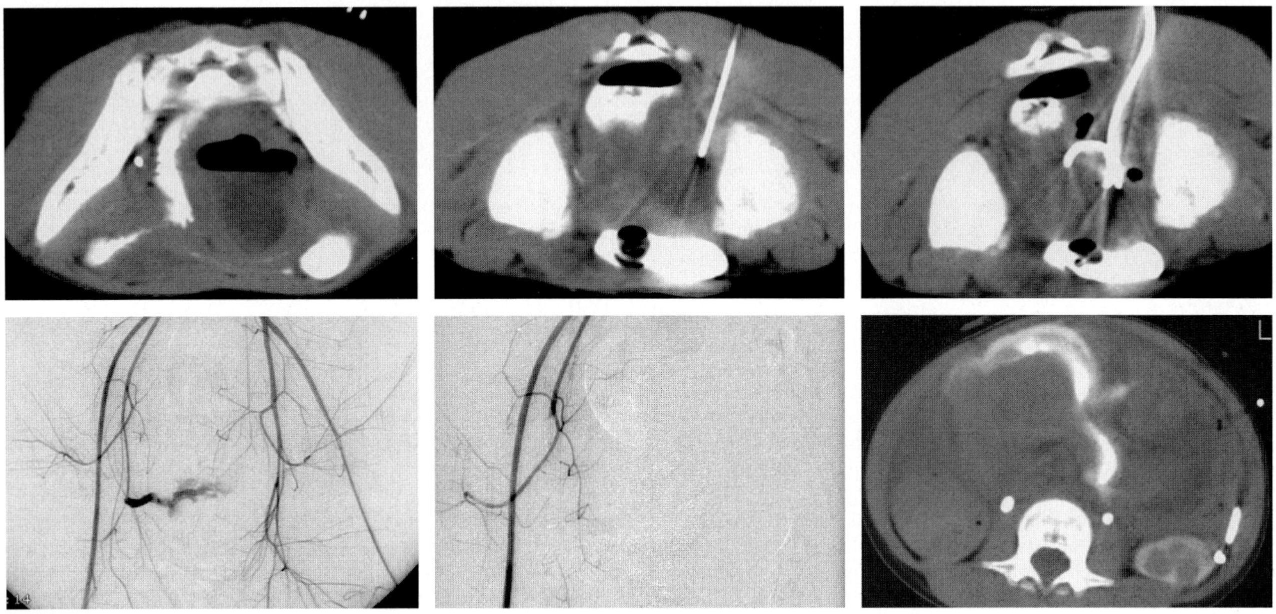

Figure 15.2.9

A: CT scan of the pelvis with the patient in the prone position shows a large fluid collection with an air-fluid level within. Note the radiopaque marker on the right buttock at the level of the iliac bone. **B:** Transgluteal puncture with an 19-gauge needle allowed access for drainage. Note that the needle was introduced more laterally than it should have been. The correct path would be closer to the sacral bone coursing just lateral to the rectum wall, to avoid the pelvic nerves and vessels. The incorrect positioning of the needle was not recognized at the time of drainage. **C:** Postdrainage CT scan shows the 8F catheter within the abscess is effectively draining the collection. After 1 week of drainage, there was improvement of the infection and the catheter was removed. Significant bleeding ensued following catheter withdrawal through the puncture hole. Significant intraperitoneal bleeding and hypotension subsequently developed, which required blood replacement and fluids. **D:** Emergency pelvic arteriography was performed, and massive bleeding from the inferior gluteal artery was identified. Immediate catheterization of the inferior gluteal artery with a microcatheter was performed, and embolization was performed using microcoils. **E:** Total occlusion of the bleeding artery was obtained, resulting in complete control of the bleeding and stabilization of the blood pressure. **F:** CT scan following embolization shows the peritoneal cavity is full of blood clots and extravasated contrast material. Laparotomy eventually was performed for blood evacuation due to development of fever 2 days after the embolization. The patient was discharged 7 days after embolization.

Comment: Faulty technique used for transgluteal pelvic abscess drainage caused this major unnecessary complication. Although it is possible that infection or catheter contact caused the arterial lesion, it is not likely in this case. The development of a pseudoaneurysm would be the more likely scenario if the infection were the cause of the vascular lesion. Acute bleeding, as presented here, more likely is related to direct puncture by the needle and catheter placement. Extreme care should be exercised when puncturing a pelvic fluid collection from the transgluteal approach. Risks are twofold: damage to the pelvic arteries, as demonstrated in this case; and neurologic injury to the sciatic nerve or branches. Careful progressive puncture through the greater sciatic foramen, just above the piriformis muscle and close to the sacral bone, is the correct technique, preferably guided by fluoroscopic CT. Note that the puncture needle is far too anterior and close to the more anterior vascular structures. The drainage catheter probably tamponaded the arterial lesion, and upon withdrawal massive bleeding ensued. Superselective embolization of the inferior gluteal artery controlled the bleeding, which otherwise would have been very difficult to treat surgically. The use of microcoils was a good option that was quick and permanent. Unfortunately, surgical evacuation of the abdominal cavity ultimately was necessary due to the persistence of fever.

The literature contains differing opinions regarding the optimal approach to deep pelvic abscesses. The transgluteal approach has been used successfully in virtually 100% of patients and obviated surgery in 81% of patients with pelvic abscess. Reported complications of CT-guided transgluteal drainage include persistent pain and venous hematoma. Arterial bleeding is rare; the only previous report in the literature reported successful treatment by arterial embolization. The potential for transvaginal and transrectal techniques is encouraging, with high success rates and low complication rates.

15.3.1 Drainage Of Pancreatic Diseases

Case 15.3.1:

A 12-year-old male patient with a history of acute pancreatic trauma who was in a bicycle accident developed a large pancreatic pseudocyst. Severe pain, nausea, and a sensation of fullness developed.

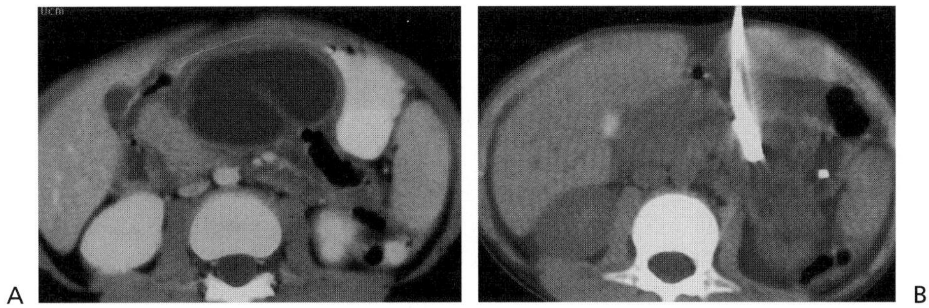

Figure 15.3.1

A: CT scan of the abdomen shows a large pancreatic pseudocyst at the level of the body of the pancreas due to a traumatic fracture. Note displacement of the stomach and surrounding soft tissues by the expansive loculated cyst. **B:** An 8F catheter was placed within the cyst, and total evacuation was performed. The catheter was kept in place for 4 weeks, and the cyst was properly drained and resolved.

Comment: Trauma is a leading cause of death in children, and abdominal trauma is common; however, there is little information on pancreatic injuries in children. The most common mechanism of injury in the developed word is the typical bicycle handlebar injury (62%); however, other common causes of blunt abdominal trauma are road traffic accidents, falls, sports, physical abuse, and contact with animals. Delays in definitive diagnosis are common due to subtle clinical signs. Increased serum amylase levels upon admission are not necessarily diagnostic for pancreatic injury. Of the 62% of patients who develop pancreatic pseudocysts, 60% to 70% undergo noninvasive management. Pancreatic trauma is rare in children, but traumatic pancreatic pseudocysts in this population is common. A high index of suspicion is required for early diagnosis. Treatment of pancreatic pseudocyst may be expectant, percutaneous drainage, or surgical drainage. The majority of pancreatic pseudocysts resolve spontaneously, and no treatment is necessary. When the pseudocyst is severely symptomatic and/or complications develop, a more invasive treatment is required.

15.3.2 Drainage Of Pancreatic Diseases

Case 15.3.2:

A 3-year-old boy with familial pancreatitis, psychiatric problems, and pancreatic insufficiency developed severe acute pancreatitis with a large pseudocyst. Severe pain, obstructive jaundice, and a sensation of abdominal fullness developed. An endoscopic biliary stent was placed but did not prove very effective.

A, B

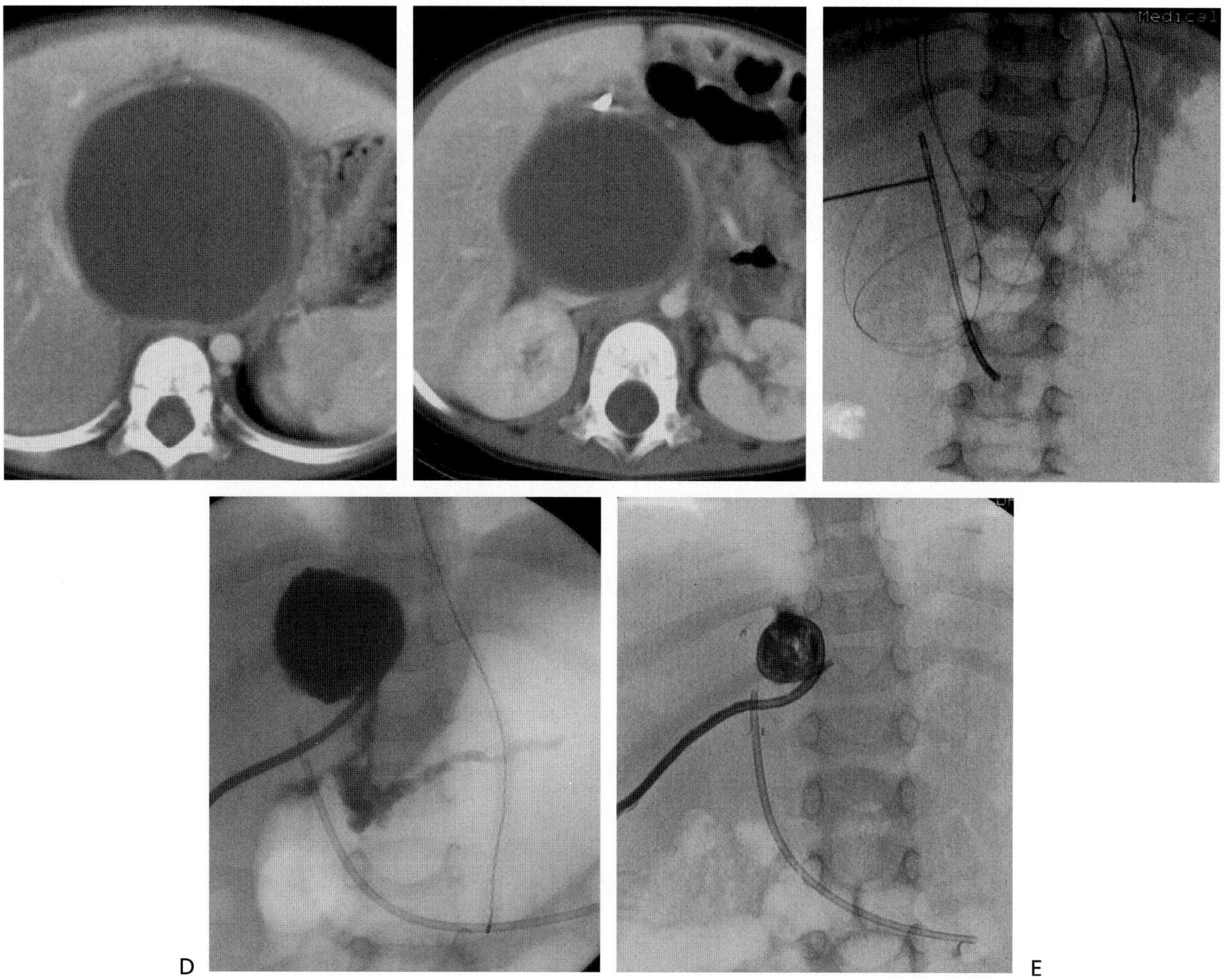

C

D

E

Figure 15.3.2

A: CT scan of the upper abdomen shows a large pancreatic pseudocyst displacing the liver and the stomach. **B:** A lower cut shows the biliary stent that was placed for biliary decompression. **C:** Percutaneous transhepatic drainage was performed. Note the biliary stent and the needle with the guidewire coiled within the large pancreatic pseudocyst. **D:** One-week follow-up sinogram shows filling of a much reduced cavity with direct communication to a very distorted pancreatic duct. Note that the biliary stent slipped into the duodenum following decompression of the pseudocyst. **E:** One-month follow-up shows resolution of the fluid collection and sealing of the fistula with the pancreatic duct. The catheter and the misplaced biliary stent were removed.

Comment: Interventional radiology has an important rote to play in the management of local complications of acute pancreatitis, such as necrosis, pseudocyst, and abscess. CT is preferred for guiding pancreatic drainages. The most common access route is through the left anterior pararenal space for pancreatic tail collections and through the gastrocolic ligament for pancreatic head and body collections. Pancreatic necrosis has a high mortality rate if infected, and the presence of infection must be determined with CT-guided needle aspiration. Careful planning of the access route to avoid the colon is important. A transhepatic window is acceptable for drainage of pseudocysts in the perihilar area of the liver. Catheter sizes of 8F to 12F usually are sufficient for pseudocyst drainage. An average of 2 to 3 weeks of drainage is required for pseudocysts without pancreatic duct communication and many more weeks to months for pseudocysts with pancreatic duct communication. Percutaneous pseudocyst drainage is associated with success rates of 80% to 90%. Pancreatic abscess drainage has reported success rates varying between 32% (infected necrosis) and 90% (true pancreatic abscess). Use of multiple catheters often is required for complete drainage of multiple fluid collections. The caliber of the drain is more dependent of the thickness of the fluid than the size of the lesion. Management of patients with severe acute pancreatitis is time consuming and labor intensive for interventional radiologists, and a team approach with close communication with the surgical team is required.

15.3.3 Drainage Of Pancreatic Diseases

Case 15.3.3:

A 41-year-old male patient with a history of nonalcoholic chronic pancreatitis underwent a Whipple procedure 6 years earlier. More recently, the patient underwent pancreatectomy because of chronic pancreatitis related to mucinous ductal ectasia. Following surgery, the patient developed a peripancreatic abscess even though a J–P (Jackson–Pratt) drain was in place. CT-guided drainage was requested.

A, B

C

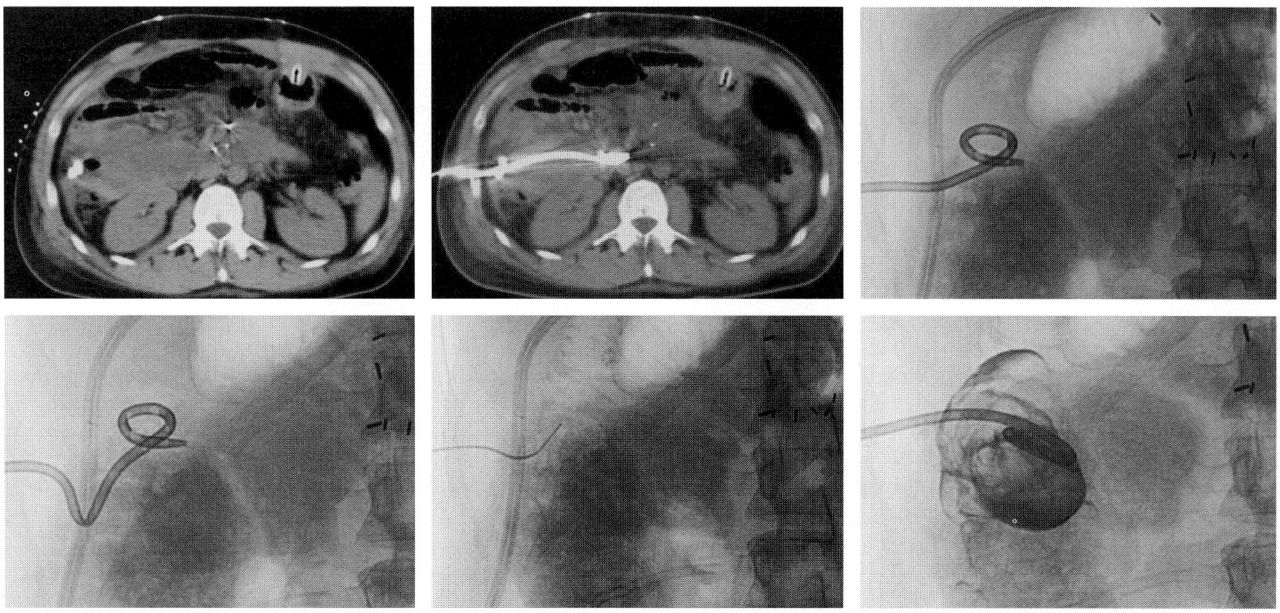

D, E

F

Figure 15.3.3

A: CT scan of the abdomen at the level of the kidneys shows a large abscess with air bubbles and a J-P drain in the periphery. **B:** CT drainage of the abscess was performed with a percutaneous 12F catheter. Note the catheter within the fluid collection, with the tip close to the inferior vena cava. There is a surgically placed jejunostomy tube on the left side of the anterior abdominal wall. **C:** The catheter was left in place for 10 days, and the patient improved. The J-P drain could not be removed by the surgeon; it appeared to be locked in place by the percutaneous drain. Initial fluoroscopic image shows the drains crossing. **D:** Pulling of the J-P drain demonstrates that the two drains are connected. Note the angle of the pigtail catheter. The initial puncture traversed the J-P drain, which is silicone made. **E:** The pigtail drain was pulled out over the wire and the wire was carefully pulled back, liberating the J-P drain. The wire was reintroduced into the cavity through the same tract and a new pigtail catheter was placed, while the J-P drain was removed. **F:** Final photograph shows the remaining cavity is filled with contrast. A biliary stricture was stented, and the patient was discharged 1 week later.

Comment: Nonalcoholic pancreatitis is encountered in 5% to 20% of patients with acute pancreatitis. Pancreatic pseudocysts occur much less frequently in nonalcoholic pancreatitis than in alcoholic pancreatitis. Spontaneous disappearance of pseudocysts is frequent; at 1 year the cumulative incidence of complications is reduced, with mortality close to zero. Postoperative complications are severe and usually related to infection, frequently in association with new bouts of pancreatitis. Bleeding due to pseudoaneurysms in peripancreatic arteries is encountered in a number of patients. Pancreatocutaneous fistula may develop in almost half of the patients treated by percutaneous drainage, but more frequently in patients with severe pancreatitis, regardless of the cause of the pancreatitis. The fistula can be used for access to the pancreatic duct and for percutaneous treatment. Cystic neoplasms of the pancreas should be ruled out.

Pseudocysts associated with chronic pancreatitis generally are intrapancreatic and associated with parenchymal disease. They tend to persist and cause complications. Morbidity was 28% and operative mortality rate was 1% in the report by Usatoff et al. Cysts in the head tend to be drained percutaneously and smaller cysts in the tail resected.

15.3.4 Drainage Of Pancreatic Diseases

Case 15.3.4:

A 55-year old male patient with alcoholic pancreatitis developed necrotizing pancreatitis. The patient presented with progressive deterioration. He was intubated and maintained under vasopressor medication. Fifteen days after admission, drainage was requested due to the development of infection.

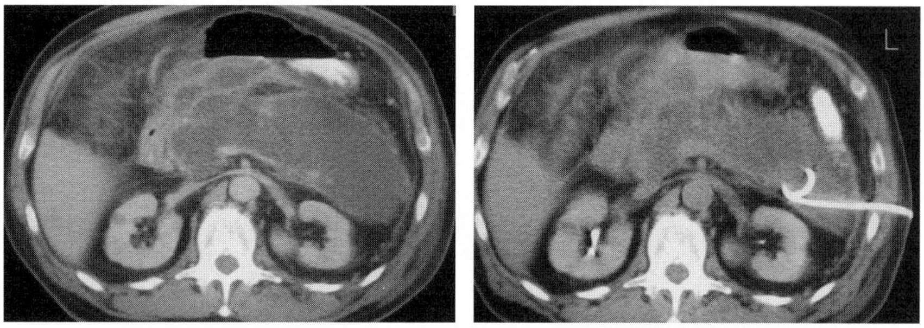

Figure 15.3.4

A: CT scan of the pancreas demonstrates a large fluid-filled cavity in the bed of the pancreas, consistent with a necrotizing pancreatic abscess. **B:** CT-guided drainage of the pancreatic abscess was performed with a 12F catheter introduced through the tail of the pancreas. The patient recovered, and he was extubated and discharged 8 days after drainage. Surgery with partial resection of the pancreas and Puestow procedure was performed 2 months later.

Comment: Pancreatic pseudocysts can be classified as (i) postnecrotic pancreatic pseudocysts produced by an attack of acute pancreatitis on a normal pancreas; (ii) postnecrotic pancreatic pseudocysts produced by an attack of acute pancreatitis superimposed on a chronic pancreatitis; (iii) chronic pancreatitis pancreatic pseudocysts ("retention cysts"); or (iv) postoperative pancreatic pseudocysts. The differential diagnosis between inflammatory and neoplastic lesions must be pursued both at the initial workup and during patient follow-up. Percutaneous drainage is one of the therapeutic options available for pancreatic pseudocysts and is indicated for (i) postnecrotic pancreatic pseudocysts produced by an attack of acute pancreatitis, which is larger than 6 cm and rapidly expanding or symptomatic; or (ii) postoperative pancreatic pseudocysts. Drainage also may be indicated for a small, highly selected group of chronic pancreatitis pancreatic pseudocysts that are symptomatic but without critical duct stenoses. Drainage in such cases may be used to decompress a retention cyst in order to improve the patient's general condition before surgery. Smaller cysts (less than 6 cm) usually can be managed without interventions. Percutaneous drainage may be technically successful in almost 100% of cases, with a morbidity of about 18% and no specific mortality, according to Mosca in 1999. Clinical success, however, may vary among different types of pancreatic pseudocysts.

Pancreatic necrosis is the most severe form of acute pancreatitis. It is diagnosed by dynamic CT scan and requires early aggressive cardiorespiratory resuscitation, nutritional support, and appropriate systemic antibiotic therapy. Development of infection is an indication for operative debridement and drainage. Percutaneous catheter drainage frequently is ineffective because there is no avenue for removal of the necrotic tissue. Freeny et al. showed a 47% cure rate by percutaneous catheter drainage only. Overall sepsis was controlled in 74% of patients, which permitted elective surgery for necrosectomy and treatment of pancreatic fistula. There was still a surgical mortality of 12%, mostly related to multiorgan failure. Percutaneous suction and debridement using a basket or snare may be attempted in selected patients, as reported by other authors, to reduce the need for surgical treatment. More recently, catheter suction with a morcellator-type device was used successfully in a number of patients (unreported experience). This expands the options available for nonsurgical management of complicated pancreatic fluid collections.

15.3.5 Drainage Of Pancreatic Diseases

Case 15.3.5:

A 36-year-old black male patient with lymphoma, chronic renal failure, neutropenia following liver transplant for choledochal cyst, and a history of alcohol abuse developed fever and pain. ERCP demonstrated occlusion of the bile ducts with intrahepatic dilatation. CT scan of the pancreas showed a small but severely symptomatic pancreatic head pseudocyst.

A, B 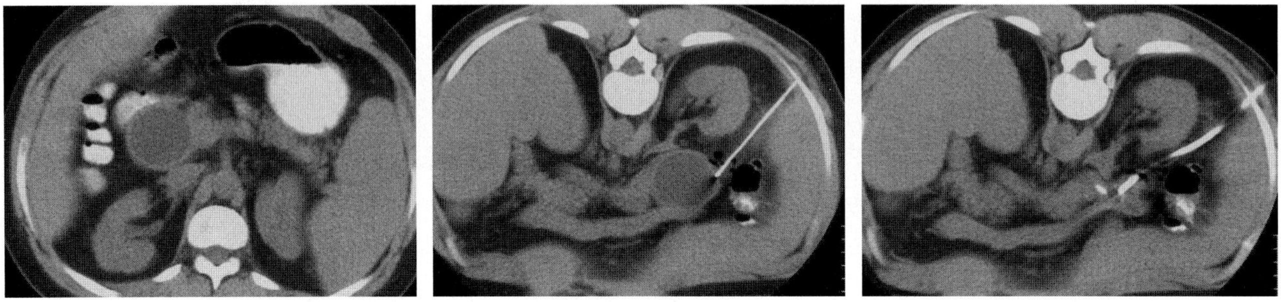 C

Figure 15.3.5

A: CT scan of the abdomen at the level of the pancreas shows a 5-cm pseudocyst in the head. **B:** The only available window was from the space between the right lobe of the liver and the right kidney. With the patient in a prone position, an 18-gauge, 15-cm, blunt needle was used to approach the lesion. **C:** Postdrainage CT scan of the pancreas shows total decompression of the pseudocyst and biliary duct. Note the biliary stent, now visible beyond the drain. Marked clinical improvement followed.

Comment: Pancreatic pseudocysts are a relatively common complication of pancreatitis. Pancreatic fluid collections are encountered in about 9% of patients with acute pancreatitis and pseudocysts in 5%, according to a recent report by Maringhini et al. Both conditions occur less frequently after biliary pancreatitis. These patients present with more serious complications than patients in the group with spontaneous disappearance, and they have higher mortality. Recent data suggest that many pseudocysts may be observed or treated successfully by percutaneous drainage. In a recent publication, Heider et al. showed that in a group of 173 patients with acute pancreatitis and diagnosis of pseudocyst, 41 were treated by observation, 66 by percutaneous drainage, and 66 by surgery. Observation was successful in 93% of patients, percutaneous drainage was successful in 42%, and surgical treatment was successful in 88% of patients. Mortality also was higher in the percutaneous group (16% vs. 0%) than in the surgical group, with higher complication rates and longer hospital stay. Although logistic regression analysis was used to identify factors responsible for the differences, it is possible that bias of selection may have assigned the more diseased patients to the percutaneous group. Those results do not hold true in many other publications.

Although the old teaching that cysts larger than 6 cm that are present for more than 6 weeks should be drained is no longer true. Current indications for drainage are presence of symptoms, progressive enlargement, complications related to infection, hemorrhage, rupture, and gastric/biliary or pancreatic duct obstruction. Percutaneous drainage should be the procedure of choice in poor-risk patients, for immature cysts, and for infected pseudocysts. Pancreatic ascites is a contraindication for percutaneous treatment. Endoscopic drainage should be reserved for mature pseudocysts, smaller pseudocysts, and pseudocysts in the head of the pancreas. In several instances, percutaneous drainage may be used as a bridge for more definitive surgical treatment, following clinical improvement, according to Pitchumoni et al.

15.3.6 Drainage Of Pancreatic Diseases

Case 15.3.6:

A 46-year-old white male patient with biliary pancreatitis initially was treated conservatively and then underwent laparoscopic cholecystectomy after his status improved. He did well for 2 weeks but then developed pancreatic pseudocysts, which were treated conservatively. As the patient's condition worsened, he was transferred to our hospital, where a CT scan showed a multiloculated pancreatic pseudocyst. Percutaneous drainage was requested.

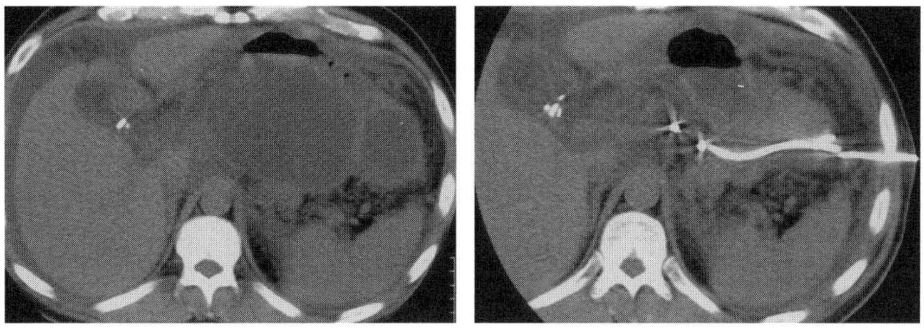

A B

Figure 15.3.6

A: CT scan of the abdomen shows a multiloculated or independent pancreatic pseudocysts. Note metal clips in the gallbladder bed, with some fluid accumulation. A left lateral window was selected for puncture. **B:** Using the same window approach, two 10F catheters were used for drainage. The more inferior catheter was located in the more superficial cyst, and the superior catheter was placed in the larger more central pseudocyst. Drainage was adequate, and the fluid collections were treated properly. With time, the more central lesion developed a fistula with the pancreatic duct (not shown). Further evaluation by ERCP and magnetic resonance imaging showed the pancreatic duct is occluded and the anatomy of the pancreas severely altered. The patient improved, and 45 days after drainage the patient underwent pancreaticojejunostomy and splenectomy, with good results.

Comment: Pancreatic collections are diverse, and the percutaneous options available reflect the complexities of those problems. Infected pancreatic pseudocysts and abscesses should be drained urgently. Noninfected pancreatic pseudocysts can be observed in a large number of cases. Indications for drainage of noninfected pseudocysts include pain, imminent leak or rupture, and obstruction of the biliary or gastrointestinal tract. Necrosis is the greatest challenge in treatment of pancreatic collections. Pancreatic abscesses are not seen until well into the course of pancreatitis, typically longer than 3 to 4 weeks. Multiple pseudocysts or multiloculated pseudocysts require an adequate number and size of catheters. Drainage in a complicated pseudocyst, as reported here, is the best option for treatment. It provides immediate relief and may cure the problem. In cases where the pancreatic duct and pancreas are unsalvageable, surgical treatment with Puestow procedure or resection must be performed, as in this case. Drainage provided immediate improvement.

15.3.7 Drainage Of Pancreatic Diseases

Case 15.3.7:

A 68-year-old white diabetic male patient with pancreatic cancer was explored for duodenal blockage. A Whipple procedure was performed. The patient gradually developed sepsis beginning 3 days postoperatively that evolved into critical conditions. He was transferred to our institution for further treatment. which consisted of surgical revision of the gastrojejunostomy and placement of G- and J-tubes. The postoperative period again was complicated by sepsis. There was an anastomotic breakdown that again was repaired surgically. Fever persisted, and a follow-up CT scan of the abdomen showed a fluid collection at the bed of the gallbladder and at the level of the resected pancreatic head. Percutaneous drainage was requested.

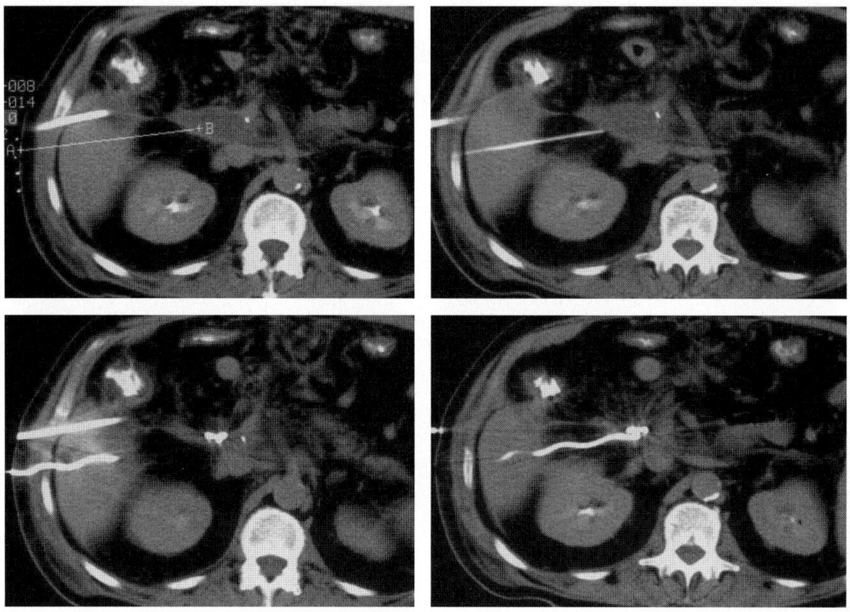

A B C D

Figure 15.3.7

A: CT scan of the abdomen shows a fluid collection at the bed of the gallbladder, which was drained. Note the 10F catheter in place. Measurements for drainage of the fluid collection in the pancreatic bed was made. **B:** Using a transhepatic window, an 18-gauge, 15-cm-long needle was used for percutaneous puncture. Note the needle traversing the liver, with the tip at the wall of the fluid collection. **C,D:** A 10F drainage catheter was placed over the wire and completely evacuated the collection. In association with aggressive antibiotic therapy, improvement of sepsis followed.

Comment: Postoperative pancreatic fluid collections are common due to the nature of pancreatic organ function, where breakdown of sutures in enteric-enteric and pancreaticoenteric anastomosis is relatively frequent. Fluid collections related to leaks at an anastomosis may lead to walling off and development of an abscess. Percutaneous drainage is indicated. As these situations usually are complex, CT guidance is preferred. The treatment strategy is to catheterize the collection and evacuate the contents. A sinogram or abscessogram is necessary to demonstrate the communication with the gastrointestinal tract and allow time for the anastomotic leak to both heal and seal. Spontaneous sealing occurs in some cases, but operation may become necessary to repair the anastomotic site. Enteric decompression and diversion of bowel contents should be performed with nasogastric or nasoenteric tubes. Decompression speeds up the healing and closing of enteric fistulas.

15.3.8 Drainage Of Pancreatic Diseases

Case 15.3.8:

A 48-year-old black male patient with necrotizing pancreatitis was septic. CT scan showed a persistent pancreatic mass with fluid and debris inside. Previous percutaneous drainage had been unsuccessful. Percutaneous suction catheter debridement was attempted.

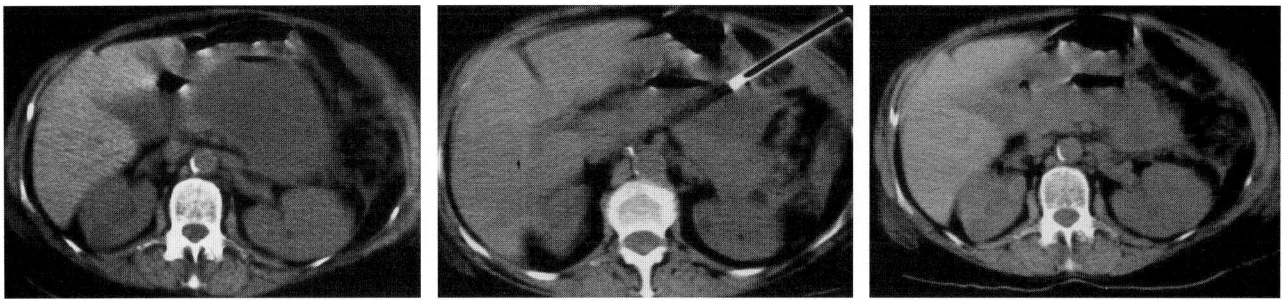

A B, C

Figure 15.3.8

A: CT scan of the abdomen after an unsuccessful attempt at catheter drainage shows a large pancreatic fluid collection resulting from infected necrotizing pancreatitis. **B:** Percutaneous large-bore catheter aspiration was performed and the lesion evacuated. Note the large sheath still in place after performing part of the procedure. There was significant clinical improvement. **C:** CT scan of the abdomen following debridement shows significant resolution of the lesion.

Comment: Pancreatic necrosis is a feared complication of acute pancreatitis because of the high morbidity and mortality when infection ensues. Only about 5% of patients develop infected necrotizing pancreatitis, but 80% of all deaths related to pancreatitis result from this process. Mortality is extremely high if infected pancreatic necrosis is left untreated. Surgical treatment still carries a mortality rate of 15% to 50%. Percutaneous catheter drainage treatment of infected pancreatic necrosis is ineffective or used only as palliation preceding surgery. Percutaneous catheter snare debridement was reported in 1994 by Dixon and in 1997 by Shonnard et al. It proved useful in a small number of cases. In 1998, Echenique et al. reported on 20 patients with necrotizing pancreatitis who were treated successfully by percutaneous catheter-directed debridement. The proposed technique uses a modified large-bore (14F) drainage catheter with the tip cut off and side holes enlarged, coupled with wall suction and abundant saline lavage fluid. The technique is time consuming, averaging 60 minutes. Multiple passes of the catheter for debris withdrawal are necessary, as are the use of metal baskets and multiple debridement sessions. The results were encouraging, with improvement in all patients despite the prolonged length of recovery and catheter drainage of most patients. Continuous vacuum aspiration drainage applied for 20 to 80 days was proposed by Migaleddu et al. as an effective alternative for treatment of chronic pancreatic pseudocysts. More recently, we developed a flexible large-bore suction catheter that works like a morcellator, sucking and cutting the more solid debris. The 14F catheter has a blunt tip and large oval side hole and it is introduced through a 14F sheath. The system includes a more rigid metal cannula with a sharp cutting tip that is introduced within the main catheter. Suction is applied to the cannula, which is manually reciprocated back and forth. The debris is sucked through the side hole, and the cannula cuts the amorphous material into smaller pieces that are pulled out through the cannula lumen. Lavage is necessary during the procedure to allow mobilization and aspiration of the more solid debris. A double-lumen suction catheter with internal irrigation also can be used to facilitate extraction of material. This technique proved useful in about 20 patients in our experience.

15.3.9 Drainage Of Pancreatic Diseases

Case 15.3.9:

A 60-year-old alcoholic male patient with necrotizing pancreatitis presented with epigastric pain and fever. Diagnosis of a large pancreatic pseudocyst fluid collection was made, and an outside percutaneous pseudocyst drainage was performed. Despite the drainage, the patient became progressively septic. The patient was transferred to our hospital. CT scan showed a large pancreatic lesion destroying the pancreatic body and tail, with fluid and debris inside, consistent with complicated pseudocyst. Percutaneous drainage was deemed unsuccessful. Percutaneous suction catheter debridement was attempted.

A, B

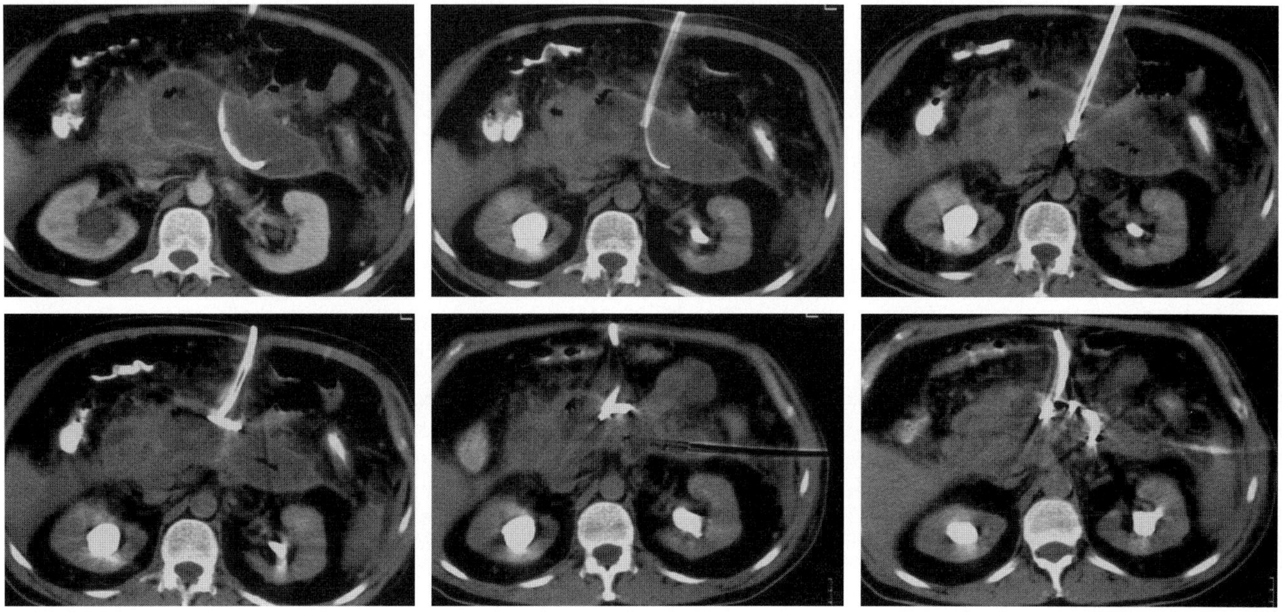

C

D, E

F

Figure 15.3.9

A: CT scan of the abdomen performed after failed percutaneous catheter drainage shows persistent pancreatic fluid collection. **B:** The catheter was exchanged over the wire for a 14F sheath in preparation for catheter-directed debridement. **C:** The morcellator suction catheter was used to evacuate the fluid and debris. **D:** Following debridement, a 12F pigtail catheter was left in place for external drainage. Residual fluid collection in the tail of the pancreas was left untreated in hopes that it would resolve with the main drain in the body of the pancreas. **E:** Despite improvement, the patient remained febrile. Five days later, a lateral left approach was used to treat the tail abscess. Note the 14F introducer sheath within the pancreatic abscess. Suction and debridement were performed. **F:** A 14F catheter was left in place for long-term drainage and aggressive treatment with antibiotics. There was significant clinical improvement. The patient subsequently underwent a partial pancreatectomy with a Puestow procedure. Total hospitalization time was 60 days.

Comment: Necrotizing pancreatitis is a life-threatening complication of acute pancreatitis. The surgical drainage is related to serious morbidity and mortality. Percutaneous catheter drainage usually is not effective or is only partially effective in alleviating symptoms and improving infection. Debridement is necessary for a more consistent response to treatment. Suction and debridement of stuff within pancreatic necrotic abscesses are mandatory to improve results of percutaneous treatment after failed catheter drainage. A 14F sheath is used to obtain access to the intrapancreatic abscess. The suction catheter is introduced within the cavity, intermittent suction is applied, and the debris is cut by the cannula. Multiple accesses, as in this case, may be necessary to treat separate loculations and compartments. Multiple sessions may be necessary and are associated with a higher chance of success. Leaving a drainage catheter in place is mandatory, because of the residual fluid and continuous inflammation within the pancreas.

15.4.1 Drainage Of Liver Collections

Case 15.4.1:

A 59-year-old alcoholic black male patient presented with exacerbation of chronic pancreatitis, recurrent pseudocyst, pain, and nausea. An endoscopic pancreatic stent was placed. He began to have fevers, with elevated white count. CT scan of the abdomen showed a peripheral hepatic abscess and a pseudocyst in the head of the pancreas.

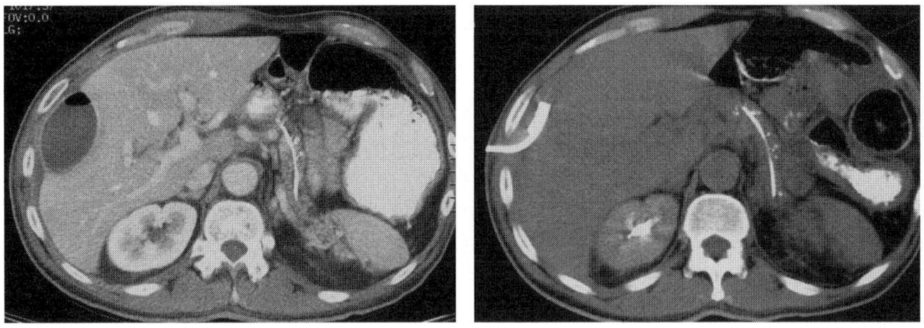

Figure 15.4.1

A: CT scan of the liver demonstrates a peripheral hepatic abscess 8 cm × 4 cm in diameter, with a small amount of gas within. **B:** Using CT guidance, the abscess was punctured with an 18-gauge needle, and a 10F pigtail catheter was placed within the abscess for drainage. Grossly purulent fluid was aspirated. Total evacuation of the abscess was performed and the patient immediately defervesced. A Whipple procedure was performed several weeks after the percutaneous drainage.

Comment: Liver abscess is more common in males and occurs more frequently in the right hepatic lobe. Most patients present with nonspecific clinical and biochemical features. An increased alkaline phosphatase level is a common biochemical abnormality found in about two thirds of patients. Chief clinical complaints are fever, pain, and jaundice. Ultrasonography is not as sensitive as CT scan in detecting abscesses. *Klebsiella pneumoniae* is a common etiologic agent detected in blood cultures and abscess aspirates. Intravenous antibiotics are the initial treatment for all patients and can be curative in a number of patients. Percutaneous catheter drainage can be the definitive treatment for most patients, up to 80% to 95%. Surgical treatment currently is used in less than 10% of patients. Prolonged hospitalization usually is associated with advanced age, degree of loculation within the abscess, concomitant diabetes, biliary fistula, and sepsis. Untreated liver abscess has a high mortality rate, but early diagnosis and antibiotic therapy in combination with percutaneous drainage reduce the mortality and morbidity to very low rates. Mortality of percutaneous drainage usually is less than 5% but may range from 5% to 13%, compared with 8% to 17% for surgical treatment. Reasons for drainage failure are tumor necrosis and tumor perforation with secondary liver abscess. In a comparative series reported by Bertel et al., the percutaneous technique was associated with a longer hospital stay (26 vs. 46 days) and higher morbidity.

15.4.2 Drainage Of Liver Collections

Case 15.4.2:

A 50-year-old cachectic, alcoholic, black male patient with a history of chronic pancreatitis, chronic abdominal pain, and multiple surgeries presented with severe nausea and vomiting for the past 36 hours. Total parenteral nutrition was started, and an open gastrostomy eventually was performed. A biliary stent was endoscopically placed. Hospital course was stormy; he developed intestinal perforation that required surgical repair. Fever and elevated white cell count persisted. CT scan of the abdomen revealed a moderate amount of perihepatic fluid and a large intrahepatic fluid-filled collection, with air-fluid level. Percutaneous drainage was requested.

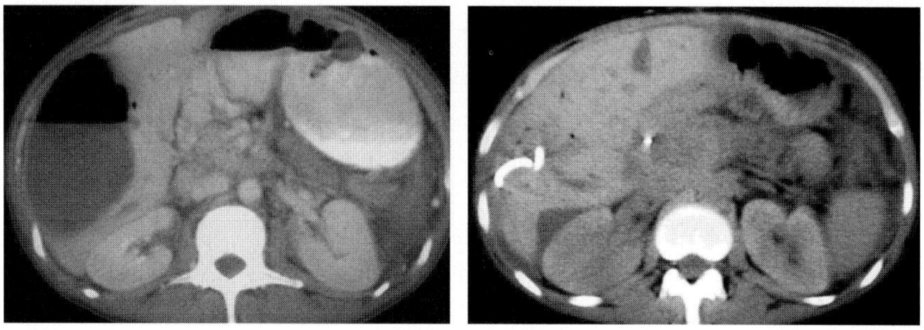

A B

Figure 15.4.2

A: CT scan of the abdomen shows a large intrahepatic fluid collection with air-fluid level. Using CT guidance, percutaneous drainage was accomplished with a 10F pigtail catheter. The patient improved and fever disappeared. Analysis of the fluid shows infection and high bilirubin content, suggesting a biloma. **B:** Nine days after drainage, follow-up CT scan demonstrates resolution of fluid collection without a significant volume of drainage. The catheter was removed.

Comment: During the approximately 20 years that imaging-guided percutaneous abscess drainage has been in use, it has had a tremendous impact on the management of patients with intraabdominal abscesses. Percutaneous drainage has become the treatment of choice for abscesses. Indications for its use continue to expand, and currently almost all fluid collections are considered amenable to percutaneous treatment. On occasion, when there is a coexisting procedure such as a bowel leak that requires surgical treatment, percutaneous drainage may be used as an adjunct procedure that provides a beneficial temporizing effect that improves the patient's condition.

Simple needle aspiration of the liver abscess can yield the etiologic agent. In a number of patients (up to 88% in some reports), it may be effective in resolving the abscess, but further catheter drainage in a second procedure may be necessary. Rapid reaccumulation of exudate within the abscess cavity, sometimes related to a biliary fistula, requires catheter drainage when needle aspiration is ineffective. In our experience, catheter drainage is a more adequate, safer, and effective treatment for hepatic abscess.

15.4.3 Drainage Of Liver Collections

Case 15.4.3:

A 55-year-old black female patient presented with right upper quadrant pain. Abdominal US revealed an incidental liver mass in the right lobe of the liver. An outside CT scan confirmed the presence of a mass, and a biopsy was attempted. During this procedure, the patient became agitated and restless. She subsequently developed signs of hypotension related to a subcapsular hematoma. The biopsy was nondiagnostic. Hemangioma was ruled out by a red cell study scan, but the patient remained symptomatic, with shortness of breath, pulmonary edema, and congestive heart failure. The patient was transferred to our institution, where a diagnostic CT scan confirmed a large subcapsular hepatic hematoma. Her heart condition was treated, and evaluation for possible drainage and biopsy was requested, as there was also a question of hematoma infection.

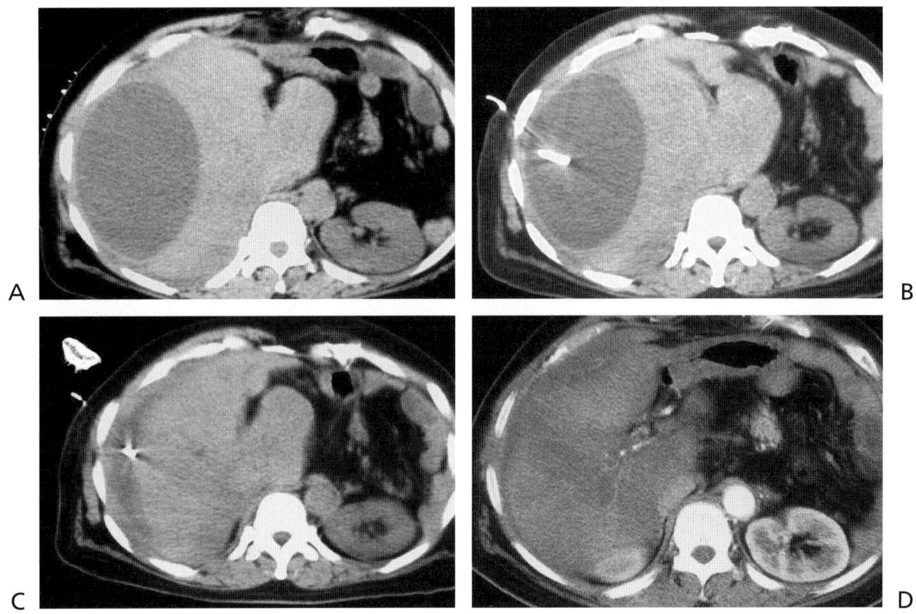

Figure 15.4.3

A: CT scan of the abdomen with intravenous contrast enhancement shows a large subcapsular hematoma in the right lobe of the liver. **B:** Percutaneous drainage with a 14F pigtail catheter was performed. Initially the hematoma did not drain well with the catheter. **C:** Active suction of the hematoma with a large-bore system was performed, and more than 200 mL of thick fluid was removed. The fluid-filled cavity collapsed, and the catheter was removed 6 days after drainage. The patient did well and was discharged. **D:** Seven weeks after drainage, the patient was reexamined with CT scan, which shows a poorly defined edge of the right lobe of the liver, a small amount of perihepatic fluid, and irregular enhancement of the liver parenchyma, suggesting either a sequela of the drained hematoma or a tumor. A needle biopsy was negative for tumor.

Comment: Fluid collections other than plain abscesses, such as hematomas, are more difficult to treat efficiently with catheter drainage, because the fluid is organized and very thick. Active suction and some form of mechanical thrombectomy may be necessary for proper treatment. Later during resolution of the hematoma, the blood will liquefy and be more easily drained; however, depending on the location, infection may ensue and require drainage. Presence of a subcapsular hematoma in the liver poses a significant risk of a localized consumptive coagulopathy with persistent life-threatening hemorrhage. Coagulopathy results from localized intraluminal activation and consumption of clotting factors. The pathogenesis is believed to involve the local release of thromboplastin, as well as contact activation of clotting factors by subendothelial procoagulant substances, locally deposited red cell fragments, and platelet aggregates. Removal of the cause reverses the coagulation abnormalities. It is unclear whether patients benefit from preoperative use of heparin or plasma. Other stasis-prone, vascular tumors, including giant hemangiomas of infancy and liver hemangiomas, may develop consumptive coagulopathy. Ischemic hepatitis from different causes can result in severe coagulopathy. Subcapsular hematoma of the liver is a rare but very serious complication of pregnancy. Spontaneous hepatic hematomas can occur during a pregnancy complicated by preeclampsia and the HELLP (hemolysis, elevated liver enzymes, and low platelet count) syndrome. The prognosis of a localized consumptive coagulopathy in the liver is reserved.

15.4.4 Drainage Of Liver Collections

Case 15.4.4:

A 67-year-old white male patient presented to the emergency room of a suburban hospital with a six-week history of weakness, weight loss, chills, fever, and syncopal episode. The patient was hypotensive and required fluid resuscitation. Abdominal US and CT scans showed a low-attenuation mass in the liver that initially was interpreted as a neoplastic process or abscess. A biopsy was performed and produced purulent material. A drain was inserted, followed by antibiotic therapy. Blood culture was positive for *Streptococcus viridans.* The hepatic drain was removed. The patient subsequently was transferred to our institution.

A 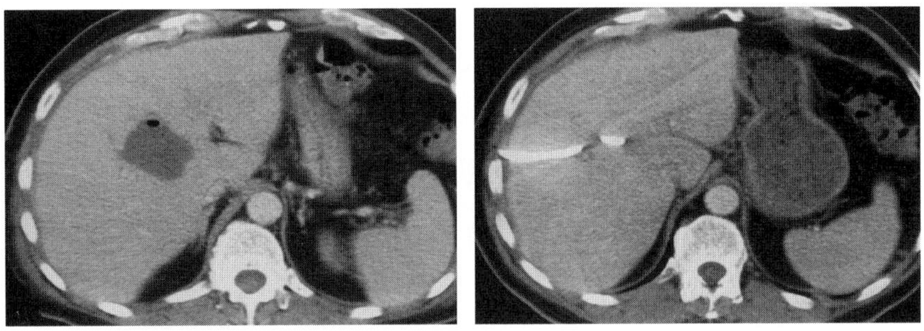 B

Figure 15.4.4

A: On admission, the patient was again febrile and endocarditis was suspected, but an echocardiogram was negative for vegetations in the heart valves (not shown). CT scan of the abdomen shows recurrence of the abscess. **B:** A new 10F catheter was placed using CT guidance. Follow-up CT scan 15 days after drainage shows total resolution of the abscess. The catheter was removed. There was permanent clinical improvement, and the patient was discharged.

Comment: Hepatic artery embolization and chemoembolization may cause hepatic abscess in about 4.5% of patients undergoing those procedures. Patients who undergo the Whipple procedure before chemoembolization and bilioenteric anastomosis have a much higher odds ratio to develop intrahepatic abscess. Other risk factors for development of pyogenic liver abscess is the presence of liver cirrhosis or Chrohn disease. Other common causes of liver abscesses include extension of gallbladder and gallstone disease, prior trauma or surgery, and seeding from sepsis (e.g., diverticulitis or endocarditis). Multiple abscesses are more difficult to treat and require multiple catheters. CT scan is the key imaging modality for identification of multiple abscesses or septated abscesses and is the preferred guidance method for placement of multiple catheters. Multiple abscesses may be juxtaposed or remote from each other. The number of catheters to be used depends basically on location. A particularly challenging liver abscess is one that is located near the dome of the diaphragm. In those cases, a combination of imaging modalities may be necessary. Clinically, virtually all liver abscesses require catheter drainage. Hepatic abscesses require a clean puncture window. No hollow bowel loops should be positioned in the path of the drain. CT scan provides the best assessment for a puncture site and safest approach. Rupture of a liver abscess into the thorax may develop a fistula into the bronchial tree and cause rapid deterioration of the patient's clinical situation. Catheter sinogram a few days after evacuation of the pus often results in demonstration of a communication to the bile ducts, particularly in trauma cases. Drainage catheters need not remain for extended periods; 3 to 5 days usually is sufficient for cure, along with antibiotic treatment.

Amebic abscesses are preferably treated with antibiotics such as metronidazole, but situations of large symptomatic lesions, poor response to antibiotic therapy, leakage, or uncertain diagnosis require percutaneous drainage.

15.4.5 Drainage Of Liver Collections

Case 15.4.5:

A 57-year-old white male patient presented with a 5-day history of bilateral lower quadrant abdominal pain and anorexia. Severe diarrhea, vomiting, and chills also were observed. A distended abdomen prompted a visit to the emergency room, and the patient was admitted to the hospital. Abdominal series revealed free intraperitoneal gas. Abdominal CT showed a pelvic abscess suggestive of perforated diverticular process. A percutaneous drain was placed in the pelvic abscess through a transgluteal access (not shown). The patient was discharged home with the catheter following remarkable improvement. One week later, the patient was readmitted to the hospital in respiratory distress, with hemoptysis, green and brown sputum, fever, and complaint of chest and abdominal pain. Possible pneumonia was considered. The patient was scheduled for a chest and abdominal CT scan on the same day, but rapidly deteriorated. He required intubation and intensive care. CT scan was performed.

A, B

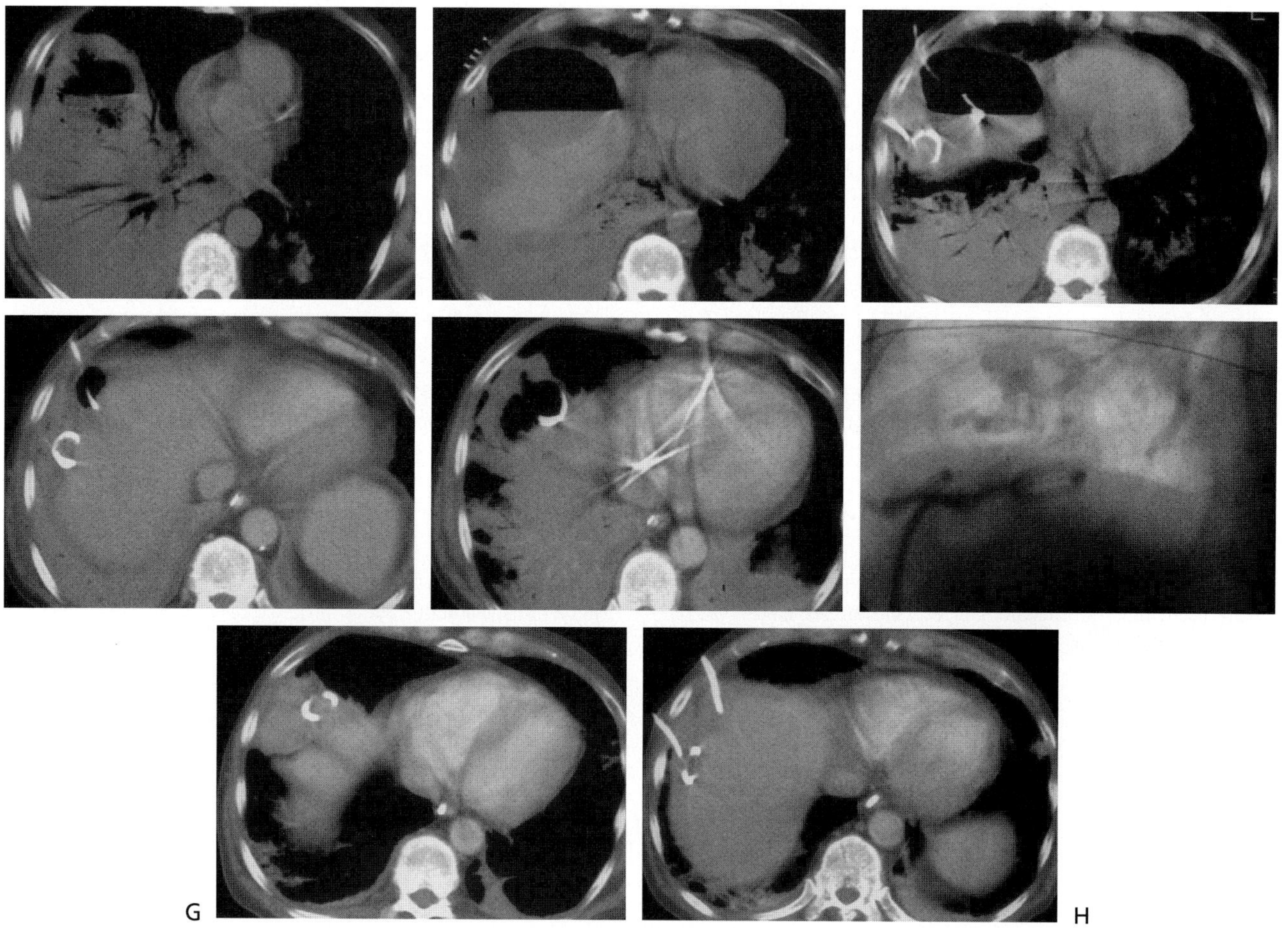

Figure 15.4.5

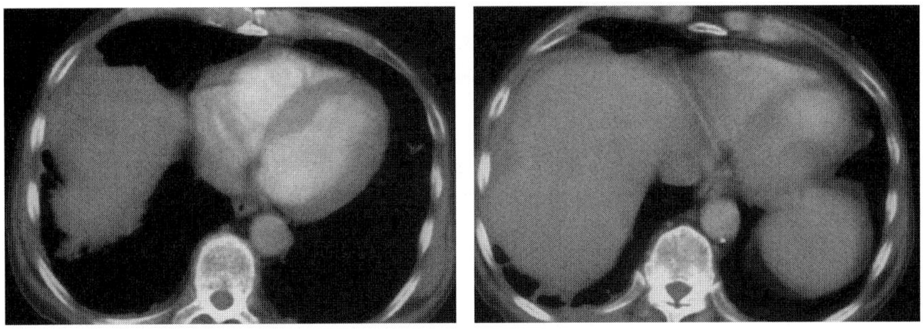

I J

Figure 15.4.5 *(continued)*

A,B: CT scan of the abdomen and base of the thorax shows a large subphrenic/intrahepatic fluid collection, with air-fluid level, associated with a collapsed right lower lobe of the lung. Note the extensive air bronchogram. CT guidance was used for drainage. **C–E:** Three catheters were used for drainage of the multiloculated fluid collection. **F:** Despite drainage, the patient continued to spit up bilious material. Follow-up chest radiography with injection of contrast material through the drains 5 days after drainage shows the presence of biliary-bronchial fistula. **G,H:** Active suction drainage for another 8 days promoted significant clinical improvement. Follow-up CT scan shows regression of the fluid collections. **I,J:** The drains were removed 2 weeks after drainage. Follow-up CT scan 30 days after drainage shows complete resolution of the hepatic abscess and bronchobiliary fistula (BBF).

Comment: BBF is a rare entity that manifests as biliptysis. It usually is a manifestation of biliary obstruction associated with severe infection and abscess formation. BBF is defined as an abnormal communication between the biliary sytem and the bronchial tree. It is an uncommon complication after hemihepatectomy, trauma, hydatid disease, choledocholithiasis, and other causes of biliary obstruction. BBFs can be minimal or massive. Usually the patients become septic, but initial symptoms can be chronic cough and dark-yellow sputum. Most patients have cholangitis and jaundice. Traditional treatment for BBF is surgical, i.e., relief of biliary obstruction and drainage of abscesses. Operative closure of the fistulous tract and diversion of the biliary stricture by a hepaticojejunal bypass usually are effective. Resection of the involved pulmonary tissue and interposition of viable tissue between the lung and the fistulous tract have been suggested as useful in selected cases of BBF. More recently, several reports of percutaneous treatment of BBF with biliary drainage and percutaneous abscess drainage demonstrated it to be successful in eradicating the fistula and reestablishing biliary flow. Percutaneous internal-external catheter drainage or internal stent placement has been used very successfully in diverting the biliary flow and allowing the fistula to seal off. Stricture balloon dilation is necessary in most patients to decompress the bile ducts. Endoscopic biliary stent placement has been very useful in treating BBF. Separate abscess drainage may be necessary. Metallic stents are useful for biliary decompression in those cases.

15.5.1 Drainage Of Splenic Collections

Case 15.5.1:

A 54-year-old male patient with transitional cell carcinoma of the bladder was treated by cystoprostatectomy and continent urinary diversion. The patient had a prolonged complicated postoperative hospital course, which included bowel anastomotic breakdown, for which he had to undergo an ileostomy. Obstructive uropathy with sepsis developed, which required bilateral percutaneous nephrostomies, tracheostomy, and intensive care for about 1 month. Deep venous thrombosis also was diagnosed. Upon transfer to the regular ward, the patient developed elevated white count and fever. CT scan of the abdomen showed a splenic abscess. Percutaneous drainage was requested.

A, B

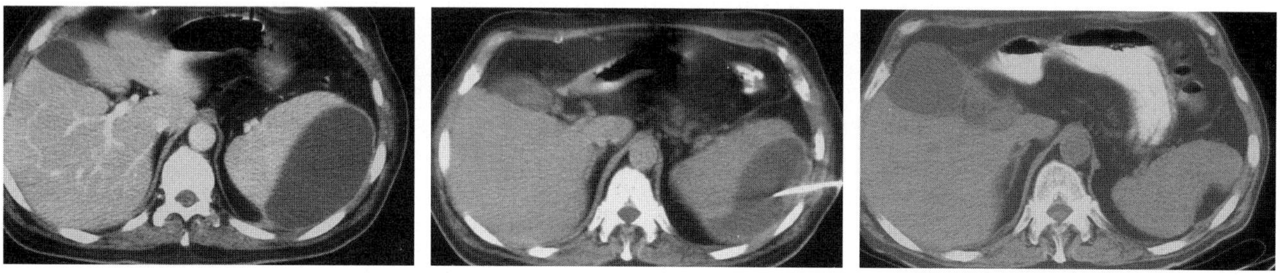

C

Figure 15.5.1

A: CT scan of the abdomen shows a large intrasplenic abscess. **B:** Using CT guidance, a 10F catheter was placed for external drainage. The patient improved clinically and the fever resolved. The catheter was pulled after 7 days. **C:** Follow-up CT scan before discharge shows a residual lesion in the spleen without clinical significance. It was decided not to treat this lesion because of the patient's much improved clinical picture.

Comment: Splenic abscesses are relatively uncommon events. A recent review found only 300 cases reported in the literature in the last 10 years, but it is a diagnostic and therapeutic challenge in most cases. The mortality of the disease is high, and the unspecific presentation of the disease usually delays the diagnosis. CT is the most sensitive study for diagnosis. Although US also is useful for diagnosis, the splenic lesion may be confused with subphrenic fluid collections, and CT scan is reputed to be more accurate and reliable in the diagnosis. Infection of the spleen with abscess formation may be related to bacterial or fungal infection. Immunosuppression frequently is related to splenic abscess development. Microorganisms and fungi more rarely cause the infection. Sepsis, bacterial endocarditis, trauma, ischemia, and sickle cell disease are common precipitating factors. Sickle cell disease may precipitate the infection following a bout of ischemia during a sickle cell crisis. Splenic tuberculosis occasionally is encountered. Several other diseases may be related to splenic infection and abscess formation. Diseases of adjacent organs may cause splenic abscess, due to invasion, rupture, and inflammatory process. Pancreatitis is a well-known cause of splenic abscess. The pancreatic pseudocysts may impinge upon the spleen and grow within the splenic parenchyma, with ensuing infection. Penetration of a left colon cancer with fistula creation is a recognized cause of splenic infection that requires splenectomy in most cases. Splenic hematomas are infrequent complications encountered in patients with acute pancreatitis. Local factors, such as thrombosis of the splenic artery or vein, intrasplenic pseudocysts, perisplenic adhesions, and enzymatic digestion, may play a role. In the absence of local factors, the etiology of nontraumatic splenic hemorrhage remains unknown. The role of diffuse microcirculatory infarction, associated with either disseminated intravascular coagulation (a localized consumption coagulopathy) or other coagulation disorders, should be considered whenever a splenic hematoma is found in a patient with acute pancreatitis.

15.5.2 Drainage Of Splenic Collections

Case 15.5.2:

A 70-year-old female patient with a medical history of breast cancer, deep venous thrombosis of the left leg, total oophorectomy/hysterectomy, and rectosigmoid resection followed by a pelvic abscess that was treated successfully by percutaneous drainage presented with severe right-sided abdominal pain for the last 2 weeks, with no significant relief from analgesics. CT scan of the abdomen showed a fluid collection in the spleen, consistent with abscess. Percutaneous drainage was requested.

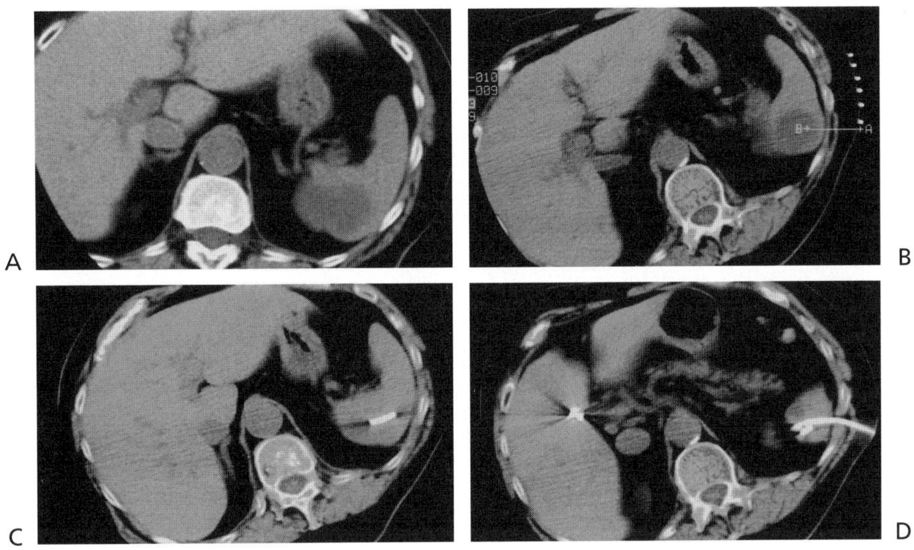

Figure 15.5.2

A: Supine CT scan of the abdomen at the level of the spleen shows a 5-cm × 3-cm splenic abscess. **B:** CT scan with a marking grid shows an adequate window of entry. **C,D:** A 10F drain was placed and the fluid collection totally evacuated. The abscess resolved and the catheter was removed. Follow-up CT scan for pelvic neoplasm evaluation about 2 weeks after catheter removal shows total resolution of the abscess, with a normal-sized spleen (not shown).

Comment: Splenic abscesses may be multiple or single. Single splenic abscess is more common. *Salmonella* and *Klebsiella* are common organisms involved. The spleen is in close proximity to the pancreas. Involvement of the spleen is relatively uncommon in acute inflammation of the pancreas, but peripancreatic pseudocysts and abscesses can perforate into the spleen. Percutaneous aspiration may yield the microorganism causing the infection. Surgical splenectomy is the gold standard treatment for splenic abscess and should be the procedure of choice when the spleen is nonfunctional, as in sickle cell disease. Most splenic abscesses can be treated successfully by US- or CT-guided catheter drainage. Antibiotic therapy and interventional percutaneous drainage have modified the therapeutic approach to splenic abscess and is now the preferred treatment for patients at high surgical risk, for unilocular lesions, or as a temporary measure even if surgical resection becomes necessary in the future. One should bear in mind, however, that splenectomy causes depressed phagocytosis and decreases serum levels of immunoglobulin M and antigen response. Subphrenic abscesses after splenectomy account for 2.5% of postoperative complications of splenectomy for trauma.

15.6.1 Treatment Of Hydatid Renal Cysts

Case 15.6.1:

A 45-year-old female patient with hepatic and renal cysts was referred for percutaneous treatment of upper quadrant pain.

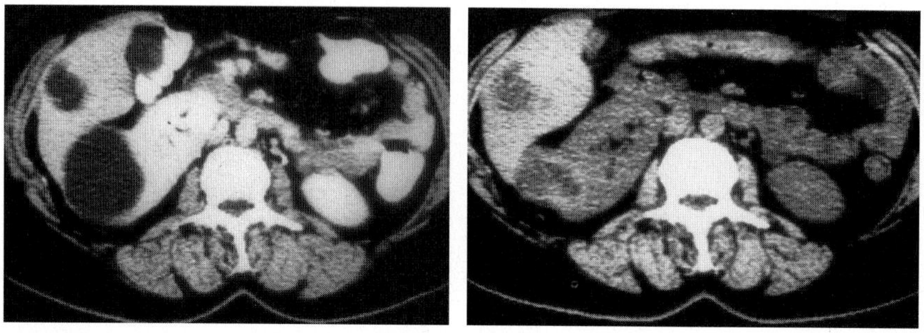

A B

Figure 15.6.1

A: CT scan shows multiple hepatic hydatid cysts. All cysts were type I. There also was a large renal cyst that was managed by catheterization technique. **B:** Follow-up CT scan study 6 months after treatment shows lesion significant resolution of the cyst. Note the renal hydatid cyst with high density and thick walls. There are two small residual cysts in segment V and in the right kidney.

Comment: Renal echinococcosis is relatively uncommon compared to liver and lung localizations. Only about 4% of the confirmed cases of hydatid disease have renal involvement. Diagnosis can be made accurately by US, CT, and immunologic tests. Presentation may be as simple as back pain, but may be as severe as flank mass, hydaturia, hematuria, infection, and hypertension. Surgical resection of the cyst is successful in most cases (75%), but nephrectomy may be necessary in as many as 25% to 40% of cases. Minimally invasive treatment includes puncture, aspiration, injection of hypertonic saline, and reaspiration [PAIR technique: *p*uncture, *a*spiration (half volume of the cyst), *i*njection (one third of the initial estimated volume of hypertonic saline solution and waiting 20 minutes), *r*einjection (all the fluid volume)], which was used in this case, with resolution of the hepatic and renal cysts. Catheterization and absolute alcohol injection should be used for cysts larger than 6 cm. Untreated renal cysts can rupture into the collecting system, leading to the possibility of urticaria and seeding of daughter lesions along the ureter and bladder.

15.7.1 Treatment Of Hydatid Liver Cyst

Case 15.7.1:

A 27-year-old male patient presented with nonspecific right upper quadrant pain and hepatomegaly. US examination showed hepatic hydatid cysts.

A

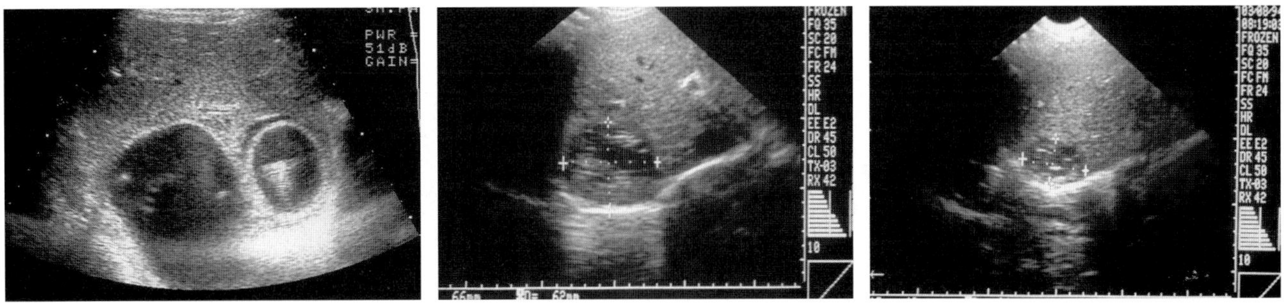

B, C

Figure 15.7.1

A: US examination shows 11-mm × 90-mm and 35-mm × 50-mm type I hydatid cysts of the right hepatic lobe. Note the needle echogenicity within the small cyst, with separation of the pericyst from the endocyst. Approximate volume of the larger cyst is 515 mL and of the smaller cyst is 36.4 mL. **B:** Three months after percutaneous treatment, dimensions are 62 mm × 66 mm, volume is 130 mL, and internal echogenicity is more solid in the larger cyst. The volume was reduced by 74%. The small cyst has disappeared, and only a scar is visible. **C:** One year follow-up shows pseudotumor appearance of the larger cyst. Dimensions are 34 mm × 48 mm, and the volume is 29 mL. The volume was reduced by 94%.

Comment: Hydatid disease caused by *Echinococcus granulosus* is endemic in Mediterranean countries, the Middle East, South America , Australia, and New Zealand. The disease is a common health problem in endemic areas and an increasing problem in Europe and North America because of immigration. Diagnostic studies such as serologic and specific antibody tests are not reliable as screening methods and follow-up modalities. Imaging techniques such as US, CT, and magnetic resonance imaging are more reliable in both diagnostic and follow-up studies. Until the development of percutaneous treatments, surgery was the treatment for hydatid cysts. There was a general concept that anaphylaxis was an extreme risk, before Muller's first percutaneous hydatid cyst treatment. No anaphylaxis was seen following percutaneous treatment procedures. Mortality, morbidity, and recurrence rates for general surgery are 0% to 6.3%, 12.5% to 80%, and 2% to 30%, respectively. Hospitalization time ranges from 14 days in uncomplicated cases to 30 days in complicated cases. The results of a recent series of 252 hydatid cysts during a 5.5-year follow-up showed 0% mortality, 12.5% complication rate, and 1.31% recurrence rate with 1-day hospital stay in uncomplicated cases and 20.4 days in complicated cases. General indication for percutaneous hydatid cyst treatment depends on sonographic cyst type, as defined by Garbhi. The Garbhi classification can be summarized as follows. Type I: pure fluid collection (Fig. 15.6.1A); type II: fluid collection with a split wall; type III: fluid collections with daughter cysts; type IV: heterogeneous echo pattern; and type V: reflecting calcified wall. Type I, type II, and some type III, as well as cysts without biliary communication, are main indications. There are mainly two percutaneous treatment methods. The first is the PAIR technique, as defined by Ben-Amor. The other technique is standard catheterization technique following the PAIR technique. Catheterization technique follows the injection period, with a 6F to 9F pigtail catheter inserted into the cavity for 24-hour free drainage. After 24 hours, a cystogram is obtained and if no communication between the cyst and biliary system is seen, a half volume of absolute alcohol of the initial volume is applied for 20 minutes for the sclerosing effect. The PAIR technique generally is used for cysts smaller than 6 cm; the catheterization technique is used for cysts larger than 6 cm. Major complications of percutaneous hydatid cyst treatment are biliary fistula development (3.2%) and infection of the cavity (1.3%). Minor complications are fever and urticaria (7.8%).

15.7.2 Treatment Of Hydatid Liver Cyst

Case 15.7.2:

A 45-year-old female patient with multiple hepatic cysts and one right renal hydatid cyst presented with nonspecific right upper quadrant pain and hepatomegaly.

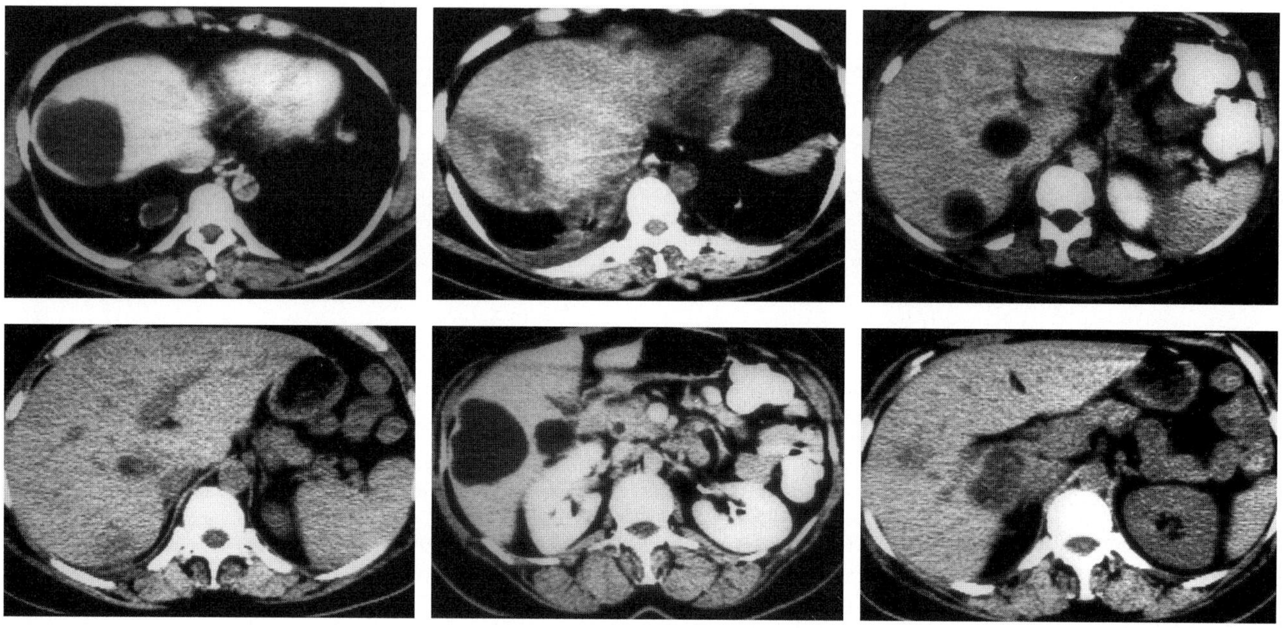

Figure 15.7.2

CT scan shows multiple hepatic hydatid cysts. All cysts were type I. Hepatic cysts (n = 8) were managed by PAIR technique **A:** Hydatid cyst at the dome of the liver. **B:** Same lesion 6 months after treatment. **C,D:** Two lesions in the middle of the liver before **(C)** and after **(D)** treatment. **E,F:** Larger lesion between segments V and VI before **(E)** and after **(F)** treatment. CT scan after treatment shows degenerative changes in the lesions.

Comment: Four different types of treatment for hydatid cyst are used: surgical, medical, endoscopic, and percutaneous. These techniques may be combined. The endoscopic approach has limitations and generally is reserved for biliary hydatid cysts. Medical therapy often is ineffective; response is observed in only 50% of patients treated with mebendazole and 27% of patients treated with albendazole. Surgery and percutaneous therapy were discussed earlier (see p. 399). This patient presented with eight hepatic cysts and one renal type I hydatid cyst. She was hospitalized for only 3 days. The renal hydatid cyst and four of the hepatic cysts were treated within the first day using percutaneous technique. The remaining hepatic cysts were treated percutaneously the following day. Excellent response was observed. There were no immediate or long-term complications.

15.7.3 Treatment Of Hydatid Liver Cyst

Case 15.7.3:

A pregnant woman with hydatid cysts was treated by percutaneous technique.

A 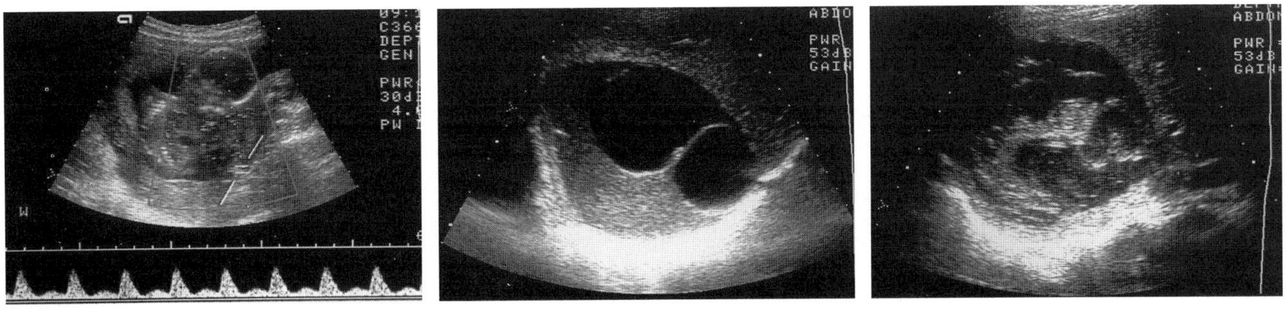 B, C

Figure 15.7.3

A: Obstetric ultrasound shows normal Doppler spectrum of the uterine artery and normal uterine perfusion. **B:** Sonographic examination of the mother's liver, which contained a type III hydatid cyst with daughter hydatid cysts. **C:** Sonographic examination after percutaneous needle treatment with alcohol shows degenerated daughter cysts.

Comment: Pregnancy complicated by hydatid cysts could present with (i) rupture of the hydatid cyst, (ii) mechanical effect of the hydatid cyst upon fetus and fetoplacental circulation; and (iii) obstruction to delivery. The traditional treatment of hydatid cysts in a pregnant woman is surgery; the preferred surgical approach is subtotal cystectomy, with administration of the antihelmintic drug albendazole. Surgery with general anesthesia is a more hazardous treatment for both the mother and the fetus compared with percutaneous treatment. Premature labor may follow successful surgery. This patient had a type III hydatid cyst with daughter cysts and a degenerated matrix. Although the catheterization technique would be more feasible for drainage of matrix, the PAIR technique were chosen because of the greater complexity of the catheterization technique compared with the PAIR technique. All daughter cysts were deactivated, and the cystic cavity was aspirated as soon as possible. Diagnostic microbiologic studies were studied in both preprocedural and postprocedural cyst aspiration. Microbiologic results showed viable hydatid cysts before treatment and nonviable hydatid cysts after treatment. Twenty-three weeks later, the patient had a healthy, 3,050-g baby without any complication.

15.8.1 Percutaneous Treatment Of Gastroenteric Fistulas

Case 15.8.1:

A 65-year-old male patient developed esophageal leak into the abdominal cavity and mediastinum after undergoing a Nissen procedure for gastroesophageal reflux. This was followed by multiple complications, including sepsis and peritonitis, which required multiple surgeries and percutaneous drainage during a 6-month hospital stay. The patient finally improved and was discharged with a large open surgical scar in the abdomen to heal on second intention with granulomatous tissue. The incision closed, but a persistent gastric fistula developed for more than 4 months. Request for a percutaneous solution was made.

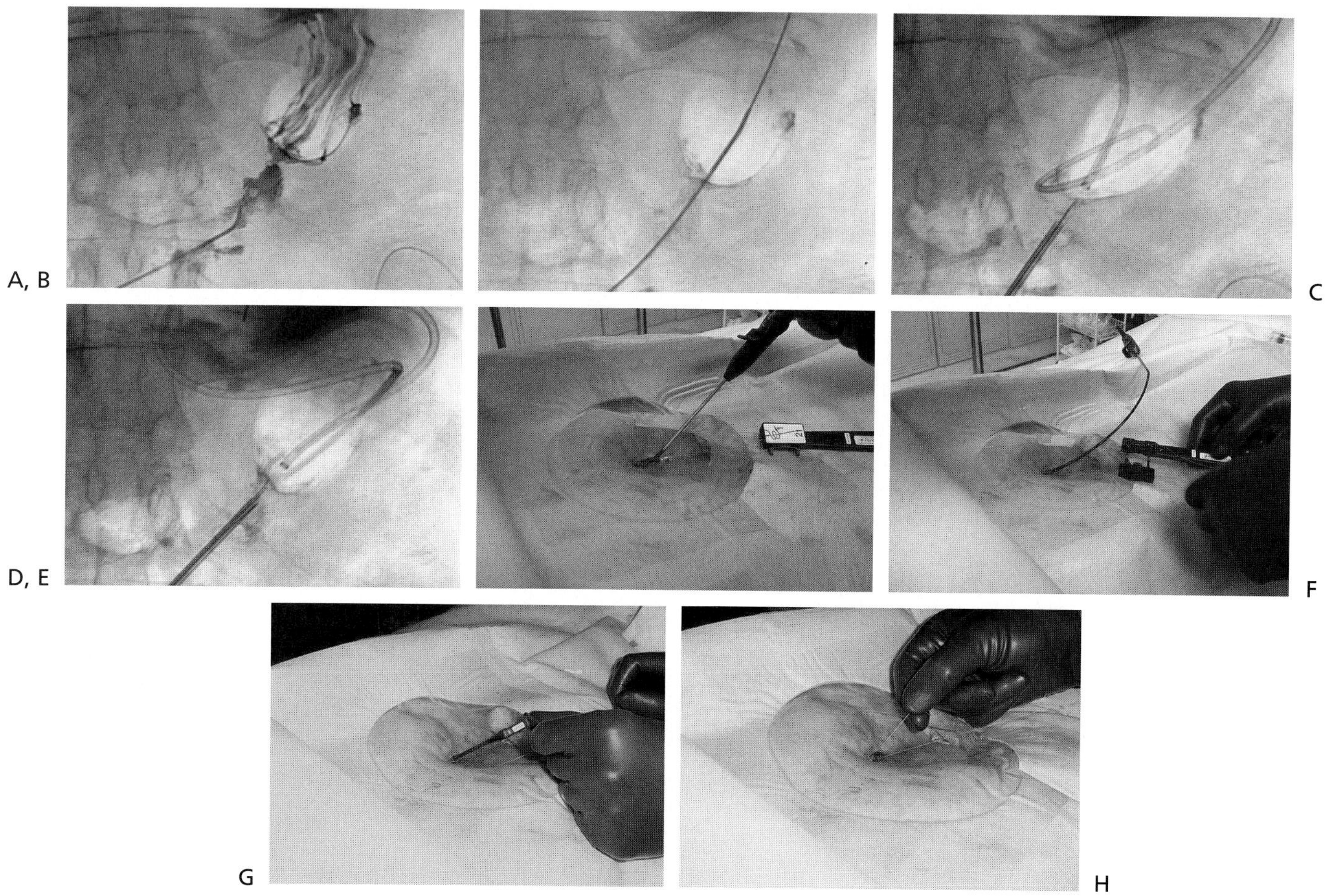

Figure 15.8.1

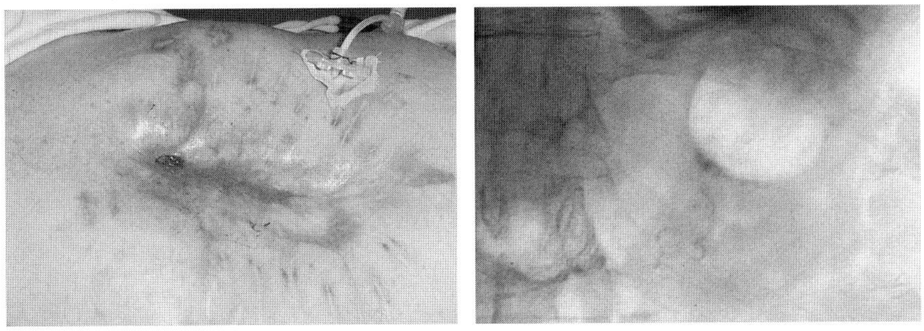

I J

Figure 15.8.1 *(continued)*

A: Retrograde injection of contrast within the fistulous tract using a KMP catheter shows a larger sinus, with an area of stenosis at the level of the gastric wall. **B:** Catheterization of the stomach was done over the wire. **C:** The Perclose device was introduced over the wire into the fistulous tract and the stomach. **D:** The needles were deployed. Note the metal needles when the foot of the device is open (not visible). **E:** The device is withdrawn and the sutures are pulled out. **F:** The Perclose device was further removed, and the (clincher) tying device was used to create the knot. **G:** The knot was slid in using the pusher. **H:** The knot was locked in place and cut. **I:** Final aspect of the fistula after suture. Note the jejunostomy catheter. **J:** Final photograph shows the stomach is full of air and contains a small amount of residual contrast. The fistula is closed at a six-month follow-up.

Comment: Suture-mediated closure devices have been available for about 10 years in Europe, but just recently have been approved for femoral artery puncture closure following percutaneous interventions, especially in patients given heparin or ReoPro and who have large access sheaths. The suture-mediated devices have potential applications in other vascular and nonvascular areas. Gastroenteric fistulas usually are chronic problems related to complicated surgeries on the gastrointestinal tract, which are left to drain until spontaneous resolution occurs. Application of a suture device, preferably at the level of the gastrointestinal wall, presents an attractive use of the device. It is possible to apply a suture to some of the fistulas using the currently available Perclose device; however, the span of the needles used for tissue capturing is not wide enough for some patients. The Perclose device can and should be improved with a longer foot, carrying the suture cups, matching wider-spread needles. There is a good chance of fistula closure if the pressure inside the hollow viscus is not too elevated. Cyanoacrylate glue can be used as an adjunct to the suture to seal the tract.

Suggested Readings

Drainage In The Chest

Aabakken L, Chittom P, McKay DC, et al. Percutaneous drainage of a mediastinal pancreatic pseudocyst: a paraspinal, extrapleural CT-guided approach. *J Vasc Interv Radiol* 1997;8:283–285.

Erasmus JJ, McAdams HP, Rossi S, et al. Percutaneous management of intrapulmonary air and fluid collections. *Radiol Clin North Am* 2000;38:385–393.

Moulton JS. Image-guided management of complicated pleural fluid collections. *Radiol Clin North Am* 2000;38:345–374.

Mwandumba HC, Beeching NJ. Pyogenic lung infections: factors for predicting clinical outcome of lung abscess and thoracic empyema. *Curr Opin Pulm Med* 2000;6:234–239.

Patankar T, Prasad S, Maniyar A, et al. Percutaneous drainage of mediastinal abscess following oesophageal perforation. *J Assoc Physicians India* 1999;47:742.

Patz EF, Goodman PC, Erasmus JJ. Percutaneous drainage of pleural collections. *J Thorac Imaging* 1998;13:83–92.

Putnam JB, Light RW, Rodriguez RM, et al. A randomized comparison of indwelling pleural catheter and doxycycline pleurodesis in the management of malignant pleural effusions. *Cancer* 1999;86:1992–1999.

van Sonnenberg E, Wittich GR, Goodacre BW, et al. Percutaneous abscess drainage: update. *World J Surg* 2001;25:362–372.

van Sonnenberg E, Wittich GR, Goodacre BW, et al. Percutaneous drainage of thoracic collections. *J Thorac Imaging* 1998;13:74–82.

White CS, Meyer CA, Templeton PA. CT fluoroscopy for thoracic interventional procedures. *Radiol Clin North Am* 2000;38:303–322.

Drainage In The Peritoneal Cavity

Barozzi L, Pavlica P, Menchi I, et al. Prostatic abscess: diagnosis and treatment. *AJR* 1998;170:753–757.

Butch RJ, Mueller PR, Ferrucci JT, et al. Drainage of pelvic abscesses through the greater sciatic foramen. *Radiology* 1986;158:487–491.

Catalano OA, Hahn PF, Hooper DC, et al. Efficacy of percutaneous abscess drainage in patients with vancomycin-resistant enterococci. *AJR* 2000;175:533–536.

Collado A, Palou J, Garcia-Penit J, et al. Ultrasound-guided needle aspiration in prostatic abscess. *Urology* 1999;53:548–552.

Fisher ME, Nisenbaum HL, Axel L, et al. Prostatic abscess due to Aspergillus fumigatus: TRUS and MR imaging finding. *J Ultrasound Med* 1998;17:181–184.

Fishman SJ, Pelosi L, Klavon SL, et al. Perforated appendicitis: prospective outcome analysis for 150 children. *J Pediatr Surg* 2000;35:923–926.

Galbis Sanjuan F, Jimenez Cidre M, Rodriguez Rodriguez R, et al. Tuberculous prostatic abscess in acquired immunodeficiency syndrome. *Arch Esp Urol* 1997;50:393–395.

Gan E. Transrectal ultrasound-guided needle aspiration for prostatic abscesses: an alternative to transurethral drainage? *Tech Urol* 2000;6:178–184.

Gervais DA, Hahn PF, O'Neill MJ, et al. CT-guided transgluteal drainage of deep pelvic abscesses in children: selective use as an alternative to transrectal drainage. *AJR* 2000;175:1393–1396.

Gerzof SG, Robbins AH, Johnson WC, et al. Percutaneous catheter drainage of abdominal abscesses: a five-year experience. *N Engl J Med* 1981;305:653–657.

Gerzof SG. Surgical and computerized tomography guided drainage for intraabdominal abscess. *Am J Surg* 1984;147:426–428.

Gonçalves LF, Rojas MV, Vitorello D, et al. Klippel-Trenaunay-Weber syndrome presenting as massive lymphangiohemangioma of the thigh: prenatal diagnosis. *Ultrasound Obstet Gynecol* 2000:15:537–541.

Haaga JR, Nakamoto D, Stellato T, et al. Intracavitary urokinase for enhancement of percutaneous abscess drainage: phase II trial. *AJR* 2000;174:1681–1685.

Huang JJ, Ruaan MK, Lan RR, et al. Acute pyogenic iliopsoas abscess in Taiwan: clinical features, diagnosis, treatments and outcome. *J Infect* 2000;40:248–255.

Jamieson DH, Chait PG, Filler R. Interventional drainage of appendiceal abscesses in children. *AJR* 1997;169:1619–1622.

Ketai L, Washington T, Allen T, et al. Is the stat Gram stain helpful during percutaneous image-guided fluid drainage? *Acad Radiol* 2000;7:228–231.

Kim BS, Sbar AD, Jatoi I. Intra-abdominal cystic lymphangioma. *Surgery* 2000;128:834–835.

Lanzieri CF, Hilar SK. Computed tomography of the sacral plexus and sciatic nerve in the greater sciatic foramen. *AJR* 1984;143:165–168.

Lim JW, Ko YT, Lee DH, et al. Treatment of prostatic abscess: value of transrectal ultrasonographically guided needle aspiration. *J Ultrasound Med* 2000;19:609–617.

Lomas DJ, Dixon AK, Thomson HJ, et al. CT-guided drainage of pelvic abscesses: the peranal transrectal approach. *Clin Radiol* 1992;45:246–249.

Ludwig M, Schoeder-Printzen I, Schiefer HG, et al. Diagnosis and therapeutic management of 18 patients with prostatic abscess. *Urology* 1999;53:340–345.

Luzzatto C, Midrio P, Tchaprassian Z, et al. Sclerosing treatment of lymphangiomas with OK-432. *Arch Dis Child* 2000;82:316–318.

Malden ES, Picus D. Hemorrhagic complication of transgluteal pelvic abscess drainage: successful percutaneous treatment. *J Vasc Interv Radiol* 1992;3:323–328.

Mueller PR, Saini S, Wittenburg J, et al. Sigmoid diverticular abscesses: percutaneous drainage as an adjunct to surgical resection in 24 cases. *Radiology* 1987;164:321–325.

Mueller PR, Simeone JF, Butch RJ, et al. Percutaneous drainage of subphrenic abscess: a review of 62 patients. *AJR* 1986;147:1237–1240.

Mueller PR, van Sonnenberg E, Ferrucci JT. Percutaneous drainage of 250 abdominal abscesses and fluid collections. *Radiology* 1984;151:343–347.

Schwartz DA, Visvesvara G, Weber R, et al. Male genital tract microsporidiosis and AIDS: prostatic abscess due to encephalitozoon hellem. *J Eukaryot Microbiol* 1994;41:61S.

Shah RD, Nardi PM, Han CC. Histoplasma prostatic abscess: rare cause in an immunocompromised patient. *AJR* 1996;166:471.

Stein M, Hsu RK, Schneider PD, et al. Alcohol ablation of a mesenteric lymphangioma. *J Vasc Interv Radiol* 2000;11:247–250.

Trambert JJ. Percutaneous interventions in the presacral space: CT-guided precoccygeal approach—early experience. *Radiology* 1999;213:901–904.

Yip SK, Cheng C, Wong MY, et al. Cryptococcal prostatic abscess in an immunocompromised patient: a case report and review of the literature. *Ann Acad Med Singapore* 1998;27:873–876.

Drainage Of Pancreatic Diseases

Adams DB, Srinivasan A. Failure of percutaneous catheter drainage of pancreatic pseudocyst. *Ann Surg* 2000;66:256–261.

Baril NB, Ralls PW, Wren SM, et al. Does an infected peripancreatic fluid collection or abscess mandate operation? *Ann Surg* 2000;231:361–367.

Dixon GD. Nitinol snare for removal of abscess debris. *J Vasc Interv Radiol* 1994;5:647–648.

Echenique AM, Sleeman D, Yrizarry J, et al. Percutaneous catheter-directed debridement of infected pancreatic necrosis: results in 20 patients. *J Vasc Interv Radiol* 1998;9:565–571.

Fotoohi M, D'Agostino HB, Wollman B, et al. Persistent pancreatocutaneous fistula after percutaneous drainage of pancreatic fluid collections: role of cause and severity of pancreatitis. *Radiology* 1999;213;573–578.

Freeny PC, Hauptmann E, Althaus SJ, et al. Percutaneous CT-guided catheter drainage of infected acute necrotizing pancreatitis: techniques and results. *AJR* 170;1998:969–975.

Heider R, Meyer AA, Galanko JA, et al. Percutaneous drainage of pancreatic pseudocysts is associated with a higher failure rate than surgical treatment in unselected patients. *Ann Surg* 1999;229:781–787.

Lee MJ, Wittich GR, Mueller PR. Percutaneous intervention in acute pancreatitis. *Radiographics* 1998;18:711–724.

Malecka-Panas E, Juszynski A, Chrzastek J, et al. Pancreatic fluid collections: diagnostic and therapeutic implications of percutaneous drainage guided by ultrasound. *Hepatogastroenterology* 1998;45:873–878.

Maringhini A, Uomo G, Patti R, et al. Pseudocyst in acute nonalcoholic pancreatitis: incidence and natural history. *Dig Dis Sci* 1999;44:1669–1973.

Migaleddu V, Strusi G, Fais G, et al. Percutaneous drainage with vacuum aspiration of pancreatic pseudocysts. *Eur Radiol* 1995;5:501–503.

Mosca F. The percutaneous drainage of pancreatic pseudocysts. *Ann Ital Chir* 1999;70:173–176.

Pitchumoni CS, Agarwal N. Pancreatic pseudocysts. When and how should drainage be performed. *Gastroenterol Clin North Am* 1999;28:615–639.

Rothlin MA, Schob O, Klotz H, et al. Percutaneous drainage of abdominal abscesses: are large-bore catheters necessary. *Eur J Surg* 1998;164:419–424.

Shonnard KM, McCarter DL, Lyon RD. Percutaneous debridement of infected pancreatic necrosis with nitinol snares. *J Vasc Interv Radiol* 1997;8:279–282.

Tsiotos GG, Sarr MG. Management of fluid collections and necrosis in acute pancreatitis. *Curr Gastroenterol Rep* 1999;1:139–144.

Tunnemann J, Easterbrook JR, Firth J, et al. Management of acute pancreatitis: a comparative audit of clinical practice against the recommendations of the British Society of Gastroenterology. *Br J Surg* 2000;87:362–373.

Usatoff V, Brancatisano R, Williamson RC. Operative treatment of pseudocysts in patients with chronic pancreatitis. *Br J Surg* 2000;87:1494–1499.

Drainage Of Liver Collections

Abdelouafi A, Ousehal A, Adil A, et al. Percutaneous treatment of liver abscess. Apropos of 34 cases. *J Radiol* 1993;74:341–346.

Al-Mezem SS, Al-jahdali HH. Chronic cough due to broncho biliary fistula. *Respiration* 1999;66:473–476.

Barrio J, Cosme A, Ojeda E, et al. Pyogenic liver abscesses of bacterial origin. A study of 45 cases. *Rev Esp Enferm Dig* 2000;92:232–239.

Berger H, Pratschke E, Berr F, et al. Percutaneous drainage treatment of primary liver abscesses. *RoFo* 1989;150:167–170.

Bertel CK, van Heerden JA, Sheedy PF. Treatment of pyogenic hepatic abscesses. Surgical vs percutaneous drainage. *Arch Surg* 1986;121:554–558.

Chan AD, Gerscovich EO. Imaging of subcapsular hepatic and renal hematomas in pregnancy complicated by preeclampsia and the HELLP syndrome. *J Clin Ultrasound* 1999;27:35–40.

Chua HK, Allen MS, Deschamps C, et al. Bronchobiliary fistula: principles of management. *Ann Thorac Surg* 2000;70:1392–1394.

Corredoira Sanchez JC, Casariego Vales E, Ibanez Alonso MD, et al. Pyogenic liver abscess: changes in etiology, diagnosis and treatment over 18 years. *Rev Clin Esp* 1999;199:705–710.

D'Albuquerque LA, Uflacker R, Genzini T, et al. Pyogenic liver abscesses: analysis of 36 cases treated by percutaneous drainage. *Rev Assoc Med Bras* 1993;39:12–16.

D'Altorio RA, McAllister JD, Sestric GB, et al. Hepatopulmonary fistula: treatment with biliary metallic endoprosthesis. *Am J Gastroenterol* 1992;87:784–786.

Dondelinger RF, Kurdziel JC, Gathy C. Percutaneous treatment of liver abscess: a critical analysis of results. *Cardiovasc Intervent Radiol* 1990;13:174–182.

Eck BD, Passinault WJ. Bronchobiliary fistula. A rare complication of chronic pancreatitis. *Int J Pancreatol* 1966;20:213–216.

Greenwood LH, Collins TL, Yrizarry JM. Percutaneous management of multiple liver abscesses. *AJR* 1982;139:390–392.

Gugenheim J, Ciardullo M, Traynor O, et al. Bronchobiliary fistulas in adults. *Ann Surg* 1988.207:90–94.

Herold G, Danz B. Endoscopic (-ERC) fibrin sealing and histoacryl sealing of an abscess induced bilio-hepatico-cutaneous and a bilio-hepatico-phrenico-bronchial fistulous system. *Z Gastroenterol* 1995;33:605–609.

Herrera-Llerandi R. Management of hepatic abscesses. *World J Surg* 1999;23:1316.

Khandelwal M, Inverso N, Conter R, et al. Endoscopic management of a bronchobiliary fistula. *J Clin Gastroenterol* 1996;23:11125–11127.

Kim W, Clark TW, Baum RA, et al. Risk factors for liver abscess formation after hepatic chemoembolization. *J Vasc Interv Radiol* 2001;12:965–968.

Levy PJ, Tabares AH, Olin JW, et al. Disseminated intravascular coagulation associated with acute ischemic hepatitis after elective aortic aneurysm repair: comparative analysis of 10 cases. *J Cardiothorac Vasc Anesth* 1997;11:141–148.

Memis A, Oran I, Parildar M. Use of histoacryl and a covered nitinol stent to treat a bronchobiliary fistula. *J Vasc Interv Radiol* 2000;11:1337–1340.

Oettl C, Schima W, Metz-Schimmerl S, et al. Bronchobiliary fistula after hemihepatectomy: cholangiopancreaticography, computed tomography and magnetic resonance cholangiography findings. *Eur J Radiol 1999;* 32:211–215.

Ogawa T, Shimizu S, Morisaki T, et al. The role of percutaneous transhepatic abscess drainage for liver abscess. *J Hepatobiliary Pancreat Surg* 1999;6:263–266.

Schwartz ML, Coyle MJ, Aldrete JS, et al. Bronchobiliary fistula: complete percutaneous treatment with biliary drainage and stricture dilation. *Radiology* 1988;168:751–752.

Scola M, Brophy M, Fiore L. Localized consumptive coagulopathy. *Circulation* 2001;104:120–121.

Unceta PR, Rodrigues MAM, Aguilar FC, et al. Hepatic abscesses: is simple aspiration puncture with echography control an alternative to catheter drainage? *Gastroenterol Hepatol* 2000;23:470–473.

van Sonnenberg E, Wittich GR, Goodacre BW, et al. Percutaneous abscess drainage: update. *World J Surg* 2001;25:362–372.

Zenda T, Kaizaki C, Sato H, et al. Irrigation of liver abscess: proposal of a novel method and possible indications. *Hepatogastroenterology* 2002;48:847–850.

Drainage In Splenic Collections

Al-Salem AH, Qaisaruddin S, Al Jam'a A, et al. Splenic abscess and sickle cell disease. *Am J Hematol* 1998;58:100–104.

Blondel C, Liard A, Bachy B, et al. US-guided percutaneous drainage of an infected epidermoid cyst of the spleen in a child. *J Radiol* 1999;80:1560–1571.

Chou YH, Tiu CM, Chiou HJ, et al. Ultrasound-guided interventional procedures in splenic abscesses. *Eur J Radiol* 1998;28:167–170.

De Bree E, Tsifitis D, Christodoulakis M, et al. Splenic abscess: a diagnostic and therapeutic challenge. *Acta Chir Belg* 1998;98:199–202.

Duggal RK, Ramachandran KA. Splenic abscess as a complication of acute pancreatitis. *J Assoc Physicians India* 1999;47:338–339.

Garduno E, Rebollo M, Asencio MA, et al. Splenic abscesses caused by Actinomyces meyeri in a patient with autoimmune hepatitis. *Diagn Microbiol Infect Dis* 2000;37:213–214.

Lebrato JC, Martinez AJL, Mas JS, et al. Splenic abscess: a case report and review of the literature. *Ann Med Intern* 1999;16:31–34.

Mrad AA, Marc SO, Bercault N, et al. Splenic abscess. A rare pathology requiring a multidisciplinary approach. *J Med Liban* 2000;48:29–33.

Murray AW, Macgregor AB. A case of multiple splenic abscesses managed non-operatively. *J R Coll Surg Edinb* 2000;45:189–191.

Nakao A, Iwagaki H, Isozaki H, et al. Portal venous gas associated with splenic abscess secondary to colon cancer. *Anticancer Res* 1999;19;5641–5644.

Salzano A, Rossi E, De Rosa A, et al. The role of computed tomography in assessing subphrenic abscesses after posttraumatic splenectomy. *Radiol Med* 1999;98:173–177.

Schaberle W, Eisele R. Percutaneous ultrasound controlled drainage of large splenic abscesses. *Chirurg* 1997;68:744–748.

Treatment Of Hydatid Renal Cysts

Akhan O, Ustunsoz B, Somuncu I, et al. Percutaneous renal hydatid cyst treatment: long-term results. *Abdom Imaging* 1998;23:209–213.

Benchekroun A, Lachkar A, Soumana A, et al. Hydatid cyst of the kidney. Report of 45 cases. *Ann Urol* 1999;33:19–24.

el Khader K, Koutani A, el Mamoun M, et al. Endoscopic percutaneous drainage of a renal echinococcal cyst during percutaneous nephrolithotomy. *Acta Urol Belg* 1998;66:43–46.

Horchani A, Nouira Y, Kbaier I, et al. Hydatid cyst of the kidney. A report of 147 controlled cases. *Eur Urol* 2000;38:461–467.

Zmerli S, Ayed M, Horchani A, et al. Hydatid cyst of the kidney: diagnosis and treatment. *World J Surg* 2001;25:68–74.

Treatment Of Hydatid Liver Cysts

Akhan O, Ozmen MN, Dinçer A, et al. Liver hydatid disease: long-term results of percutaneous treatment. *Radiology* 1996;198:259–264.

Al Karawi MA, Mohamed ARE, Yasawy MI. Advances in diagnosis and management of hydatid disease. *Hepatogastroenterology* 1990;37:327–331.

Belli L, del Favero E, Marni A, et al. Resection versus pericystectomy in the treatment of hydatidosis of the liver. *Am J Surg* 1983;145:239–242.

Ben Amor N, Gargouri M, Gharbi HA, et al. Traitment du kyste hydatique du foie du mouton par ponction sous echographie. *Tunis Med* 1986;64:325–331.

Bilge A, Sozuer EM. Diagnosis and surgical treatment of hydatid disease. *Surgery* 1994;8:77–81.

Filice C, Di Perri G, Strosselli M, et al. Parasitologic findings in percutaneous drainage of human hydatid liver cysts. *J Infect Dis* 1990;161:1290–1295.

Gargouri M, Ben Amor N, Chehida FB, et al. Percutaneous treatment of hydatid cysts. *Cardiovasc Intervent Radiol* 1990;13:169–173.

Gharbi HA, Hassine W, Brauner MW, et al. Ultrasound examination of the hydatid liver. *Radiology* 1981;139:459–463.

Kain KC, Keystone JS. Recurrent hydatid disease during pregnancy. *Am J Obstet Gynecol* 1988;159:1216–1217.

Khuroo MS, Zargar SA, Mahajan R. Echinococcus granulosus cysts of the liver: management with percutaneous drainage. *Radiology* 1991;180:141–145.

Mottaghian H, Saidi F. Postoperative recurrence of hydatid disease. *Br J Surg* 1978;65:237–242.

Mueller PR, Dawson SL, Ferruci JT, et al. Hepatic echinococcal cyst: successful percutaneous drainage. *Radiology* 1985;155:627–628.

Rahman MS, Rahman J, Lysikiewicz A. Obstetric and gynecological presentations of hydatid disease. *Br J Obstet Gynaecol* 1982;89:665–670.

Ulualp DM, Aydemir I, Senturk H, et al. Management of intrabiliary rupture of hydatid cyst of the liver. *World J Surg* 1996;19:720–724.

Percutaneous Treatment Of Gastroenteric Fistulas

Chamberlin JR, Lardi AB, McKeever LS, et al. Use of vascular sealing devices (VasoSeal and Perclose) versus assisted manual compression (FemoStop) in transcatheter coronary interventions requiring abciximab (ReoPro). *Catheter Cardiovasc Interv* 1999;4:143–147.

Duda SH, Wiskirchen J, Erb M, et al. Suture-mediated percutaneous closure of antegrade femoral arterial access sites in patients who have received full anticoagulation therapy. *Radiology* 1999;210:47–52.

Hahn U, Betsch A, Wiskirchen J, et al. A new device for percutaneous suture-mediated closure of arterial puncture sites using exteriorized needles: initial experience. *J Invasive Cardiol* 2001;13:456–459.

Sesana M, Vaghetti M, Albiero R, et al. Effectiveness and complications of vascular access closure devices after interventional procedures. *J Invasive Cardiol* 2000;12:400–401.

CHAPTER 16

Percutaneous Nonvascular Interventions

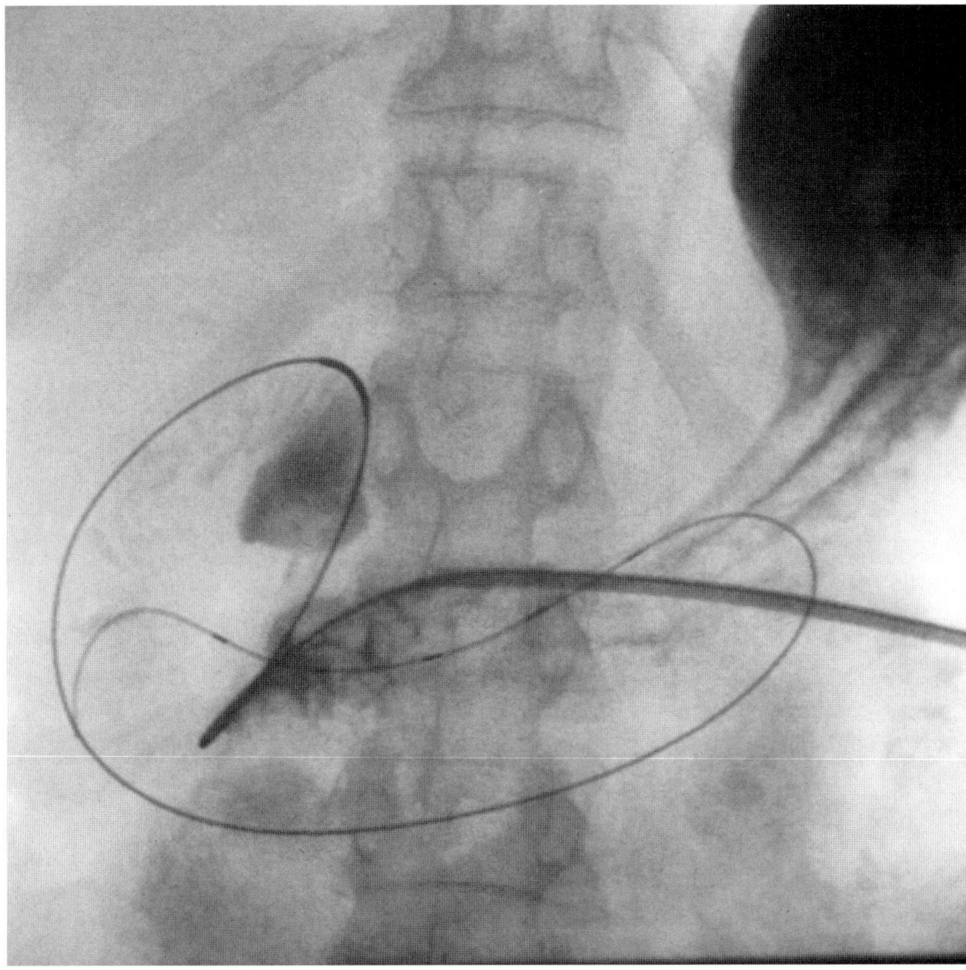

16.1.1 Tracheal Stenting And Bronchial Stenting

Case 16.1.1:

A 65-year-old male patient presented with iatrogenic benign stricture of the trachea following heart surgery that required postoperative prolonged intubation. Severe breathlessness, wheezing, stridor, and recurrent infection developed over a 6-month period. Balloon plasty and stent placement were requested.

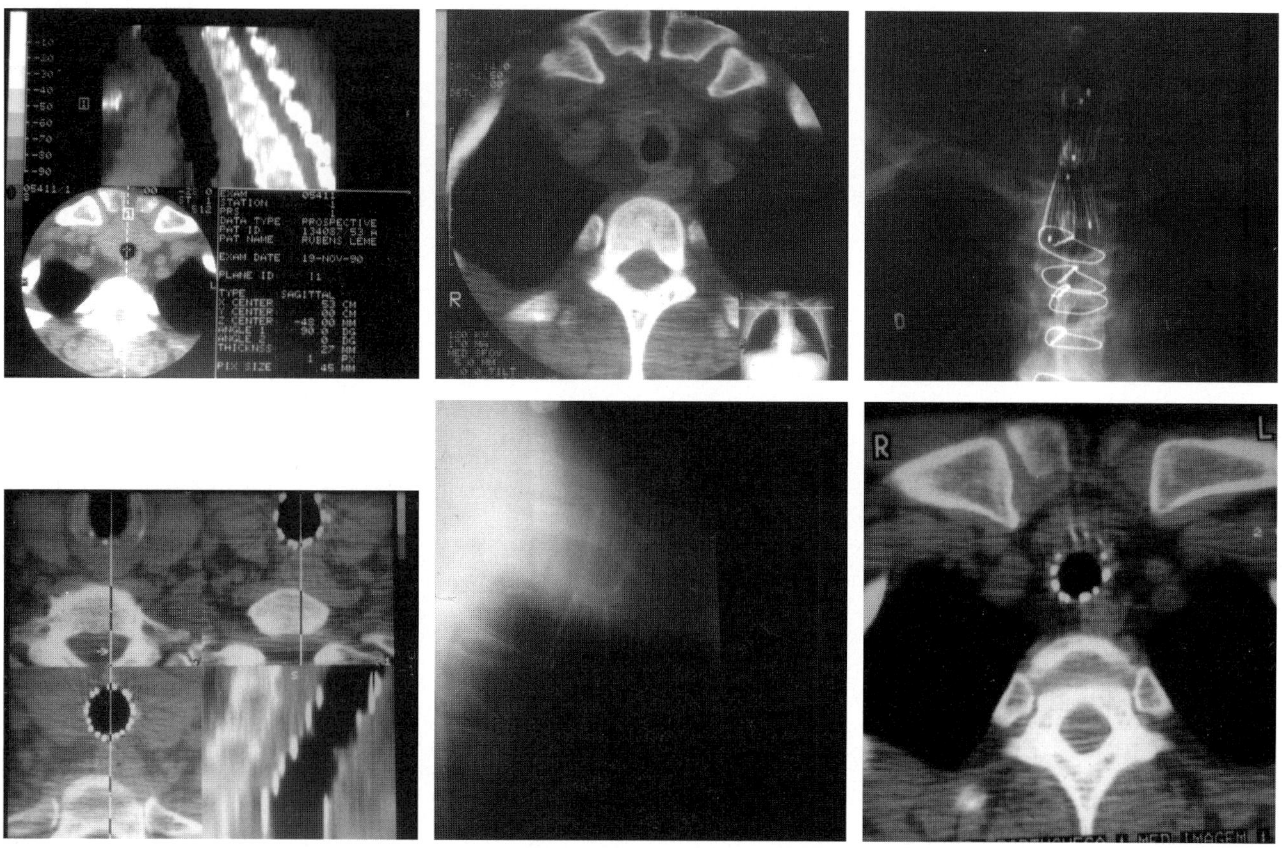

A, B C D, E F

Figure 16.1.1

A: Lateral view of the two-dimensional reconstruction of the computed tomographic (CT) scan of the trachea shows a narrowing. The axial view demonstrates the stricture is more severe than initially thought. **B:** Axial view of the trachea just below the greatest area of stenosis shows thick walls and narrowed lumen. **C:** Balloon plasty was performed (not shown), followed by placement of a large, double-body Z-stent. Axial views and two-dimensional reconstruction CT scan shows patency of the trachea. **D:** Axial view of the CT scan below the main stenosis shows the open stent and a larger lumen. **E,F:** Anteroposterior and lateral radiographs of the neck show the expanded stent with a narrowed segment in the center. At that time, the Z-stent was not connected by sutures but through a metal rod from top to bottom. There was marked clinical improvement, with resolution of the dyspnea and recurrent infections.

Comment: The majority of benign strictures of the trachea are iatrogenic. Multiple complications may derive from the stricture, but the main symptoms are dyspnea and recurrent infections. Short circumscribed strictures are best treated by surgery. Longer and severe strictures are more difficult to manage surgically, and balloon dilation and stenting are adequate alternatives for most of the situations. Balloon or bougie dilation techniques are not effective in providing long-term palliation for those patients. Balloon dilation may have an important role in neonates and infants as a temporizing measure to allow growth of the child until a more definitive procedure can be considered. Balloon dilation should precede stent placement. For many years, the larger Z-stent was the only alternative available. The initial design did not connect adequately the two bodies of the stent; a gap was maintained between the two stents, which were connected by a metal rod. The more recent device is connected by sutures, and the segments are *solidaire* and aligned with each other. More recently, the larger tracheal Wallstents that have become available are more flexible. Potential problems with metal stents placed in the trachea include ingrowth of granulation or tumor tissue through the stent mesh, which leads to recurrent airway obstruction. The stents become incorporated into the wall of the airway within 4 to 6 weeks and are difficult to remove without surgery. Covered stents are now available.

16.1.2 Tracheal Stenting And Bronchial Stenting

Case 16.1.2:

A 32-month-old male child with postpartum cerebral palsy had been intubated for most of his life, due to past severe respiratory difficulties. When not intubated, he developed tracheomalacia and respiratory dysfunction, due to collapse of the tracheal walls. To discharge the patient, a decision was made to use a stent to support the trachea in an attempt to improve respiratory function.

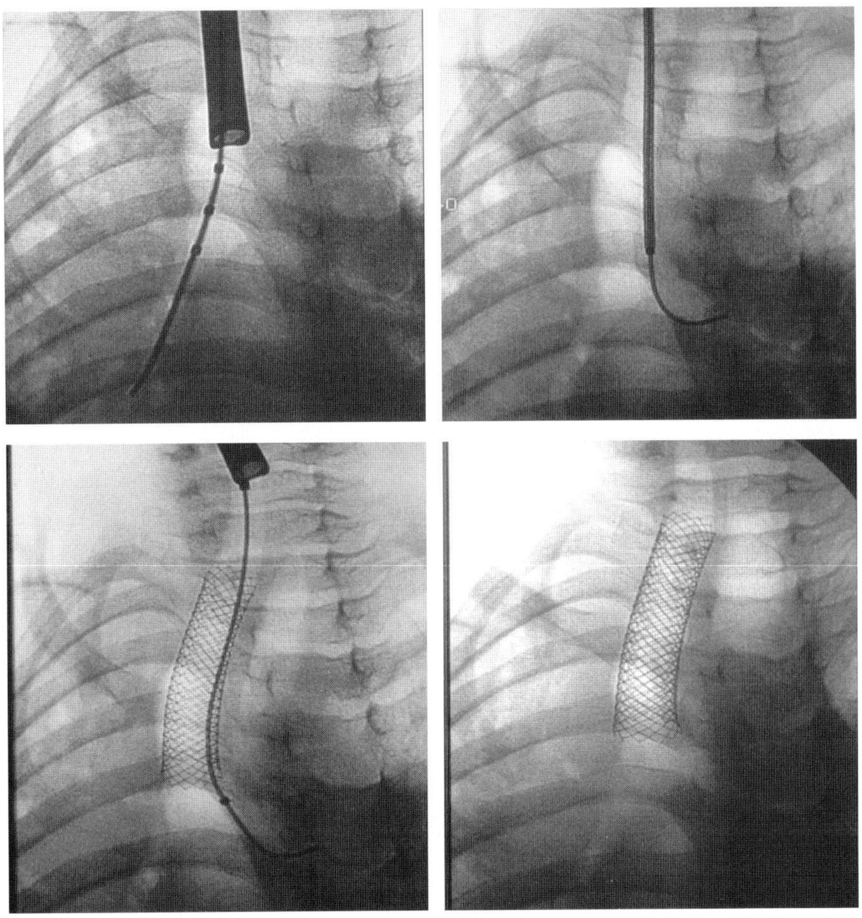

A B C D

Figure 16.1.2

A: Bronchoscopy reveals severe tracheomalacia. Note the irregularity and dilation of the trachea. Through the bronchoscope, a graduated guidewire was introduced into the trachea and right bronchus to obtain measurements. **B:** After measurement, a 10-mm × 40-mm Wallstent was selected and introduced over the wire into the trachea. **C:** The stent was deployed above the carina into the trachea to support the tracheal walls. Note the delivery system is still in place. **D:** Follow-up chest x-ray film shows the stent is fully expanded and is supporting the tracheal walls. There was marked improvement of respiratory function, and the patient was discharged a couple of days after the stenting procedure. Follow-up is now more than 12 months, and the patient is asymptomatic with regard to respiratory status.

Comment: The Wallstent tracheobronchial endoprosthesis is a flexible, self-expanding metal mesh having a cylindrical design. The delivery system is similar to the vascular device; it includes a sleeve that constrains the device and radiopaque markers that show the limits of the stent in the constrained status. There is a considerable foreshortening in length. The final diameter of the stent selected should be larger than the target area of the airway to assure stability of the device within the trachea or bronchus by the radial force of the stent. Although a Wallstent with less radial force than the Z stent is available, the device is fairly effective in keeping bronchial and tracheal stenoses open. In cases of tracheomalacia, the support provided by the device is more to prevent collapse of the tracheal walls than to keep open a stenosis. The flexibility provided by the Wallstent allows precise placement, and the compliance of the walls permits coverage of all irregularities. Granulation tissue growth through the stent mesh occurs in about 20% of patients and can be managed by repeated balloon plasty and/or endoscopic resection. If the stent migrates and covers the orifice of a main stem bronchus or a branch, the wall of the stent can be opened up with laser cautery to improve patency.

16.1.3 Tracheal Stenting And Bronchial Stenting

Case 16.1.3:

A 45-year-old male patient with α_1-antitrypsin–related chronic pulmonary disease required a unilateral right lung transplant. Following the lung transplant, recurrent infection and shortness of breath due to segmentary bronchomalacia in the right main bronchus and bronchus of the right lower lobe were verified by bronchoscopy.

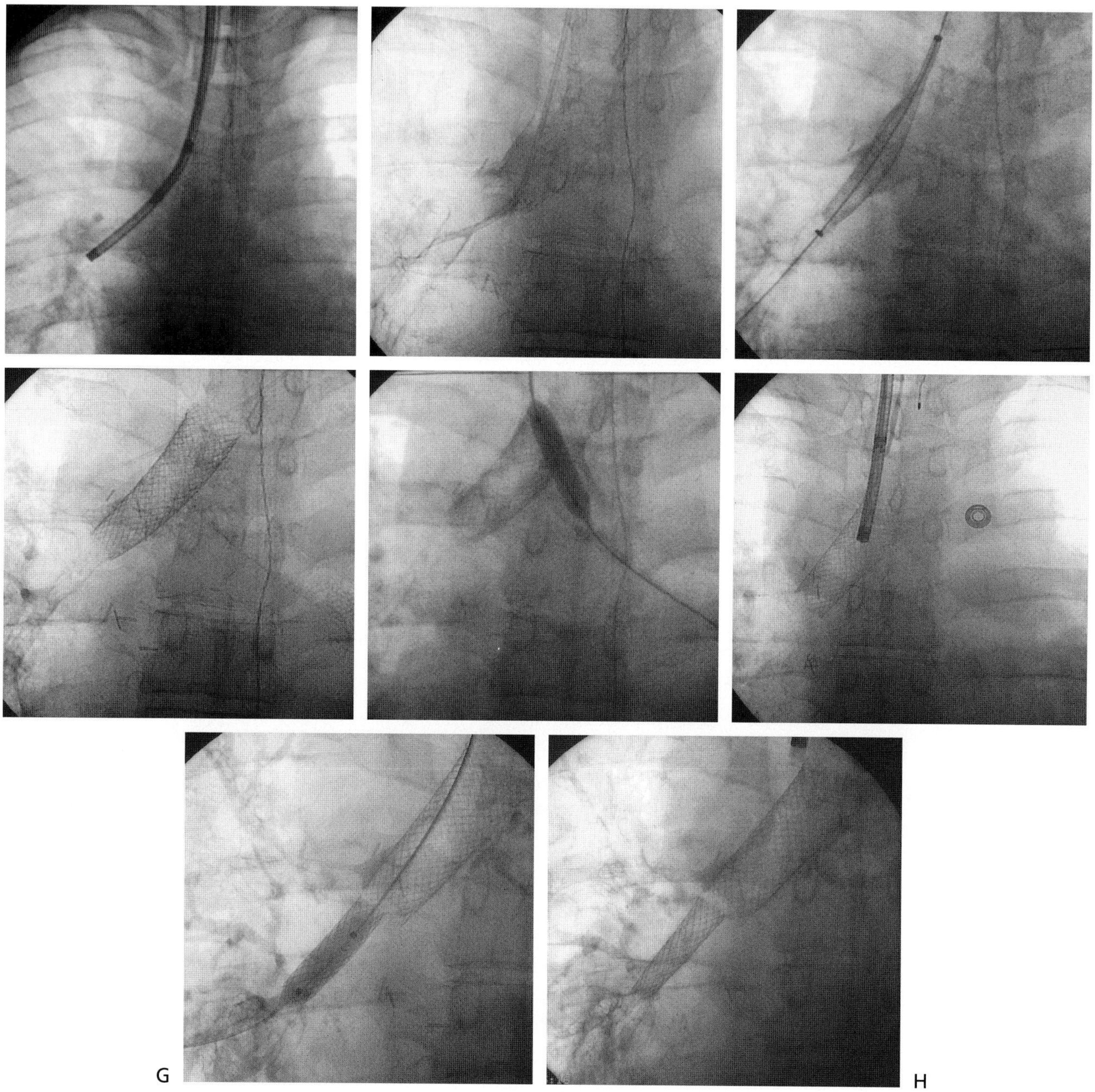

A, B C D, E F G H

Figure 16.1.3

A: With the patient under general anesthesia, bronchoscopy was performed to identify the character of the lesions to be treated. **B:** A guidewire was advanced through the bronchoscope into the right bronchus. A KMP catheter was advanced into the right bronchus for a contrast bronchography, which demonstrated collapse of the right bronchus during inspiration (not shown). **C:** A large 14-mm × 30-mm Wallstent was introduced into the right main bronchus and deployed. **D:** Digital radiography shows the final position of the stent within the right bronchus. The stent extends into the trachea and crosses the orifice of the left bronchus. **E:** The stent segment mesh wall covering the orifice of the left bronchus initially was opened up with an 8-mm balloon, which did not work well. **F:** Catheter laser beam was used to open up the stent wall to reduce the chances of mucus clogging the stent mesh. Note the discontinuity of the stent wall as observed by bronchoscopy. **G:** Several weeks later, the patient still experienced difficulty in expanding the right lower lobe properly. A new procedure was performed to place a Wallstent in the right lower lobe bronchus. Note the stent was already placed beyond the main bronchus stent by dilation with an 8-mm balloon. **H:** Final photograph shows the stents in place and maintaining the lower lobe expanded. The patient experienced severe rejection and other complications, and he died about 6 months after stent treatment.

Comment: Following stent placement, there usually is significant clinical improvement. The overall technical success rate of stent treatment of bronchial strictures and malacias is close to 100%, but clinical success is closer to 80%. Indications for bronchial stenting usually are related to failure to wean from a ventilator or lifestyle-limiting shortness of breath. Although the follow-up reported in the literature is relatively short, up to 3 years, several different problems are known to develop following bronchial stent placement. Growth of granulation tissue is common in up to 20% of the patients and may require repeated treatment. The literature reports a relatively limited survival of this population with bronchial problems requiring stent treatment, but longer survival increases the chances of restenosis.

16.1.4 Tracheal Stenting And Bronchial Stenting

Case 16.1.4:

A 31-year-old female patient with α_1-antitrypsin–related chronic pulmonary disease required a bilateral lung transplant. Following the lung transplants, progressive shortness of breath developed due to segmentary stenosis in the right lower lobe bronchus. Balloon plasty was requested.

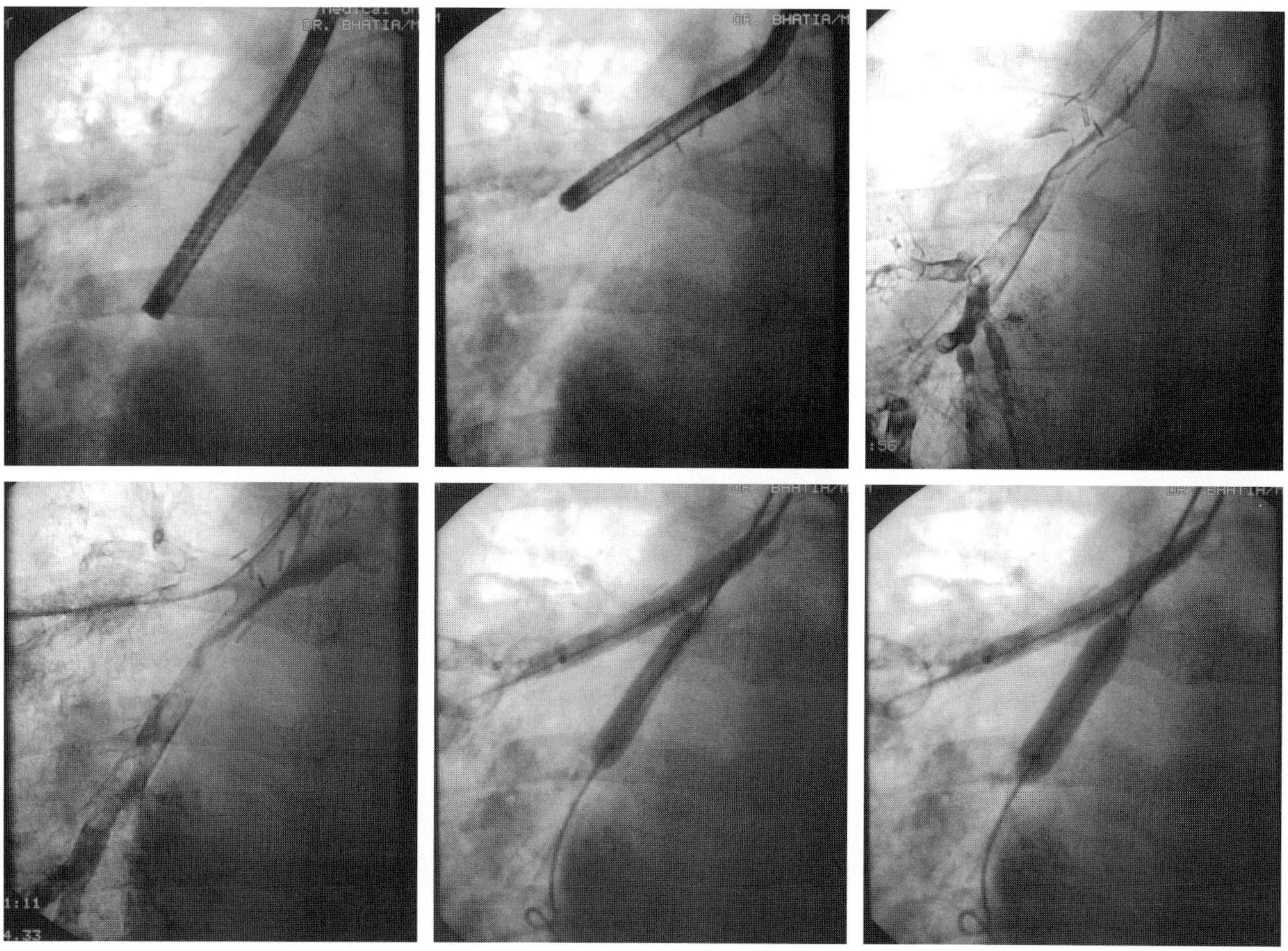

A, B C
D, E F

Figure 16.1.4

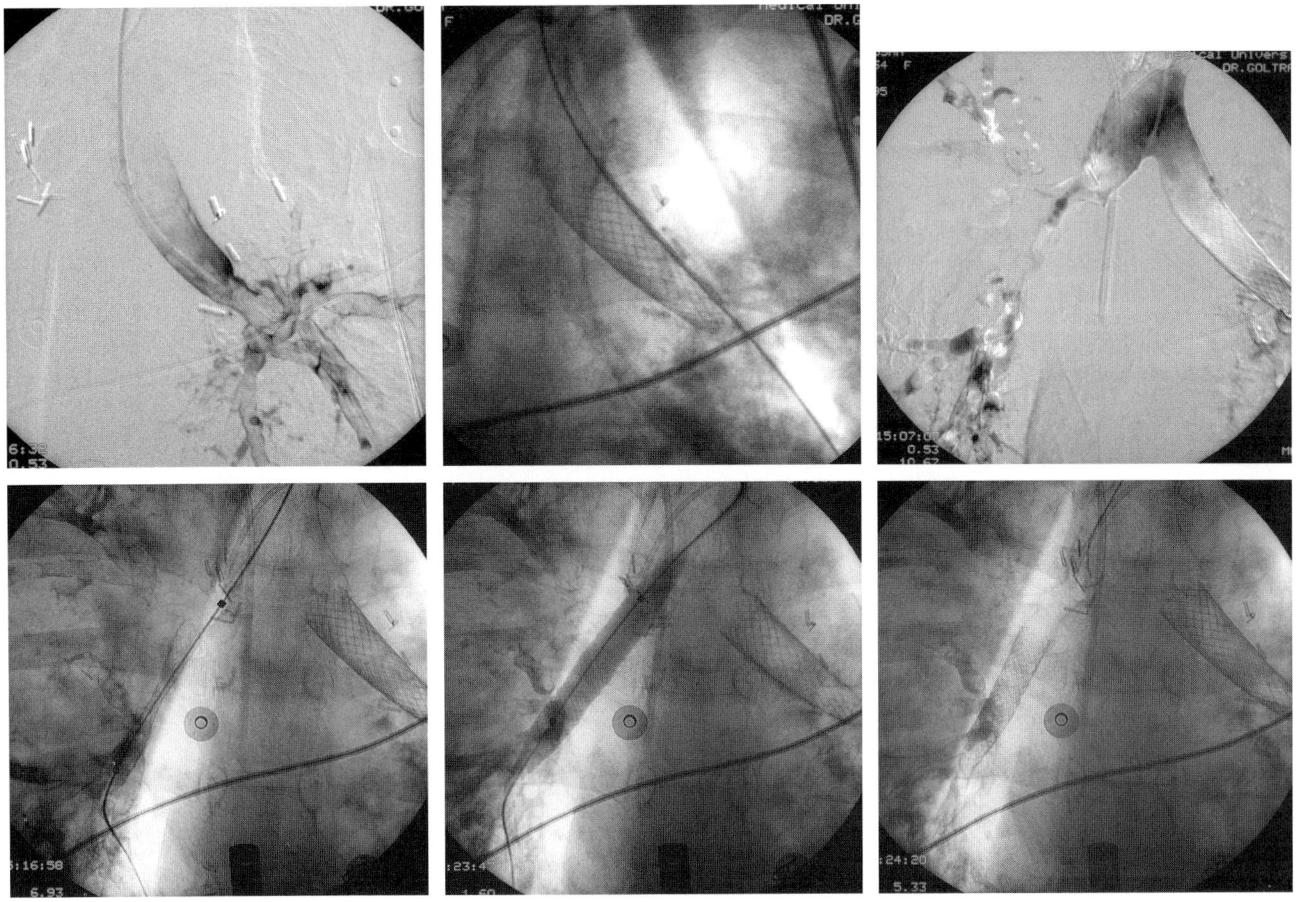

Figure 16.1.4 *(continued)*

A,B: With the patient under general anesthesia, bronchoscopy reveals the presence of stenosis in the right lower lobe bronchus. **C,D:** Bronchogram of the right lower lobe shows severe stenosis of the right lower lobe bronchus segment. **E,F:** Balloon dilation was performed with 10-mm and 7-mm kissing balloons. **G:** About 1 month after balloon dilation, the right bronchial stenosis recurred and a new severe stenosis developed in the left main bronchus. **H:** A 14-mm Wallstent was placed to treat the left bronchial stenosis. **I:** Right bronchography shows severe recurrence of the lesion on the right side. **J:** A 10-mm Wallstent was placed within the stenosis in the right bronchus. **K:** Dilation of the stent was performed with a 10-mm balloon. **L:** Final position of the stents achieved a good clinical result, with improvement in dyspnea.

Comment: Treatment of bronchial stenosis with bare stenting is very challenging, and there is a significant rate of occlusion or restenosis. More recently, silicone-covered Wallstents have become available. The primary indication for use is to treat strictures or obstructions secondary to tumoral lesions or to exclude fistulas. The main limitation of the covered stents is related to occluding side branches of the bronchial tree, which may cause lung collapse and infection. Great care must be exercised to reduce this type of complication. Tumor ingrowth is avoided effectively by the stent cover. As demonstrated in this case, balloon dilation often fails to maintain the bronchus open for a significant period of time. Although stents are effective in keeping the strictures open, there is significant impairment of the mucociliary clearance, leading to accumulation of secretions and even lung collapse, mostly with plastic stents. The metal stents present a significant advantage over the plastic stents due to the lower profile and smaller amount of material in contact with the bronchial wall. Cryotherapy, laser ablation, and balloon plasty are effective in treating tumor ingrowth and mucosal hyperplasia, but they require repeated procedures in some patients. The silicone cover of the new stents inhibits tumor ingrowth but potentially adversely affects the mucociliary function of the bronchial wall.

16.2.1 Percutaneous Gastrostomy

Case 16.2.1:

A 44-year-old male patient with esophageal cancer that extended into the stomach and esophageal obstruction was unable to maintain nutrition with oral intake. He required enteral feeding through a gastrostomy.

A, B C D, E F G, H I

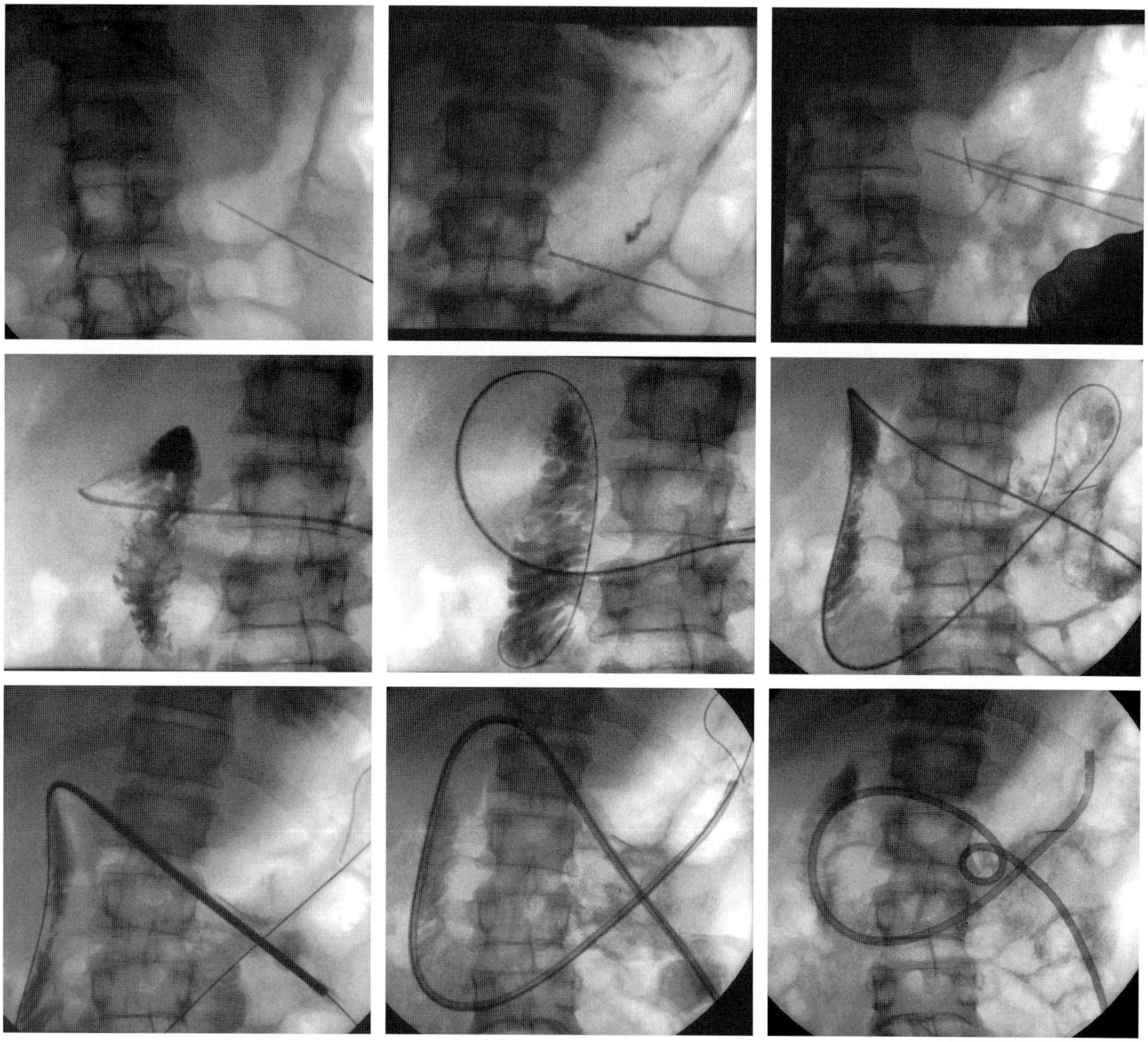

Figure 16.2.1

A: Following oral intake of effervescent pearls, the stomach was slightly distended with gas. After selection of an appropriate puncture site under fluoroscopy, a 15-cm, 19-gauge trocar needle was inserted with the tip angled toward the pylorus. **B:** The stomach was further insufflated with air and a small amount of contrast medium for better demonstration of the pylorus and outline of the stomach rugae. **C:** A single retention suture was introduced into the stomach and then pulled up to bring the anterior stomach against the abdominal wall. A second puncture was made with an 18-gauge needle through the same incision, adjacent to the suture anchor needle, with the retention suture held taut. **D:** A super-stiff guidewire was introduced and the tract dilated. A KMP catheter was advanced into the antrum and pylorus. Contrast injection shows the duodenum. **E:** A Lunderquist guidewire was advanced through the catheter into the duodenum and used to further advance the catheter, thus assuring access to the jejunum. **F:** A super-stiff guidewire was advanced into the proximal jejunum. **G:** Holding the retention suture under gentle traction, progressively larger Teflon dilators were used to enlarge the entrance hole. **H:** A 12F peel-away introducer sheath was placed and a Shetty gastrojejunostomy tube (Cook) with a stiffener was inserted over the wire. Once the tube reached the jejunum, the peel-away sheath was removed. **I:** The catheter sling thread was pulled back and the Cope retention loop formed in the stomach, holding it in place. Initially the catheter was stitched to the skin with a 2–0 silk suture. As the tract becomes established, the suture can be removed.

Comment: Patients who are unable to maintain nutrition with oral intake require either enteral or parenteral feeding. The most common causes are neurologic circumstances that cause the inability to swallow or upper gastrointestinal obstructive malignancy. Because enteral feeding is always preferable, surgical gastrostomy techniques were used, but they have the disadvantages of higher costs and increased morbidity and mortality. More recently, gastrostomy techniques have been developed, including endoscopic procedures, fluoroscopic placement of gastric tubes, and CT fluoroscopy guidance for stomach puncture, which render the surgical technique almost obsolete. Technical success rate ranges from 98% to 100%, and there is a low rate of complications (5% major and 5% minor). Procedure-related mortality is about 1%, mostly because of the type of population treated. Agitated and uncooperative patients are more prone to complications and mortality due to accidental catheter removal and peritonitis. Percutaneous gastrostomy is rather straightforward, inexpensive, and can be accomplished with local anesthesia and mild or no sedation. Percutaneous endoscopic gastrostomy (PEG) is more costly, requires two operators, and usually necessitates heavy intravenous sedation. Mortality and major complication rates attributable to PEG are similar to those of the percutaneous approach; however, there appears to be a higher incidence of wound infection and aspiration due to the heavier sedation and the need for oral access. Placement of the gastrostomy catheter in the stomach cavity may cause esophageal reflux, especially in patients with severe neurologic problems. It appears reasonable to place the tip of the catheter into the jejunum of most patients or to create a gastrojejunostomy. Nowadays, we seldom perform a simple gastrostomy; in most of our patients we place a gastrojejunostomy. Percutaneous gastrostomy and gastrojejunostomy are simple, safe, and cost-effective techniques and should be the preferred choices of treatment for these patients.

16.3.1 Percutaneous Gastroenterostomy

Case 16.3.1:

A 71-year-old male patient with severe neurologic impairment requiring enteral nutrition presented with esophageal reflux several months after undergoing PEG. The patient was referred for conversion to a percutaneous gastroenterostomy.

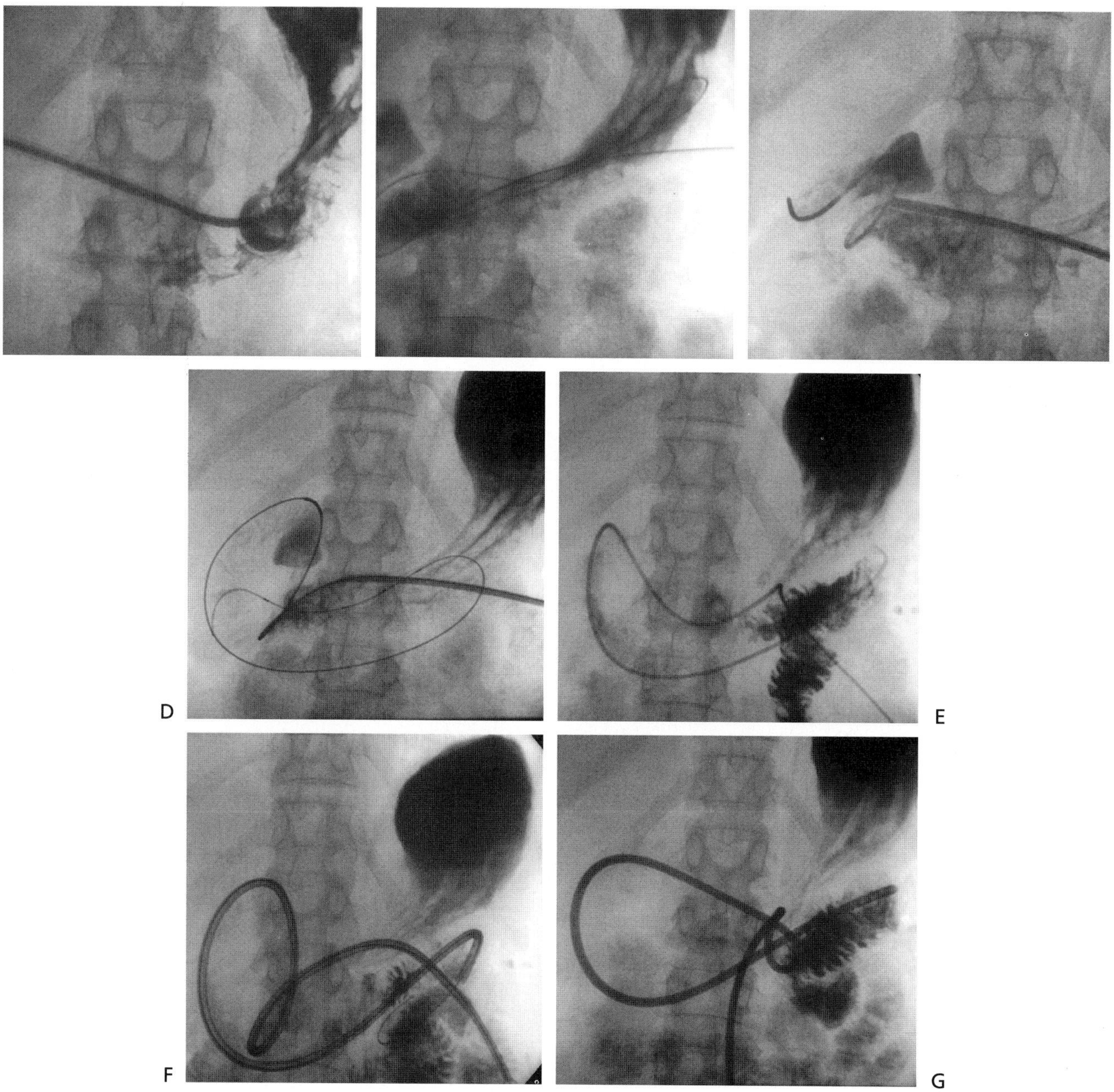

Figure 16.3.1

A: Contrast injection through the PEG catheter shows the retention ring within the stomach cavity. **B:** An extra stiff guidewire was placed within the PEG catheter, and the catheter was pulled out. The guidewire was directed toward the antrum, but it buckled back into the stomach. **C:** A KMP catheter was introduced through the pylorus. **D:** A steerable Lunderquist guidewire was advanced into the duodenum. **E:** The multipurpose catheter was advanced into the jejunum and a super-stiff wire was advanced. **F:** The Shetty gastrojejunostomy was introduced through a pell-away sheath up to the proximal jejunum. **G:** The Cope retention loop was formed inside the stomach. Note how far the tip of the catheter was introduced into the jejunum.

Comment: Most patients who require gastrojejunostomy are elderly or have severe disabilities. The more frequent indications are stroke-related neurologic conditions that cause dysphagia, malignancies, a number of chronic neurologic/psychiatric disorders (multiple sclerosis, senile dementia, Alzheimer disease, and Parkinson disease), severe burns, chronic pancreatitis, Crohn disease, and bowel decompression.

16.3.2 Percutaneous Gastroenterostomy

Case 16.3.2:

A 24-year-old female patient presented with multiple problems, which included surgically treated congenital heart disease and esophageal atresia that was treated by colonic interposition, food aspiration, gastroesophageal reflux, and a poorly functioning surgical gastrostomy that had been removed. Due to difficulties in feeding and weight loss, percutaneous placement of a gastroenterostomy tube was requested.

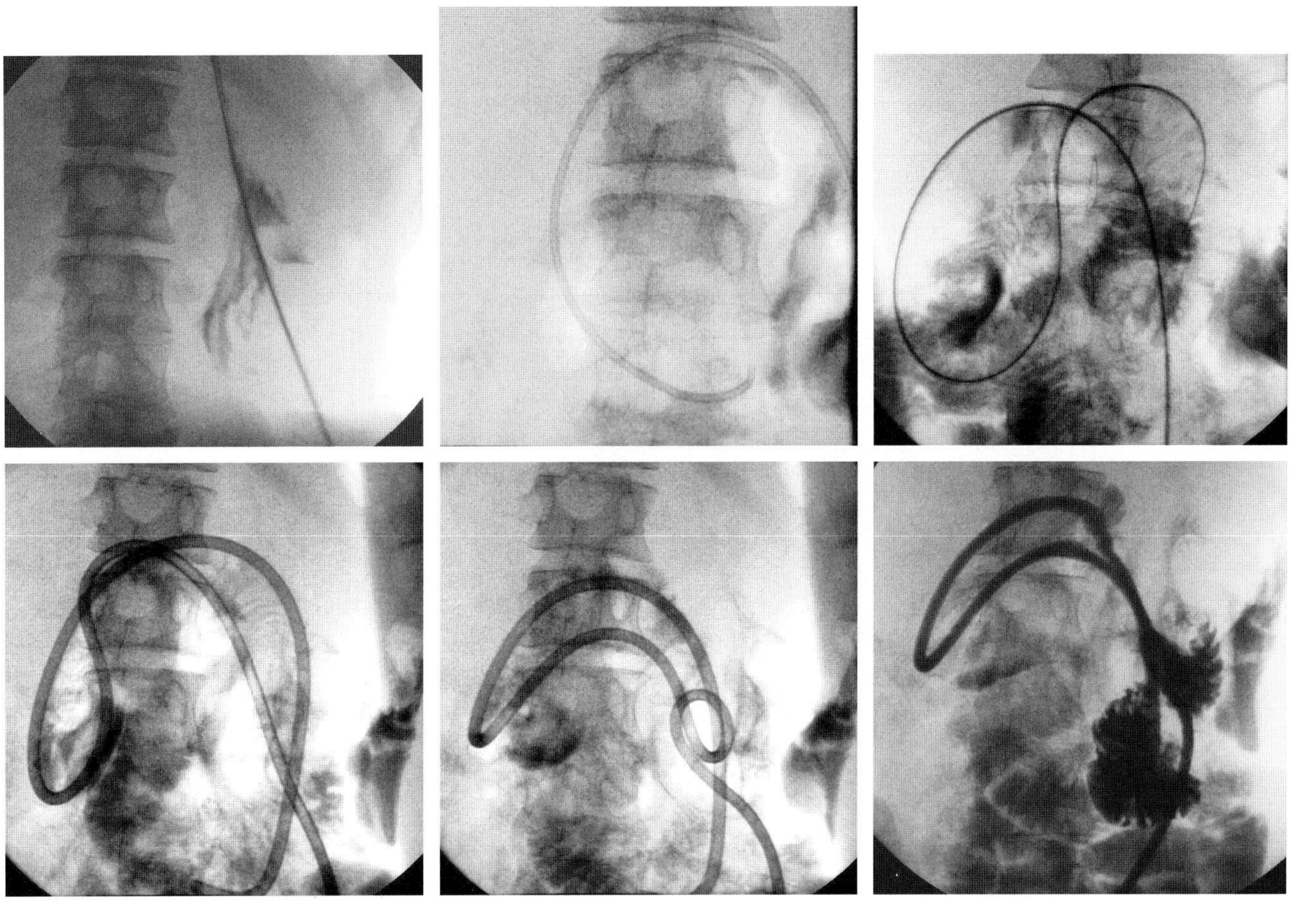

A B, C D E, F

Figure 16.3.2

A: With the patient under general anesthesia, a small catheter was advanced into the stomach and a small amount of contrast material was injected to guide the percutaneous puncture. Note the 18-gauge trocar and the guidewire directed toward the fundus. The guidewire was placed directly into the interposed colon. **B:** A Cobra catheter was advanced into the duodenum. **C:** A super-stiff guidewire was passed into the jejunum. **D:** The puncture hole was dilated to 12F, and through a peel-away sheath the gastrojejunostomy catheter was placed with its tip in the jejunum. **E:** The catheter sling was pulled back and the Cope loop was closed into the stomach. **F:** Injection of contrast material shows good placement within the proximal jejunum. The catheter has been in place for 10 months, and the patient has gained weight.

Comment: Almost 80% of patients can be treated with local anesthesia and sedation; 11% with local anesthesia; and 11% with general anesthesia. Percutaneous gastrostomies were performed more frequently in the past. Gastrojejunostomies now are preferred, because they reduce reflux and permit enteral nutrition, which is more physiologic. We have seen an increasing number of patients with gastrostomies to be converted to gastrojejunostomies. Well-positioned, uncomplicated gastrojejunostomies last for long periods of time (more than 1 year). Skin irritation is relatively common during the initial period. Recurrent infection can develop and is related to lack of proper care in some patients. Management of the tubes is an ongoing challenge and requires a multidisciplinary approach for maintenance.

16.4.1 Esophageal Balloon Dilation, Stenting, And Foreign Body Retrieval

Case 16.4.1:

A 65-year-old male patient presented with squamous cell carcinoma of the esophagus. Palliative treatment with esophageal stenting was requested.

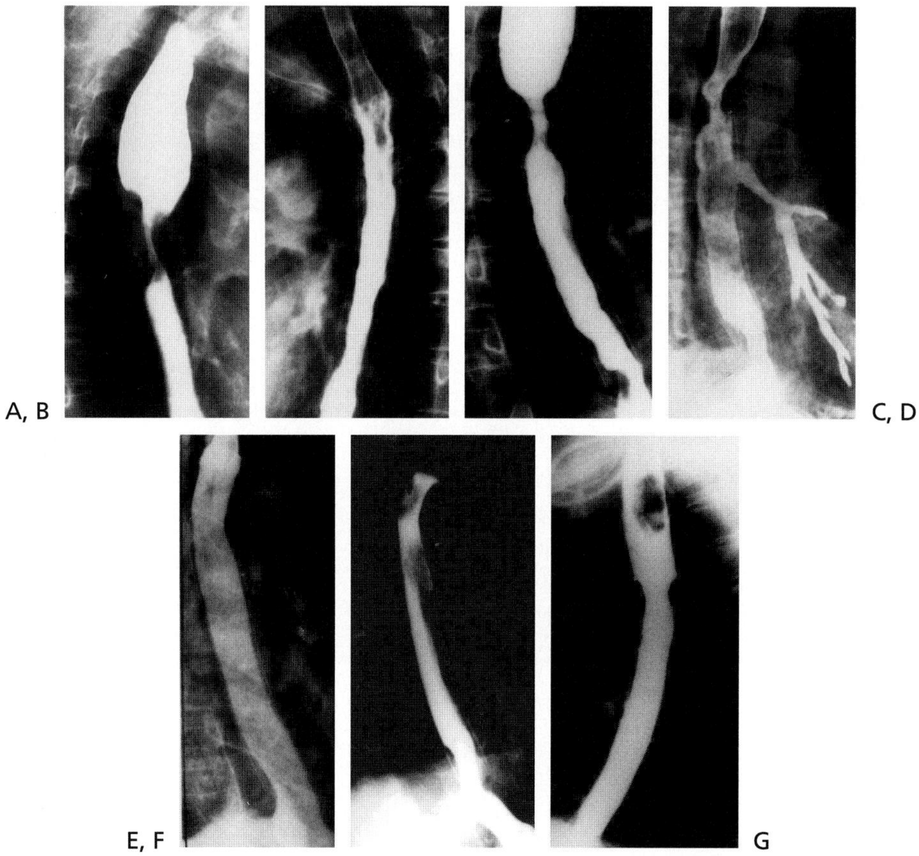

Figure 16.4.1

A: Upper gastrointestinal barium contrast study shows stricture due to squamous cell carcinoma of the esophagus. **B:** A bare Strecker stent was placed to open the esophageal lumen and facilitate swallowing. **C:** Follow-up esophagram at 11 months shows narrowing of the stent lumen due to ingrowth and overgrowth of the tumor. The patient was tolerant to both liquid and solid diet, and no stenting was performed. **D:** The patient developed dysphagia, fever, and cough while feeding. Follow-up esophagogram at 14 months shows restenosis at the proximal site of the stent and esophagotracheal fistula at the middle level of the stent. **E:** A covered Strecker stent was deployed into the first stent. **F,G:** Follow-up esophagograms obtained 1 week and 1 month after placement of the second covered stent show a normal-sized lumen.

Comment: The main symptom of malignant esophageal strictures is dysphagia. Almost all dysphagias occur after 60% luminal reduction in the diameter of the esophagus. Therefore, about 50% of patients have advanced disease at the time of diagnosis, and they require only palliative treatment. The main palliative procedures are surgical bypass, which has a mortality rate of 5% to 60%; and radiation therapy, which palliates dysphagia in around 40% of patients. Laser therapy has low morbidity and high efficacy, but it is not inexpensive and requires repeated treatments. Conventional rigid endoprosthesis has 20% morbidity and mortality rates due to the rigidity of the materials used in the device. Use of the self-expanding esophageal stent is a relatively new, highly efficient technique associated with very low morbidity and mortality rates. Both covered and uncovered metallic stents can be used for palliation of malignant strictures, but only covered stents can be used for treatment of esophagobronchial fistulas. The complications of self-expanding metallic stents include fistula formation (5%), stent torsion (5%), esophageal ulceration (7%), and incomplete expansion of the device (2%) in one published article in the literature. The presented case had a 70% stricture and mediastinal metastasis at the time of diagnosis. The patient's main complaint was dysphagia. Initial treatment just after the diagnosis was performed with a bare, self-expanding Strecker stent. The patient improved and gained more than 5 kg up to the time of a esophagotracheal fistula development. The patient died 5 months after fistula management due to advanced disease and metastasis.

16.4.2 Esophageal Balloon Dilation, Stenting, And Foreign Body Retrieval

Case 16.4.2:

A 3-month-old male child presented with recurrent stenosis of the esophagus after surgical correction of congenital stenosis. Esophageal balloon dilation was requested.

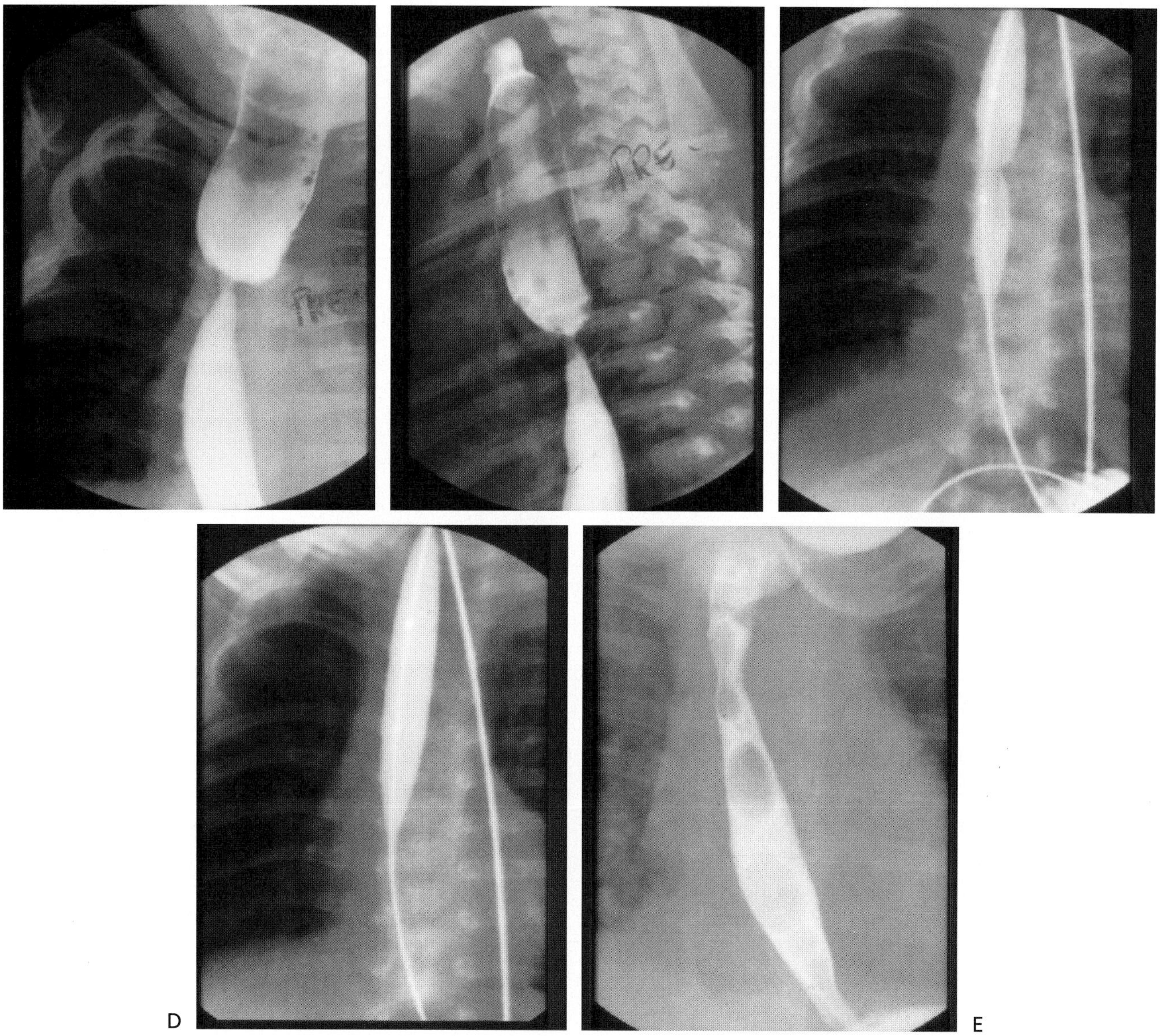

Figure 16.4.2

A: Barium esophagogram obtained to define the location and character (length, diameter, mucosal surface) of the stricture lesion in the mid-proximal esophagus. **B:** Lateral view of the barium esophagogram does not show any fistula or ulceration. **C:** Dilation with 10-mm balloon angioplasty was performed. Note the balloon waist localizing the site of the stricture. **D:** After total expansion of the balloon, dilation of the stenosis was achieved. **E:** Postdilation esophagogram shows adequate dilation, excellent barium flow, and excluded perforation.

Comment: Causes of benign esophageal strictures in adults and children include atresia, reflux esophagitis, caustic material ingestion, inflammatory diseases, webs, achalasia, spasm, and recurrent strictures in surgical anastomoses. The stricture typically manifests itself as dysphagia or other symptoms of esophageal obstruction, such as aspiration and odynophagia. Nonoperative dilation of esophageal strictures using bougies has been performed for more than a century. The bougienage technique was standard until the early 1980s, when the balloon technique was described. Balloons apply radial forces to the esophageal wall, thus reducing the risks of rupture, mucosal injury, and recurrent stenosis. Fluoroscopically guided balloon dilation of esophageal strictures is safer and easier than comparative endoscopic procedures. In children, a 6-mm balloon should be used initially, followed by a larger balloon as necessary, usually within the range from 8 to 10 mm. In adults, larger balloons with diameters of 20 to 25 mm may be necessary. Tight strictures should be approached with smaller balloons first. Longer balloons are necessary for stability during the procedure. Sedation and neuroleptic analgesia usually are necessary. Results are encouraging. Recent publications reported 47% permanent relief of symptoms after only one dilation. Some patients may require two to seven additional dilations for long-lasting results. In general, patients with achalasia or anastomotic strictures respond better than patients with strictures caused by reflux esophagitis, caustic substance ingestion, or malignancies. In one reported series, relief initially was obtained in 98% of patients, decreased to 81% at 6 months, and leveled off at 71% after 9 months. Potential complications include bleeding, esophageal perforation, and infection.

16.4.3 Esophageal Balloon Dilation, Stenting, And Foreign Body Retrieval

Case 16.4.3:

A 2-year-old female child with a metallic foreign body (a quarter coin) in the esophagus presented to the hospital emergency room. Retrieval of the foreign body was requested.

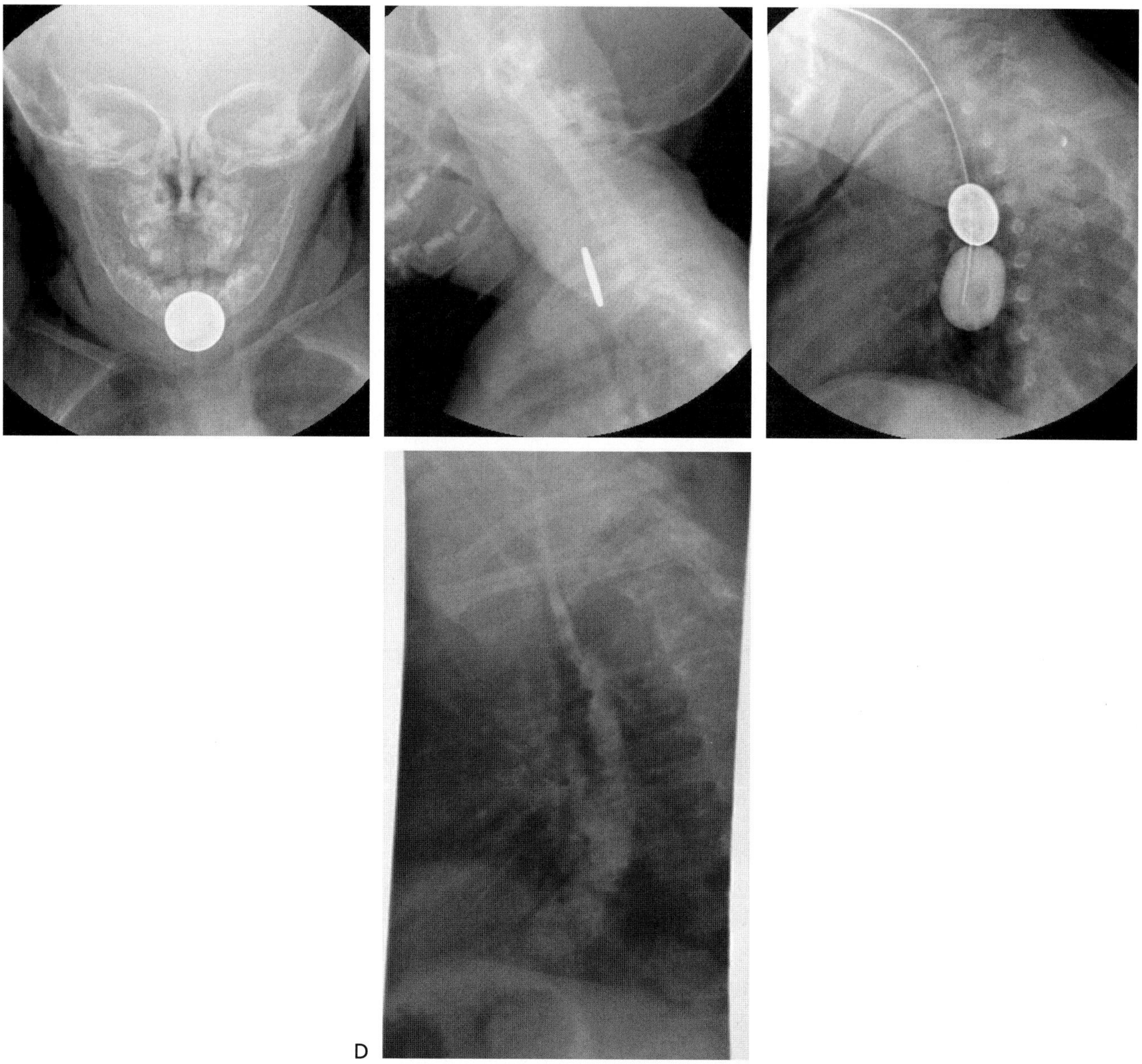

A, B

C

D

Figure 16.4.3

A: Lateral view of the upper chest shows the coin. A Foley catheter was advanced beyond the coin, the balloon was inflated, and the coin was pulled out. **B:** Postretrieval esophagogram shows patency of the esophagus, but some degree of spasm.

Comment: Most swallowed foreign objects pass through the gastrointestinal tract spontaneously; 10% to 20% must be removed by a nonoperative procedure; and about 1% requires surgery. Coins are swallowed very frequently by children, whereas adults have problems with impaction of food and bones. Esophagograms are initially indicated if the foreign body is not radiopaque. Plain radiographs are the initial studies for radiopaque foreign bodies, such as coins. Treatment depends on the symptoms, nature and location of the swallowed object, and length of time since ingestion. Larger coins usually stop in the proximal esophagus, and a balloon catheter is successful for management. Treatment must be performed under fluoroscopic guidance to reduce the chances of esophageal perforation. If the foreign body is ferromagnetic, endoscopy or a fluoroscopically guided magnet attached to the end of a catheter may be used successfully. Restraint devices should be used with young children to increase safety. Acute airway obstruction is a possibility that should be monitored carefully during the procedure.

16.4.4 Esophageal Balloon Dilation, Stenting, And Foreign Body Retrieval

Case 16.4.4:

A 15-month-old female patient swallowed a coin. Retrieval of the foreign body was requested.

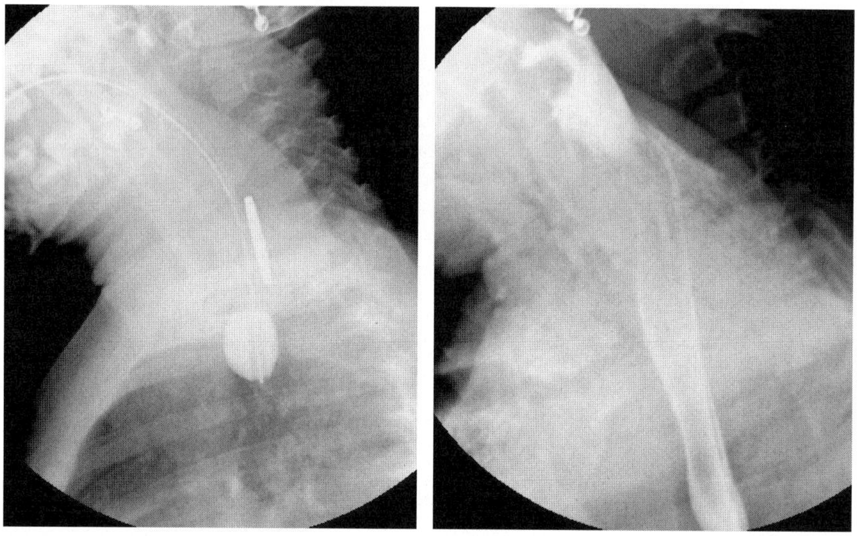
A B

Figure 16.4.4

A,B: Anteroposterior and lateral views of the chest show a large coin in the proximal esophagus of the small child. **C:** A Foley catheter was advanced into the esophagus, and the coin migrated more distally. The balloon was inflated, and the coin was pulled out. **D:** Postprocedure esophagogram shows diffuse spasm of the esophagus. No complications ensued.

Comment: There is a certain risk of pushing a foreign body further down into the esophagus. Forced distal migration should be carefully avoided due to the risk of laceration and esophageal rupture. Retrieval may be very difficult in cases of large foreign bodies. Sharp objects cannot be pulled out with a balloon or a grasping forceps. Open safety pins are especially difficult challenges, because the sharp ends of the pins can perforate the esophagus and/or stomach and create fistulas and abscesses. Vascular perforations are not rare and can be lethal when pins, bones, or open safety pins are swallowed.

16.5.1 Treatment Of Colonic And Enteric Strictures With Stents

Case 16.5.1:

A 55-year-old male patient with a history of abdominal pain and worsening of nausea and vomiting was seen in the emergency room. Clinical history and x-ray examination revealed bowel obstruction. Colonoscopic examination was attempted, but access could not be achieved through colonic stricture.

A 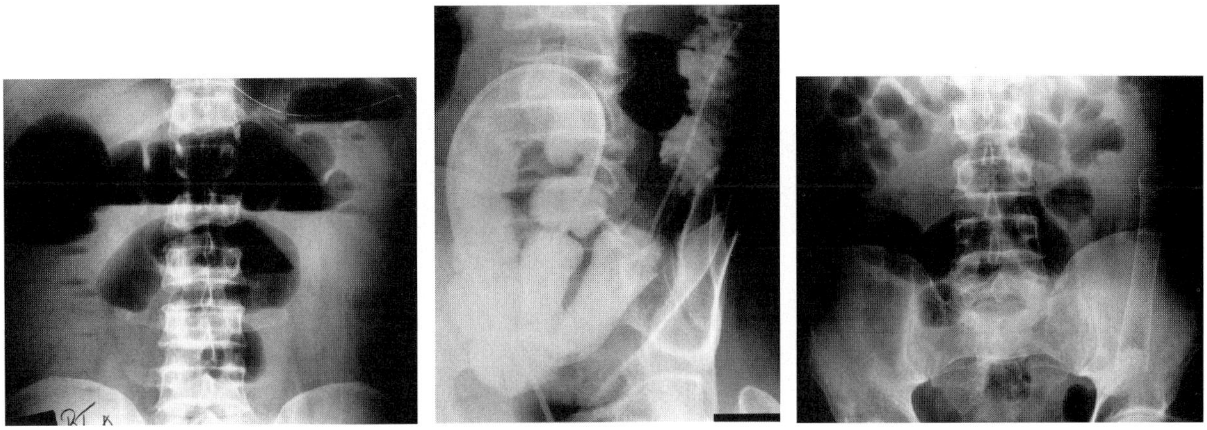 B, C

Figure 16.5.1

A: Initial upright abdominal x-ray film reveals marked dilation of the small and large bowel, with numerous air-fluid levels consistent with clinical diagnosis of bowel obstruction. **B:** Gastrografin injected proximally and distally to the lesion reveals high-grade stenosis in the descending colon that was responsible for the patient's acute colonic obstruction. Technique: Initial Gastrografin enema is used to determine point of obstruction. Using a transanal approach with the patient in a prone position, a diagnostic catheter (7F or 8F multipurpose) is carefully advanced with the use of a steerable wire, either an angled, floppy 0.035-inch wire or a hydrophilic coated wire. Occasionally, a long sheath or guiding catheter is used for additional support. The wire is carefully advanced through lesion, then the catheter is advanced over the wire past the lesion. **C:** A large 22-mm × 60-mm Wallstent was deployed across the obstructing lesion. Technique: With the angiographic catheter placed past the lesion, an Amplatz super-stiff guidewire was advanced and the catheter removed. An appropriate tracheobronchial Wallstent is used to bridge the obstruction. The length (35, 45, or 70 mm) and diameter (20, 22, or 24 mm) of the Wallstent vary; the best length and diameter are selected. The stent is advanced under fluoroscopic guidance and deployed with the middle of the stent covering the lesion site. If the lesion is long, a second stent may be needed, with approximately one half of the stent overlapping the first. Follow-up plain abdominal film is obtained 24 hours after placement to assess decompression and confirm stent position. Stent migration is a potential problem, especially for lesions located in the rectosigmoid colon. If migration occurs, the stent can easily be retrieved under fluoroscopic guidance.

Comment: The alternative approach for treatment of colonic obstruction with an expandable metallic stent using the Tejero-Mainar technique is becoming more popular. Under fluoroscopic guidance, access is easily obtained through high-grade stenotic and clinically occluded segments. This technique allows the opportunity for quick decompression in patients who often are elderly and debilitated. Then, if necessary, these patients can undergo resuscitation and bowel preparation prior to elective surgical resection. With this technique, the patient can avoid colostomy. If surgery is not advisable, the stents can remain in place as a long-term palliative device.

16.5.2 Treatment Of Colonic And Enteric Strictures With Stents

Case 16.5.2:

A 65-year-old terminally ill female patient with metastatic gastric carcinoma presented with pyloric obstruction. A gastrostomy tube had been placed earlier, but it could not be directed through the obstruction.

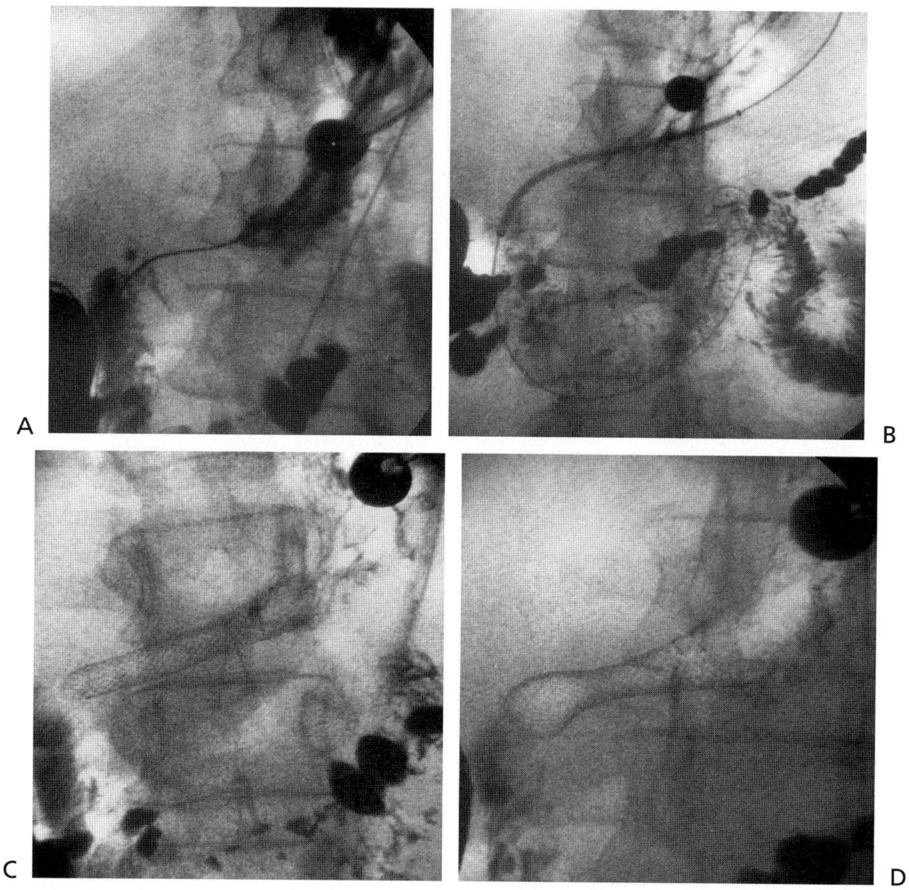

Figure 16.5.2

A: Thin barium was injected through the gastrostomy and revealed near-complete occlusion of the pylorus. After spraying topical anesthetic into the mouth and tongue, access through the oropharynx was obtained with a 5F headhunter catheter and 0.035-inch stiff, angled glidewire. The catheter and wire were advanced carefully past the obstruction and into the duodenum. The glidewire was exchanged for a super-stiff Amplatz 260 guidewire. The diagnostic catheter then was exchanged for an 8F guiding catheter in which thin barium could be injected to better define the lesion and its length. **B:** The guiding catheter was removed, and a tracheobronchial Wallstent (22 × 70 mm) was advanced over the stiff guidewire. During the first attempt, the patient bit down on the stent delivery system, thus rupturing the thin plastic membrane and necessitating exchange for new stent. The photograph depicts the stent prior to deployment. **C,D:** Postdeployment images show the stents are fully expanded and contracting with peristaltic pulsation of the stomach and pylorus. Decompression of the stomach was achieved, and she could be fed through the gastrostomy tube. The patient died two months later from complications of the cancer.

Comment: The long-term patency of self-expandable metallic stents in treating pyloric stenoses is limited because of the undigested food content. Unlike esophageal stents, metallic stents cannot be easily removed. Hence, these stents are still highly experimental and should be reserved for terminal patients. An alternative procedure would have been dilation and advancement of a gastrojejunostomy catheter past the pyloric lesion.

16.6.1 Celiac Block For Pain Control

Case 16.6.1:

Percutaneous anterior approach for celiac plexus block was used in a 67-year-old male patient with pancreatic carcinoma and severe abdominal pain.

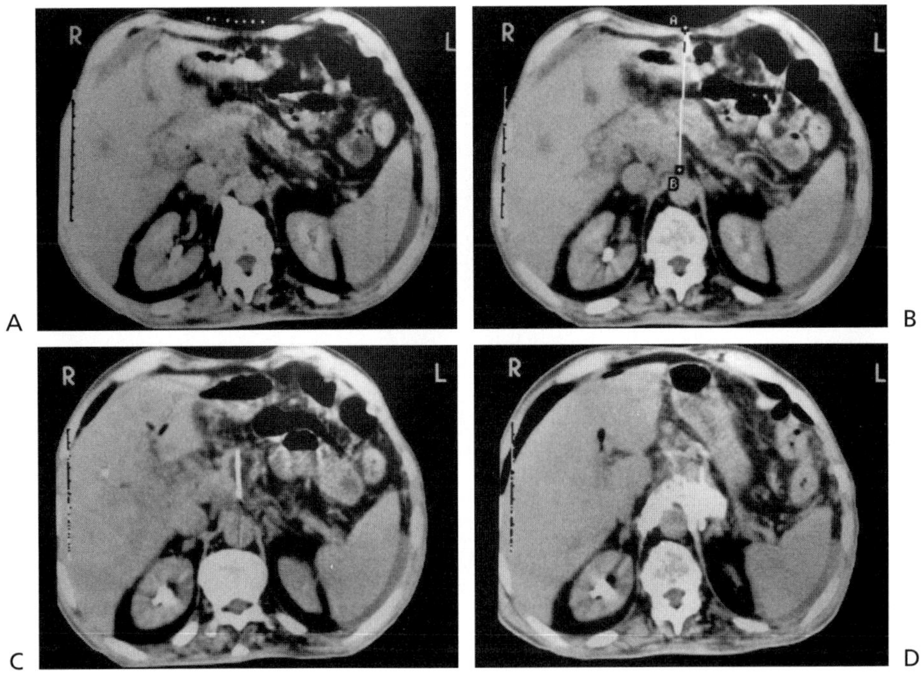

Figure 16.6.1

Percutaneous anterior approach to celiac plexus neurolysis. **A:** Abdominal CT scan of the patient with pancreatic carcinoma. Note markers on the skin in the anterior wall of the abdomen. **B:** Distance measurement from the skin to the abdominal aorta near the celiac artery. Note that a central reference point was selected. **C:** A 21-gauge needle was placed just anterior to the abdominal aorta. A small amount of lidocaine (0.2 to 0.4 mL/kg) was given to locate the celiac plexus and to elicit an anesthetic effect for the final procedure. Immediate response to local anesthetic is a good sign for both the success and the proper localization of the needle. **D:** Contrast medium was given. Dispersement of the contrast within the anterior compartment of the aorta, near the celiac artery, demonstrates that the compartment is blocked. Following the localization procedure, 50 mL of 50% alcohol solution was injected for neurolysis.

Comment: The celiac plexus is located near and around the celiac artery interconnecting the celiac ganglia. Celiac plexus block is reserved for relieving pain produced by malignancy or by pancreatitis after failed systemic analgesia. The neurolysis procedure can be done either intraoperatively or with percutaneous techniques. Intraoperative techniques have been found to be slightly less effective than percutaneous techniques, and they are more invasive. Alcohol injected intraoperatively disperses in the operative bed. Percutaneously injected alcohol remains restrained around the celiac plexus. The anterior approach with a 21-gauge or 22-gauge needle is safe and causes no significant injury to hollow organ viscera. There are two main percutaneous approaches: anterior and posterior. Both CT scan and ultrasound can be used for guidance. The posterior approach technique risks injuring the sympathetic and lumbar plexus, which is located in the area around the spine and aorta. The transaortic approach sometimes is required to reach the plexus using the posterior approach. Complications with the percutaneous approach are paraplegia in about 1% of patients (with posterior approach), diarrhea, increased peristalsis and retroperitoneal pain, orthostatic hypotension, reactive pleurisy, and transient hematuria. The average success rate of the technique is between 58% and 98% according to published series, and 71% in a study using the anterior approach.

16.6.2 Celiac Block For Pain Control

Case 16.6.2:

Percutaneous posterior approach for celiac plexus block was used in a 60-year-old male patient with pancreatic carcinoma and severe abdominal pain.

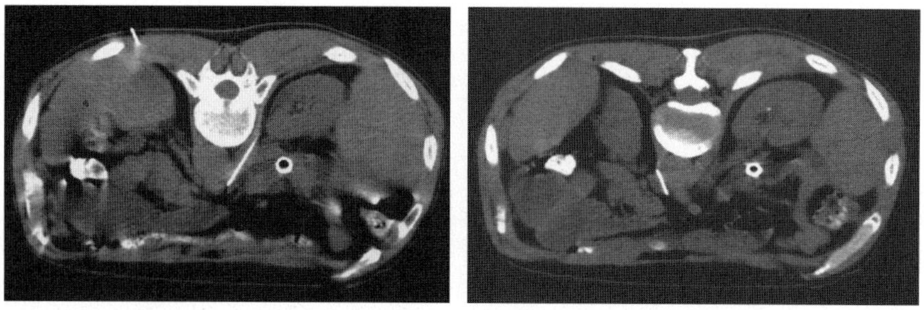

A B

Figure 16.6.2

A: Prone abdominal CT scan used to guide neurolysis of the celiac plexus. A 21-gauge needle was placed just lateral to the abdominal aorta on the right side. A small amount of lidocaine (0.2 to 0.4 mL/kg) was given to locate the celiac plexus and to elicit an anesthetic effect for the final procedure. Following the localization procedure, 50 mL of 50% alcohol solution was injected for neurolysis. **B:** The same procedure was performed on the left side.

Comment: The celiac plexus is located around the celiac artery interconnecting the celiac ganglia. Celiac plexus block is used for palliation of pain produced by malignancies. The neurolysis procedure can be done through either an anterior or a posterior approach using a percutaneous technique. Percutaneously injected alcohol remains around the celiac plexus and causes ablation of the celiac plexus. There are two main percutaneous approaches: anterior and posterior. The posterior approach technique is associated with a slight risk of injuring the sympathetic and lumbar plexus, which is located on the side of the spine and aorta. Complications with the percutaneous approach are paraplegia in about 1% of patients (with posterior approach), diarrhea and retroperitoneal pain, orthostatic hypotension, reactive pleurisy, and transient hematuria. Note that the needle in the posterior approach may cross the pleural space and the kidney substance. Progressive advancement of the needle under CT guidance prevents vascular damage or puncture.

16.7.1 Axillary Brachial Plexus Block

Case 16.7.1:

Case report of axillary brachial plexus block is demonstrated in a 45-year-old female patient.

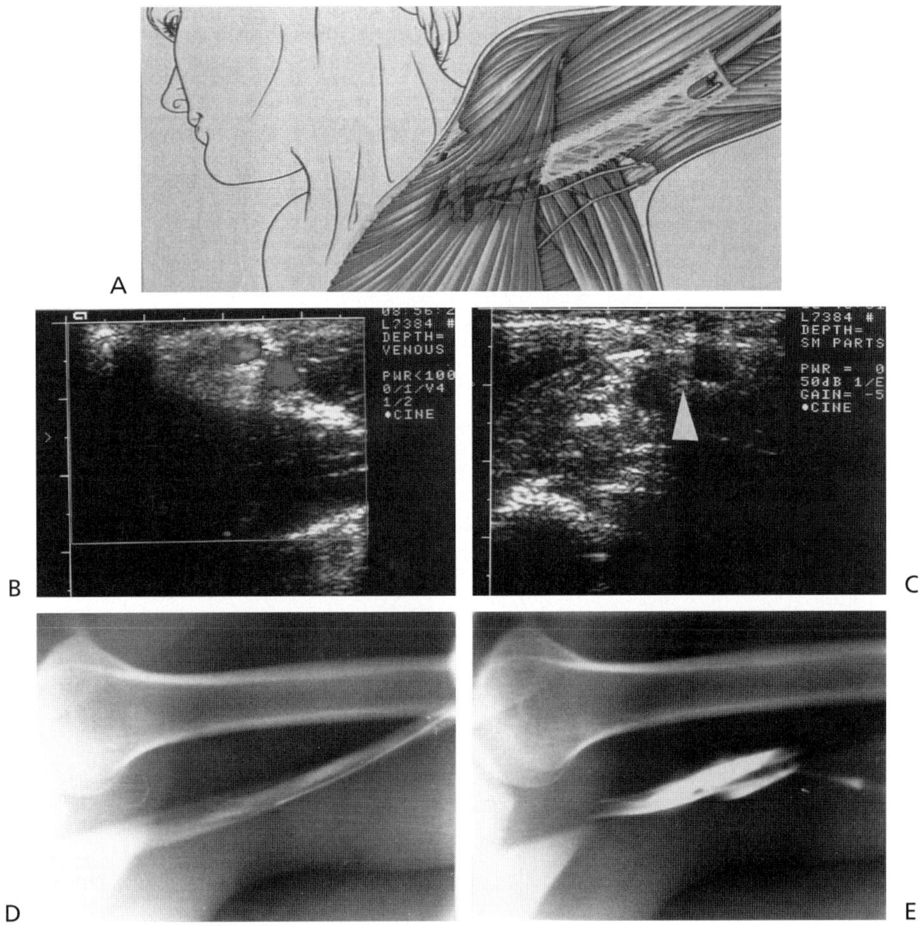

Figure 16.7.1

A: Axillary neurovascular bundle. **B:** Transverse image of the axillary artery and vein. **C:** Transverse image showing tip of the sheathed needle *(arrow)*. **D:** Control contrast study of the neurovascular bundle and guidewire. The guidewire is parallel to the axillary vein. **E:** Relationship between the axillary vein and the catheter in the neurovascular bundle. Technique: The axillary region is visualized with the patient in the supine position, as shown in Fig. 16.7.1A. After skin preparation, a 7.5-MHz linear transducer is covered with a sterile disposable plastic drape. After a 45-degree distal sloping of the probe, a 18-gauge sheathed needle is directed proximal to the axilla from the anesthetized skin region to the area between the axillary artery and vein, as shown in Fig. 16.7.1D–E. Following this step, a small catheter (0.45 × 0.85 mm, 40 cm long) is placed over a guidewire for local anesthesia.

Comment: Brachial plexus block through an axillary route may be desired for purposes of regional anesthesia and continuous analgesia. Single-dose applications may be useful for minor surgical or nonsurgical interventions. However, single-dose applications are not adequate for long-term or continuous blockage. Several approaches for continuous axillary blockage have been described, including forearm venography-guided axillary blockage. As previously reported, ultrasound guidance for axillary blockage has some advantages, such as no risk of pneumothorax, no need to use contrast material to guide the axillary sheath, and no need to use the angiography suite. In addition, the ultrasound approach may be done as a bedside procedure using a portable ultrasound machine.

16.8.1 Fallopian Tube Recanalization

Case 16.8.1:

A 31-year-old woman presented with infertility and a history consistent with salpingitis of indeterminate etiology producing proximal tubal obstruction.

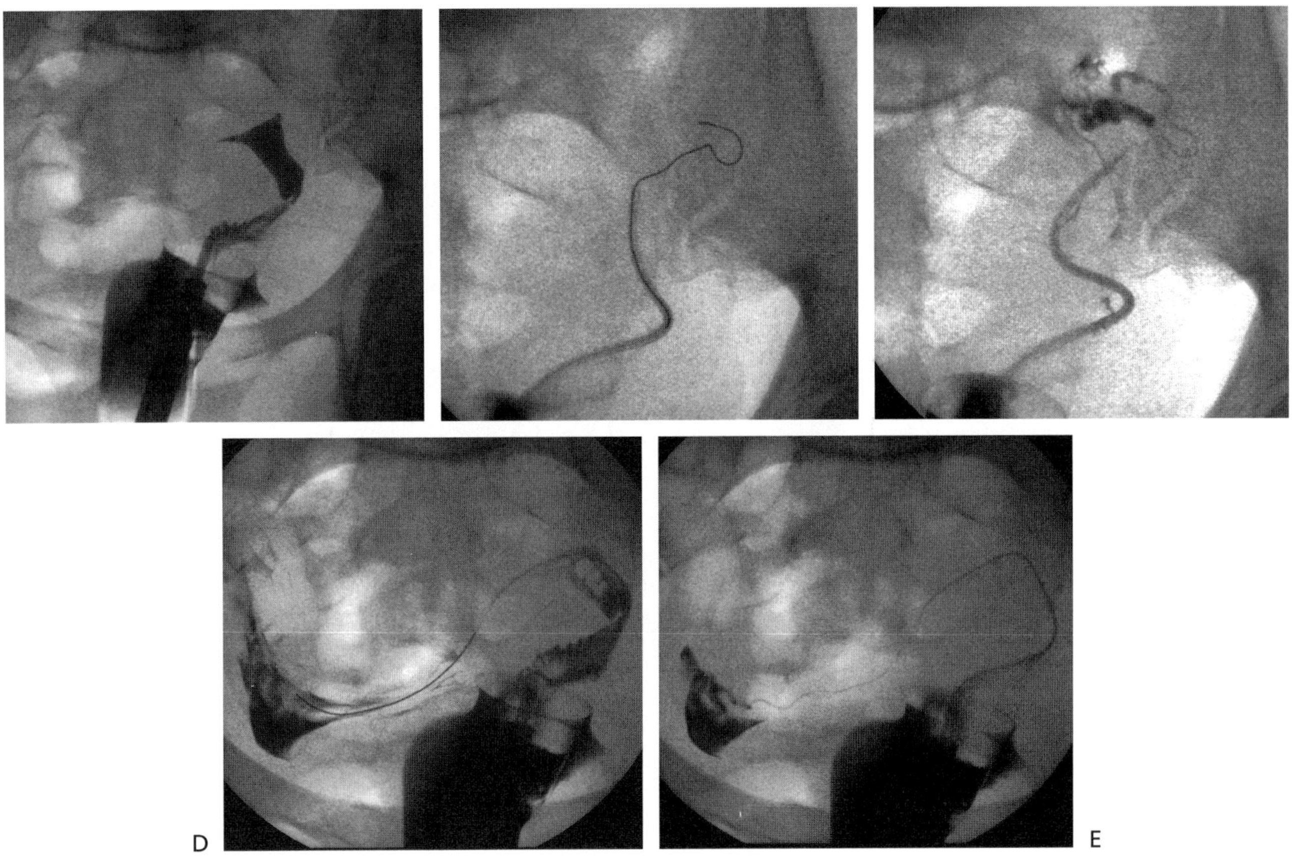

A B, C D E

Figure 16.8.1

A: Hysterosalpingography shows proximal tubal obstruction. **B:** Following catheterization of the proximal tortuous tube, a 0.018-inch guidewire was advanced into the tube for recanalization. **C:** Forceful injection of contrast material into the left ostium shows filling of the tube and contrast spill. Note some irregularities in the tubal contour. **D:** Recanalization of the right tube with the guidewire. **E:** Injection of contrast material into the proximal fallopian tube shows smooth tubal appearance and free intraperitoneal spill of contrast. The patient conceived 6 months after the procedure.

Comment: Proximal obstruction of the fallopian tube causes infertility in approximately 20% of women with tubal disease. Tubal disease is the single most common cause of female infertility, accounting for 25% to 35% of involuntary infertility. It is a difficult problem to treat. Tubal microsurgery is associated with a 30% to 50% pregnancy rate after 2 years; *in vitro* fertilization has a 10% to 15% pregnancy rate. Both procedures are associated with significant morbidity and expense. Fluoroscopic transcervical fallopian tube catheterization for recanalization was developed in the last 10 years. It provides a method to open the tubes without surgery and thus allows the patient to conceive naturally. The procedure has reduced morbidity/mortality and is less costly compared with surgical and *in vitro* techniques. Unilateral or bilateral fallopian tube recanalization is successful in 71% to 96% of cases. Postprocedure conception reported in the literature ranges from 7% to 47%. Possible complications are related to tube perforation and subintimal injection, but some authors also consider ectopic pregnancies, which may occur in up to 9% of patients, as possible adverse events related to the technique.

16.9.1 Percutaneous Vertebroplasty

Case 16.9.1:

A 91-year-old female patient with rheumatoid arthritis, multiple lumbar vertebral fractures, and massive osteoporotic compression fracture of the vertebral body of T12 and L1 could not walk and presented with untreatable pain. The patient was referred for vertebroplasty using methylmethacrylate.

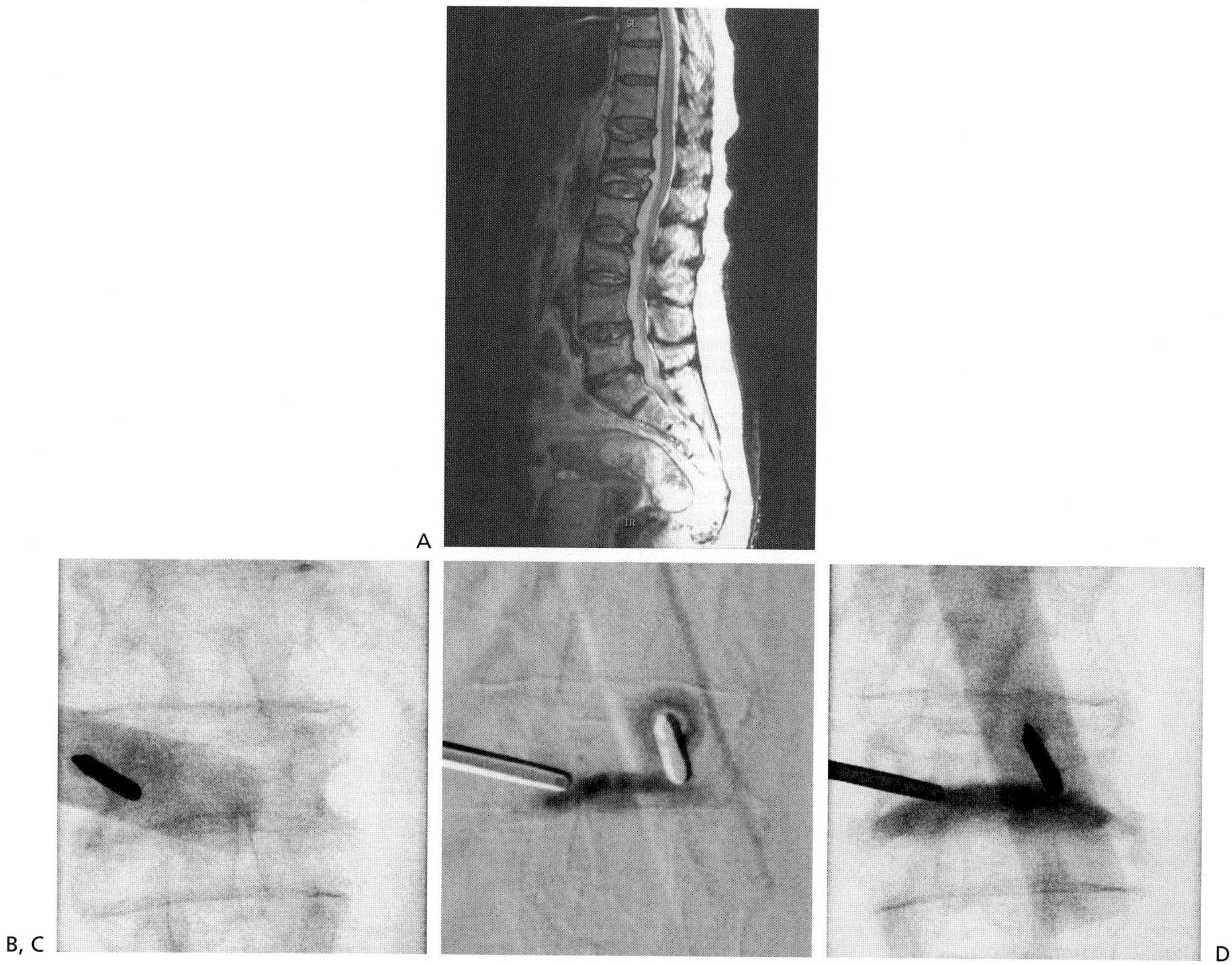

Figure 16.9.1

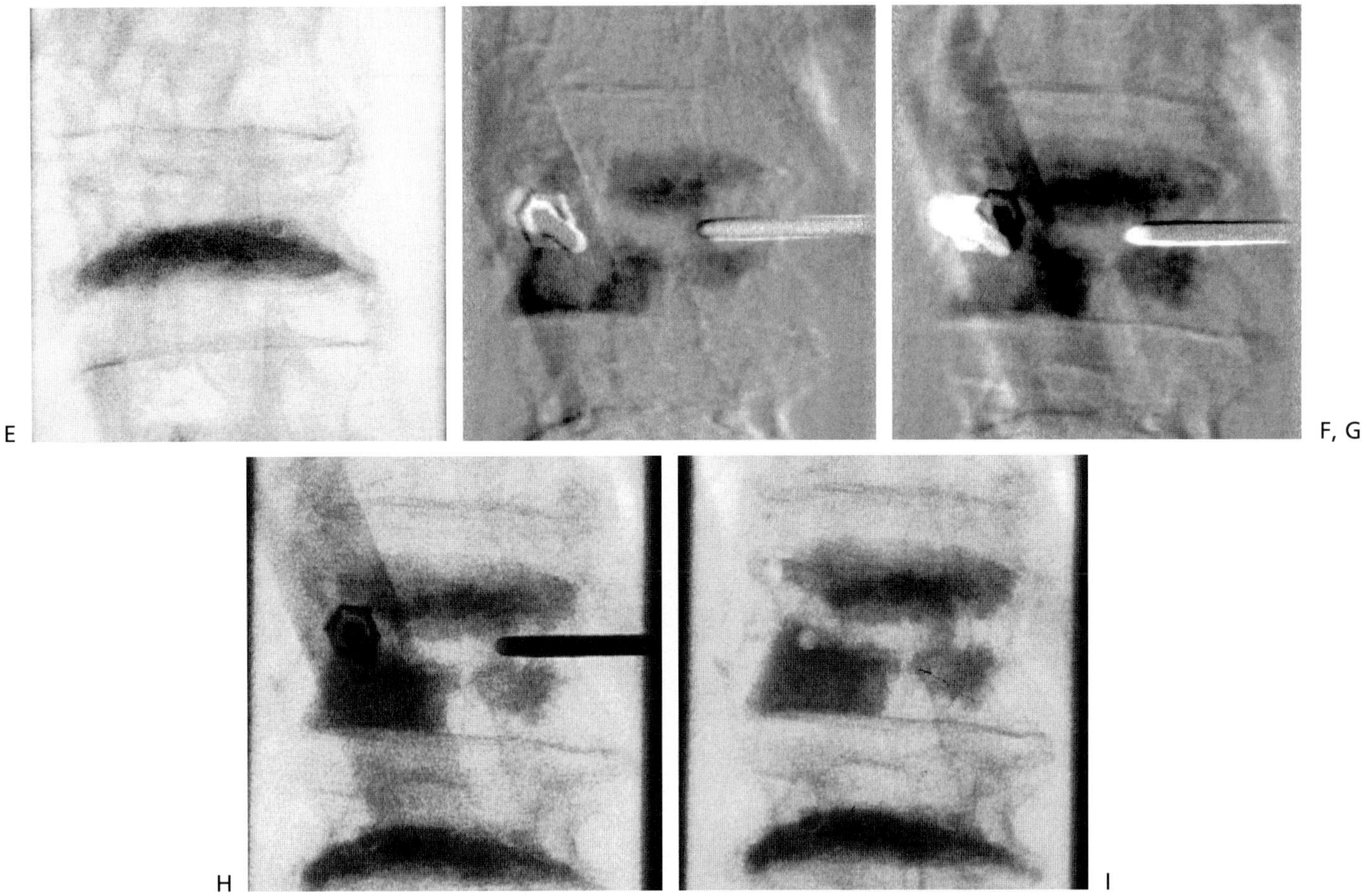

Figure 16.9.1 *(continued)*

A: Magnetic resonance imaging of the spine shows signs of fracture and collapse of the vertebral body of L1 and fracture of the vertebral body of T12. **B:** Spot radiograph at the level of L1 shows the trocar needle in the vertebral body through the left pedicle of L1. **C:** Right-side trocar in place while a venogram was obtained. No drainage was observed in the subtracted pictures. **D:** Spot radiograph obtained during injection of methylmethacrylate shows the density within the collapsed vertebral body. **E:** Final spot radiograph shows the material within the vertebral body. At the end of the procedure, the patient presented with tachycardia and hypertension. The procedure for T12 was aborted. **F:** The next day, T12 was approached in the same manner with bilateral puncture. The venogram from the left side shows the contrast material mostly contained within the vertebral body but with filling of the left paraspinal ascending vein. **G:** Venogram performed from the right side shows the same aspect as in **F**. **H:** Bilateral injection of methylmethacrylate material shows filling of the vertebral body without extravasation. **I:** Spot radiograph of both T12 and L1 vertebral bodies shows the material well located within the bone. There was marked improvement in the 48 hours following the procedure. Although the patient still was in pain, she was able to walk again.

Comment: With the aging of the world population, increasing numbers of elderly persons are sustaining vertebral compression fractures due to osteopenia. Other patients suffer fractures as a result of chronic steroid use. The vertebral fractures frequently cause persistent often excruciating pain, with impairment of mobility and quality of life. Multiple treatments may be necessary, such as external bracing, common analgesics, and narcotics, which may be more lifestyle altering than the fracture itself. Malignant and benign tumoral vertebral compression fractures have been treated in the past by surgical decompression and injection of polymethylmethacrylate cement. More recently, percutaneous vertebroplasty performed through a transpedicular or paravertebral approach using CT and/or fluoroscopic guidance has been developed. The procedure is performed under strict sterile conditions. Biplane fluoroscopy is recommended to allow simultaneous imaging of the stylet tip position in two planes. Following local anesthesia and through a small skin incision, the 11-gauge Jamshidi needle is advanced through the cortex of the bone into the pedicle with simultaneous imaging in both planes, and finally introduced into the middle third of the vertebral body. Before injecting the methylmethacrylate, a vertebral venography is performed to ascertain the location of the vertebral venous plexus and the containment of contrast within the bony trabeculae. The methylmethacrylate is added to a mixture of sterile tungsten powder and sterile barium sulfate powder. Once the desired toothpaste consistency is achieved, the material is injected. The injection pressure required to push the material increases over time as the vertebral body fills and the methylmethacrylate polymerizes. If filling of the venous system is visualized, injection is slowed or halted while the material thickens. Injection is continued until hemivertebral or holovertebral filling is achieved. The material will cure in about 3 hours, and the patient is kept in the hospital overnight.

16.9.2 Percutaneous Vertebroplasty

Case 16.9.2:

An 87-year-old male patient with full fracture of the vertebral body of L2 suffered in a fall was unresponsive to narcotic analgesics and epidural injections. Percutaneous vertebroplasty was requested.

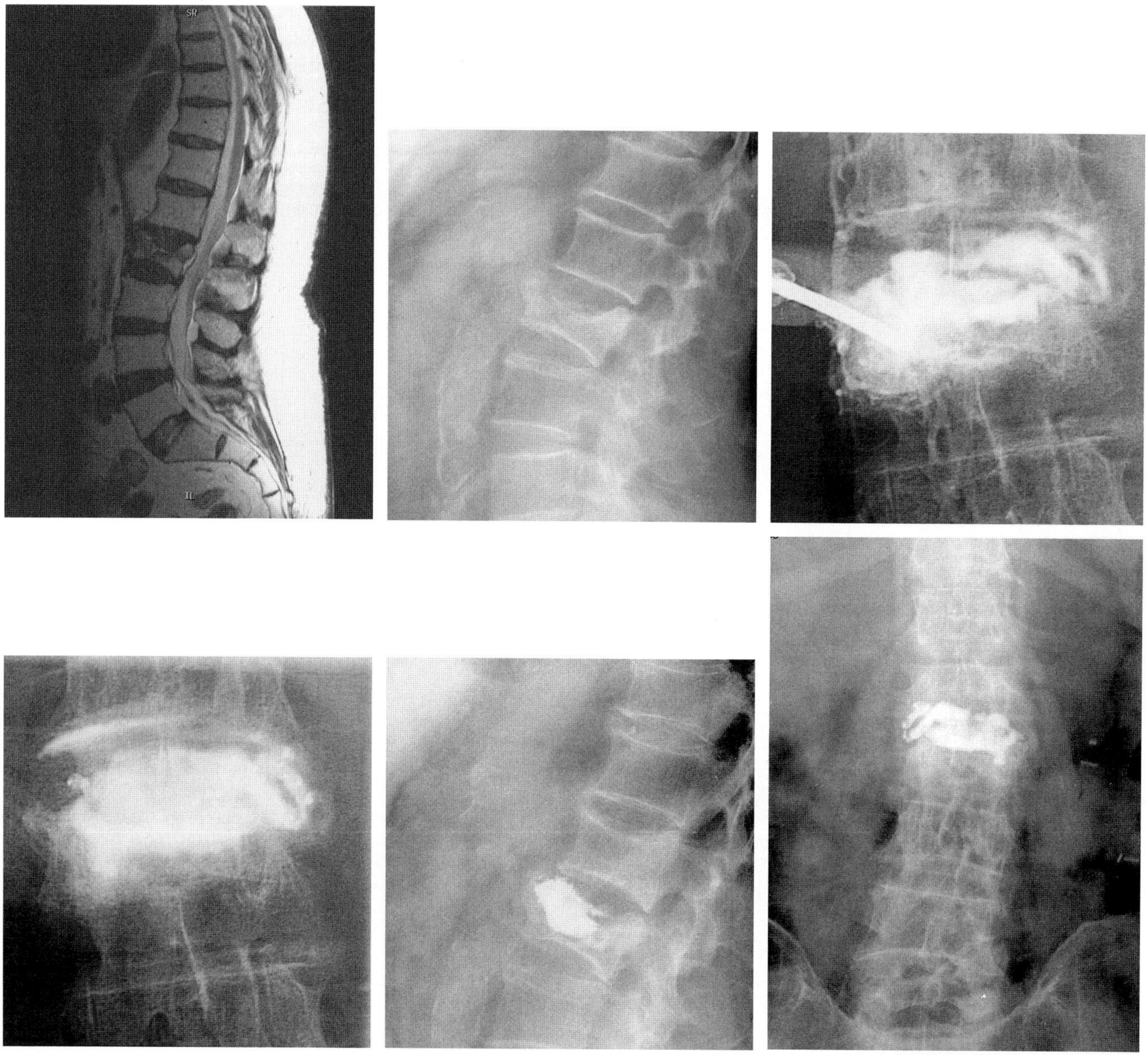

A, B C D, E F

Figure 16.9.2

A: Magnetic resonance imaging of the spine shows fracture of L2. **B:** Lumbar spine radiograph in the lateral view shows severe collapse of L2 and marked osteoporosis. Note the aortic calcifications. **C:** Following puncture of the left vertebral pedicle with an 11-gauge trocar, venogram shows the contrast material contained within the vertebral body, with drainage through the left ascending lumbar vein. **D:** Spot radiograph following injection of methylmethacrylate shows adequate filling of the vertebral body. **E,F:** Two months after the procedure, lumbar spine radiographs in the lateral and anteroposterior views show filling of the vertebral body with the methylmethacrylate material, supporting the spine. There was marked improvement of pain and mobility.

Comment: Indications for vertebroplasty use are osteolytic vertebral metastasis and myeloma, vertebral hemangioma, and painful osteoporotic vertebral collapse. Vertebroplasty can be technically successful in most or all patients. Resolution or relief of pain is achieved in 90% of patients within 24 hours after treatment. Mobility also is improved. Most patients who require parenteral narcotics can be switched to oral analgesics. A few patients will report no improvement of the pain and will require pretreatment medical regimen. No worsening of pain has been reported. Complications reported in the limited series available range from 0% to 10%, including transient dysphagia and radiculopathy. No infection has been reported. Potential risks of methylmethacrylate toxicity have been described and include decreased pulmonary function and drop in arterial pressure. The long-term outcome of this treatment is still subject to analysis, but it has proved a valuable new tool in the treatment of osteoporotic vertebral compression fractures and osteolytic metastatic disease, providing pain relief and early mobility in appropriate patients.

Suggested Readings

Tracheal Stents And Bronchial Stents

Kishi K, Fujimoto HK, Somura T, et al. A dedicated Z-stent for acquired Saber-Sheath tracheobronchomalacia. *Cardiovasc Intervent Radiol* 1997;20:462–465.

Lehaman JD, Gordon RL, Kerlan RK, et al. Expandable metallic stents in benign tracheobronchial obstruction. *J Thorac Imaging* 1998;13:105–115.

Rafanan AL, Mehta AC. Stenting of the tracheobronchial tree. *Radiol Clin North Am* 2000;38:395–408.

Percutaneous Gastrostomy

Bell SD, Carmody EA, Yeung EY, et al. Percutaneous gastrostomy and gastrojejunostomy: additional experience in 519 procedures. *Radiology* 1995;194:817–820.

Chait PG, Weinberg J, Connolly BL, et al. Retrograde percutaneous gastrostomy and gastrojejunostomy in 505 children: a 4 1/2-year experience. *Radiology* 1996;201:691–695.

Watkinson AF, Fache JS, Burhenne HJ. Percutaneous gastrostomy and gastrojejunostomy experience in 100 cases. *Eur Radiol* 1995;5:13–18.

Wills JS, Oblesby JT. Percutaneous gastrostomy. *Radiology* 1983;149:449–453.

Percutaneous Gastrojejunostomy

Ho CS, Young EY. Percutaneous gastrostomy and transgastric jejunostomy. *AJR* 1992;158:251–257.

Esophageal Stents

Acunas B, Rozanes L, Akpinar S, et al. Palliation of malignant esophageal strictures with self-expanding nitinol stents: drawbacks and complications. *Radiology* 1996;199:648–652.

Albertson M, Ewers SB, Widmark H, et al. Evaluation of palliative effect of radiotherapy for esophageal carcinoma. *Acta Oncol* 1989;28:267–270.

Bethge N, Sommer A, Gross U, et al. Human tissue responses to metal stents implanted in vivo for the palliation of malignant stenoses. *Gastrointest Endosc* 1996;43:596–601.

Bethge N, Sommer A, Vakil N. Treatment of esophageal fistulas with a new polyurethane-covered, self-expanding mesh stent: a prospective study. *Am J Gastroenterol* 1995;90:2143–2146.

Cwikiel M, Cwikiel W, Albertsson M. Palliation of dysphagia in patients with malignant esophageal strictures. *Acta Oncol* 1996;35:75–79.

De Palma GD, Galloro G, Sivero L, et al. Self-expanding metal stents for palliation of inoperable carcinoma of the esophagus and gastroesophageal junction. *Am J Gastroenterol* 1995;90:2140–2142.

Dougenis D, Petsas T, Bouboulis N, et al. Management of nonresectable malignant esophageal stricture and fistula. *Eur J Cardiothorac Surg* 1997;11:38–45.

Feins RH, Johnstone DW, Baronos ES, et al. Palliation of inoperable esophageal carcinoma with the Wallstent endoprosthesis. *Ann Thorac Surg* 1996;62:1603–1607.

Garcia M, D'Altorio RA, Glowacki D. Palliative treatment of malignant esophageal obstruction with metallic Wallstent. *Dig Dis Sci* 1994;39:2685–2688.

Loizou LA, Grigg D, Atkinson M, et al. A prospective comparison of laser therapy and intubation in endoscopic palliation for malignant dysphagia. *Gastroenterology* 1991;100:1303–1310.

Nelson DB, Axelrad AM, Fleischer DE, et al. Silicone-covered Wallstent prototypes for palliation of malignant esophageal obstruction and digestive-respiratory fistulas. *Gastrointest Endosc* 1997;45: 31–37.

Raijman I, Walden D, Kortan P, et al. Expandable esophageal stents: initial experience with a new nitinol stent. *Gastrointest Endosc* 1994;40:614–621.

Saxon RR, Morrison KE, Lakin PC, et al. Malignant esophageal obstruction and esophagorespiratory fistula: palliation with a polyethylene-covered Z-stent. *Radiology* 1997;202:349–354.

Song HY, Do YS, Han YM, et al. Covered, expandable metallic stent tubes: experiences in 119 patients. *Radiology* 1994;193:689–695.

Song HY, Park SI, Do YS, et al. Expandable metallic stent placement in patients with benign esophageal strictures: results of long-term follow-up. *Radiology* 1997;203:131–136.

Watkinson A, Ellui J, Entwisle K, et al. Plastic covered metallic endoprostheses in the management of oesophageal perforation in patients with oesophageal carcinoma. *Clin Radiol* 1995;50:304–309.

Watson A. Surgery for carcinoma of the oesophagus. *Postgrad Med J* 1988;64:860–864.

Winkelbauer FW, Schoff R, Niederle B, et al. Palliative treatment of obstruction of esophageal cancer with nitinol stents. *AJR* 1996;166:79–84.

Treatment Of Colonic And Enteric Strictures With Stents

Canon CL, Baron TH, Morgan DE, et al. Treatment of colonic obstruction with expandable metal stents: radiological features. *AJR* 1997;168:199–205.

Mainar A, Tejero E, Maynar M, et al. Colorectal obstruction: treatment with metallic stents. *Radiology* 1996;198:761–764.

Pinto LT. Malignant gastric and duodenal stenosis: palliation by peroral implantation of a self-expanding metallic stent. *Cardiovasc Intervent Radiol* 1997;20:431–434.

Saunders BP, Bartram C. Self expanding metal stents for malignant colonic obstruction. *Clin Radiol* 1998;53:237–238.

Wholey MH, Ferral H, Reyes R, et al. Retrieval of migrated colonic stent from the rectum. *Cardiovasc Intervent Radiol* 1997;20:477–480.

Celiac Block For Pain Control

Gimenez A, Martinez-Noguera A, Donoso L, et al. Percutaneous neurolysis of the celiac plexus via the anterior approach with sonographic guidance. *AJR* 1993;161:1061–1063.

Ischia S, Ischia A, Polati E, et al. Three posterior percutaneous celiac plexus block techniques. *Anesthesiology* 1992;76:534–540.

Lieberman RP, Nance PN, Cuka DJ. Anterior approach to celiac plexus block during interventional biliary procedures. *Radiology* 1988;167:562–564.

Matamala AM, Lopez FV, Martinez LI. The percutaneous anterior approach to the celiac plexus using CT guidance. *Pain* 1988;34:285–288.

Myhre J, Hilsted J, Tronier B, et al. Monitoring of celiac plexus block in chronic pancreatitis. *Pain* 1989;38:269–274.

Sherman S, Kopecky K, et al. Percutaneous celiac plexus block with botulinum toxin A did not help the pain of chronic pancreatitis. *J Clin Gastroenterol* 1995;20:343–344.

Axillary Nerve Block

Koyobash I, Takahashi H, Hatakeyama Y, et al. Ultrasound guided supraclavicular approach to brachial plexus. *Anesthesiology* 1994;81[3A]:A906.

Moore DC. *Axillary approach for block of the brachial plexus: regional block,* fourth ed. Springfield, IL: Charles C. Thomas, 1979:443–456.

Pham-Dang C, Kick O, Bourelli B, et al. Continuous axillary brachial plexus block: a new method of catheter insertion. *Anesthesiology* 1994;81[3A]:A905.

Fallopian Tube Recanalization

Hayashi N, Kimoto T, Sakai T, et al. Fallopian tube disease: limited value of treatment with fallopian tube catheterization. *Radiology* 1994;190:141–143.

Hovsepian DM, Bonn J, Eschelman DJ, et al. Fallopian tube recanalization in an unrestricted patient population. *Radiology* 1994;190:137–140.

Kumpe DA, Zwerdlinger SC, Rothbarth LJ, et al. Proximal fallopian tube occlusion: diagnosis and treatment with transcervical fallopian tube catheterization. *Radiology* 1990;177:183–187.

Thurmond AS, Rösch J. Nonsurgical fallopian tube recanalization for treatment of infertility. *Radiology* 1990;174:371–374.

Percutaneous Vertebroplasty

Cotten A, Boutry N, Cortet B, et al. Percutaneous vertebroplasty: state of the art. *Radiographics* 1998;18:311–320.

Gangi A, Dietemann J-L, Mortazavi R, et al. CT-guided interventional procedures for pain management in the lumbosacral spine. *Radiographics* 1998;18;621–633.

Gangi A, Kastler BA, Dietemann J-L. Percutaneous vertebroplasty guided by a combination of CT and fluoroscopy. *AJNR* 1994;15:83-86.

Jensen ME, Evans AJ, Mathis JM, et al. Percutaneous polymethylmethacrylate vertebroplasty in the treatment of osteoporotic vertebral body compression fractures: technical aspects. *AJNR* 1997;18:1897–1904.

Mathis JM, Petri M, Naff N. Percutaneous vertebroplasty treatment of steroid-induced osteoporotic compression fractures. *Arthritis Rheum* 1998;41:171–175.

Weill A, Chiras J, Simon JM, et al. Spinal metastases: indications for an results of percutaneous injection of acrylic surgical cement. *Radiology* 1996;199:241–247.

INDEX

C